Chronic Diseases and Cancer

Chronic Diseases and Cancer

Edited by **Robert Miller**

hayle
medical

New York

Published by Hayle Medical,
30 West, 37th Street, Suite 612,
New York, NY 10018, USA
www.haylemedical.com

Chronic Diseases and Cancer
Edited by Robert Miller

International Standard Book Number: 978-1-63241-081-8 (Hardback)

Printed in China.

Contents

	Preface	**IX**
Part 1	**Dynamics of Immune System and Inflammatory Diseases**	**1**
Chapter 1	**Inflammation, Aging and Cancer: Friend or Foe?** Mahin Khatami	**3**
Chapter 2	**The Innate Immune Response Mediated by TLRs in Atherosclerosis** Luis Chávez-Sánchez, Karina Chávez-Rueda, María Victoria Legorreta-Haquet, Eduardo Montoya-Díaz and Francisco Blanco-Favela	**31**
Chapter 3	**The Impact of Macrophage Membrane Lipid Composition on Innate Immune Response Mechanisms** Julia Schumann	**53**
Chapter 4	**Autoimmunity, Atherosclerosis and Apoptotic Cell Clearance** Tamar Aprahamian	**75**
Chapter 5	**The Platelet as an Immunomodulator: The Old Thespian with New Roles in Atherosclerosis, Sepsis and Autoimmune Disease** Omar L. Esponda, Yaliz Loperena, Gladiany Ramos and A. Valance Washington	**97**
Chapter 6	**Inflammation, Immunity and Redox Signaling** Joshua Jabaut and Karina Ckless	**121**
Chapter 7	**Regulatory T Cells and Viral Disease** Tanya LeRoith and S. Ansar Ahmed	**137**

Chapter 8 **The Role of Chemokines and Cytokines in the Pathogenesis of Periodontal and Periapical Lesions: Current Concepts** 161
Gustavo P. Garlet, Andreza M.F. Aranha, Elcia M. Silveira, Andreia Espindola Vieira, Celso M. Queiroz-Junior, Mila F.M. Madeira, Sandra Y. Fukada and Tarcilia A. Silva

Chapter 9 **Complement Receptors in Inflammation** 207
Priyanka Pundir and Marianna Kulka

Chapter 10 **Parasitic Infections and Inflammatory Diseases** 251
Joziana M.P. Barçante, Thales A. Barçante, Ana Paula Peconick, Luciano J. Pereira and Walter S. Lima

Chapter 11 **Involvement of Microglial Cathepsin B in Pro-Interleukin-1β Processing and Persistent Pain** 265
Hiroshi Nakanishi

Chapter 12 **"Suppressor of Cytokine Signalling" Molecules in Infection and Inflammation** 273
Berit Carow and Martin E. Rottenberg

Chapter 13 **Review of Cytomegalovirus Anterior Uveitis** 301
C. E. Pang

Chapter 14 **Role of the Neutrophil NADPH Oxidase and S100A8/A9 in the Pathophysiology of Chronic Inflammation** 307
Sabrina Bréchard, Véronique Schenten and Eric J. Tschirhart

Part 2 **Medical and Pharmacological Aspects of Inflammatory Diseases** **331**

Chapter 15 **Malnutrition and Inflammation** 333
Jorge R. Mujico, Fátima Pérez-de-Heredia, Sonia Gómez-Martínez and Ascensión Marcos

Chapter 16 **Inflammation in COPD and New Drug Strategies** 351
Liam Heaney and Izhaq Masih

Chapter 17 **Ocular Involvement in Behçet's Disease** 375
Yonca Aydın Akova and Sirel Gür Güngör

Chapter 18 **Anti-CXCL13 and Anti-TNFα Monoclonal Antibodies Combinatorial Treatment Inhibits Autoimmune Disease in a Murine Model of Systemic Lupus Erythematosus** **401**
Debra B. Gardner, Patricia Rafferty, Peter Bugelski and Bailin Liang

Chapter 19 **Biologic Agents for Inflammatory Bowel Disease (The Current, the Future and the Controversy)** **417**
Iyad A. Issa

Permissions

List of Contributors

Preface

This book consists of brilliant reviews and perspectives contributed by experts in the multidisciplinary field of basic science, clinical studies, and treatment options for a broad extent of acute and chronic inflammatory diseases or cancer. The aim of this book is to show that persistent or chronic (unresolved or subclinical) inflammation is an ordinary denominator in the genesis, progression and manifestation of various diseases and/or cancers, especially during the aging process. Considering the elementary basis of shared and interrelated immunological characteristics of unresolved inflammation in initiations and progression of chronic illnesses or cancer are expected to hold real promises, when the designs of cost-effective approaches are contemplated for diagnosis, prevention or treatment of various age-associated diseases such as autoimmune and neurodegenerative diseases as well as many cancers.

Significant researches are present in this book. Intensive efforts have been employed by authors to make this book an outstanding discourse. This book contains the enlightening chapters which have been written on the basis of significant researches done by the experts.

Finally, I would also like to thank all the members involved in this book for being a team and meeting all the deadlines for the submission of their respective works. I would also like to thank my friends and family for being supportive in my efforts.

Editor

Part 1

Dynamics of Immune System and Inflammatory Diseases

1

Inflammation, Aging and Cancer: Friend or Foe?

Mahin Khatami
National Cancer Institute (NCI), The National Institutes of Health (NIH), Bethesda, Maryland, USA

1. Introduction

Rudolph Virchow, in the 19th century noted that *"the signs of inflammation are four; redness, and swelling, with heat & pain"*. Since this historical observation, the role of inflammation in the genesis and progression of many acute diseases (e.g., sepsis, pneumonia, meningitis or major trauma), allergies (e.g., asthma, emphysema, skin and ocular inflammatory diseases), age-associated chronic, neurodegenerative, autoimmune and other inflammatory diseases (e.g., hypertension, colitis, gastritis, hepatitis, nephritis, prostatis, pancreatitis, appendicitis, opthalmitis, Bechet's, esophagitis, neuritis, diabetes and cardiovascular complications, stroke, rheumatoid arthritis, atherosclerosis, lupus, psoriasis, Alzheimer's, multiple sclerosis) and many cancers (e.g., lung, colon/rectal, breast, prostate, bladder, liver, gall bladder, appendix, ovarian, pancreas, brain, lymphoid tissue) has been reported in literature. However, the mechanisms of inflammatory responses in the induction of a wide range of inflammatory diseases or cancer that are manifested in tissues as site- specific conditions are not understood. For example, the ongoing debates and controversies in literature whether inflammation is protective in preventing carcinogenesis or it is a cause of cancer demonstrate lack of understanding in differentiating the role of acute and chronic inflammatory responses in preventing or inducing cancer. Consequently, despite heavy public investment for over four decades on cancer war, too many expensive and out-of-focus clinical trials that use potent drugs which are pro-inflammatory mediators or inhibitors of growth factors (poisons) have caused serious and life-threatening side-effects for cancer patients (reviewed in Khatami 2011 a, b).

This chapter will provide a brief overview of recent definitions for acute and chronic inflammation and the role that inflammation plays in the induction of acute and age-associated chronic diseases, with emphasis on cancer. Attempts were made to demonstrate that self-terminating natural property of immune system (immune surveillance) in acute inflammation is protective to the body ('Friend'). However, unresolved and persistent inflammation (oxidative stress) could change the dynamics of immune responses creating an immunological chaos or 'immune tsunami' that would cause loss of architectural integrity and function in susceptible tissues leading to initiation, progression and manifestation of a wide range of chronic conditions or cancer ('Foe') that are very likely interrelated and potentially preventable (Khatami, 2008, 2009, 2011 a, b). Evaluation of current approaches in 'targeted' therapies will be summarized. Outlines of a framework for future designs of clinical trials based on a concept that inflammation is a common denominator in the genesis and manifestation of a wide range of age-associated chronic diseases and cancer will also be presented.

2. Acute inflammation: Protective, self-terminating property of immune system: Body's immune surveillance

During evolutionary process, inflammation became an inherent protective and self-limiting property of immune system to guard the body against harmful elements that the body recognizes as foreign elements (stimuli or irritants). Briefly, effective immunity is provided through natural pleiotropy or duality (polarity) of immune cells via acute inflammation to facilitate the organ systems the ability to return to normal physiological function after encountering internal or external foreign elements [e.g., microorganisms (e.g., viruses, bacteria, parasites), allergens, biological, chemical or environmental hazards, carcinogens, useless or non-functional proteins/enzymes, genetic and epigenetic defects (e.g., mutated DNA/RNA, hypo- hypermethylated genetic components), useless cells (e.g., polyclonal B cell complexes, senescent and cancerous cells), oxidized metabolites (e.g., crystalline uric acid)], so that the body can survive and thrive throughout life (Khatami, 2008, 2009, 2011 a, b).

Acute inflammatory process was recently defined as the balance between two highly regulated and biologically opposing arms termed 'Yin' (apoptosis, growth-arresting, pro-inflammatory or tumoricidal) and 'Yang' (wound healing, growth-promoting, anti-inflammatory, tumorigenic) responses of immune cells with intimate participation of vasculature (Khatami, 2008) (Figure 1).

Stimuli-induced local or systemic immune responses or cell mediated and humoral immunity (CMI, HI), are provided by a highly sophisticated and precise communications between activated innate immune cells [e.g., natural killer cells (NKs), macrophages (MΦs), dendritic cells (DCs), mast cells (MCs)] and their counterparts in the adaptive immune cells [e.g., T and B cells, and subpopulations (cytotoxic T cells, Th1, Th2, Treg)], vasculature and neuroendocrine system to initiate and transmit danger signals within cellular compartments for the purpose to destroy and eliminate the foreign elements as well as terminate and resolve inflammatory responses (Abraham and John 2010, Bonasio and von Andrian 2006, Bosch et al, 2002, Corthay 2006, Crotzer and Blum 2010, Davalos et al, 2010, Fischetti and Tedesco 2006, Gurish and Boyce 2006, Kabelitz and Medzhitov 2006, Khatami 2008, 2009, 2011, a, b, Lodoen and Lanier 2006, Serbina et al, 2008, Serhan and Savill 2005, Thompson et al, 2006, Wagner and Frenette 2008).

The principal mission of acute inflammation (immune surveillance) is two folds:

1. Encounter (sense), process/digest, destroy and eliminate intrinsic or extrinsic foreign elements and infected/injured host tissue,
2. Resolve and terminate inflammation and repair and construct or remodel the target/injured host tissue.

The major outcome of an acute inflammation is lymphocyte-derived clonal expansion, increased synthesis of allergen- or pathogen-specific antibodies and plasma and memory T and B cells (Khatami 2008, 2009, 2011 a, b).

Simply described, apoptosis ('Yin') is responsible for production of death signals and oxidants to destroy the enemy and injured host cells, while wound healing ('Yang') is required to counteract apoptosis and neutralize and remove the toxic 'debris' from the 'battle field' and to reconstruct and repair the host and resolve or terminate inflammation.

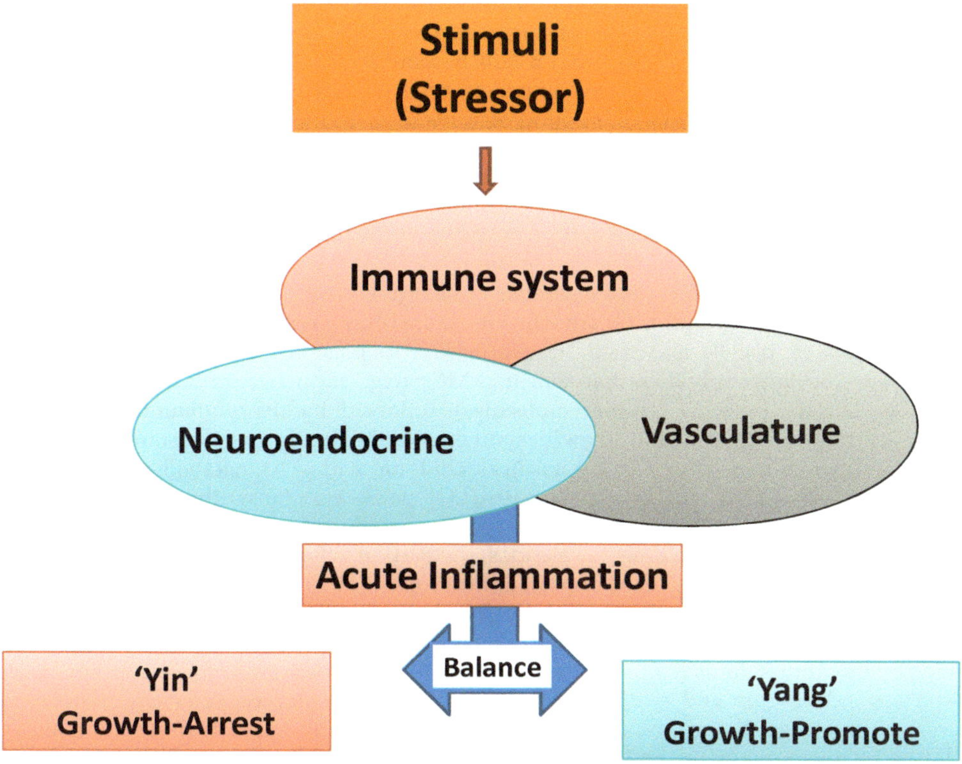

Fig. 1. Schematic representation of 'Yin' and 'Yang' in acute inflammation. Stimuli- (stressor-) induced a well balanced signals between 2 biologically opposing arms, 'Yin' (growth-arresting) and 'Yang' (growth-promoting) processes through elaborate cross-talks between immune and non-immune systems (e.g., vasculature and neuroendocrine) to combat and destroy foreign elements and injured host tissue and to neutralize, resolve and terminate inflammation and to repair and reconstruct the damaged target tissues.

3. Specialized and complementary features of cell mediated and humoral immunity (CMI, HI): Antigen presenting and effector cells

Crucial shared and special features of host defense mechanisms are recognition, uptake and clearance of a wide variety of external or internal foreign elements or hazardous materials (stimuli) by resident and/or infiltrated/recruited mononuclear phagocytes and their subpopulations within innate immune cells [e.g, MΦs, NKs, DCs, MCs, eosinophils (Eos)] and their counterparts in adaptive immune cells (T and B cells)]. The host defense system has also tolerance and remembrance capacities to develop memory and regulatory T or B cells when encountering specific foreign elements including cancerous cells (Khatami 2005 a, 2007, 2008, 2009, 2011 a).

In general, CMI that are mediated by MΦs (classical M1 or alternative M2) and DCs [classical/immature DC1, mature DC2, or their tissue lineage subset population (e.g., $CD11^-$ CD4+ $CD45RA^+$, phenotypes plasmacytoid) or neuronal myeloid] play key roles in combating viruses and bacteria. CMI that mediates through NKs and/or cytotoxic T cells (CTs) is essential for elimination of virus-infected cells and neoplastic cells (internal microorganisms). On the occasions that B cells become antigen presenting cells (APCs) [e.g., stimuli-induced activation of conjunctival-associated lymphoid tissues (CALTs), gut-associate lymphoid tissues (GALTs), lung airways, etc], B cells are responsible for sensing and processing microorganisms or allergens/antigens; activation and biosynthesis of specific antibodies that determine which innate immune cells are required for processing, digestion and destruction of hazardous elements and how pathogen-host interactions are directed to induce appropriate responses including induction of memory B and T cells. For example, CMI mediated by MCs and eosinophils (Eos) are involved in elimination of helminth (parasitic infections) and clearance of allergens/antigens. Under these conditions, B cells function as APCs and MCs are effector cells within innate immunity. Activation and differentiation of B cells and their transformation to plasma cells induce expression of antigen-specific IgE antibodies that sensitize MCs (e.g., induction of antigen-specific Fcε receptors, surface proteins adaptor molecules), followed by degranulation of MCs and release of potent preformed or newly synthesized mediators [e.g., histamine, heparin, oxidants, enzymes (e.g., chymase, tryptase), arachidonic acid (AA) metabolism, activation of cyclo-oxygenase (COX) and lipo-oxygenase (LO) pathways, biosynthesis and release of prostaglandins and cytokines/chemokines, etc], induction of vascular hyperpermeability, activation of blood complement cascades, activation of membrane metalloproteases (MMPs), cell adhesion molecules (CAMs), infiltrations of other inflammatory cells (e.g., Eos) to the site of injury. These events include simultaneous expression of anti-inflammatory mediators, hormones and growth factors (e.g., NFkB, interleukins, VEGF, FGF, cortisol, etc) enzymes and antioxidants [e.g., catalase, superoxide dismutases (SODs)]. The inflammatory responses induce pain and swelling (e.g., perhaps through binding of histamine-receptor-nerves within target tissue vasculatures) or tearing that would facilitate destruction and/or dilution of microorganisms and injured cells as well as termination of inflammation and tissue repair and reconstruction (Abraham and John 2010, Akhiani 2005, Bonetti et al, 2003, Boon et al, 2006, Diz et al, 2008, Drayton et al, 2006, Fischetti and Tedesco 2006, Helleboid et al, 1991, Khatami etal, 1984, 1985, Khatami 2005 a, b, 2008, 2009, Khazaie et al, 2011, Serhan and Savill 2005, Smith and Popmihajlov 2008, Soehnlein and Lindbom 2010, Spite and Serhan 2010, Vasto et al, 2007).

These interdependent and complex immunobiological cross talks are examples of numerous other sophisticated bilateral communications between immune and non-immune systems that are orchestrated during acute inflammatory responses to maintain and protect the psychophysiological and architectural integrity of organ systems throughout life.

Communications errors between CMI and HI due to oxidative stress-induced over-, or under expression of immune or non-immune responses, aberrations in chromosomal, genetic and epigenetic components, enzymes, antibodies, receptors/adaptors or surface molecules are implicated in a variety of chronic allergies, neurodegenerative and autoimmune diseases, non-Hodgkin lymphoma, Sjogren's disease, and/or tumorigenesis and cancer (Berosbaken et al, 2009, Booman et al, 2008, Culmsee and Landshamer 2006, D'Amato et al, 2007, Davis et al, 2011, Drayton et al, 2006, Dvorak 1986, Harvey et al, 2008, Kabelitz and Medzhitov 2006, Khatami 2005 a, b, 2008, 2009).

Polarization of Immune Cells: As shown in Table 1, inflammatory mediators with known dual (polarization) properties include toll-like receptors (TLRs 1-9), tumour necrosis factor-α and receptor (TNF-α/TNFR), MCP-1-CCL2, macrophage colony-stimulating factor (M-CSF), transforming growth factor-β(TGF-β), granulocyte M-CSF (GM-CSF), histamine, heparin, membrane metaloproteases (MMPs), prostaglandins (e.g., PGF1α/PGI-2 to PGE2), cytokine suppressor molecules (e.g., S100 family of calcium-binding proteins), enzymes (e.g., tryptase/chymase, neutrophil-derived serine proteases, indolamine 2, 3-dioxygenase),

Factor/Mediator	Immune Cell	Major Effects/Function
Toll-like receptors (TLRs 1-9)	DC1/DC2/TADC M1/M2/TAMs MCs (granulated) LMCs (partially granulated), TAMCs (?)	AI: Signal transduction, 'Yin'-'Yang' CI: decoy receptors in tumour microenvironment
TNF-a/TNFR	DCs/TADCs, MFs/TAM MCs/LMCs/TAMCs	AI: induction of apoptosis, CI: decoy receptor, intracellular, growth promotion, tumourigenic
TGF-β	MFs, DCs, MCs(?)	AI: immune regulation CI: decoy receptor, tumorigenic
Histamine	MCs, LMCs, TAMCs	AI: vasoactive, IgE Fc-dependent receptor binding; CI: independent of IgE-Fc receptor, tumorigenic
Macrophage colony stimulating factor-(MCSF)	M1, M2, TAMs	AI: apoptosis/wound healing; CI: decoy receptor, immune suppressor
Indolamine 2, 3-dioxygenase (IDO)	DC1/DC2/TADC MCs/MΦs (?)	AI : Wound healing CI: Local immune-privileged, carcinogen
Prostaglandins (PGs)	DCs, MCs, MΦs, T and B cells	AI: PGF1α/PGI 2, tumoricidal CI: PGE2, tumorigenic
Other factors Interleukins (ILs) Chemokines, Cytokines, Enzymes, Genetic/epigenetic	MΦs (M1/M2) or TAMs DCs, T and B cells (?) MCs (?)	AI: TNF-α, IL-1, IL-12, INF-γ, iNOS (arginine), constitutive CXCL1/NFkB, apoptosis-wound healing; endogenous lymphotrophic hormones (ILs); negative control of immune response; etc CI: IL-1RA (decoy), TNF-a/TNFR (decoy), IL-3, IL-4-Eotaxin-2/CCL24, CCL-18, arginase/ornithine-polyamine; CXCl inducible CCL2; Ser/ Thr Ks; PGs/PGE2; MAPKs, PI3K; etc

Table 1. Inherent polarization of immune cells. Acute inflammation induces bilateral and balanced responses between apoptotic ('Yin') and wound healing ('Yang') pathways. Immune response dynamics alter under chronic inflammation. [AI, acute inflammation; CI, chronic inflammation. Modified from Khatami 2011 b, Cell Biochem Biophys with permission]

cytokines, chemokines, endogenous lymphotrophic hormone-like interleukins (ILs, e.g., IL-2, IL-3, IL-5, IL-10, IL-12, IL-13) and receptor molecules that are involved in feedback or negative control (switching off the positive driving force of immune response after antigen clearance or oxidative stress, or auto-antigens, tumour antigens, infections or allografts), interferons (IFNs, e.g., IFN-γ), eosinophils chemotactic factor of anaphylaxis (ECFA), SCF, c-kit, antibodies (e.g., IgE, IgG isotypes, IgA, IgM), platelet-derived growth factor (PDGF) and gene activation pathways, mutated DNA, hypo-hyper-methylation and expression of abnormal proteins that are identified in cancer research (e.g., p53, p27, p70, MAPKs, KRAS, BRAF, ALK, Myc, BCR, ABL, MGMT, TKIs, PI3ks, tyr/ser Ks, etc) or surface antigens, adaptor molecules or cell recognition molecules (CDs, e.g., CD2, CD11, CD18, CD22, CD25, CD26, CD40, CD 50, CD54, CD63, CD69, CD88, CD154, etc) (Al-Sarireh and Eremin 2000, D'Amato et al, 2007, Diz et al, 2008, Fischetti and Tedesco 2008, Gordon 2005, Gounaris etal, 2007, 2009, Gurish and Boyce 2006, Khatami 2008, 2009, 2011 a, b, Lee et al, 2002, Mackawa and Watanabe 2007, Nishioka et al, 2011, Peerschke et al, 2006, Ribatti et al, 2003, Smith and Popmihajlov 2008, Soehnlein and Lindbom 2010, Suzuki et al, 1998, Thompson et al, 2006, Quezada et al, 2004, Valencia et al, 2011, Wagner 2008). (Table 1, Figure 2).

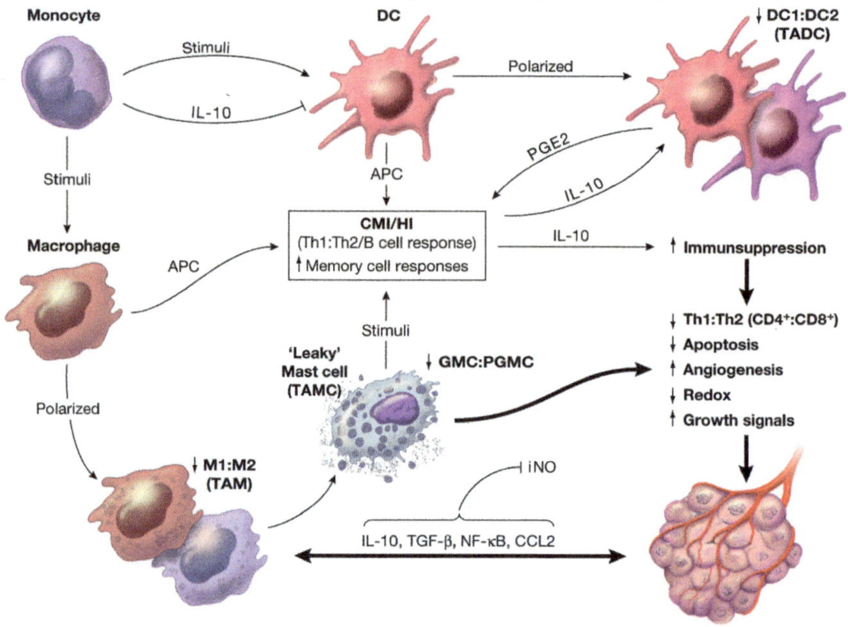

Fig. 2. Pleiotropic roles of immune responses and oxidative stress-induced immune suppression. Oxidative stress can decrease ratios of (DC1/DC2), M1/ M2 (tumour-associated MΦs-TAMs), and/or granulated mast cells (GMC) to partially granulated ('leaky' or TAMCs). These immune response changes could contribute to altered function of cell mediated and humoral immunity (CMI/HI), B- and T- or memory cell responses (e.g., decrease in Th1/Th2 (CD4/CD8 ratios), expression of PGE2, IL-10, NFkB, CCL2, in the direction of immune suppression, reduced apoptosis, redox potential, and increased growth signals for tumor growth and angiogenesis. [Reproduced from Khatami 2008, Exp Opin Biol Ther, 2008 with permission].

4. Unresolved inflammation: 'Immune tsunami' and loss of architectural integrity in immune-responsive and immune-privileged tissues

Unresolved inflammation was defined as the loss of balance between 'Yin' and 'Yang' of acute inflammation. Briefly, acute inflammation provides immunity (immune surveillance) and protection of target tissues via two major mechanisms (reviewed in Khatami 2009, 2011 a):

a. Immune-responsive tissues, the sites of initial contact and processing of internal or external stimuli include squamous and grandular epithelial tissues, epithelial-associated mucosal surfaces (e.g., goblet cells), endothelial, stroma, fibroblasts, lymphoid tissues and vasculatures.
b. Immune-tolerant (privileged) tissues including avascular cornea, neuroretina, retinal pigment epithelium (RPE), blood brain barrier (BBB), central nervous system (CNS), hair follicles, testis or uterus, prohibit the processing and spread of pathogen- or stimuli-induced inflammation because these episodes threaten the delicate integrity and function of these stress-sensitive tissues. Immune surveillance in the immune-privileged tissues (self tolerance or ignorance) is provided by presence of one or a combination of barriers [e.g., limited or absence of vasculature, few APCs or recognition molecules such as major histocompatibility class molecules (MHC) class I or II or HLA].

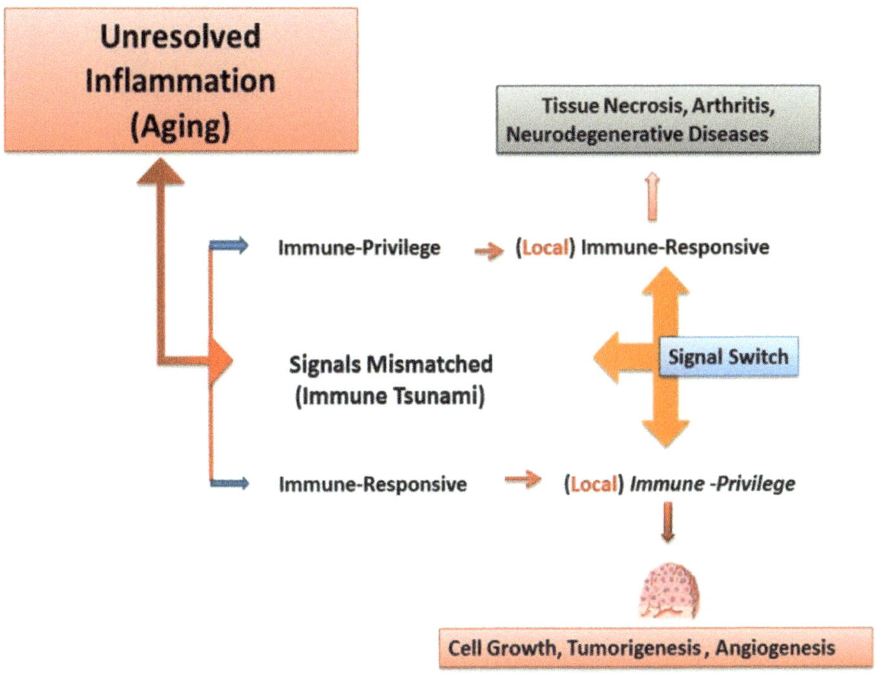

Fig. 3. Unresolved inflammation and altered immune signals in susceptible target tissues. Inflammation and aging could create immune dysfunction (immune tsunami) that cause signal switches by inducing local immune-responsiveness in tissues that are naturally immune-privileged causing tissue necrosis and neurodegenerative disorders. Chronic inflammation can also cause loss of integrity in immune-responsive tissues by induction of local immune-privilege to satisfy increased growth requirements of cancerous cells leading to cancer metastasis and angiogenesis.

Oxidative stress or continuous exposure to irritants could damage immune surveillance (protection) in either or both immune-responsive and immune-privileged tissues (Figure 3). Oxidative stress could induce exaggerated co-expression of apoptotic and/or wound healing factors in target tissues and create an 'immunological chaos' ('immune tsunami') that would erode the architectural integrity and function of naturally immune-responsive or immune-privileged tissues (Khatami 2011 a) leading to the induction of a wide range of allergies, chronic infections, autoimmune or neurodegenerative diseases as well as cell growth, neoplasia, cancer metastasis and angiogenesis (Abrahams et al, 2003, Culmsee and Landshamer 2006, Ferguson and Griffith 2007, Hamrah et al, 2003, Karman et al, 2004, Khatami 2009, 2011 a, Kwidzinski et al, 2003, Niederkorn 2006, O'Brien et al, 2008, Schneider et al, 2011, Siffrin et al, 2007, Streilein et al, 2002, Widera et al, 2008, Zamiri et al, 2007) (Figure 3).

5. Acute inflammatory diseases

Severe acute inflammatory diseases (e.g., sepsis, respiratory diseases, meningitis, major trauma, etc), and perhaps anti-cancer drug-induced cachexia, anorexia and sarcopenia, often lead to multiple organ failure (MOF) (Coss et al, 2011, Hall et al, 2011, Harrois et al, 2009, Hotamisisligil 2006, Khatami 2011 a, b, Lyman 2011, Okamoto 2002, Suzuki et al, 2011, Terrabui et al, 2007). In severe acute inflammatory conditions, potent pathogens and their products (e.g., endotoxins, pneumonia, meningitis, etc) can induce rapid destruction of vascular integrity allowing pathogens to gain direct access to host tissues at multiple sites and inducing expression of massive quantities of apoptotic factors and toxins ('cytokine storm' or 'immune tsunami') such as TNF-α, ILs, strong oxidants (e.g., peroxynitriles) that can rapidly shift the balance between apoptosis and wound healing pathways in favor of growth-arresting properties of immune cells and causing severe damage to important host cellular components (e.g., mitochondrial oxidative damage, interruption in electron transfer system, changes in oxido-redux ratios, accumulation of free radicals and severe toxicity to intracellular and/or cytoplasmic membrane components) leading to increased risk of organ failure in lung, kidney, brain, central nervous system and/or heart, in a matter of hours or days (Akamizu et al, 2010, Aubert and Lansdorp 2008, Braun and Marks 2010, Khatami 2011 a, b, Suzuki et al, 2011, Terrabui et al, 2007).

The end results of long-term inflammatory conditions (unresolved inflammation) during the aging process were suggested to be similar to those described for acute inflammatory diseases that lead to organ dysfunction and the genesis of chronic conditions such as neurodegenerative and autoimmune diseases and cancer (Khatami 2011 a, b). Therefore, while acute inflammation is considered a 'friend' that protects the body against harmful elements, chronic or persistent inflammation becomes a 'foe' that destroys the tissue integrity and function.

6. Inflammation and age-associated diseases

Biology of aging is a complex process involving declines, slow-down or alterations in expression or function of multiple important hormones (e.g., estrogen, testosterone, DHA, insulin, cortisol) and altered metabolism or transport of nutrients and metabolites (e.g., vitamin C, glucose, myo-inositol, etc) that would lead to biological rearrangements in organs/tissues (biological senescence). Aging process is also associated with minor or major changes in immune response profiles and co-expression and co-existence of mismatched or misdirected inflammatory mediators (e.g., TNF-α, IL-6, IFN-α,β, IFNs, PGE2, etc) features that are characteristics of immunoscenescence involved in a wide range of chronic diseases (Davalos et al 2010, Ginaldi et al, 2005, Chung et al., 2008, Khatami 2008, 2009, 2011a, Nagai et al, 2010, Ren et al, 2009, Romanyukha and Yashin 2003, Sansoni et al, 2008, Sedivy et al, 2008, Serbina et al, 2008, Siffrin et al, 2007, Zhang 2010) (Figures 3 and 4).

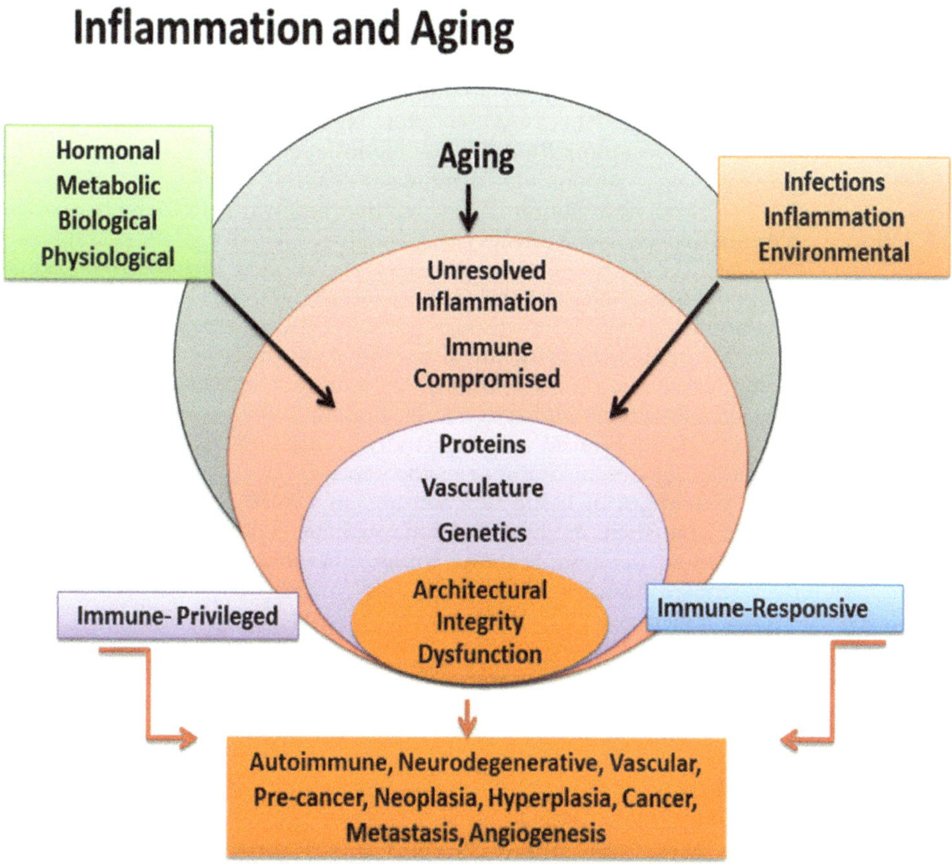

Fig. 4. Schematic representation of chronic (persistent) inflammation and aging as co-morbidity and co-mortality risk factors in the genesis and progression of chronic diseases. Unresolved inflammation could induce shifts in immune responses in naturally immune-privileged and/or immune-responsive tissues and initiating damage to the cellular components such as proteins, genes and vasculature that would lead to destruction of architectural integrity and function of susceptible tissues and induction of chronic diseases such as autoimmune or neurodegenerative conditions, cardiovascular conditions or tumour growth, cancer metastasis and angiogenesis.

Briefly, low grade (unresolved or subclinical) inflammation and longevity are known as co-morbidity and co-mortality risk factors in the genesis and progression of nearly all chronic illnesses. Accumulation of confluent, complex and useless cells is considered additional sources of oxidative stress that would maintain activation of immune cells and unresolved inflammation. However, longevity and the rate of functional capacities of organ systems and susceptibility to chronic diseases vary in individuals, due to a combination of genetics, immunological or biological factors and the frequency of exposure to diverse environmental hazards. In an attempt to find a common forum on enormous amount of fragmentary information on the biology of chronic diseases that are linked to inflammation, highlights of major molecular theories of aging are outlined in the following (reviewed in Khatami 2009):

a. **Oxidative Stress:** Aging and stress-induced alterations in redox state of cells is likely a major cause of progressive damage to the biological systems. Oxidative stress is associated with activation of NADPH and NADH oxidases and peroxisome proliferators-activated receptors (PPARs) that could lead to the declines in host tissue reducing powers [e.g., superoxide dismutases (SODs), catalase, NADH/NAD+ reductases, GSH/GSSG and vitamin E regeneration pathways, etc]. The peroxidation-induced accumulation of free radicals [e.g., reactive oxygen species (ROS), reactive nitrogen species (RNS)] could damage extracellular and intracellular signaling pathways, inducing interruption of the electron transfer activities and detoxifying and reducing enzymes (e.g., cytochrome p450, SODs, etc), declines in energy out put (e.g., reduced ATP/ADP ratios), impairment of oxidative metabolism in mitochondria, as well as inducing abnormal protein bindings to chromosomal components (e.g., fos, c-jun, c-myc, b actin, etc) and altered activities of immune and non-immune cell response profiles. Oxidative stress-induced altered activity of immune cells would lead to co-expression of inflammatory mediators causing tissue necrosis and/or growth. These immunobiological changes in tissue function are implicated in a wide range of age-associated conditions such as hypertension, asthma, multiple sclerosis, arthritis, diabetes and cardiovascular complications, stroke, atheroma, emphysema, autoimmune and neurodegenerative diseases, Alzheimer's, and cancer (Deng et al, 2008, Ginaldi et al, 2005, Goronzy and Wevand 2005, Khatami 2009, 2011 a, Nagai et al, 2010, Siffrin et al, 2007, Vasto et al, 2008, Zhang 2010).
b. **Immunoscenescence:** Immunoscenescence is the results of readjustment (remodeling) of immune cell functions, a basis for hyper- or hypo-sensitivity (skewing) responses toward new or self-antigens and an overall defects in lymphohematopoetic progenitor competence. Aging and atrophy of thymus is associated with dysfunction of stem cells (manufacturers of hematopoietic cells) and the declines in total number of T lymphocytes subpopulation (CD3+, CD4+, CD8+), decreases in generation and/or exhaustion of naïve/virgin T cells (T0 or CD95-), Th1/Th2 ratios, increases in activities of cytotoxic T cells (CTs) and NKs, declines in B cells function, clonal expansion of CD28+ T and memory B cells. Defects in stem cells function are associated with increased severity of cardiovascular pathology, increased production of low density lipoproteins (LDL) and arteriosclerosis plaque formation, as well as up-regulation of pro- (e.g., IL-2, TNF-α, histamine, NO) (or anti- (e.g., IL-4, IL-5, IL-6, IL-8, IL-10, PGE2) inflammatory mediators in arthritis, atherosclerosis, multiple sclerosis, neurological disorder, dementia/Alzheimer's, osteoporosis, diabetes, lymphoid hypertrophy or cancer. Other contributing factors in changes of immune competency include alterations in bone marrow remodeling and regenerative processes. Age-induced declines in T cell repertoire and accumulation of memory effector cells and oligoclonal complexes (megaclones) result in tissue vulnerability toward infectious agents. Oxidative stress

also influences immune response modifications of MHC-binding regions (epitopes), alterations of antigen processing, accumulation of terminally differentiated effector T cells and skewed lymphocytes polyclonal complexes that could be a basis for inability of immune and non-immune systems to properly respond to new antigenic challenges (e.g., viral, bacterial, neoplastic cells or vaccines) and enhanced vulnerability toward chronic illnesses or cancer (Campisi 2011, Chidgev et al, 2007, Chung et al, 2008, Davalos et al, 2010, Deng et al, 2008, Gounaris et al, 2006, 2009, Khatami 2008, 2009, 2011 a, Klein et al, 2009, Montavani et al, 2004, 2008, O'Brien et al, 2008, Romanyukha and Yashin 2003) (Figures 3 and 4).

c. **Hormones, Metabolites and Lipids in Biology of Aging:** Aging process is associated with altered functions of important hormones (e.g., estrogen, progesterone, insulin, glucagon, androgen, andosterone, testosterone, thyroxine, glucocorticoids, epinephrine, cortisol, mineralcorticoids, dehydroepiandosterone-DHEA, etc) and hormone-like growth factors (e. g., IGF-1, FGF, EGF, VEGF, etc). The influence of these hormones and growth factors on multiple organs and sub-cellular systems (e.g., CNS and brain cognition, stem cells, mitochondrial function, neurogenesis and myelination, traumatic injury, wound healing responses) in reproductive and non-reproductive, immune and non-immune systems and their association in the development of chronic diseases or cancer have been the topic of extensive studies (Davis et al, 2011, Deng et al, 2008, Khatami 2009, Mikkola and Clakson 2002, Pisani 2008, Piatkliewicz and Czech 2011, Poulsen and Kruger 2006, Rauvala and Rouhianen 2001, Ren et al, 2009, Schwarts and Pashko 2004).

For example, steroids or insulin play important roles not only in the function of reproductive organs and regulation of fluid homeostasis and/or metabolic pathways and immune responses to stress, but they are also involved in physiology, function and remodeling of bone, neuronal function, myelination and neurogeneration of brain and CNS and/or membrane-associated fatty acid metabolism (Bosch et al, 2002, Brunello et al, 2011, Campisi 2011, Chung et al, 2011, Goronzy and Wavand 2005, Hotamisisligil 2006, Khatami 1990, 2009, Li et al, 1986, Mikkola and Clarkson 2002, Sansoni et al, 2008, Simon and Balkau 2010, van Kruijsdijk et al, 2009). Insulin deficiency, insulin-resistance or hyper- insulinimia, or glucose toxicity and hyperglycemia of diabetes-induced increased glycosylation of proteins (advanced glycation end-products-AGE and their receptors RAGE) are associated with disturbances in transport and metabolism of important nutrients (e.g., ascorbic acid, pyridoxal phosphate, myo-inositol, etc), increased oxidative stress, accumulation of ROS, and co-expression of pro- and anti- inflammatory mediators such as NF-kB, VEGF, TNF-α, IL-1a, IL-6, IL-8, IL-12, and Ikappa B kinase (IKK-β), platelets' CD40L, VCAM-1, in endothelial, hepatocytes or myeloid cells and/or tissues that are insulin-dependent (e.g., muscle, liver, adipocytes) or insulin-independent (e.g., vasculature, kidney, nerves, retina, RPE, lens) for glucose transport or metabolism (Khatami 1988, 1990, 2009, Li et al, 1986, Park et al, 2005, Pisan 2008, Piatkiewicz and Czech 2011, Simon and Balkau 2010, Stern et al, 2002).

The relationship between diabetes, inflammation and production of AGE/RAGE and the increased risk of certain cancers has been the topic of many recent studies (Piatkiewicz and Czech 2011, Simon and Balkau 2010, Simon et al, 2010, Zhang and Hu 2010). It should also be noted that chronic inflammation in patients with neurodegenerative diseases, asthma or diabetes are reported to increase the risks for certain site-specific cancers (e.g., lung cancer in asthmatic patients, or liver and pancreas in diabetics) and decreased risk for certain other cancers (e.g., prostate in diabetics) (Brunello and Kappor 2011, Khatami 2011 b, Piatkkiewicz and Czech 2011, Stern et al, 2002, Vena et al, 1985, Vesterinen et al, 1993, Vingeri et al. 2009,

Zhang and Hu 2010, manuscript in preparation). It is possible that expression and release of abnormal inflammatory factors into circulation would induce growth-arresting or growth-promoting impact at site-specific susceptible/accessible tissues.

Lipids: Long-chain polyunsaturated fatty acids or essential fatty acids (FAs) including membrane arachidonic acid (AA) metabolites, prostaglandins (e.g., PGI2/PGF-1α, PGD, PGE2) and leukotrienes (e.g., LT4, LTC), phosphatidylinositol (PI), phosphatidylserine (PS), and associated enzymes (e.g., COX, LO, phospholipases A, B and C) play critical roles in metabolism, integrity and function of tissues, including signal transduction, immune responses, vascular toning, bone remodeling and function (Al-Sarireh et al, 2000, Bosch et al, 2002, Baso 2008, Helleboid et al, 1991, Khatami 2005, 2007, 2009, Parks et al, 2005, Plourde et al, 2008, Poulsen and Kruger 2006, Spite and Serhan 2010, Wagner and Frenette 2008). Aging, oxidative stress and certain life styles (e.g., smoking or heavy alcohol consumption) are associated with decreases in capacity to metabolize and convert precursor of FAs into polyunsaturated FAs, decreases in bone mass, resorption and remodeling and impaired calcium balance, alterations in osteoblastogenesis, osteoclastogenesis, and functions of osteoblast and osteoclast during menopause, as well as rheumatoid arthritis. Bone remodeling and function is regulated by activation of a sophisticated signal transduction in cellular membrane-lipid complexes and intracellular soluble form of ligands and inflammatory mediators (e.g., nuclear-kappa B ligand binding, RANK to RANKL, decoy receptor proteins and bone-specific osteoprotegerin-OPG) that are essential for differentiation and activation of osteoclasts (Basu 2008, Khatami 2009, Plourde et al, 2008, Poulsen and Kruger 2006, Spite and Serhan 2010).

d. **Inflamm-Aging and Genetic and Epigenetic Damage:** Inflammation is considered a precancerous state of cells that initiates genetic mutations, epigenetic abnormalities, and accumulation of genetic errors, impaired regulation of gene expression. Epigenetics modification events (e.g., methylation, DNA binding proteins, histone proteins, repair and related enzyme modifications) or telomere-telomerase pathways are sensitive to oxidative stress. Aging and chronic inflammation can cause alterations of multiple genomic functions including mutations of suppressor genes (e.g., p25, p35, p38, or p53), instability in somatic maintenance and repair, proliferative control of gene expression, DNA damage response and hypo- or hypermethylation, alterations in polymorphism and contact inhibition regulation, cell cycle regulation and cyclin-dependent kinases (e.g., ser-thr kinases), or telomere shortening. Furthermore, mitogen-activated protein kinase (MAPK) pathways (p38 suppressor genes) are involved in regulation of extracellular-signal regulated kinase (ERK), c-Jun N-terminal kinase (JNK) and inactivation or mutations in suppressor gene pathways that could cause enhancement of cellular transformation and disruption in the induction of senescence concurrent with tumor development. In addition, abnormalities in DNA methylation of CpG islands which are important checkpoints in gene expression events potentially influence healthy aging, carcinogenesis, inflammation and viral infection (Aubert and Lansdorp 2008, Bannar and Gerner 2011, Barber 2011, Khatami 2009, 2011 b, Mackawa and Watanabe 2007, Osborne et al, 2004, Shames et al, 2007, Song and Rudolph 2009, Vasto et al, 2008, Yung and Julius 2008, Zingg et al, 2008).

7. Cancer immunobiology

Cancer cell may be viewed as an evolutionary opportunistic defective cell, inherently possessing independent oncogenic properties like viruses, parasites or bacteria, which coexist within multi-cellular layers of host tissues. As such, cancer cell, like viruses or bacteria is a foreign entity whose growth is routinely monitored and arrested by body's effective immune system (immune surveillance). Due to its inherent oncogenic and stem cell-like features, cancer cell has the potential to become independent (atavistic metamorphosis) and behave like single-celled viruses, parasites or bacteria to grow and multiply and feed itself at the cost of destroying the host organ (Arguella 2011, Khatami 2009, 2011 b).

Carcinogenesis is a multistep progressive erosion of interactions between activating and deactivating immune and non-immune biological activities of host tissue that result in progressive destruction of integrity of susceptible primary and/or secondary tissues (metastasis). The microenvironments of malignant and non-malignant cells (e.g., stroma or vasculature) are cluttered by chaotic, heterogeneous and misdirected communications between normal and mutant cell populations, expressing inappropriate growth arresting and growth promoting factors in the direction of cell growth and selective apoptosis to benefit cancer invasiveness. In the microenvironments of tumor cells, exaggerated or inappropriate expression of apoptotic and wound healing (growth) factors, derived from genetic errors, DNA mutations and epigenetic components (e.g., TNF-α, MMPs, proteases or ROSs, kinases, telomerase, VEGF, etc) are required for tumor growth and proliferation, as well as membrane degradation and invasion to the neighboring tissues and migration through vasculature and lymphatic channels during metastasis (Al-Sarireh and Ermin 2000, Arguello 2011, Booman et al, 2008, Davalos et al, 2010, Dryaton et al, 2006, Ferrantini et al, 2008, Dvorak 1986, Gounaris et al, 2007, Ibrahim et al, 2006, Innocenti et al, 2011, Khatami 2007, 2008, 2009, 2011a, b, Kimura et al, 2007, Meeker 2006, Montavani et al, 2004, 2008, Muller et al, 2008, Nardin and Abastado 2008, Nyakern et al, 2006, Osborne et al, 2004, Peggs et al, 2008, Risques et al, 2007, Rodriguez et al, 2005, Rook and Dalgleish 2011, Sethi et al, 2008, Shames et al, 2007, Vena et al, 1985, Vire et al, 2011, Zitvogel et al, 2008).

The following is a list of major interrelated immunobiological features in carcinogenesis:

a. Destruction of immune surveillance (loss of balance in 'Yin' and 'Yang' of acute inflammation) in the microenvironment of susceptible target tissues. In order to satisfy their enhanced growth requirements cancer cells induce decoy receptors [e.g., TNFR (d), IL-1R (d), M-CSF-R (d)] that cause misguided oxidative signals and abnormal growth activation pathways (e.g., MAPKs, IP3Ks, PKC, PGE2, ILs, etc), genetic and epigenetic modifications that would further impair immune responses (Figures 2 and 4). The weakened or loss of immune competency and altered tumoricidal vs tumorigenic ratios of immune system, particularly during aging process, is perhaps the first essential opportunistic events for cancer cell to impose its oncogenic features on host machinery for its enhanced growth requirements, like any other opportunistic pathogen;
b. Decline/loss of cell contact inhibition perhaps due to oxidative stress-induced damage to extracellular/intracellular communication signals causing under-, or over-expression of receptor molecules or enzymes or other factors (e.g., MMPs, ECM, CAMs, collagen type IV, fibronectin, cell surface proteins/enzymes and antigens, oxidases, antibodies, cytokines/chemokines, etc) that would further facilitate cancer growth and motility;
c. Capability of cancer cells to grow under hypoxic conditions perhaps due to increased ratios of neovascularization (angiogenesis) to vascular cell number and/or damage to mitochondria oxidative metabolism and declines in energy output (ATP/ADP) accompanied by increased anaerobic glycolysis. Having enhanced glucose utilization requirements, cancer cell could also interfere with active transport (ATP-dependent) or

facilitated diffusion of glucose or other important metabolites (e.g., ascorbate or myo-inositol) which share or compete with glucose transporters into epithelial or endothelial tissues (Khatami, 1988, manuscript in preparation);

d. Loss of vascular integrity that would lead cancer cell clumps to access to other tissues (secondary sites);
e. Invasion of cancer cells in lymphoid organs and circulation and access to bone structures;
f. Metastasis and multiple organ failure (MOF) (Khatami 2009, 2011 a, manuscript in preparation.

8. Association between inflammation and cancer

8.1 Circumstantial evidence

Observations by Ehrlich (1909) that tumor cells are recognized and eliminated by immune system were later evolved to the theory of immune surveillance or killing of cancer cells by immune system (Burnet 1957). However, while numerous reports on circumstantial evidence for an association between chronic inflammation and many cancers (e.g., lung, breast, colon, prostate, gastric, liver, bladder, pancreas, esophagus, ovarian) have accumulated for more than a century (reviewed in Khatami 2005 a, 2007, 2008, 2009, 2011 a, b), except for our 'accidental' discoveries in 1980's (Khatami et al, 1989), little/no evidence demonstrated a direct link between inflammation and tumorigenesis. In addition, except for our publication (Khatami 2005 a) no other data demonstrated time course kinetics of inflammation-induced identifiable developmental phases of immune dysfunction that would lead to tumorigenesis and angiogenesis.

8.2 Direct evidence: Models of acute and chronic inflammatory diseases

In 1980s/90's, our research team at the University of Pennsylvania, established experimental models of acute and chronic inflammatory diseases in conjunctival-associated lymphoid tissues (CALTs) in guinea pigs, by topical (unilateral and/or bilateral) application of fluoresceinyl-ovalbumin (FLOA, antigen), in the presence or absence of infective agents (e.g., A Suum and its extracts), adjuvant or tumour promoting agents (TPAs) for up to 30 months (Khatami et al, 1984, 1985, 1989, Haldar et al 1990, Helleboid et al 1991, Khatami 2005 a, 2008). At least three distinct developmental phases of inflammatory responses were identified:

1. **Acute phase:** Clinical and histopathological findings; initiated 9 days after topical immunization and challenges induced strong or weak acute (type 1) clinical reactions including tearing, conjunctival edema, milky secretions in tears, IgE-dependent mast cells (MCs) degranulation, release of histamine and prostaglandin (PGs) and vascular hyperpermeability. Time course kinetics of histamine and PGs (6-keto-PGF-1α; or PGI2) release in tears suggested that histamine was a primary mediator that activated arachidonic acid metabolism and cyclooxygenase pathways and the synthesis and release of prostanoids via constituent and/or infiltrating inflammatory cells. No correlation was found between circulating homocytotropic-IgE and the degree of clinical reactions. Preliminary observations suggested tight binding (high affinity) of IgE-MCs-Fc-ε receptor molecules in CALTs and other tissues (e.g., lung MCs, or maternal/paternal antibody transfer to new-born babies).
2. **Intermediate phase (down-regulation phenomenon):** Occurring within 2 months of repeated sensitization and challenge, involved minimal tearing or tissue edema, loss

(exhaustion) of mast cell function, increased infiltration of eosinophils into subepithelium and mucus secreting GCs and neovascularization.

3. **Chronic response phase (tumorigenesis):** Occurring between 12 to 30 months of continuous challenges with antigen, involved induction of tumor-like lesions in conjunctival tissues, angiogenesis, massive lymphoid hyperplasia, follicular formation with germinal centers, activated macrophages, increased swollen GCs, degranulated-partially granulated ('leaky') MCs, involvement of lymphatic channels, extensive epithelial thickening (growth) and/or thinning (necrosis) that often observed in the same tissue sections. Cross-sectional areas of massive hyperplastic lymphoid nodules from animals that were continuously challenged with antigen were at least five times greater than lymphoid tissues in normal-untreated animals (Figures 5 and 6).

Animals treated with a mixture of FLOA and TPAs showed development of tumor-like lesions within 6 months after commencement of sensitization suggesting shifts in time course kinetics of immune response alterations through activation of protein kinase C (PKC) and/or other related tumor growth pathways.

From a total of 400 eyes that were examined, 12/40 (30%) of eyes from animals that were not sacrificed during earlier immunization periods developed tumor-like lesions or hyperplasia of CALTs. Tumor development in CALTs primarily occurred in animals that produced minimal early type 1 responses toward antigen challenge. Monitoring percentage of tumor-like lesions developed with strong or weak responses during the entire course of immunization is perhaps among the important knowledge gaps that awaits future investigations.

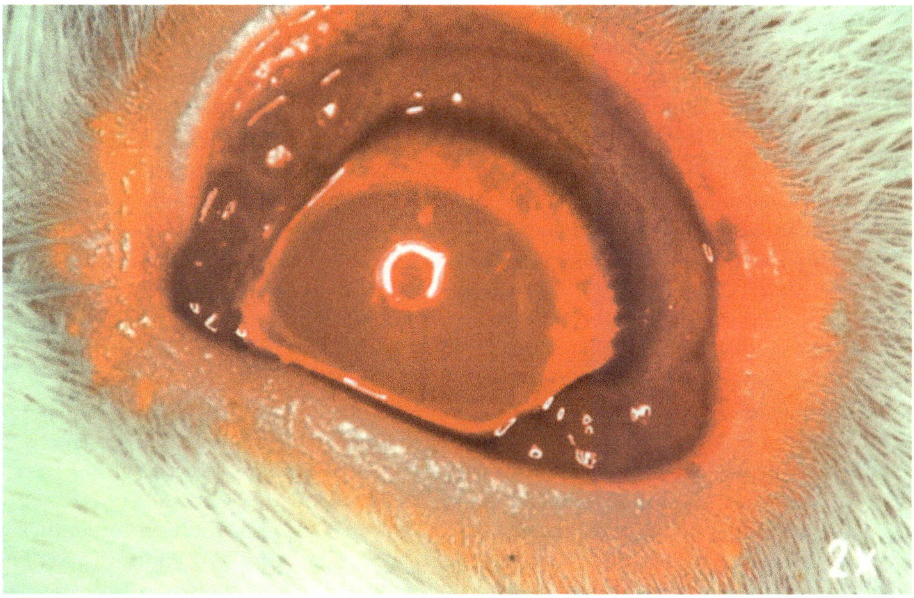

Fig. 5. Inflammation-induced tumour-like lesions in guinea pigs. Multiple round follicular lymphoid masses originating from upper and lower conjunctiva, 18 months after repeated topical (conjunctival) immunization and challenge with FLOA. [Reproduced from Khatami et al, 1989. Copyright American Medical Association @1989. All rights reserved.]

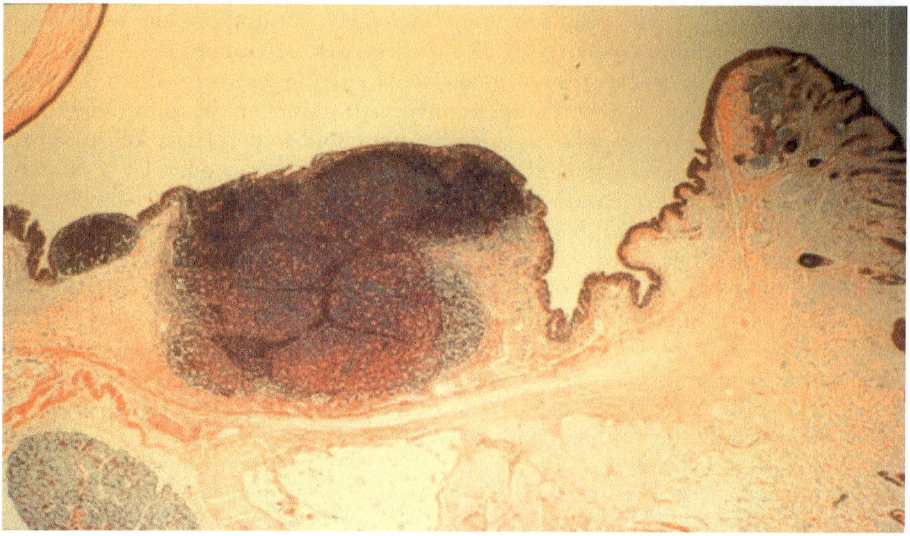

Fig. 6. Histopathological section of eyelid in an animal that was repeatedly immunized and challenged with FLOA, showing hyperplasia of CALTs. [Reproduced from Khatami et al 1989. Copyright American Medical Association @1989. All rights reserved.]

Antibody Isotypes: Comparison of antibody profiles (i.e., IgG1/IgG2 isotypes) in ocular and/or splenic tissues in highly sensitized animals during the course of immunization suggested that chronic inflammation-induced site-specific/local (CALTs) alterations in B-plasma cells (or memory cells) expression profiles of immunoglobulin subclass (e.g., IgG1/IgG2 ratios). Stimuli-induced B-plasma cell-derived expression of Ig isotype specificities and profiles and binding to respective receptors [e.g., FcεR (IgE), FCγR1 (IgG1), FcγRII (IgG2), FcγRIII (IgG3), FcαR (IgA) or FcμR (IgM)] have been identified in a number of inflammatory and infectious disease processes, tumorigenesis and cancer including conjunctival associated lymphoid hyperplasia, gut-associated lymphomas, asthma, polyps, chronic lymphocytic leukemia, Sjogren's disease, squamous cell carcinoma in atopic eczema of conjunctiva (Akhiani 2005, D'Amato et al, 2007, Drayton et al, 2006, Diz et al, 2008, Gouranis et al, 2007, Gurish 2006, Haldar et al, 1988, Heinz et al, 2003, Khatami et al, 1989, Khatami 2005 a, Vire et al, 2011).

Role of Mucus Secreting Goblet Cells. Mucus secreting GCs seemed to play a role in developmental phases of immune dysfunction and genesis of tumor-like lesions in CALTs. Heavy eosinophil infiltration into GCs was identified during the intermediate stage of immune responses. The number of swollen GCs also increased in massive hyperplastic tissues (Khatami et al, 1985, 1989, Khatami 2005 a, 2008, 2009). Others reported a role for mucosal immunity and GCs in human inflammatory diseases such as appendicitis and neoplasia of endocrine system or carcinomas (Hanson et al, 2004, Henson and Alborez-Saavedra 2001, Leiper et al, 2001).

These studies are suggestive of the first evidence for a direct link between inflammation and tumor development and a first report on developmental phases of inflammation-induced immune dysfunction that would lead to tumorigenesis and angiogenesis. Confirmation and identification of inflammation-induced developmental phases of immune dysfunction in different tissues/organs and expression of various mediators that are produced during acute, intermediate and chronic phases of inflammatory responses that would lead to tumor growth are perhaps among the first essential steps in understanding the mechanisms of inflammatory diseases or cancer.

Since 1998, at the National Cancer Institute (NCI), during author's involvement in review of major expensive clinical studies, such as prostate-lung-colorectal-ovarian (PLCO) Cancer Screening Trials, it was suggested that inflammatory mediators are ideal targets for diagnosis, prevention and therapy of several cancers. The design of a cohort clinical study was developed based on a framework that inflammation is a basis for induction of many chronic illnesses and cancer. Furthermore, cancer biomarkers criteria were standardized by creating data elements as a foundation of a database tracking system and M-CSF was used as a prototype to test the data elements (e.g., comparison of superior specificity and sensitivity with conventional biomarkers (Khatami 1999, 2005 a, b, 2007, NCI-Invention-Federal Register, 2005, NCI proposals 1999, 2004, 2006). Over the last decade, the number of funded projects that are focused on the role of various inflammatory mediators in cancer has significantly increased within and outside NCI/NIH. The Omics fields of proteomics, glycomics, metabolomics, lipidomics or genomics and related technologies/ nanotechnologies, symposia, networks and applications of a wide range of 'targeted' therapies and clinical trials have flourished in cancer research. However, these fragmented approaches have created more chaos in selection of 'personalized' or 'targeted' therapies for site-specific cancers (see the following section). Furthermore, cancer community has resisted to systematically study the role of oxidative stress or unresolved inflammation, in the loss of balance between tumoricidal vs tumorigenic ('Yin' and 'Yang') properties of immune system and the developmental phases of immune response dysfunction that participate in the many simultaneous events involved in carcinogenesis, particularly during aging process (Khatami 2011 b).

9. Evaluation of current 'targeted' therapies or 'personalized' medicine

Majority of current approaches in 'targeted' therapies or 'personalized' medicine focus on utilization of potent apoptosis-inducing factors (poisons) to inhibit specific events in numerous growth pathways that are involved in support of tumorigenesis (Alberts et al, 2011, Arguello 2011, Bannar and Gerner 2011, Boon et al, 2006, Cataldo et al, 2011, Chen et al, 2011, Coss et al, 2011, Del Fabbro et al, 2011, Florescu et al, 2011, Innocenti et al, 2011, Khatami 2011 a, b, Lesterhuis etal, 2011, Nishioka et al, 2011, Nyakern et al, 2006, Osborne et al, 2004, Ramsdale et al, 2011, Rove and Flaig 2010, Zitvogel et al, 2008). These drugs [e.g., apoptotic factors (TNF-α), monoclonal antibodies against growth factors or enzymes (e.g., VEGF, kinases), mutated genes, epigenetic modifications, etc] introduce additional oxidative stress ('immune tsunami') to an already immune-compromised body, causing additional damage not only to the primary target tissue, but also to other tissues, resulting in devastating side effects, such as cancer-associated cachexia, anorexia, sarcopenia, severe inflammation, venous thromoembolism, diarrhea, excessive loss of appetite and weight, drug-resistance and cancer relapse and multiple organ failure (MOF). Mechanisms of drug-induced cancer cachexia are very likely the results of significant systemic shifts in the balance between 'tumoricidal' and 'tumorigenic' properties of the immune system, features that are shared by potent pathogens-(e.g., endotoxins, meningitis or pneumonia viruses) induced 'cytokine storm' or 'immune tsunami' in severe acute inflammatory diseases such as sepsis, pneumonia, or meningitis and MOF (Khatami 2011 a, b) (Figure 7). These drugs could induce simultaneous production of oxidants (e.g., superoxide-$O2^-$, nitric oxide-NO and peroxynitrite) that would disrupt and damage electron chain transport and detoxifying enzymes (e.g., cytochrome C electron carriers, glutathione-GSSG/GSH, NAD^+/NADH and/or vitamin E regeneration pathways) and impair mechanisms of removal of reactive oxygen species (ROS), reactive nitrogen species (RNS), peroxides and byproducts of the citric acid cycle. Furthermore, drug-induced oxidative damage to mitochondrial integrity and function could further impact catabolism of muscle proteins that would induce sarcopenia, and oxidation of adipose tissues, leading to excessive loss of appetite and weight and MOF (Akamizu and Kangawa 2010, Alberts et al, 2011, Blum et al, 2011, Chen et al, 2011, Del Fabbro et al, 2011, Hall et al, 2011, Khatami 2011 a, b, Okamoto 2002, Suzuki et al, 2011, Terrabui et al, 2007, manuscript in preparation).

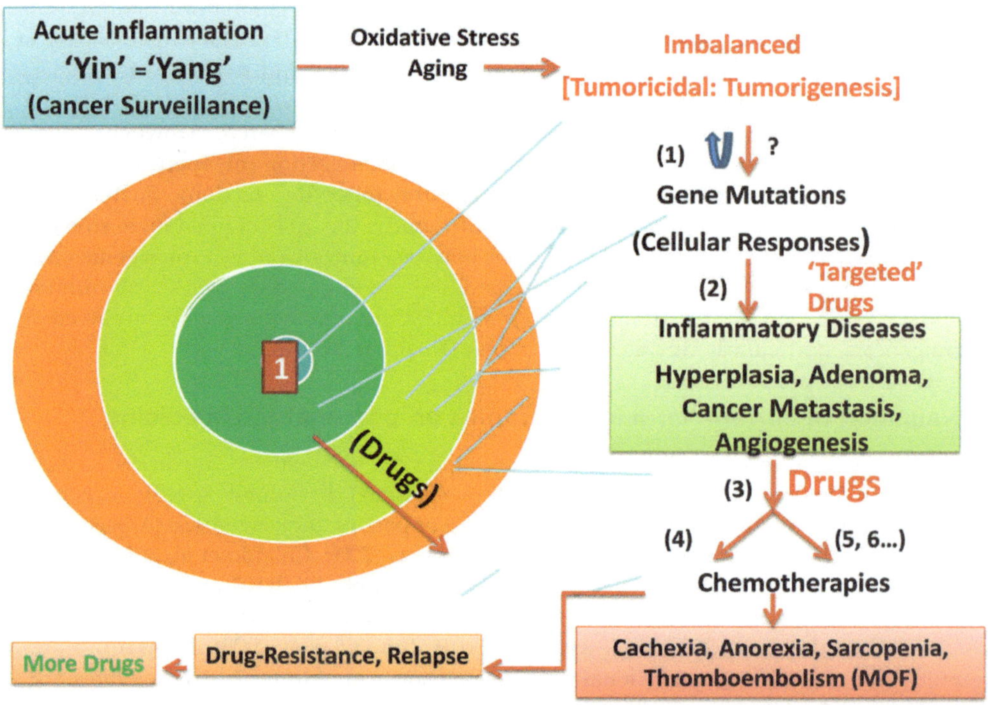

Fig. 7. Dartboard representation of current 'targeted' therapies. The figure schematically shows where we are and where we should be in 'targeting' cancer therapies. Correct/actual target is the loss of balance between tumoricidal and tumorigenic ability of immune system or loss of cancer surveillance (marked as [1]) shown at the center of dartboard. However, the claimed 'targeted' therapies for site-specific cancers are inhibitors of one or few specific genes or factors from hundreds or thousands of other molecular components that are routinely identified in pathways at multi-stages in tumorigenesis. [Modified from Khatami 2011 b, Cell Biochem. Biophys. All Right Reserved]

While the isolated molecular components, identified and/or used for 'targeted' therapies, are part (s) of the molecular pathways identified in cancer biology, they should not be considered as 'target' for therapy as they have little/no value on their own for translational purposes in treating or preventing cancer. Investigators using such approaches in 'targeted' or 'personalized' medicine fail to consider that pathways involved in cell growth-arrest ('Yin') or growth-promote ('Yang') are inherently capable of activating or deactivating alternative and interdependent pathways in immune and non-immune systems (e.g., vasculature and neuroendocrine). Several recent studies demonstrated increased risks of metastasis (cancer relapse) and additional immune suppression after radiotherapy and 'targeted' therapies in site-specific cancers (e.g., hepatic carcinoma, colon, lung, prostate, lymphoid tissues, etc). The life-threatening side effects of such 'targeted' therapies include development of cachexia, aneroxia, arterial hypertension, secondary interstitial pneumonia and diffuse alveolar damage and pulmonary edema, broncopneumonia, lung hemorrhage, pulmonary and venus thromboembolism, metastasis and cancer relapse, as well as depression and fatigue ('sickness behaviors') (Blum et al, 2011, Braun and Marks 2010, Del Fabbro et al, 2011, Elamin 2011, Hall et al, 2011, Khatami 2011 a, b, Lukaszewicz and Payen 2010, Lyman 2011, Ranmsdale et al, 2011, Suzuki et al, 2011, Terrabui et al, 2007). In addition, 'targeted' therapy-induced cancer cachexia and associated involuntary excessive loss of weight and appetite in patients are accompanied by significant declines in nutritional intake (e.g., zinc, vitamin B, anti-oxidants, etc) that contribute to the metabolic abnormalities and conditions such as hypothyroidism,, hypoadrenalism, and hypogonadism as well as induction of systemic inflammation and excessive expression of inflammatory mediators (e.g., IL-6, IL-1β, IL-8 and TNF-α, potent oxidants, etc). These drug-induced metabolic and inflammatory conditions are catabolic forces in driving the tissues toward hyper metabolism and destruction of adipocytes and muscle integrity and function that would lead to multiple organ failure or cancer relapse (manuscript in preparation).

In this section it is appropriate to remember the 1959 statement made by Peyton Rous (Nobel Laureate in Physiology or Medicine 1966) that "*A hypothesis is best known by its fruits. What have been those of the somatic mutation hypothesis? It has resulted in no good thing as concerns the cancer problem, but in much that is bad . . . . Most serious of all the results of the somatic mutation hypothesis has been its effect on research workers. It acts as a tranquilizer on those who believe in it.*" This statement was made over fifty years ago, well before the genetic study in cancer was put on steroids! (Khatami 2011 b).

10. Concluding remarks and future direction

Maintenance of immune or cancer surveillance, or the balance between 'Yin' and 'Yang' of acute inflammation is a key to healthy aging. Proposed future studies in the designs of effective diagnostic, preventive or therapeutic measures, based on the concept that unresolved inflammation is a common denominator in the genesis and progression of many age-associated diseases or cancer are summarized in the following.

1. Systematic studies on the role of unresolved inflammation in the loss of balance between inherent 'tumoricidal' vs 'tumorigenic' ('Yin' and 'Yang') protective properties of immune cells as primary focus in understanding the cancer biology and/or other chronic diseases.
2. Role of unresolved inflammation or oxidative stress in the induction of immune dysfunction in tissues that are naturally immune-privileged or immune-responsive and could cause neurodegenerative and autoimmune diseases or cancer.

3. Tissue susceptibility toward oxidative stress in immune-responsive and immune-privileged tissues, and in insulin-dependent or insulin-independent tissues for glucose transport.
4. Tissues susceptibility in immune-responsive, immune-privileged, insulin-dependent or insulin-independent tissues for glucose transport, toward oxidative stress-induced damage to genetic modifications of immune and non-immune systems.
5. Pathogen-host interaction profiles that include identification of principal response features on pathogen-, allergen-, oxidative stress-induced activation of resident or recruited immune cells in target tissues.
6. Potential reversibility of early stages of inflammation-induced immune dysfunction [e.g., pathways identified between a (acute) and b (intermediate) phases in our studies described above] that include identification of altered initial immune responses and cellular chromosomal/genetic material that would lead to cellular growth and induction of hyperplasia, neoplasia/precancer or cancer-malignancy deserve detailed studies. Outcomes of these studies are anticipated to lay a foundation for translational approaches in designs of effective prevention, diagnosis and/or therapy of cancer and many age-associated chronic diseases.
7. Potential health benefits of antioxidants, anti-inflammatory agents, or sulfhydryl-containing agents (e.g., Amifostine, isothiocyanate, mercaptoethanol, N-acethylcysteine or captopril) or precursors of glutathione on redox-sensitive transcription factors (e.g., NF-kB), leukocyte adherence to be examined at early stages of immune dysfunction for potential promotion and/or stabilization of innate and adaptive immune cells.

Promotion and/or stabilization of inherent ability of immune system toward healthy aging, that include identifying the features of pathogen-host interactions in susceptible organ systems bring their own intellectual and technical challenges but the outcomes are expected to hold serious promises in understanding how cancer cells become a threat to body and how effectively translate biology of cancer into effective clinical studies.

11. Acknowledgement

Laboratory studies were established at the University of Pennsylvania, Department of Ophthalmology, Scheie Eye Institute with supportive team of John H. Rockey, M.D., Ph.D.

12. References

Abraham AN, St. John AL: Mast cell-orchestrated immunity to pathogens. Nature Rev. Immunology, 2010, 10: 440-452.

Abrahams VM, Kamsteeg M, Mor G: The Fas/Fas ligand system and cancer: immune privilege and apoptosis. Mol Biotechnology, 2003, 25: 19-30.

Akamizu T, Kangawa K: Gherin for cachexia. J Cachexia Sarcopenia Muscle, 2010, 1: 169-176.

Alberts SR, Reid JM, Morlan BW, Farr GH, et al: Gemcitabine and Docetaxel for hepatocellular carcinoms: A phase II North Central Cancer Treatment Group Clinical Trials. Am J Clin Oncology, 2011 [Epub, ahead of print].

Akhiani AA: The role of type-specific antibodies in colonization and infection by Helicobacter pylori. Curr Opin Infect. Dis. 2005, 18: 223-227.

Al-Sarireh B, Eremin O: Tumour-associated macrophages (TAMS): disordered function, immune suppression and progressive tumour growth. J R Coll Surg Edinb 2000, 45L 1-16.

Arguello F: Atavistic Metamorphosis: a new and logical explanation for the origin and biological nature of cancer, Book -ISBN: 1460968999, 2011.

Aubert D, Lansdorp PM: Telomers and aging. Physiol Rev, 2008, 88: 557-579.

Bannar N, Gerner EW: Targeting polyamines and inflammation for cancer prevention. Recent Results Cancer Res. 2011, 188:49-64.

Barber GN: Innate immune DNA sensing pathways: STING, AIMII and the regulation of interferon production and inflammatory responses. Current Opin Immunology, 2011, 23: 10-20.

Basu S: F2-isoprostanes in human health and diseases: From molecular mechanisms to clinical implications. Antioxidants Redox Signaling, 2008, 10: 1405-1434.

Berosbaken T, Fink SL, Cookson BT: Pyroptosis: host cell death and inflammation. Nat Rev. Microbiology, 2009, 7: 99-109.

Bishop NC and Gleeson M: Acute and chronic effects of exercise on markers of mucosal immunity. Front Bioscience, 2009, 4444-4456.

Blum D, Omlin A, Baracos VE, Solheim TS, etal: Cancer cachexia: a systematic literature review of items and domains associated with involuntary weight loss in cancer. Crit Rev Oncol Hematology, 2011, 80: 114-144.

Bonasio R, von Andrian U: Generation, migration and function of circulating dendritic cells. Curr Opin Immunology, 2006, 18: 503-511.

Bonetti B, Valdo P, Ossi G, De Toni L, et al: T-cell cytotoxicity of human Schwann cell: TNF-alpha promotes fasL-mediated apoptosis and IFN gamma perforin-mediated lysis. Glia, 2003, 43: 141-148.

Booman M, Suzuhai K, Rosenwald A, Hartman E, et al: Genomic alterations and gene expression in primary diffuse large B-cell lymphomas of immune-privileged site: the importance of apoptosis and immunomodulatory pathways. J Pathology, 2008, 216: 209-217.

Boon T, Coulie PG, Van denFynde BJ, van der Bruggen P: Human T cell responses against melanoma. Ann Rev Immunology, 2006, 24: 175-208.

Bosch JA, Ring C, de Geus EJ, Veerman EC, Amerongen AV: Stress and secretory immunity. Int Rev Neurobiology, 2002, 52: 213-253.

Braun TP, Marks DL: Pathophysiology and treatment of inflammatory anorexia in chronic disease. J Cachexia Sarcopenia Muscle, 2010, 1: 135-145.

Brunello A, Kapoor R, Extermann M: Hyperglycemia during chemotherapy for hematologic and solid tumours is correlated with increased toxicity. Am J Clin Oncology, 2011, 34: 292-296.

Burnet M: Cancer; a biologic approach. I. The processes of control. Br. Med Journal, 1957, 779-786.

Campisi J: Cellular senescence; putting the paradox in perspective. Curr Opin Genet Development, 2011, 21: 107-112.

Cataldo VD, Gibbons DL, Perez-Soler R, Quintias-Cardama A: Treatment of non-small cell cancer with erlotinib or gefinitib. N Engl J Medicine, 2011, 364: 947-955.

Chen Y, Xie Y, Chen T, Sami A, et al: Adjuvant effect of HER-2/neu-specific adenoviral vector stimulating CD8(+) T and natural killer cell responses on anti-HER-2/neu antibody therapy for well-established breast tumors in HER-2/neu transgenic mice. Cancer Gene Therapy, 2011 [Epub, ahead of print]

Chidgev A, Dudakov J, Seach N, Boyd R: Impact of niche aging on thymus regeneration and immune reconstitution. Semin Immunology, 2007, 19: 331-340.

Chung Y, Norieva R, Eshashi E. Wang YH, et al: A critical role of costimulation during intrathymic development of invariant NK T cells. J Immunology, 2008, 180: 2276-2283.

Corthay A: A three-cell model for activation of naïve T helper cells. Scand J Immunology, 2006, 64:93-96.

Coss CC, Bohl CE, Dalton JT: Cancer cachexia therapy: a key weapon in the fight against cancer. Current Opin Clin Nutr Metab Care, 2011, 14: 268-273.

Crotzer VL, Blum JS: Cytosol to lysosome transport of intracellular antigens during immune surveillance. Traffic, 2010, 9: 10-16.

Culmsee C, Landshamer S: Molecular insights into mechanisms of the cell death program: role in the progression of neurodegenerative disorders. Curr. Alzheimer Research, 2006, 3: 269-283.

Davis BK, Wen H, Ting JP: The inflammasome NLRs in immunity, inflammation and associated disease. Ann Rev Immunology, 2011, 29: 707-735.

D'Amato G, Salzillo A, Piccolo A, D'Amato M, Liccardi G: A review of anti-IgE monoclonal antibody (omalizumab) as add on therapy for severe allergic (IgE-mediated) asthma. Ther Clin Risk Management, 2007, 3: 613-619.

Davalos AR, Coppe JP, Campisi J, Desprez PY: Senescent cells as a source of inflammatory factors for tumor progression. Cancer Metastasis Reviews, 2010, 29: 273-283.

Del Fabbro E, Hui D, Dalal S, Dev R: Clinical outcomes and contributors to weight loss in a cancer cachexia clinic. J Palliat Medicine, 2011, 14: 1004-1009.

Deng Y, Chan SS, Chang S: Telomere dysfunction and tumor suppression: the senescence Connection. Nat Rev Cancer, 2008, 8: 450-458.

Diz R, McCray SK, Clarke SH: B cell receptor affinity and B cell subset identity integrate to define the effectiveness, affinity threshold, and mechanism of anergy. J Immunology, 2008, 181: 3834-3840.

Drayton DL, Liao S, Mounzer RH, Ruddle NH: Lymphoid organ development: from ontology to neogenesis. Nature Immunology, 2006, 7: 344-353.

Dvorak HF: Tumors: wounds that do not heal. Similarities between tumor stroma generation and wound healing. N Engl J Medicine, 1986, 315:1650-1659.

Elamin E: Dietary and pharmacological management of severe catabolic conditions. Am J Med Science, 2011 (Epub ahead of print).

Ehrlich P, Uber den jetzigen Stand der Karzinomforschung. Ned Tijdschr Geneeskd 1909, 5: 273-90.

Ferguson TA, Griffith TS: The role of Fas ligand and TNF-related apoptosis-inducing ligand (TRAIL) in the ocular immune response. Chem. Immunol Allergy, 2007, 92: 140-54.

Ferrantini M, Capone I, Belardelli F: Dendritic cells and cytokines in immune rejection of cancer. Cytokine and Growth Reviews, 2008, 19: 93-107.

Fischetti F, Tedesco F: Cross-talk between the complement system and endothelial cells in physiologic conditions and vascular diseases. Autoimmunity, 2006, 39: 417-428.

Florescu A, Amir E, Bouganim N, Clemons M: Immune therapy for breast cancer in 2010-hype or hope? Curr Oncology, 2011, 18:e9-e18.

Ginaldi L, Martinis MD, Monti D, Franceschi C: Chronic antigenic load and apoptosis in immunosenescence. Trends in Immunology, 2005, 28: 79-84.

Gordon S: Alternative activation of macrophages. Nat Rev Immunology, 2005, 5: 953-964.

Goronzy JJ, Wevand CM: T cell development and receptor diversity during aging. Curr Opin Immunology, 2005, 17: 468-475.

Gounaris E, Blatner NR, Dennis K, Mahnusson F, et al: T-regulatory cells shift from a protective anti-inflammatory to a cancer-promoting proinflammatory phenotype in polyposis. Cancer Research, 2009, 69: 5490-5497.

Gounaris E, Erdman SE, Restanio C, Gurish MF, et al: Mast cells are an essential hematopoietic component for polyp development. PNAS, 2007, 104: 19977-19982.

Gurish F, Boyce JA: Mast cells: Ontogeny, homing, and recruitment of a unique innate effector cell. J Allerg Clin Immunology, 2006, 117: 1285-91.

Haldar JP, Khatami M, Donnelly, JJ; Rockey JH: Experimental allergic conjunctivitis: production of different isotypes of antibody by conjunctival-associated lymphoid tissue in culture. Regional Immunology, 1988, 1: 92-99.

Hall DT, Ma JF, Marco SD, Gallouzi IE: Inducible nitric oxide synthase (iNOS) in muscle wasting syndrome, sarcopenia and cachexia. Aging (Albany NY), 2011, 3: 702–715.

Hamrah P, Hug SO, Liu Y, Zhang Q, Dana MR: Corneal immunity is mediated by heterogenous population of antigen-presenting cells. J Leukocyte Biology, 2003, 74: 172-178.

Hanson A, Gosemann M, Pruss A, et al: Abnormalities in peripheral B cell memory of patients with primary Sjogren's syndrome. Arthritis and Rheumatism, 2004, 50: 1897-1908.

Harrois A, Huet O, Duranteau J: Alterations of mitochondrial function in sepsis and critical illness. Curr Opin Anesthesiology, 2009, 22: 143-149.

Harvey BP, Quan TF, Rudenga BJ, Roman RM, et al: Editing antigen presentation: antigen transfer between B lymphocyte and macrophages mediated by Class A Scavenger receptors. J Immunology, 2008, 181: 4043-4051.

Heinz C, Fanihagh F, Steuhl KP: Squamous cell carcinoma of the conjunctiva in patients with atopic eczema. Cornea, 2003, 22: 135-137.

Helleboid L, Khatami M, Wei Z-G, Rockey JH: Histamine and prostacyclin: Primary and secondary release in allergic conjunctivitis. Invest Ophthalmol Vis Science, 1991, 32: 2281-2289.

Henson DE, Alborez-Saavedra J (Eds). In pathology of incipient neoplasia. 3rd edition, 2001, Oxford: Oxford University Press.

Hotamisisligil GS: Inflammation and metabolic disorders. Nature, 2006, 444: 860-867.

Ibrahim R, Frederickson H, Parr A, Ward Y, et al: Expression of FasL in squamous cell carcinomas of the cervix and cervical intraepithelial neoplasia and its role in tumor escape mechanism. Cancer, 2006, 106: 1065-1077.

Innocenti F, Cox NJ, Dolan ME: The use of genomic information to optimize cancer chemotherapy. Semin Oncology, 2011, 38: 186-195.

Kabelitz D, Medzhitov R: Innate immunity-cross-talk with adaptive immunity through pattern recognition receptors and cytokines. Curr Opin Immunology, 2006, 19: 1-3.

Kardon R, Price RF, Julian J, Lagow E, et al: Bacterial conjunctivitis in Muc1 null mice. Invest. Ophthalmol. Vis Science, 1999, 40: 1328-1335.

Karman J, Ling C, Sauder M, Fabry Z: Initiation of immune responses in brain is promoted by local dendritic cells. J Immunology, 2004, 173: 2353-2361.

Khatami M: Na^+-Linked active transport of ascorbate into cultured bovine retinal pigment epithelial cells: Heterologous inhibition by glucose. Memb Biochemistry, 1988, 7: 115-130.

Khatami M: Inhibition of nonenzymatic glycosylation by pyridoxine, pyridoxal phosphate and aminoguanidine; a potential antivitamin B6 agent. In Current Status of Prevention and Treatment of Diabetes Complications (N Sakamoto, KGMM Alberti and N Hotta eds). 1990, pp. 649-654.

Khatami M: Inositol transport into young and old RPE cells: In vitro models of diabetes and aging. Gerontological Society of America, 51st Annual Scientific Meeting, Philadelphia, PA. Nov. 1998.

Khatami M: Induction of conjunctival-associated lymphoid hyperplasia by antigen and tumor promoting agents. Targeting mediators of inflammatory responses as biomarkers for early detection of tumor/cancer. Am Assoc Cancer Research; Special Conference Proceedings: The Biology and Genetics of Early Detection and Chemoprevention of Cancer. Bal Harbour, Fl., 1999.

Khatami M, Donnelly JJ, John T, Rockey JH: Vernal conjunctivitis. Model studies in guinea pigs immunized topically with fluoresceinyl ovalbumin. Arch. Ophthalmology, 1984, 102: 1683-1688.

Khatami M, Donnelly JJ, Rockey JH: Induction and down-regulation of conjunctival type-1 hypersensitivity reactions in guinea pigs sensitized topically with fluoresceinyl ovalbumin. Ophthalmic Research, 1985, 17:139-147.

Khatami M, Donnelly JJ, Haldar JP, Rockey JH: Massive follicular lymphoid hyperplasia in experimental chronic recurrent allergic conjunctivitis. Arch. Ophthalmology, 1989, 107:433-438.

Khatami M: Developmental phases of inflammation-induced massive lymphoid hyperplasia and extensive changes in epithelium in an experimental model of allergy. Implications for a direct link between inflammation and carcinogenesis. Am J Therapeutics, 2005 (a), 12: 117-128.

Khatami M: Cyclooxygenase inhibitor Ketorolac or mast cell stabilizers: immunological challenges in cancer therapy. Letters to the Editor. Clin Cancer Research, 2005 (b), 11: 1350-1352.

Khatami M: Standardizing cancer biomarkers criteria: data elements as a foundation for a database. Inflammatory mediator/M-CSF as model marker. Cell Biochem. Biophysics, 2007, 47: 187-198.

Khatami M: "Yin and Yang" in inflammation: Duality in innate immune cell function and tumorigenesis. Exp Opin Biol Ther. 2008, 8: 1461-1472.

Khatami M: Inflammation, Aging and Cancer: Tumoricidal vs Tumorigenesis of Immunity: A Common Denominator Mapping Chronic Diseases. Cell Biochem. Biophysics, 2009, 55: 55-79.

Khatami M: Unresolved inflammation: 'immune tsunami' or erosion of integrity in immune-privileged and immune-responsive tissues and acute and chronic inflammatory diseases or cancer. Exp Opin Biol Ther. 2011 (a), 11:1419-1432.

Khatami M: Unresolved inflammation and cancer: loss of natural immune surveillance as the correct 'target' for therapy! Seeing the 'elephant' in the light of logic. Cell Biochem. Biophysics (Commentary), 2011 (b) (Epub, ahead of print).

Khazaie K, Blantner NR, Khan MW, Gounari E, et al.: The significant role of mast cells in cancer. Cancer Metastasis Reviews, 2011, 30: 45-60.

Kimura YN, Watari K, Fotovati A, Hosoi F, et al: Inflammatory stimuli from macrophages and cancer cells synergistically promote tumor growth and angiogenesis. Cancer Science, 2007, 98: 2009-2018.

Klein L, Hinterberger M, Wirnsberger G, Kyewski B: Antigen presentation in the thymus for positive selection and central tolerance induction. Nature Rev. Immunology, 2009, 9: 833-844.

Kwidzinski E, Mutlu LK, Kovac AD, Burse J, Goldmann J, et al: Self-tolerance in the immune privileged CNS: lessons from the entorhinal cortex lesion model. J Neural Transm Suppl., 2003, 65: 29-49.

Lee HO, Herndon JM, Barreiro R, Ferguson TA: TRAIL: a mechanism of tumor surveillance in an immune privileged site. J Immunology, 2002, 169: 4739-4747.

Leiper K, Cambell BJ, Jenkinson MD, Milton, et al: Interaction between bacterial peptides, neutrophils and goblet cells. A possible mechanism for neutrophil recruitment and goblet cell depletion in colitis. Clinical Science (London), 2001, 101: 395-402.

LesterhuisWJ, Haanen JB., Punt CJ: Cancer immunotherapy-revisited. Nat Rev Drug Discovery, 2011, 10: 591-600.

Li W, Chan LS, Khatami M, Rockey JH: Non-competitive inhibition of myo-inositol transport in cultured bovine retinal capillary pericytes by glucose and reversal by sorbinil. Biochim. Biophys. Acta, 1986, 857: 198-208.

Lodoen M B, Lanier LL: Natural killer cells as an initial defense against pathogens. Curr. Opin Immunology, 2006, 18: 391-398.

Lukaszewicz AC, Payen D: The future is predetermined in severe sepsis, so what are the implications? Crit Care Medicine, 2010, 38:S512-S517.

Lyman GH: Venus thromboembolism in the patient with cancer: focus on burden of disease and benefits of thromboprophylazis. Cancer, 2011, 117: 1334-1349.

Mackawa M, Watanabe Y: Epigenetics: relationship to disease and laboratory findings. Current Medicinal Chemistry, 2007, 14: 2642-2653.

Mantovani A, Sica A, Sozzani S, Allavena P, et al: The chemokine system in diverse forms of macrophage activation and polarization. Trends Immunology, 2004, 25: 677-686.

Montovani A, Romero P, Palucka AK, Marincola FM: Tumour immunity: effector response to tumour and role of the microenvironment. Lancet, 2008, 371:771-783.

Meeker AK: Telomeres and telomerase in prostatic intraepithelial neoplasia and prostate cancer biology. Urol Oncology, 2006, 24: 122-130.

Mikkola TS, Clarkson TB: Estrogen replacement therapy, atherosclerosis and vascular function Cardiovasc Research, 2002, 53: 605-619.

Muller AJ, Sharma MD, Chandler PR, Duhadaway JB, et al: Chronic inflammation that facilitate tumor progression create local immune suppression by inducing indoleamine 2, 3 dioxygenase. Proc Natl Acad Science, 2008, 105: 17073-17078.

Nardin A, Abastado JP: Macrophages and cancer. Front Bioscience, 2008, 13: 3494-3505.

Nagai M, Hoshide S, Kairo K: Hypertension and dementia. Am. J. Hypertension, 2010, 23: 116-124.

Niederkorn JY: See no evil, hear no evil, do no evil: the lessons of immune privilege. Nature Immunology, 2006, 7: 354-359.

Nishioka Y, Aono Y, Sone S: Role of tyrosine kinase inhibitors in tumor immunology. Immunotherapy, 2011, 3: 107-116.

Nyakern M, Cappellini A, Mantovani I, Martelli AM: Synergistic induction and apoptosis in human leukemia T cells by the Akt inhibitor perifosine and etoposide through activation of intrinsic and Fas-mediated extrinsic cell death pathways. Mol Cancer Ther., 2006, 5: 1559-70.

O'Brien K, Fitzgerald DC, Nailken K, Alugupalli KR, Rostami AM, Gran B: Role of the innate immune system in autoimmune inflammatory demyelination. Curr. Med. Chemistry, 2008, 15: 1105-1115.

Okamoto T: NSAID zaltoprofen improves the decrease in body weight in rodent sickness behavior models: proposed new applications of NSAIDs (Review). Int J Mol Medicine, 2002, 9:369-372.

Osborne C, Wilson P, Tripathy D: Oncogenes and tumor suppressor genes in breast cancer: potential diagnostic and therapeutic applications Oncologist, 2004, 9: 361-377.

Park HS, Park JY, Yu R: Relationship of obesity and visceral adipocity with serum concentrations of CRP, TNF-a and IL-6, Diab Res Clin Practice, 2005, 69: 29-35.

Peerschke EI, Yin W, Griggs SE, Ghebrehiwere B: Blood platelets activate the classical pathways of human complement. J Thromb Harmost., 2006, 4:2035-2042.

Peggs KS, Quezada SA, Allison JP: Cell intrinsic mechanisms of T cell inhibition and application to cancer therapy. Immunol Reviews, 2008, 224: 141-165.

Piatkiewicz P, Czech A: Glucose metabolism disorders and the risk of cancer. Arch Immunol Ther Exp (Warsz), 2011, 59: 215-230.

Pisani P: Hyper-insulimia and cancer, meta-analyses of epidemiological studies. Arch Physiol Biochemistry, 2008, 114:63-70.

Plourde M, Jew S, Cunnane SC, Jones PJ: Conjugated linoleic acids: why the discrepancy between animal and human studies. Nutrition Reviews, 2008, 66: 415-421.

Poulsen RC, Kruger MC: Detrimental effect of eicosapentanoic acid supplementation on bone following ovariectomy in rats. Prostaglandins Leukotriens and Essential fatty acids, 2006, 75: 419-427.

Quezada SA, Jarvinen LZ, Lind EF, Noelle RJ: CD40/CD154 interactions at the interface of tolerance and immunity. Ann Rev Immunology, 2004, 22: 307-328.

Ramsdale E, van Bensien K, Smith SM: Personalized treatment of lymphoma: promise and reality. Semin Oncol., 2011, 38: 225-235.

Ren J-L, Pan J-S, Lu Y-P, Sun P, Han J: Inflammatory signaling and cellular senescence. Cellular Signal., 2009, 21: 378-383.

Ribatti D, Ennas MD, Vacca A et al; Tumour vascularity and tryptase-positive mast cells correlate with a poor prognosis in melanomas. Eur J Clin Investigations, 2003, 33: 420-425.

Risques RA, Vaughan TL, Li X, Odze RD,et al: Leukocyte telomere length predicts cancer risk in Barrett's esophagus. Cancer Epidemiol Biomarkers Prevention, 2007, 16: 2649-2655.

Rodriguez PC, Hernandez CP, Quiceno D, Dubinett SM,et al: Arginase 1 in myeloid suppressor cells is induced by COX-2 in lung carcinoma J Exp. Medicine, 2005, 202:931-939.

Romanyukha AA, Yashin AI: Age related changes in population of peripheral T cells: towards a model of immunoscenescence. Mech Ageing Development, 2003, 124: 433-443.

Rook GA, Dalgleish A: Infection, immuneregulation, and cancer. Immunol. Reviews, 2011, 240: 141-159.

Rove KO, Flaig TW: A renaissance in the medical treatment of advanced prostate cancer, Oncology -Williston Park, 2010, 24:1308-1318.

Sansoni P, Vescovoni R, Fagnoni F, Biasini C, et al: The immune system in extreme longevity. Exp Gerontology, 2008, 43: 61-65.

Schneider R, Mohebiany AN, Ifergan I, Beauseigle, at el: B cell-derived IL-15, enhances CD8 T cell cytotoxicity and is increased in multiple sclerosis patients. J Immunology, 2011, 187: 4119-4128.

Schwartz AG, Pashko LL: Dehydroepiandostone, glucose-6-phosphate dehydrogenase, and longevity. Ageing Res Reviews, 2004, 3: 171-187.

Sedivy JM, Banumathy G, Adams PD: Aging by epigenetics-A consequence of chromatin damage? Experimental cell Research, 2008, 314: 1909-1917.

Serbina NV, Jia T, Hohl TM, Pamer EG: Monocyte-mediated defense against microbial pathogens. Ann Rev Immunology, 2008, 26: 421-452.

Serhan CN, Savill J: Resolution of inflammation: the beginning programs to end. Nature Immunology, 2005, 6:1191-1197.

Sethi G, Sung B, Aggarwal BB: TNF: A master switch for inflammation and cancer. Front Bioscience, 2008, 13: 5094-5107.

Shames DS, Minna JD, Gazdar AF: DNA methylation in health, disease, and cancer. Current Molecular Medicine, 2007, 7: 85-102.

Siffrin V, Brandt AU, Herz J, Zipp F: New insights into adaptive immunity in chronic neuroinflammation. Adv. Immunology, 2007, 96: 1-40.

Simon D, Balkau B, Diabetes mellitus, hyperglycemia and cancer. Diabetes and Metabolism, 2010, 36: 182-191.

Smith KA, Popmihajlov Z: The quantal theory of immunity and the interleukin2-dependent negative feedback regulation of the immune response. Immunol Reviews, 2008, 224: 124-140.

Soehnlein O, Lindbom L: Phagocyte partnership during the onset and resolution of inflammation. Nature Rev. Immunology, 2010, 10: 427-439.

Song Z, Ju Z, Rudolph KL: Cell intrinsic and extrinsic mechanism of stem cell aging depend on telomere status. Experimental Gerontology, 2009, 44: 75-82.

Spite M, Serhan CN: Novel lipid mediators promote resolution of acute inflammation: impact of aspirin and statin. Circ Research, 2010, 107: 1170-1184.

Stern D, Yan SD, Yan SF, Schmidt AM: Receptor for advanced glycation end products: a multiligand receptor magnifying cell stress in diverse pathologic settings. Adv Drug Delivery Reviews, 2002, 54: 1615-1625.

Streilein JW, Masli S, Takeuchi M, Kezuka T: The eye's view of antigen presentation. Hum Immunology, 2002, 63: 435-443.

Suzuki H, Asakawa A, Li JB, Tsai M, et al: Zinc as an appetite stimulator-the possible role of zinc in the progression of diseases such as cachexia and sarcopenia. Recent Pat Food Nutr Agri., 2011 (Epub ahead of print).

Suzuki M, Kobayashi H, Ohwada M, et al: Macrophage-colony stimulating factor as a marker for malignant germ cell tumors of the ovary. Gynecol Oncology, 1998, 68: 35-37.

Thompson LJ, Koluman GA, Thomas S, Murali-Kirshna K: Innate inflammatory signals induced by various pathogens differentially dictate the IFN-1 dependence of CD8 T cells for clonal expansion and memory formation. J Immunology, 2006, 177: 1746-1754.

Terrabui JAA, Parra ER, Farhat C, Capelozzi VL: Autopsy-proven causes of death in lung of patients immunocompromised by secondary interstitial pneumonia. Clinics (Sao Paulo), 2007, 62: 69-76.

Valencia J, Hernandez-Lopez C, Martinez VG, Hildago L, et al: Wnt5a skews dendritic cell differentiation to an unconventional phynotype with tolerogenic features. J Immunology, 2011, 187: 4129-4139.

van Kruijsdijk RCM, van der Wall E, Visseren FLJ: Obesity and cancer: the role of dysfunctional adipose tissue. Cancer Epidemiol. Biomarkers Prevention, 2009, 18: 2569-2578.

Vanden Eynde M, Baurain JF, Mazzeo F, Machiels JP: Epidermal growth factor receptor targeted therapies for solid tumors. Acta Clin Belg., 66: 10-17, 2011.

Vena JE, Bona JR, Byers TE, Middleton E Jr, et al: Allergy related diseases and cancer: an inverse association Am. J Epidemiology, 1985, 122: 66-74.

Vasto S, Candore G, Listi F, Balisteri CR, et al: Inflammation, genes and zinc in Alzheimer's disease. Brain Res. Reviews, 2008, 58: 96-105.

Vesterinen E, Pukkala E, Timonen T, Aromaa A: Cancer incidence among 78,000 asthmatic patients. Int J Epidemiology, 1993, 22: 976-982.

Vire B, David A, Wiestner A: TOSO, the Fc {micro} Receptor, is highly expressed on chronic lymphocytic leukemia B cells, internalizes upon IgM binding, shuttles to the lysosome, and is downregulated in response to TLR activation. J Immunol.ogy, 2011, 187: 4040-4050.

Wagner DD, Frenette PS: The vessel wall and its interactions. Blood, 2008, 111:5271-5281.

Widera D, Kaus A, Kaltschmidt C, Kaltschmidt B: Neuronal stem cell, inflammation and NF-kB: basic principle of maintenance and repair or origin of brain tumours?. Neuroscience Rev. Series, 2008, 12: 459-470.

Yung RL, Julius A: Epigenetics, aging and autoimmunity. Autoimmunity, 2008, 41: 329-335.

Zamiri P, Sugita S, Streilein JW: Immunosuppressive properties of the pigmented epithelial cells and the subretinal space. Chem Immunol Allergy, 2007, 92: 86-93.

Zhang K: Integration of ER stress, oxidative stress and the inflammatory response in health and disease. Int. J Clin Exp Med. 2010, 3: 33-40.

Zhang W, Hu R: Why does diabetes offer protective effects against prostate cancer? The possible role of its microvascular complications. Med Hypotheses, 2010, 74: 242-243.

Zingg JM, Azzi A, Meydani M: Genetic polymorphisms as determinants for disease-preventive effects of vitamin E. Nutr. Reviews, 2008, 66: 406-414.

Zitvogel L, Apetoh L, Chiringhelli F, Kroemer G: Immunological aspects of cancer chemotherapy. Nat. Rev. Immunology, 2008, 8: 59-73.

2

The Innate Immune Response Mediated by TLRs in Atherosclerosis

Luis Chávez-Sánchez, Karina Chávez-Rueda,
María Victoria Legorreta-Haquet, Eduardo Montoya-Díaz
and Francisco Blanco-Favela
Unidad de Investigación Médica en Inmunología de la UMAE, Hospital de Pediatría, Centro Médico Nacional SXXI, Instituto Mexicano de Seguro Social
México

1. Introduction

The average life expectancy increased in the 20th Century, implying that important changes in disease and causes of death worldwide have occurred. Longevity increase and risk factors for chronic diseases have been combined to turn cardiovascular diseases into one of the main causes of death in the world (Libby, 2011). Heart disease and stroke are the first and third leading causes of death, respectively, in the United States. In 2006, cardiovascular disease was responsible for 31.7% of all deaths: 26.0% from heart disease and 5.7% from stroke (Heron et al., 2009). Deaths from coronary heart disease (425,425 deaths) comprise 67.4% of all deaths from heart disease (631,636 deaths) (Keenan et al., 2011). In developing countries such as Mexico, cardiovascular disease is the leading cause of death (Inegi, 2009). Atherosclerosis is a disease characterized by the accumulation of lipids, fibrous elements, cell proliferation and an inflammatory response that results in changes to the arterial wall (Libby, 2002). This disease has been observed in man throughout history, having been identified and reported in Egyptian mummies 3500 years old (Allam et al., 2009).

2. Risk factors associated with cardiovascular diseases

The risk factors associated with cardiovascular disease include the following: age, male gender, high serum levels of low-density lipoproteins (LDL), cholesterol, high-density lipoproteins, high serum cholesterol levels, diabetes mellitus, hypertension, smoking, family history of premature cardiovascular disease and infections by microorganisms such as *Chlamydia pneumoniae*. Furthermore, the combination of these risk factors is associated with a higher risk of cardiovascular disease (Ross, 1999, Garg, 2011).

3. Low-density lipoprotein structure

LDL is a spherical particle with a 22 nm diameter and a molecular weight of 2500 kDa. The particle consists of a hydrophobic nucleus of about 1600 cholesterol ester molecules and 170 triglyceride molecules surrounded by a superficial monolayer of 700 phospholipids molecules (mainly phosphatidylcholine) and 600 molecules of free cholesterol. Apolipoprotein B-100 (apoB-100) is found embedded in a monolayer; it consists of 4536 residues of amino acids, with a molecular weight of 500 kDa (figure 1). The average half-life of circulating LDL is 2.5 days (Segrest et al., 2001). The main disposal mechanism for LDL in the blood is by endocytosis of nucleated cells through the LDL receptor, which is also the primary source of cholesterol used to maintain cell membranes (Jeon & Blacklow, 2005).

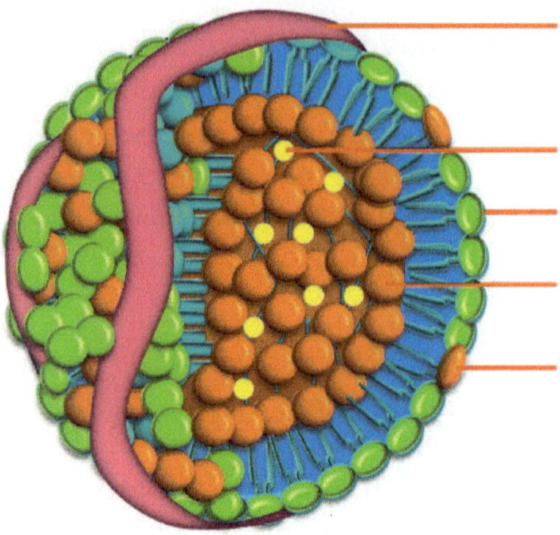

Fig. 1. Low-density lipoprotein structure. The LDL is a spherical particle consisting of the cholesterol ester, triglycerides, phospholipids, free cholesterol and apolipoprotein B-100.

4. Contribution of the low-density lipoprotein in atherosclerotic lesion development

An increase in plasma LDL levels leads to an increase in the adherence of circulating monocytes to arterial endothelial cells and, at the same time, to an increased rate of entry of LDL into the intima, resulting in a higher steady state concentration of LDL in the intima. Once incorporated, the LDL can undergo oxidative modification by endothelial cells, smooth muscle cells, or macrophages and this oxidation is a key step in the development of an atherosclerotic lesion (Steinberg, 1997). There is evidence demonstrating that oxidized LDL (oxLDL) is present in atherosclerotic plaques. Immunohistochemical analysis using antibodies against oxLDL has revealed oxLDL in atherosclerotic lesions of humans and hyperlipidemic rabbits (Damasceno et al., 2006). Likewise, oxLDL has also been obtained from atherosclerotic plaques of human arteries, and this molecule (oxLDL) presents the same properties and characteristics as oxLDL observed *in vitro*: a high electrophoretic mobility, high free cholesterol content, and a high proportion of sphingomyelin and lysophosphatidylcholine in the phospholipid fraction (Ylä-Herttuala et al., 1989). LDL may suffer a minimal oxidation and is known as minimally modified LDL (mmLDL) or complete (oxLDL); mmLDL increases adherence and penetration of monocytes, in part by stimulating the release of MCP-1 from endothelial cells (Cushing et al., 1990). mmLDL can also stimulate the release of macrophage colony-stimulating factor, which can induce differentiation of the monocyte into a cell with the phenotypic pattern of a tissue macrophage, including increased expression of the scavenger receptor (SR) (Rajavashisth et al., 1990), which does not recognize mmLDL (Berliner et al., 1990). In contrast, oxLDL is itself directly chemotactic for monocytes and is the major ligand for SR and other receptors on the arterial macrophage that contribute to foam cell formation. These may be the basis for the contribution that cells make to the foam cell population. A centrally important point is that the fatty streak lesion, while being clinically silent itself, is the precursor of the more complex lesions that cause stenosis and limited blood flow. These complex lesions ultimately represent the sites of thrombosis leading to myocardial infarction (Steinberg, 1997).

5. Atherosclerotic plaque development

The atherogenic process starts with endothelial dysfunction, recently, have shown that endothelial dysfunction may be caused by increased production of free radicals causing oxidative damage in vascular endothelial cells, which may be due to unresolved inflammatory response or the loss of balance between tumorigenic [apoptosis ('Yin')] and tumoricidal [wound healing or resolution ('Yang')] of the acute inflammatory process, which represents one of the first stages in the pathogenesis of atherosclerosis (Khatami M, 2008, 2009, 2011). The first phase consists of a loss of homeostatic functions in the endothelium (anti-adhesive, anti-aggregating, anti-proliferative, anti-thrombotic, antioxidant, and vasomotor tone regulator), as well as an increase in the endothelial permeability to LDL, which retain the extracellular matrix (figure 2A) (Ross, 1999). The LDL is modified by lipoperoxidation in the sub-endothelial space by oxygen-derived compounds produced by endothelial cells (Steinberg, 1997, Libby, 2002). The increase of LDL particles in the sub-endothelial space initiates the formation of the atherosclerotic plaque (Ross, 1999, Steinberg, 1997, Libby, 2002). The lipolysis of LDL by phospholipase A2 and lipoperoxidation generates lysophosphatidylcholine, which increases the pro-inflammatory effect in the artery intima (Mehrabian & Allayee, 2003). As a consequence, the expression of adhesion molecules are increased, including platelet/endothelial cell adhesion molecule (PECAM)-1, intercellular cell adhesion molecule (ICAM)-1, and vascular cell adhesion molecule (VCAM)-1 (Davies et al., 1993). These adhesion molecules permit the interaction of T cells and circulating monocytes with endothelial cells (Ross, 1999, Libby, 2002).

Moreover, the endothelial and smooth muscle cells synthesize and secrete chemoattractants, such as monocyte chemotactic protein (MCP)-1 (Ross, 1999, Libby, 2002), thereby stimulating the migration and accumulation of monocytes to the lesion site (figure 2A) (Osterud & Bjorklid, 2003). Other cells that participate in the atherosclerotic plaque include macrophages and platelets, which adhere to proteins of the extracellular matrix, such as von Wilebrand factor and exposed collagen. The adherence of platelets to the exposed matrix is considered the first stage in the formation of a clot (Ross, 1999). Subsequently, activated platelets release vasoactive mediators that lead to the formation of a pro-inflammatory state during clot development (Shi & Morrell, 2011). The smooth muscle cells then migrate to the lesion (figure 3B), stimulated by growth factors, such as fibroblast growth factor, among other stimuli. In addition, T cells are recruited (figure 2B) and secrete tumor necrosis factor (TNF)-α, IL-2, and other molecules (Ross, 1999, Libby, 2002).

Monocytes and macrophages participate in the innate immune response and are essential effector cells during atherosclerosis. These cells express the cell surface scavenger receptors

(SR A type I and II, and CD36), which identify and internalize oxLDL particles (Mazzone, 2000). Upon internalization, oxLDL induces monocyte transformation into foam cells (figure 2B). These events precede the formation of the advanced lesion (figure 2C), which tends to form a fibrous cover in the walls of the lumen. The fibrous cover is characterized by an extracellular growth of lipids, especially cholesterol, cholesterol esters, and matrix proteins derived from smooth muscle cells. These lesions extend to the shoulders of the plaque (Ross, 1999). As a result, the activated macrophages in the plaque secrete pro-inflammatory cytokines (Takahashi et al., 2002), among which are interleukin (IL) -1β, IL-8, TNF-α, macrophage colony-stimulating factor, and MCP-1, resulting in further monocyte/macrophage recruitment and their accumulation (Ross, 1999). Within the plaque, macrophages increase their expression of the co-stimulatory molecules CD80/CD86 (Buono et al., 2004), CD40 (Phipps, 2000), and major histocompatibility (MHC) type II molecules, which modulate T cell activation (Buono et al., 2004). The activation of T cells favors the secretion of interferon-gamma and TNF-α, which act to amplify the inflammatory response. However, apoptosis or necrosis may be generated by the accumulation of lipids, promoting the advance of the necrotic nucleus to the plaque (figure 2C) (Ross, 1999). Moreover, damage to the lesion may be augmented by macrophages that produce TNF-α, IL-1β, and metalloproteinases (Ross, 1999, Libby, 2002). The atherosclerotic lesion may suffer a rupture in the fibrous layer (figure 2D) or ulceration, which leads to unstable angina syndromes or myocardial infarction (Ross, 1999). The vulnerability of the plaque originates from a thinning of the shoulders of the lesion, which happens when macrophages degrade the matrix of the fibrous layer by means of interstitial collagenase, gelatinase, and stromelysin. In addition, there is an inhibition in the secretion of the matrix proteins from smooth muscle cells by IFN-γ secreted by T cells. Degradation of the fibrous layer may lead to a hemorrhage (figure 2D). Alternatively, the activated platelets adhere to the injured artery and cause the formation of the clot and occlusion of the artery. These changes may also be accompanied by the production of pro-coagulant tissue factors, which enhances the possibility of thrombosis (Ross, 1999, Libby, 2002).

6. TLRs

Several lines of evidence have demonstrated that toll-like receptors (TLRs) play an essential role in inflammatory responses (Medzhitov, 2001, Trinchieri & Sher 2007) and may be important for the progression of atherosclerotic disease. The gene that encodes the Toll receptor was discovered early in the 1980s as an essential component in the path that establishes the dorsoventral axis in the early *Drosophila melanogaster* embryo (Anderson et al., 1985). In 1996, Lemaitre et al. documented the first Toll-like receptor involved in the anti-fungal immune response in *D. melanogaster*, and the discovery of the first human TLR4 was performed in 1997 by Medzhitov et al., which has since been identified as a crucial component of the innate and adaptive immune responses. In mammals, 13 TLRs have been described, (11 in humans), which are located at the cellular surface and in intracellular vesicles (Kawai, et al., 2010). The TLRs form a family of receptors that have been phylogenetically conserved, exhibiting three structural characteristics: 1) they have an extracellular region that is rich in leucine-rich repeats; 2) they have a short transmembrane region; and 3) they have a cytoplasmic region that is homologous to the IL-1 receptor, also called Toll/interleukin-1–receptor (TIR), which is required to initiate signaling cascades (Medzhitov, 2001).

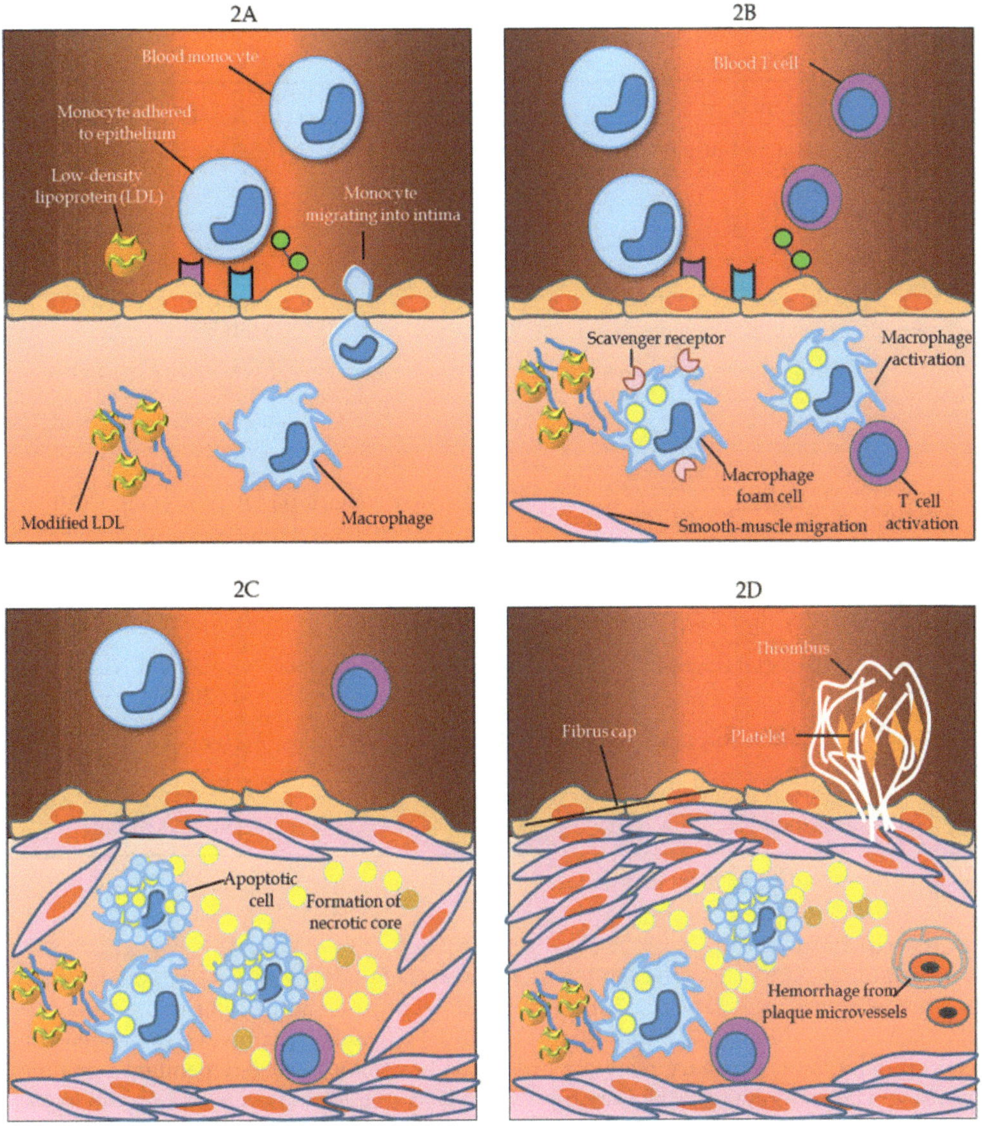

Fig. 2. Development of the atherosclerotic plaque. (2A) The lesion originates when damage to the endothelium increases the endothelial permeability and promotes leukocyte migration and adhesion. (2B) In the following stage of the lesion, smooth muscle cells migrate to the lesion, macrophages transform into foam cells, T cells are activated, platelets adhere to and accumulate at the lesion, and leukocytes continue to arrive. (2C) In the lesion, an accumulation of macrophages occurs, which subsequently die by apoptosis or necrosis, generating the necrotic nucleus and forming the fibrous layer. (2D) In the final stages, the lesion exhibits a thinning of the fibrous cap, and plaque rupture and bleeding of microvessels can ensue.

TLRs participate in the innate immune response, recognizing pathogen-associated molecular patterns (PAMPs), which are described in Table 1.

TLR	Ligand	Source ligand	
TLR1/TLR2	Tri-acyl lipopeptides	*Mycobacterium tuberculosis*	(Takeda et al., 2002)
TLR2	Peptidoglycan	*Staphylococcus aureus*	(Schwandner et al., 1999)
	Lipoarabinomannan	*Mycobacterium tuberculosis*	(Tapping & Tobias 2003)
	Phospholipomannan	*Candida albicans*	(Netea et al., 2002b)
TLR3	dsRNA	Viruses	(Alexopoulou et al., 2001)
TLR4	LPS	Gram-negative bacteria	(Chow et al., 1999)
	Envelope F protein	Respiratory syncytial virus	(Kurt-Jones et al., 2000)
	Glycoinositolphospholipids	*Trypanosoma cruzi*	(Oliveira et al., 2004)
TLR5	Bacterial flagellin	*Salmonella typhimurium*	(Andersen-Nissen et al., 2007)
TLR6/TLR2	Lipoteichoic acid	Group B streptococcus	(Henneke et al., 2005)
TLR7	ssRNA	Viruses	(Diebold et al., 2004)
TLR8	ssRNA	Viruses	(Heil et al., 2004)

Table 1. TLRs and some of their ligands

6.1 TLRs signaling

The activation of TLRs involves their dimerization, heterodimerization, or collaboration with other receptors, as well as a redistribution and aggregation at the cell surface (Husebye et al., 2006, Trianrafilou et al., 2006). Most TLRs use signaling pathways dependent on myeloid differentiation primary response protein 88 (MyD88). MyD88-dependent signaling starts in the TIR region, which then recruits the MyD88 adaptor molecule and promotes the association of IRAK (IL-1RI-associated protein kinase) 4 and IRAK1. During the formation of this complex, IRAK4 activates and phosphorylates IRAK1, which in turn interacts with TRAF (TNF receptor-associated factor) 6, thereby generating the IRAK1-TRAF6 complex that can interact with other molecules and induce the activation of the IKK complex. The IKK complex consists of IKKα and IKKβ, which catalyze phosphorylation of IkB. Phosphorylated IkB is then ubiquitinated and degraded by the proteosome, allowing the liberation and further translocation of NF-κB to the nucleus. The MyD88 independent pathway involves the TRIF protein (Toll/interleukin-1-receptor (TIR)-domain-containing adaptor protein inducing interferon (IFN)-β), which associates with the TANK-binding kinase (TBK) 1. TBK1, in turn, induces the phosphorylation of the interferon-regulatory factor (IRF) 3 transcription factor and allows its translocation to the nucleus. Thus, the activation of TLR signaling pathways induces NF-κB and IRF translocation, which activate multiple inflammatory genes such as TNF-α, IL-1β, IL-6, IFN-β, CD80, CD86, ICAM-1, VCAM-1, IL-8, and MIP1-α, among other molecules (figure 3) (Akira et al., 2006, Medzhitov, 2001).

7. TLRs Expression in atherosclerosis

In human and mouse atherosclerotic lesions, TLR1, TLR2, and TLR4 have been shown to be over-expressed in endothelial cells and monocytes/macrophages (Edfeldt et al., 2002). For example, endothelial cells located within the atherosclerotic lesion express high levels of TLR1, TLR2, and TLR4, whereas endothelial cells from a normal artery exhibit lower expression levels of these TLRs (Edfeldt et al., 2002). *In vivo,* the endothelial cells of the coronary artery increase TLR2 expression under hyperlipidemia. This increase is also observed in regions where blood flow is altered, suggesting that TLR2 participates in the initial pro-inflammatory events and contributes to the early processes of atherosclerosis (Mullick et al., 2008).

Circulating monocytes in peripheral blood from patients with unstable angina and myocardial infarction express higher levels of TLR4 than patients with stable angina or healthy subjects (Methe et al., 2005). Monocytes from patients with cardiovascular disease present higher levels of TLR2 when compared to monocytes from healthy controls. Indeed, high TLR2 levels in patients are considered a risk factor for atherogenesis (Kuwahata et al., 2010) and reflect levels of infiltrated macrophages, which also predominantly overexpress TLR2 and TLR4, in the atherosclerotic plaque of humans (Edfeldt et al., 2002).

7.1 The role of TLRs in the development of atherosclerosis

The participation of TLRs in the development of atherosclerosis has been clearly demonstrated in studies using animal models. In Apo $E^{-/-}$/$TLR4^{-/-}$ mice, a reduction in atherosclerotic plaques has been found, and it has been associated with decreased levels of pro-inflammatory cytokines, such as IL-12 or MCP-1, as well as an alteration in the plaque composition, characterized by a decrease in the macrophage infiltrate in the lesion area (Michelsen et al., 2004). In a similar study using $LDLR^{-/-}$/$TLR2^{-/-}$ mice fed a diet high in fat, under pathogen-free conditions, TLR2-deficient mice exhibited a considerable decrease in atherosclerotic lesions when compared with $LDLR^{-/-}$/$TLR2^{+/+}$ control mice. These studies clearly establish a role for TLR2 in the development of atherosclerosis, suggesting the possibility that endogenous ligands activate TLR2. Another study demonstrated that the bone marrow (BM) from $TLR2^{+/+}$ or $TLR2^{-/-}$ mice did not impact the cellular expression of TLR2 in the aortic lesion when transplanted into $LDLR^{-/-}$ mice. This effect is attributed to the resident cells, such as endothelial cells, or cells from the smooth muscle and fibroblasts, but not to cells derived from the BM, such as monocytes and macrophages. Finally, it was found that the specific *in vivo* activation of TLR2 results in an increase in the formation of the atherosclerotic plaque in control mice (Mullick et al., 2005). Other studies that support the participation of TLRs in the development of atherosclerotic lesions have demonstrated that MyD88-deficient mice are somewhat protected from the development of atherosclerosis and have a reduction in the development of the atherosclerotic plaques, accompanied by a decrease in circulating levels of pro-inflammatory cytokines, such as IL-12 and MCP-1 (Michelsen et al., 2004, Björkbacka et al., 2004).

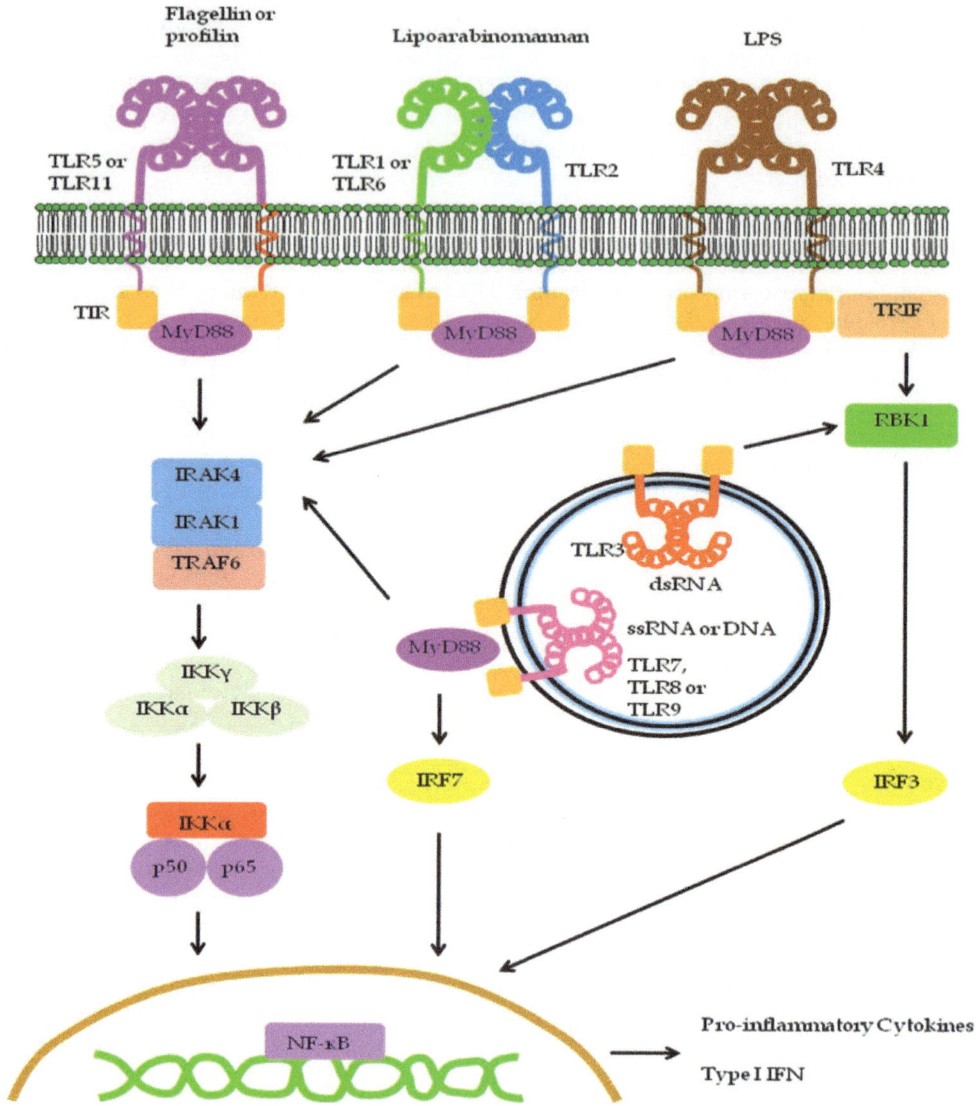

Fig. 3. Schematic representation of the TLR signaling pathway. The signaling of TLRs starts when they recognize their specific ligands. The TLRs signal through a MyD88-dependent pathway to initiate a complex signaling cascade that involves diverse proteins and culminates in the activation of NF-κB, which facilitates the expression of pro-inflammatory cytokines such as IL-1β, IL-6, and TNF-α, among others. Similarly, the MyD88-independent signaling pathway involves TRIF proteins, which are associated with the TANK binding kinase (TBK1); this induces phosphorylation of the transcription factor IRF3 and facilitates the expression of type I interferon. IkB, inhibitor of NF-κB; IRF, interferon-regulatory factor; MyD88, myeloid differentiation primary-response gene 88; TBK1, TANK-binding kinase; TRIF, Toll/interleukin-1-receptor (TIR)-domain-containing adaptor protein inducing interferon (IFN)-β.

7.2 TLR polymorphisms in atherosclerosis

The Asp299Gly polymorphism in TLR4 attenuates signaling of the receptor and decreases the inflammatory response to Gram-negative pathogens, which have been associated with a decrease in the risk for atherosclerosis (Kiechl et al., 2002). Some studies have reported this polymorphism as associated with cardiovascular disease (Ameziane et al., 2003, Boekholdt et al., 2003), although other groups have not found this association (Yang et al., 2003, Netea et al., 2004).

Some functional studies have shown that the Arg753Gln polymorphism in TLR2 results in a weak response to bacterial peptides (Lorenz et al., 2004), and it is associated with protection during restenosis (Hamann et al., 2005). However, there was no association with myocardial infarction (Labrum et al., 2007, Balistreri et al., 2008), similar to observations of the Thr1237Cys and Thr1486Cys polymorphisms from the TLR9 promoter, which suggested that these polymorphisms were not associated with atherogenesis or restenosis (Hamann et al., 2006).

7.3 The role of TLRs in response to infectious agents in atherosclerosis

One of the possible causes of inflammation in atherosclerosis is lipopolysaccharide exposure, which is a glycolipid present in the external wall of Gram-negative bacteria (Bryant et al., 2010), such as *C. pneumoniae* (Kuo et al., 1993), *Porphyromonas gingivalis* (Dorn et al., 1999), and *Helicobacter pylori* (Ameriso et al., 2001). These bacteria have been associated with atherosclerosis. Likewise, cytomegalovirus (CMV) has been associated with cardiovascular disease (Nieto et al., 1996).

For example, *C. pneumoniae* has been isolated from coronary arteries in patients with acute coronary syndrome (Saikku et al., 1988), and in experimental studies, it has been found that infection with *C. Pneumoniae* increases atherosclerotic plaque size in Apo $E^{-/-}$ mice compared to the controls. It has also been reported that the size of the aortic lesion and the expression of pro-inflammatory cytokines, such as MCP-1, IL-12p40, TNF-α, and IL-6, are reduced in $ApoE^{-/-}TLR2^{-/-}$, $ApoE^{-/-}TLR4^{-/-}$ and $ApoE^{-/-}MyD88^{-/-}$ mice when compared with the $ApoE^{-/-}$ controls infected with *C. Pneumoniae* (Naiki et al., 2008). Other studies have reported that HSP60 of *C. Pneumoniae* (cHSP60) reduces the expression and activity of nitric oxide synthase in the endothelial cells of the human coronary artery, which has also been associated with endothelial dysfunction. Moreover, the effect of cHSP60 on endothelial nitric oxide synthase deregulation is inhibited by blocking TLR2 and TLR4 (Chen et al., 2009). Additionally, the endogenous cHSP60 stimulates the proliferation of vascular smooth muscle cells (Hirono et al., 2003). Other studies have shown that *C. Pneumoniae* induces the formation of foam cells in the presence of oxLDL through TLR2 (Cao et al., 2007) and that this occurs through both MyD88-dependent or –independent pathways (Chen et al., 2009). Finally, infection of vascular smooth muscle cells with *C. Pneumoniae* mediates the persistent release of MCP-1 through the activation of TLR2 (Yang et al., 2005), and infection of mononuclear cells with *C. Pneumoniae* induces TLR2- dependent TNF and IL-1β secretion (Netea et al., 2002a), which may also contribute to the formation of the plaque.

Infection of $ApoE^{-/-}$ mice with *P. gingivalis* demonstrated an increase in the atherosclerotic plaque, characterized by an increase in levels of lipids, macrophages, and T cells (Hayashi et al., 2011). Moreover, *P. gingivalis* induced the expression of TLR2-dependent inflammatory mediators, such as IFN-γ, IL-1β, IL-6 and TNF-α (Hayashi et al., 2010). Another study demonstrated that *P. gingivalis* LPS increased TLR2 expression and induced IL-6 and TNF-α secretion in vascular secretion cells. It was also found in this study that a heterotypic receptor complex is formed, comprised of TLR2, TLR1, CD36, and CD11b/CD18 (Triantafilou et al., 2007), resulting in an overregulation of ICAM-1 and VCAM-1 in endothelial cells, which facilitates the adhesion of mononuclear cells (Nakamura et al., 2008). Other data have demonstrated that the infection by CMV increases the size atherosclerotic plaque in ApoE$^{-/-}$ mice (Hsich et al., 2001). However, to date, no data exists regarding the role of the TLRs in response to a CMV infection in the context of atherosclerosis. It is important to mention that TLR7 and TLR9 may exhibit redundant roles in the production of IFN-α/β, IL-12p40, and TNF-α by plasmacytoid dendritic cells (pDC) during CMV infection (Zucchini et al., 2008). Likewise, pDCs infected with CMV are capable of triggering the proliferation of B cells and the production of antibodies in the presence of T cells (Varani et al., 2008). This evidence suggests that a role for CMV in the pathogenesis of atherosclerosis may exist, particularly because the atherosclerotic plaque contains pDC (Van Vré et al., 2011).

TLRs participate in the innate immune response in atherosclerosis, recognizing infectious agents, which are described in Table 2.

TLR	Ligand	Infectious agent	
TLR2		*C. pneumoniae*	(Naiki et al., 2008)
	HSP60	*C. Pneumoniae*	(Chen et al., 2009)
	LPS	*P. gingivalis*	(Nakamura et al., 2008)
TLR4	HSP60	*C. Pneumoniae*	(Chen et al., 2009)

Table 2. TLRs and some of their ligands in infectious agents.

7.4 Role of TLRs in response to PAMP in atherosclerosis

It has been clearly established that PAMPs promote various processes in atherosclerosis. Among these are endothelial cell activation, foam cell formation and the development of an atherosclerotic plaque (Erridge, 2008).

The endothelium maintains the vascular tone and blood flow with little or no expression of pro-inflammatory factors under homeostatic conditions (Hadi et al., 2005). However, LPS induces cell activation resulting in an increase in the expression of TLR2 and TLR4, as well as the secretion of IFN-γ, TNF-α (Faure et al., 2001), and MCP-1 (Yumoto, et al., 2005) in vascular endothelial cells. Cell activation also results in the expression of adhesion molecules, such as E-selectin, VCAM-1 and ICAM-1, which are involved in the adhesion of monocytes and T cells to the endothelium (Jersmann et al., 2001). In addition, LPS and histamine (acting via H1 receptors) synergistically induce the production of prostaglandin and IL-6 in endothelial cells (Raveendran et al., 2011). Coronary artery endothelial cells activation through TLR2 with lipoteichoic acid exocytose Weibel-Palade bodies is accompanied by the release of von Willebran factor, P-selectin, and IL-8 (Into et al., 2007). Additionally, TLR3 activation of endothelial cells impairs endothelium-dependent vasodilation, increases the production of reactive oxygen species, reduces re-endothelialization after carotid artery damage, and increases atherosclerotic plaque formation in ApoE$^{-/-}$ mice (Zimmer et al., 2011).

Macrophages play key roles in lipid metabolism and immune responses. However, macrophages are converted into foam cells during early and late stages of atherosclerosis and contain massive amounts of cholesterol esters (Glass & Witztum, 2001). Stimulation of RAW264.7 macrophages through TLR2 with the ligand Pam3Cys in the presence of LDL leads to the formation of foam cells, and this effect is not observed in TLR2-deficient macrophages (Cao et al., 2007). The accumulation of cholesterol ester during atherogenesis reflects a balance between the internalization of lipids by scavenger receptors and cholesterol efflux. Alterations in this balance favoring the removal of lipids by efflux could limit the formation of foam cells, whereas interference with the efflux pathway would exacerbate the lesion. In this context, activation of macrophages with poly I:C, the ligand for TLR3, and lipid A, a TLR4 ligand, inhibit cholesterol efflux-dependent apoAI (Castrillo et al., 2003). These data suggest that signaling via TLR2, TLR3, or TLR4 is potentially an important modulator of cardiovascular disease, which is supported by studies in animal models that have revealed the role of PAMPs in the development of atherosclerosis. The administration of the TLR2 ligand PamCys to LDLR$^{-/-}$ mice, which are susceptible to developing atherosclerosis, showed a dramatic increase in the severity of atherosclerotic plaques (Mullick et al., 2005), while PamCys induced intimal hyperplasia in arteries of C57BL/6 mice (Schoneveld et al., 2005).

7.5 Role of TLRs in response to endogenous ligands during atherosclerosis

Most studies have focused on determining the involvement of TLRs in response to microorganisms or PAMPs. However, there is growing evidence showing that TLRs can signal through endogenous ligands, which are classified as damage-associated molecular patterns and are able to mount an inflammatory response in the absence of exogenous antigens (Chen & Nuñez, 2010).

During atherosclerosis, several endogenous ligands have the potential to activate TLRs. Initial studies indicate that the activation of macrophages with oxLDL induces the up-regulation of TLR4 mRNA in a dose-dependent manner, suggesting that a mechanism connecting lipids and TLRs exists (Xu et al., 2001). Subsequently, it was determined that mmLDL is capable of binding to CD14 and that, through the TLR4/MD2 complex, mmLDL causes actin polymerization and membrane spreading in macrophages (Miller et al., 2002). However, it has been shown that mmLDL induces secretion of pro-inflammatory cytokines, such as IL-1β, IL-6, and TNF-α, in human monocytes and macrophages through CD14 (Chávez-Sánchez et al., 2010a, Chávez-Sánchez et al., 2010b), which is corroborated by the fact that the blockade of CD14 with anti-CD14 antibodies significantly reduces the concentration of pro-inflammatory cytokines, including IL-1β and IL-6, produced by macrophages in response to oxLDL (Pasini et al., 2007). The stimulation of human monocytes and macrophages with mmLDL induces the secretion of IL-1 β, IL-6, and TNF-α through a TLR4-dependent mechanism (Chávez-Sánchez et al., 2010a, Chávez-Sánchez et al., 2010b), which is similar to the mechanism by which end products of LDL glycosylation lead to the production of TNF-α (Hodgkinson et al., 2008a). Another study showed that mmLDL induces the secretion of MIP-2 in mice and that this secretion is TLR4/MyD88 dependent in mouse macrophages, whereas the secretion of MCP-1, TNF-α, and IL-6 was shown to be independent of TLR4/MyD88 (Miller et al., 2005). Discrepancies across these studies could be due to different types of mmLDL or differences in the types of cells that were used in each study. For example, Chávez-Sánchez et al. used copper-modified LDL whereas Miller et al. used LDL modified by fibroblasts that overexpressed 15-lipoxygenase.

mmLDL has also been shown to activate TLR2 and induce the secretion of IL-1β, IL-6, and TNF-α in human monocytes and macrophages (Chávez-Sánchez et al., 2010a, Chávez-

Sánchez et al., 2010b). Moreover, the stimulation of monocytes with mmLDL causes a redistribution of CD14 and TLR4 on the cell surface, as well as the colocalization of CD14 and TLR4. mmLDL also caused the redistribution and patching of TLR2 on the cell surface, suggesting that there is a close association between these cell surface receptors (Chávez-Sánchez et al., 2010a). Similar data show that TLR2 and TLR4 colocalized with oxLDL (Su et al., 2011). Notably, mmLDL increases the expression of TLR2, rather than the expression of TLR4, in human monocytes and macrophages (Chávez-Sánchez et al., 2010a), suggesting that mmLDL may induce cross-talk between the TLR2 and TLR4 pathways of activation, resulting in amplified secretion of pro-inflammatory cytokines (Fan et al., 2006). Similarly, it has been shown that oxLDL, which can induce foam cell transformation, can increase TLR2 and TLR4 transcript expression (Holvoet et al., 2006). Surprisingly, mmLDL induces mRNA synthesis of IL-10 (Bae et al., 2009) and the secretion of this cytokine in monocytes and macrophages (Chávez-Sánchez et al., 2010b), indicating that the activation of TLR2 and TLR4 also initiates regulatory mechanisms, including the production of anti-inflammatory cytokines such as IL-10 (Liew et al., 2005).

Endogenous ligands have been associated with atherosclerosis in recent studies, including elevated serum amyloid A , which can predict cardiovascular events (Kosuge et al., 2007) and has been postulated as a shared mediator of inflammation and cardiovascular disease (Wilson et al., 2008). Serum amyloid A can induce cellular activation through TLR2 (Cheng et al., 2008), and activation of smooth muscle cells by serum amyloid A lead to an increase in the incorporation of sulfate proteoglycan, which causes an increase in glycosaminoglycan chain size and a greater binding affinity of LDL (Wilson et al., 2008).

Another acute phase protein that is involved in cardiovascular disease is fibrinogen, which induces the secretion of MCP-1 in macrophages (Smiley et al., 2001), IL-8 in monocytes (Kuhns et al., 2007), and TNF-α, IL-6, MMP-1, and MMP-9, among other molecules (Hodgkinson et al., 2008b), through the activation of TLR4.

In mice and humans, atherosclerotic plaque-resident macrophages and foam cells express fibronectin with an extra domain A (EDA) (Tan et al., 2004). This EDA domain may act as a ligand for TLR4 (Okamura et al., 2001) and TLR2, which feeds back to increase the expression of TLR2, TLR4 and CD11b (Schoneveld et al., 2008). In the development of atherosclerosis, there is a marked increase in the number of macrophages producing high mobility group box 1 (HMGB1) protein (Kalinina et al., 2004). HMGB1 can activate the

TLR	Ligand	
TLR2	mmLDL	(Chavez-Sanchez et al., 2010)
	Serum amyloid A	(Cheng et al., 2008)
	EDA	(Okamura et al., 2001)
	HMGB1	(Park et al., 2004)
TLR4	mmLDL	(Miller et al., 2002, Chavez-Sanchez et al., 2010)
	AGE-LDL	(Hodgkinson et al., 2008)
	Fibrinogen	(Hodgkinson et al., 2008)
	EDA	(Okamura et al., 2001)
	HMGB1	(Park et al., 2004) (Yang et al., 2010)

Table 3. TLRs and some of their ligands in atherosclerosis.

receptor for advanced glycation end products, and it induces secretion of TNF following activation of TLR2 and TLR4 and downstream NF-κB (Park et al., 2004). HMGB1 in endothelial cells increases the expression of ICAM-1 and E-selectin, whereas the inhibition of TLR4 leads to a suppression of these molecules plus NF-κB (Yang et al., 2010).
TLRs participate in the innate immune response in atherosclerosis, recognizing endogenous ligands, which are described in Table 3.

7.6 The TLRs as therapeutic targets

TLR4 and TLR2 have a pathogenic role in cardiovascular disease; their ability to initiate and propagate inflammation makes them attractive therapeutic targets. Therefore, blocking antibodies directed against these TLRs and pharmacological inhibitors of their signaling pathways have been considered as potential therapeutics.
Eritoran (E5564) is an antagonist of lipid A that interferes with TLR4/MD2/LPS complex formation and attenuates the inflammatory response in myocardial ischemic reperfusion, as evidenced by a reduction in infarct size and a decrease in the expression of TNF-α, IL-1β, IL-6, MIP-1α, MIP-2, and MCP-1 (Shimamoto et al., 2006). This compound is in phase III clinical trials for sepsis, and its administration in patients undergoing surgery cardiac causes no cytotoxicity, but significantly reduces the incidence of any adverse action or postoperative systemic inflammation/organ dysfunction endotoxin (Bennett-Guerrero et al., 2007).
Similarly, the blockade of TLR2 with anti-TLR2 antibody (OPN-301) reduces myocardial ischemia-reperfusion and preserves cardiac function in vivo. OPN-301 prevents the activation of NF-κB and reduces the production of TNF-α, CD11b, and proapoptotic signals, as well as stinting the infiltration of leukocytes. Thus, OPN-301 is a good candidate for adjuvant therapy in patients undergoing percutaneous transluminal coronary angioplasty (Arslan et al., 2010).

8. References

Alexopoulou L, Holt AC, Medzhitov R, Flavell RA. (2001). Recognition of double-stranded RNA and activation of NF-kappaB by Toll-like receptor 3. *Nature* 413(6857),732-738.

Allam AH, Thompson RC, Wann LS, Miyamoto MI, Thomas GS. (2009). Computed tomographic assessment of atherosclerosis in ancient Egyptian mummies. *JAMA* 302(19), 2091-2094.

Ameriso SF, Fridman EA, Leiguarda RC, Sevlever GE. (2001). Detection of Helicobacter pylori in human carotid atherosclerotic plaques. *Stroke* 32(2),385-391.

Ameziane N, Beillat T, Verpillat P, Chollet-Martin S, Aumont MC, Seknadji P, Lamotte M, Lebret D, Ollivier V, de Prost D. (2003). Association of the Toll-like receptor 4 gene Asp299Gly polymorphism with acute coronary events. *Arterioscler Thromb Vasc Biol* 23(12),e61-e64.

Andersen-Nissen E, Smith KD, Bonneau R, Strong RK, Aderem A. (2007). A conserved surface on Toll-like receptor 5 recognizes bacterial flagellin. *J Exp Med* 204(2),393-403.

Anderson KV, Jurgens G, Nsslein-Volhard C. (1985). Establishment of dorsalventral polarity in the Drosophila embryo: genetic studies on the role the *Toll* gene product. *Cell* 42(3), 779-789.

Arslan F, Smeets MB, O'Neill LA, Keogh B, McGuirk P, Timmers L, Tersteeg C, Hoefer IE, Doevendans PA, Pasterkamp G, de Kleijn DP. (2010). Myocardial ischemia/reperfusion injury is mediated by leukocytic toll-like receptor-2 and reduced by systemic administration of a novel anti-toll-like receptor-2 antibody. *Circulation* 121(1),80-90.

Bae YS, Lee JH, Choi SH, Kim S, Almazan F, Witztum JL, Miller YI. (2009). Macrophages generate reactive oxygen species in response to minimally oxidized low-density lipoprotein: toll-like receptor 4- and spleen tyrosine kinase-dependent activation of NADPH oxidase 2. *Circ Res* 104(2),210-218.

Balistreri CR, Candore G, Mirabile M, Lio D, Caimi G, Incalcaterra E, Caruso M, Hoffmann E, Caruso C. (2008). TLR2 and age-related diseases: potential effects of Arg753Gln and Arg677Trp polymorphisms in acute myocardial infarction. *Rejuvenation Res* 11(2),293-296.

Bennett-Guerrero E, Grocott HP, Levy JH, Stierer KA, Hogue CW, Cheung AT, Newman MF, Carter AA, Rossignol DP, Collard CD. (2007). A phase II, double-blind, placebo-controlled, ascending-dose study of Eritoran (E5564), a lipid A antagonist, in patients undergoing cardiac surgery with cardiopulmonary bypass. *Anesth Analg* 104(2),378-383.

Berliner JA, Territo MC, Sevanian A, Ramin S, Kim JA, Bamshad B, Esterson M, Fogelman AM. (1990). Minimally modified low density lipoprotein stimulates monocyte endothelial interactions. *J Clin Invest* 85(4),1260-1266.

Björkbacka H, Kunjathoor VV, Moore KJ, Koehn S, Ordija CM, Lee MA, Means T, Halmen K, Luster AD, Golenbock DT, Freeman MW. (2004). Reduced atherosclerosis in MyD88-null mice links elevated serum cholesterol levels to activation of innate immunity signaling pathways. *Nat Med* 10(4),416-421.

Boekholdt SM, Agema WR, Peters RJ, Zwinderman AH, van der Wall EE, Reitsma PH, Kastelein JJ, Jukema JW; REgression GRowth Evaluation Statin Study Group. (2003). Variants of toll-like receptor 4 modify the efficacy of statin therapy and the risk of cardiovascular events. *Circulation* 107(19),2416-2421.

Bryant CE, Spring DR, Gangloff M, Gay NJ. (2010). The molecular basis of the host response to lipopolysaccharide. *Nat Rev Microbiol* 8(1),8-14.

Buono C, Pang H, Uchida Y, Libby P, Sharpe AH, Lichtman AH. (2004). B7-1/B7-2 costimulation regulates plaque antigen-specific T-cell responses and atherogenesis in low-density lipoprotein receptor-deficient mice. *Circulation* 109(16),2009-2015.

Cao F, Castrillo A, Tontonoz P, Re F, Byrne GI. (2007). Chlamydia pneumoniae--induced macrophage foam cell formation is mediated by Toll-like receptor 2. *Infect Immun* 75(2),753-759.

Castrillo A, Joseph SB, Vaidya SA, Haberland M, Fogelman AM, Cheng G, Tontonoz P. (2003). Crosstalk between LXR and toll-like receptor signaling mediates bacterial and viral antagonism of cholesterol metabolism. *Mol Cell* 12(4),805-816.

Chávez-Sánchez L, Chávez-Rueda K, Legorreta-Haquet MV, Zenteno E, Ledesma-Soto Y, Montoya-Díaz E, Tesoro-Cruz E, Madrid-Miller A, Blanco-Favela F. (2010a). The activation of CD14, TLR4, and TLR2 by mmLDL induces IL-1β, IL-6, and IL-10 secretion in human monocytes and macrophages. *Lipids Health Dis* 14(9),117.

Chávez-Sánchez L, Madrid-Miller A, Chávez-Rueda K, Legorreta-Haquet MV, Tesoro-Cruz E, Blanco-Favela F. (2010b). Activation of TLR2 and TLR4 by minimally modified low-density lipoprotein in human macrophages and monocytes triggers the inflammatory response. *Hum Immunol* 71(8),737-744.

Chen C, Chai H, Wang X, Lin PH, Yao Q. (2009). Chlamydia heat shock protein 60 decreases expression of endothelial nitric oxide synthase in human and porcine coronary artery endothelial cells. *Cardiovasc Res* 83(4):768-777.

Chen GY, Nuñez G. (2010). Sterile inflammation: sensing and reacting to damage. *Nat Rev Immunol* 10(12),826-837.

Cheng N, He R, Tian J, Ye PP, Ye RD. (2008). Cutting edge: TLR2 is a functional receptor for acute-phase serum amyloid A. *J Immunol* 181(1),22-26.

Chow JC, Young DW, Golenbock DT, Christ WJ, Gusovsky F. (1999). Toll-like receptor-4 mediates lipopolysaccharide-induced signal transduction. *J Biol Chem* 274(16),10689-10692.

Cushing SD, Berliner JA, Valente AJ, Territo MC, Navab M, Parhami F, Gerrity R, Schwartz CJ, Fogelman AM. (1990). Minimally modified low density lipoprotein induces monocyte chemotactic protein 1 in human endothelial cells and smooth muscle cells. *Proc Natl Acad Sci U S A* 87(13),5134-5138.

Damasceno NR, Sevanian A, Apolinario E, Oliveira JM, Fernandes I, Abdalla DS. (2006). Detection of electronegative low density lipoprotein (LDL(-)) in plasma and atherosclerotic lesions by monoclonal antibody-based immunoassays. *Clin Biochem* 39(1),28-38.

Davies MJ, Gordon JL, Gearing AJ. (1993). The expression of the adhesion molecules ICAM-1, VCAM-1, PECAM and E-selectin in human atherosclerosis. *J Pathol* 171(3),223-229.

Diebold SS, Kaisho T, Hemmi H, Akira S, Reis e Sousa C. (2004). Innate antiviral responses by means of TLR7-mediated recognition of single-stranded RNA. *Science* 303(5663),1529-1531.

Dorn BR, Dunn WA Jr, Progulske-Fox A. (1999). Invasion of human coronary artery cells by periodontal pathogens. *Infect Immun* 67(11),5792-5798

Edfeldt K, Swedenborg J, Hansson GK, Yan ZQ. (2002). Expression of Toll-like receptors in human atherosclerotic lesions. A possible pathway for plaque activation. *Circulation* 105(10),1158-1161.

Erridge C. (2008). The roles of pathogen-associated molecular patterns in atherosclerosis. *Trends Cardiovasc Med* 18(2),52-56.

Fan J, Li Y, Vodovotz Y, Billiar TR, Wilson MA. (2006). Hemorrhagic Schock-activated neutrophils augment TLR4 signaling-induced TLR2 upregulation in alveolar macropahges: Role in hemorrhage-primed lung inflammation. *Am J Physiol Lung Cell Mol Physiol* 290(4),L738–L746.

Faure E, Thomas L, Xu H, Medvedev A, Equils O, Arditi M. (2001). Bacterial lipopolysaccharide and IFN-gamma induce Toll-like receptor 2 and Toll-like receptor 4 expression in human endothelial cells: role of NF-kappa B activation. *J Immunol* 166(3),2018-2024.

Garg A. (2011). What is the Role of Alternative Biomarkers for Coronary Heart Disease?. *Clin Endocrinol* 10.1111/j.1365-2265.

Glass CK, Witztum JL. (2001). Atherosclerosis. the road ahead. *Cell* 104(4),503-516.

Hadi HA, Carr CS, Al Suwaidi J. (2005). Endothelial dysfunction: cardiovascular risk factors, therapy, and outcome. *Vasc Health Risk Manag* 1(3),183-198.

Heil F, Hemmi H, Hochrein H, Ampenberger F, Kirschning C, Akira S, Lipford G, Wagner H, Bauer S. (2004). Species-specific recognition of single-stranded RNA via toll-like receptor 7 and 8. *Science* 303(5663),1526-1529.

Hamann L, Glaeser C, Hamprecht A, Gross M, Gomma A, Schumann RR. (2006). Toll-like receptor (TLR)-9 promotor polymorphisms and atherosclerosis. *Clin Chim Acta* 364(1-2),303-307.

Hamann L, Gomma A, Schröder NW, Stamme C, Glaeser C, Schulz S, Gross M, Anker SD, Fox K, Schumann RR. (2005). A frequent toll-like receptor (TLR)-2 polymorphism is a risk factor for coronary restenosis. *J Mol Med* 83(6),478-785.

Hayashi C, Madrigal AG, Liu X, Ukai T, Goswami S, Gudino CV, Gibson FC 3rd, Genco CA. (2010). Pathogen-mediated inflammatory atherosclerosis is mediated in part via Toll-like receptor 2-induced inflammatory responses. *J Innate Immun* 2(4),334-343.

Hayashi C, Viereck J, Hua N, Phinikaridou A, Madrigal AG, Gibson FC 3rd, Hamilton JA, Genco CA. (2011). Porphyromonas gingivalis accelerates inflammatory atherosclerosis in the innominate artery of ApoE deficient mice. *Atherosclerosis* 215(1),52-59.

Henneke P, Morath S, Uematsu S, Weichert S, Pfitzenmaier M, Takeuchi O, Müller A, Poyart C, Akira S, Berner R, Teti G, Geyer A, Hartung T, Trieu-Cuot P, Kasper DL, Golenbock DT. (2005). Role of lipoteichoic acid in the phagocyte response to group B streptococcus. J Immunol. 174(10),6449-6455.

Heron M, Hoyert DL, Murphy SL, Xu JQ, Kochanek KD, Tejada-Vera B. (2009). Deaths: final data for 2006. Hyattsville, MD: US Department of Health and Human Services, CDC, National Center for Health Statistics. *National Vital Statistics Report*, 57,(14) Available from http://www.cdc.gov/nchs/data/nvsr/nvsr57/nvsr57_14.pdf

Hirono S, Dibrov E, Hurtado C, Kostenuk A, Ducas R, Pierce GN. (2003). Chlamydia pneumoniae stimulates proliferation of vascular smooth muscle cells through induction of endogenous heat shock protein 60. *Circ Res* 93(8),710-716.

Hodgkinson CP, Laxton RC, Patel K, Ye S. (2008a). Advanced glycation end product of low density lipoprotein activates the toll like 4 receptor pathway implications for diabetic atherosclerosis. *Arterioscler Tromb Vasc Biol* 28(12),2275-2281.

Hodgkinson CP, Patel K, Ye S. (2008b). Functional Toll-like receptor 4 mutations modulate the response to fibrinogen. *Thromb Haemost* 100(2),301-307.

Holvoet P, Davey PC, De Keyzer D, Doukouré M, Deridder E, Bochaton-Piallat ML, Gabbiani G, Beaufort E, Bishay K, Andrieux N, Benhabilès N, Marguerie G. (2006). Oxidized low-density lipoprotein correlates positively with toll-like receptor 2 and interferon regulatory factor-1 and inversely with superoxide dismutase-1 expression: studies in hypercholesterolemic swine and THP-1 cells. *Arterioscler Thromb Vasc Biol* 26(7),1558-1565.

Hsich E, Zhou YF, Paigen B, Johnson TM, Burnett MS, Epstein SE. (2001). Cytomegalovirus infection increases development of atherosclerosis in Apolipoprotein-E knockout mice. *Atherosclerosis* 156(1),23–28.

Husebye H, Halaas Ø, Stenmark H, Tunheim G, Sandanger Ø, Bogen B, Brech A, Latz E, Espevik T. (2006). Endocytic pathways regulate Toll-like receptor 4 signaling and link innate and adaptive immunity. *EMBO J* 25(4),683-692.

Inegi Available from

http://www.inegi.org.mx/inegi/contenidos/espanol/prensa/contenidos/estadisticas/2009/corazon09.asp?s=inegi&c=2740&ep=21

Into T, Kanno Y, Dohkan J, Nakashima M, Inomata M, Shibata K, Lowenstein CJ, Matsushita K. (2007). Pathogen recognition by Toll-like receptor 2 activates Weibel-Palade body exocytosis in human aortic endothelial cells. *J Biol Chem* 282(11),8134-8141.

Jeon H, Blacklow SC. (2005). Structure and physiologic function of the low density lipoprotein receptor. *Annu Rev Biochem* 74,535-562.

Jersmann HP, Hii CS, Ferrante JV, Ferrante A. (2001). Bacterial lipoplysaccharide and tumor necrosis factor alpha synergistically increase expression of human endothelial adhesion molecules through activation of NF-kappa B and p38 mitogen-activated protein kinase signaling patways. *Infect Immun* 69(3),1273-1279.

Kalinina N, Agrotis A, Antropova Y, DiVitto G, Kanellakis P, Kostolias G, Ilyinskaya O, Tararak E, Bobik A. (2004). Increased expression of the DNA-binding cytokine HMGB1 in human atherosclerotic lesions: role of activated macrophages and cytokines. *Arterioscler Thromb Vasc Biol* 24(12),2320-2325.

Kawai T, Akira S. (2010). The role of pattern-recognition receptors in innate immunity: update on Toll-like receptors. *Nat Immunol* 11(5),373-384.

Keenan NL, Shaw KM; Centers for Disease Control and Prevention (CDC). (2011). Coronary heart disease and stroke deaths - United States, 2006. *MMWR Surveill Summ* 14(60) 62-66.

Kiechl S, Lorenz E, Reindel M, Wiedermann CJ, Oberhollenzer F, Bonora E, Willeit J, Schwartz DA. (2002). Toll-like receptors 4 polymorphisms and atherogenesis. *N Engl J Med* 347(3):185-192.

Kosuge M, Ebina T, Ishikawa T, Hibi K, Tsukahara K, Okuda J, Iwahashi N, Ozaki H, Yano H, Kusama I, Nakati T, Umemura S, Kimura K.(2007). Serum amyloid A is a better predictor of clinical outcomes than C-reactive protein in non-ST-segment elevation acute coronary syndromes. *Circulation Journal* 71(2),186–190.

Kuhns DB, Priel DA, Gallin JI. (2007). Induction of human monocyte interleukin (IL)-8 by fibrinogen through the toll-like receptor pathway. *Inflammation* 30(5),178-188.

Kumar H, Kawai T, Akira S. (2009). Pathogen recognition in the innate immune response. *Biochem J* 420(1),1-16.

Kuo CC, Gown AM, Benditt EP, Grayston JT. (1993). Detection of Chlamydia pneumoniae in aortic lesions of atherosclerosis by immunocytochemical stain. *Arterioscler Thromb* 13(10),1501-1504.

Kurt-Jones EA, Popova L, Kwinn L, Haynes LM, Jones LP, Tripp RA, Walsh EE, Freeman MW, Golenbock DT, Anderson LJ, Finberg RW. (2000). Pattern recognition receptors TLR4 and CD14 mediate response to respiratory syncytial virus. *Nat Immunol* 1(5),398-401.

Kuwahata S, Fujita S, Orihara K, Hamasaki S, Oba R, Hirai H, Nagata K, Ishida S, Kataoka T, Oketani N, Ichiki H, Iriki Y, Saihara K, Okui H, Ninomiya Y, Tei C. (2010). High expression level of Toll-like receptor 2 on monocytes is an important risk factor for arteriosclerotic disease. *Atherosclerosis* 209(1),248-254.

Khatami M. (2009). Inflammation, aging, and cancer: tumoricidal versus tumorigenesis of immunity: a common denominator mapping chronic diseases. *Cell Biochem Biophys* 55(2),55-79.

Khatami M. (2011). Unresolved inflammation: 'immune tsunami' or erosion of integrity in immune-privileged and immune-responsive tissues and acute and chronic inflammatory diseases or cancer. *Expert Opin Biol Ther* [Epub ahead of print].

Khatami M. (2008). 'Yin and Yang' in inflammation: duality in innate immune cell function and tumorigenesis. *Expert Opin Biol Ther* 8(10),1461-1472.

Labrum R, Bevan S, Sitzer M, Lorenz M, Markus HS. (2007). Toll receptor polymorphisms and carotid artery intima-media thickness. *Stroke* 38(4),1179-1184.

Lemaitre B, Nicolas E, Michaut L, Reichhart JM, Hoffmann JA. (1996). The dorsoventral regulatory gene cassette spätzle/Toll/cactus controls the potent antifungal response in Drosophila adults. *Cell* 86(6),973-983.

Libby P. (2002). Inflammation in atherosclerosis. *Nature* 420(6917), 868-874.

Libby P. (2011). The vascular biology of atherosclerosis, In: *Fundamentals of cardiovascular disease*, pp. Libby, Peter, Bonow, Robert O., Mann, Douglas L., Zipes, Douglas P., Braunwald, Eugene, pp. 985-1002, Saunders; 9 edition, ISBN 1416041079, Estados Unidos.

Liew FY, Xu D, Brint EK, O'Neill LA. (2005). Negative regulation of toll-like receptor-mediated immune responses. *Nat Rev Immunol* 5(6),446-458.

Lorenz E, Mira JP, Cornish KL, Arbour NC, Schwartz DA. (2000). A novel polymorphism in the toll-like receptor 2 gene and its potential association with staphylococcal infection. *Infect Immun* 68(11),6398-6401.

Mazzone T. (2000). Scavenger receptors in atherosclerosis: new answers, new questions. *Arterioscler Thromb Vasc Biol* 20(12),2506-2508.

Medzhitov R. (2001). Toll-like receptors and innate immunity. Nat Rev Immunol. Vol. 1, pages 135-145.

Medshitov R, Preston-Hurlburt P, Janeway CA Jr. (1997). A human homologue of the *Drosophila* Toll protein signals activation of adaptive immunity. *Nature* 388(6640):394-397.

Mehrabian M, Allayee H. (2003). 5-lipoxygenase and atherosclerosis. *Curr Op Lipid* 14(5),447-457.

Methe H, Kim JO, Kofler S, Weis M, Nabauer M, Koglin J. (2005) Expansion of circulating Toll-like receptor 4-positive monocytes in patients with acute coronary syndrome. *Circulation* 111(20),2654–2661.

Michelsen KS, Wong MH, Shah PK, Zhang W, Yano J, Doherty TM, Akira S, Rajavashisth TB, Arditi M. (2004). Lack of Toll-like receptor 4 or myeloid differentiation factor 88 reduces atherosclerosis and alters plaque phenotype in mice deficient in apolipoprotein E. Proc Natl Acad Sci U S A. 101(29),10679-10684.

Miller YI, Viriyakosol S, Binder CJ, Feramisco JR, Kirkland TN, Witztum JL. (2003). Minimally modified LDL binds to CD14, induces macrophage spreading via TLR4/MD-2, and inhibits phagocytosis of apoptotic cells. *J Biol Chem* 278(3),1561-1568.

Miller YI, Viriyakosol S, Worrall DS, Boullier A, Butler S, Witztum JL. (2005). Toll-like receptor 4-dependent and -independent cytokine secretion induced by minimally oxidized low-density lipoprotein in macrophages. *Arterioscler Thromb Vasc Biol* 25(6),1213-1219.

Mullick AE, Soldau K, Kiosses WB, Bell TA 3rd, Tobias PS, Curtiss LK. (2008). Increased endothelial expression of Toll-like receptor 2 at sites of disturbed blood flow exacerbates early atherogenic events. *J Exp Med* 205(2),373-383.

Mullick AE, Tobias PS, Curtiss LK. (2005). Modulation of atherosclerosis in mice by toll-like receptor 2. *J Clin Invest* 115(11),3149-3156.

Naiki Y, Sorrentino R, Wong MH, Michelsen KS, Shimada K, Chen S, Yilmaz A, Slepenkin A, Schröder NW, Crother TR, Bulut Y, Doherty TM, Bradley M, Shaposhnik Z, Peterson EM, Tontonoz P, Shah PK, Arditi M. (2008).TLR/MyD88 and Liver X Receptor α Signaling Pathways Reciprocally Control *Chlamydia pneumoniae*-Induced Acceleration of Atherosclerosis *J Immunol* 181(10),7176-7185.

Nakamura N, Yoshida M, Umeda M, Huang Y, Kitajima S, Inoue Y, Ishikawa I, Iwai T. (2008). Extended exposure of lipopolysaccharide fraction from Porphyromonas gingivalis facilitates mononuclear cell adhesion to vascular endothelium via Toll-like receptor-2 dependent mechanism. *Atherosclerosis* 196(1),59-67.

Netea MG, Hijmans A, van Wissen S, Smilde TJ, Trip MD, Kullberg BJ, de Boo T, Van der Meer JW, Kastelein JJ, Stalenhoef AF. (2004). Toll-like receptor-4 Asp299Gly polymorphism does not influence progression of atherosclerosis in patients with familial hypercholesterolaemia. *Eur J Clin Invest* 34(2),94-99.

Netea MG, Kullberg BJ, Galama JM, Stalenhoef AF, Dinarello CA, Van der Meer JW. (2002). Non-LPS components of Chlamydia pneumoniae stimulate cytokine production through Toll-like receptor 2-dependent pathways. *Eur J Immunol* 32(4),1188-1195.

Netea MG, Van Der Graaf CA, Vonk AG, Verschueren I, Van Der Meer JW, Kullberg BJ. (2002). The role of toll-like receptor (TLR) 2 and TLR4 in the host defense against disseminated candidiasis. *J Infect Dis* 185(10),1483-1489.

Nieto FJ, Adam E, Sorlie P, Farzadegan H, Melnick JL, Comstock GW, Szklo M. (1996). Cohort study of cytomegalovirus infection as a risk factor for carotid intimal-medial thickening, a measure of subclinical atherosclerosis. *Circulation* 94(5),922-927.

Okamura Y, Watari M, Jerud ES, Young DW, Ishizaka ST, Rose J, Chow JC, Strauss JF 3rd. (2001). The extra domain A of fibronectin activates Toll-like receptor 4. *J Biol Chem* 276(13),10229-10233.

Oliveira AC, Peixoto JR, de Arruda LB, Campos MA, Gazzinelli RT, Golenbock DT, Akira S, Previato JO, Mendonça-Previato L, Nobrega A, Bellio M. (2004). Expression of functional TLR4 confers proinflammatory responsiveness to Trypanosoma cruzi glycoinositolphospholipids and higher resistance to infection with T. cruzi. *J Immunol* 173(9),5688-5696.

Osterud B, Bjorklid E. (2003). Role of monocytes in atherogenesis. *Physiol Rev* 83(4),1069-1112.

Park JS, Svetkauskaite D, He Q, Kim JY, Strassheim D, Ishizaka A, Abraham E. (2004). Involvement of toll-like receptors 2 and 4 in cellular activation by high mobility group box 1 protein. *J Biol Chem* 279(9),7370-7377.

Pasini AF, Anselmi M, Garbin U, Franchi E, Stranieri C, Nava MC, Boccioletti V, Vassanelli C, Cominacini L. (2007). Enhanced levels of oxidized low-density lipoprotein prime monocytes to cytokine overproduction via upregulation of CD14 and toll-like receptor 4 in unstable angina. *Arterioscler Thromb Vasc Biol* 27(8),1991-1997.

Phipps RP. (2000). Atherosclerosis: the emerging role of inflammation and the CD40-CD40 ligand system. *Proc Natl Acad Sci U S A* 97(13),6930-6932.

Rajavashisth TB, Andalibi A, Territo MC, Berliner JA, Navab M, Fogelman AM, Lusis AJ. (1990). Induction of endothelial cell expression of granulocyte and macrophage colony-stimulating factors by modified low-density lipoproteins. *Nature* 344(6263),254-257.

Raveendran VV, Tan X, Sweeney ME, Levant B, Slusser J, Stechschulte DJ, Dileepan KN. (2011). Lipopolysaccharide induces H1 receptor expression and enhances histamine responsiveness in human coronary artery endothelial cells. *Immunology* 132(4),578-588.

Ross R. (1999). Mechanisms of Disease: Atherosclerosis - An Inflammatory Disease. *New Engl J Med* 340(2),115-126.

Saikku P, Leinonen M, Mattila K, Ekman MR, Nieminen MS, Mäkelä PH, Huttunen JK, Valtonen V. (1988). Serological evidence of an association of a novel Chlamydia, TWAR, with chronic coronary heart disease and acute myocardial infarction. *Lancet* 2(8618),983-986.

Schoneveld AH, Hoefer I, Sluijter JP, Laman JD, de Kleijn DP, Pasterkamp G. (2008). Atherosclerotic lesion development and Toll like receptor 2 and 4 responsiveness. *Atherosclerosis* 197(1),95-104

Schoneveld AH, Oude Nijhuis MM, van Middelaar B, Laman JD, de Kleijn DP, Pasterkamp G. (2005). Toll-like receptor 2 stimulation induces intimal hyperplasia and atherosclerotic lesion development. *Cardiovasc Res* 66(1),162-169.

Schwandner R, Dziarski R, Wesche H, Rothe M, Kirschning CJ. (1999). Peptidoglycan- and lipoteichoic acid-induced cell activation is mediated by toll-like receptor 2. *J Biol Chem* 274(25),17406-17409.

Segrest PJ, Jones MK, Hans De Loof, Dashti N. (2001). Structure of apolipoprotein B-100 in low density lipoproteins. *J Lipid Res* 42(9),1346-1367.

Shi G, Morrell CN. (2011). Platelets as initiators and mediators of inflammation at the vessel wall. *Thromb Res* 127(5),387-390.

Shimamoto A, Chong AJ, Yada M, Shomura S, Takayama H, Fleisig AJ, Agnew ML, Hampton CR, Rothnie CL, Spring DJ, Pohlman TH, Shimpo H, Verrier ED. (2006). Inhibition of Toll-like receptor 4 with eritoran attenuates myocardial ischemia-reperfusion injury. *Circulation* 114(1 Suppl),I270-I274.

Smiley ST, King JA, Hancock WW. (2001). Fibrinogen stimulates macrophage chemokine secretion through toll-like receptor 4. *J Immunol* 167(5),2887-2894.

Steinberg D. (1997). Low density lipoprotein oxidation and its pathobiological significance. *J Biol Chem* 272(74),20963-20966.

Su X, Ao L, Shi Y, Johnson TR, Fullerton DA, Meng X. (2011). Oxidized low density lipoprotein induces bone morphogenetic protein-2 in coronary artery endothelial cells via Toll-like receptors 2 and 4. *J Biol Chem* 286(14),12213-12220.

Takeda K, Takeuchi O, Akira S. (2002). Recognition of lipopeptides by *Toll-like receptors. J Endotoxin Res* 8(6),459-463.

Takahashi K, Takeya M, Sakashita N. (2002). Multifunctional roles of macrophages in the development and progression of atherosclerosis in humans and experimental animals. *Med Electron Microsc* 35(4),179-203.

Tan MH, Sun Z, Opitz SL, Schmidt TE, Peters JH, George EL. (2004). Deletion of the alternatively spliced fibronectin EIIIA domain in mice reduces atherosclerosis. *Blood* 104(1),11-18.

Tapping RI, Tobias PS. (2003). Mycobacterial lipoarabinomannan mediates physical interactions between TLR1 and TLR2 to induce signaling. *J Endotoxin Res* 9(4),264-268.

Trianrafilou M, Gamper FG, Haston RM, Mouratis MA, Morath S, Hartung T, Triantafilou K. (2006). Membrane sorting of toll-like receptor (TLR)-2/6 and TLR2/1 heterodimers at the cell surface determines heterotypic associations with CD36 and intracellular targeting. *J Biol Chem* 281(41),31002-31011.

Triantafilou M, Gamper FG, Lepper PM, Mouratis MA, Schumann C, Harokopakis E, Schifferle RE, Hajishengallis G, Triantafilou K. (2007). Lipopolysaccharides from atherosclerosis-associated bacteria antagonize TLR4, induce formation of TLR2/1/CD36 complexes in lipid rafts and trigger TLR2-induced inflammatory responses in human vascular endothelial cells. *Cell Microbiol* 9(8),2030-2039.

Trinchieri G, Sher A. (2007). Cooperation of Toll-like receptor signals in innate immune defence. *Nat Rev Immunol* 7(3),179-190.

Van Vré EA, Bosmans JM, Van Brussel I, Maris M, De Meyer GR, Van Schil PE, Vrints CJ, Bult H. (2011). Immunohistochemical characterisation of dendritic cells in human atherosclerotic lesions: possible pitfalls. *Pathology* 43(3):239-247.

Varani S, Cederarv M, Feld S, Tammik C, Frascaroli G, Landini MP, Söderberg-Nauclér C. (2007). Human cytomegalovirus differentially controls B cell and T cell responses through effects on plasmacytoid dendritic cells. *Immunol* 179(11),7767-7776.

Wilson PG, Thompson JC, Webb NR, de Beer FC, King VL, Tannock LR. (2008). Serum amyloid A, but not C-reactive protein, stimulates vascular proteoglycan synthesis in a pro-atherogenic manner. *American Journal of Pathology* 173(6),1902–1910.

Xu XH, Shah PK, Faure E, Equils O, Thomas L, Fishbein MC, Luthringer D, Xu XP, Rajavashisth TB, Yano J, Kaul S, Arditi M. (2001). Toll-like receptor-4 is expressed by macrophages in murine and human lipid-rich atherosclerotic plaques and upregulated by oxidized LDL. *Circulation* 104(25),3103-3108.

Yang IA, Holloway JW, Ye S; Southampton Atherosclerosis Study (SAS) Group. (2003). TLR4 Asp299Gly polymorphism is not associated with coronary artery stenosis. *Atherosclerosis* 170(1),187-190.

Yang J, Huang C, Yang J, Jiang H, Ding J. (2010). Statins attenuate high mobility group box-1 protein induced vascular endothelial activation : a key role for TLR4/NF-κB signaling pathway. *Mol Cell Biochem* 345(1-2),189-195.

Yang X, Coriolan D, Schultz K, Golenbock DT, Beasley D. (2005). Toll-like receptor 2 mediates persistent chemokine release by Chlamydia pneumoniae-infected vascular smooth muscle cells. *Arterioscler Thromb Vasc Biol* 25(11),2308-2314.

Ylä-Herttuala S, Palinski W, Rosenfeld ME, Parthasarathy S, Carew TE, Butler S, Witztum JL, Steinberg D. (1989). Evidence for the presence of oxidatively modified low density lipoprotein in atherosclerotic lesions of rabbit and man. *J Clin Invest Vol* 84(4),1086-1095.

Yumoto H, Chou HH, Takahashi Y, Davey M, Gibson FC 3rd, Genco CAYumoto H, Chou HH, Takahashi Y, Davey M, Gibson FC 3rd, Genco CA. (2005). Sensitization of human aortic endothelial cells to lipopolysaccharide via regulation of Toll-like receptor 4 by bacterial fimbria-dependent invasion. Infect Immun. 73(12),8050-8059.

Zimmer S, Steinmetz M, Asdonk T, Motz I, Coch C, Hartmann E, Barchet W, Wassmann S, Hartmann G, Nickenig G. (2011). Activation of Endothelial Toll-Like Receptor 3 Impairs Endothelial Function. *Circ Res* 108(11),1358-1366.

Zucchini N, Bessou G, Traub S, Robbins SH, Uematsu S, Akira S, Alexopoulou L, Dalod M. (2008). Cutting edge: Overlapping functions of TLR7 and TLR9 for innate defense against a herpesvirus infection. *J Immunol* 180(9),5799-5803.

3

The Impact of Macrophage Membrane Lipid Composition on Innate Immune Response Mechanisms

Julia Schumann
Institute of Physiological Chemistry, Faculty of Veterinary Medicine, University of Leipzig
Germany

1. Introduction

Most microorganisms that are encountered in the daily life of a healthy individual are detected and destroyed within minutes or hours by the defence mechanisms of the innate immunity. Macrophages play a key role in innate immunity because they can recognize, ingest and destroy many pathogens without the aid of an adaptive immune response. Macrophages recognize pathogens via cell-surface receptors that can discriminate between the surface molecules displayed by pathogens and those of the host (Bryant & Fitzgerald, 2009). Binding of bacteria to macrophage receptors stimulates phagocytosis and uptake of pathogens into intracellular vesicles, where they are destroyed (Groves et al., 2008). Upon phagocytosis macrophages produce a variety of toxic products that help to kill the engulfed microorganisms. The most important of these are antimicrobial peptides, nitric oxide (NO), the superoxide anion (O_2^-), hydrogen peroxide (H_2O_2), the hydroxyl radical ($^{\cdot}OH$), hypochlorite (OCl^-) and hypobromide (OBr^-), which are directly toxic to bacteria (Pourova et al., 2010; Robinson, 2009). In addition, activation of macrophage receptors triggers the production of pro-inflammatory cytokines and chemokines (including IL-1β, IL-6, TNF-α and CXCL8) (Hamilton et al., 1999) and the expression of co-stimulatory molecules such as B7.1 and B7.2 (Glaros et al. 2009), which orchestrates immune responses.

Fatty acids are indispensable to life for all organisms. They serve as a source of metabolic energy providing twice the energy density compared to carbohydrates or proteins. In addition, fatty acids are an integral part of cellular membranes. The heterogeneity of fatty acids in the membrane contributes to membrane fluidity as well as to the physical and chemical properties of various membrane domains (Stillwell & Wassall, 2003; Wassall & Stillwell, 2008). Numerous cellular functions critically rely on the dynamic characteristics of the membranes. Thus, fatty acids are important for signalling mechanisms as well as catalytic processes by membrane-associated enzymes (Stillwell & Wassall, 2003; Wassall & Stillwell, 2008). The oxygenated derivatives of some fatty acids include prostaglandins, prostacyclins, thromboxanes and leukotrienes, lipoxins, resolvins, protectins and marensins (Bannenberg & Serhan, 2010; Kohli & Levy, 2009; Löffler et al., 2007; Norling & Serhan, 2010). This group of biological messenger substances mediate numerous and diverse actions especially in the immune system (Bannenberg & Serhan, 2010; Kohli & Levy, 2009; Löffler et al., 2007; Norling & Serhan, 2010).

Diseases occur when a microorganism succeeds in evading or overwhelming innate host defences to establish a local site of infection, and then replicates there to allow its further transmission within the body. Immunocompromised individuals are in special danger in developing serious illness (Kamboj, et al., 2005; Prescott, 1991; Trautmann et al., 2005). Immune cell activity depends on numerous external as well as internal stimuli. One important factor modulating immune function is the diet. In particular, nutritional fatty acids have an impact on membrane fatty acid composition. Basic properties of membranes, including fatty acid chain order, phase behaviour, elastic compressibility, ion permeability, fusion, rapid flip-flop as well as protein function are determined by the lipid composition (Stillwell & Wassall, 2003; Wassall & Stillwell, 2008). Accordingly, changes in membrane fatty acid pattern may impact cell signalling pathways and membrane-associated enzymes via modulating membrane fluidity (Stillwell & Wassall, 2003; Wassall & Stillwell, 2008). The interrelation between dietary fatty acids, membrane composition and macrophage function provides a link between dietary fatty acid uptake, inflammation and immunity.

1.1 Innate immunity

The innate immunity is the frontline in the host`s immune response. After infection the innate immunity detects and destroys invading microorganisms within minutes or hours. Only if the pathogen overwhelms the innate immunity an adaptive immune response is needed.

A typical attribute of the innate immunity is its efficiency in fighting a wide variety of pathogens. The differentiation between self and non-self is based on a limited and invariant repertoire of pattern recognition receptors (PRRs) (Bryant & Fitzgerald, 2009). These receptors bind evolutionary conserved regular molecular structures, the so called pathogen-associated molecular patterns (PAMPs) (Bryant & Fitzgerald, 2009). In general, PAMPs represent typical structures on the surface of microorganisms, which are not found on host cells. This includes peptidoglycane, lipopolysaccharide (LPS), mannose-rich oligosaccharides and un-methylated GC-rich DNA (Mogensen, 2009).

The innate immunity is based on leucocytes of the myeloide cell line: macrophages, granulocytes (neutrophil, eosinophil, basophil), mast cells and dendritic cells. Macrophages and neutrophil granulocytes are predominantly phagocytes. They engulf pathogens and destroy them inside (Silva, 2010). Premature dendritic cells are phagocytes as well (Miloud et al., 2010). After maturing dendritic cells function as antigen presenting cells (Miloud et al., 2010). Eosinophil and basophil granulocytes as well as mast cells are characterized by a great amount of secretory granula (Boyce et al., 2009). Eosinophils are thought to play an important role in the immune defence against parasites (Boyce et al., 2009). Mast cells promote locale inflammation in tissues (Boyce et al., 2009).

1.2 Macrophages

Macrophages (figure 1) are migrating mononuclear phagocytes, which appear throughout the body. In particular, macrophages can be found in high numbers in connective tissue, in the submucosa of the intestinal tract, in the lung, in the liver, in the spleen and along specific blood vessels (Varol et al., 2009). Macrophages function as pathogen-recognitive and antigen-presentating scavenger cells (Russel et al., 2009). In addition, macrophages serve as a source of pro-inflammatory cytokines as IL-1β, IL-6, TNF-α and CXCL8 (Hamilton et al., 1999). The cells are crucial for engulfment and killing of invading microorganisms and for orchestrating the immune response (Russel et al., 2009). At this, macrophages trigger the initiation of inflammatory processes via secretion of pro-inflammatory signal proteins, which activates further immune cells (Hamilton et al., 1999). A special function of macrophages is the clearance of the body from dead cells and cell debris (Russel et al., 2009).

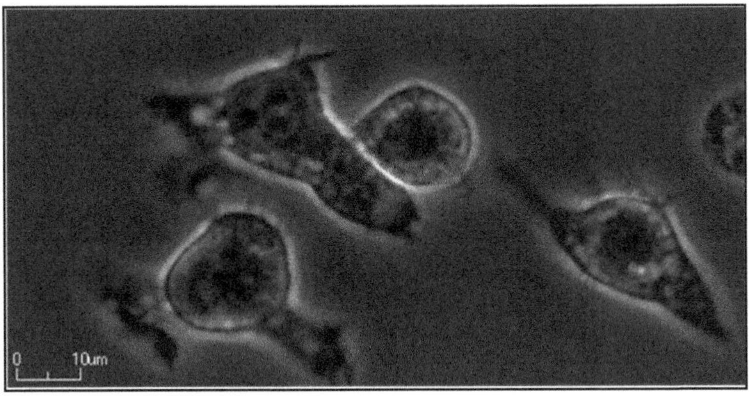

Fig. 1. Macrophages of the murine cell line RAW264.7 (phase-contrast).

Macrophages express several cell-surface receptors, which can discriminate numerous bacterial components as bacterial carbohydrates (mannose receptor, glucan receptor), bacterial lipids (LPS receptors) as well as other structures typically found on pathogen surfaces (Toll-like receptors, scavenger receptors) (Bryant & Fitzgerald, 2009). The binding of a bacterium to a macrophage receptor stimulates the engulfment of the pathogen into intracellular vesicles, a process known as phagocytosis (Groves et al., 2008) (figure 2). The phagocytosis is an active process. Initially, the receptor-bound pathogen is surrounded by the membrane of the phagocyte. This is followed by an internalisation of the pathogen into an intracellular vesicle, the so called phagosom. The destruction of the microorganism in the phagosom occurs via lowering of the pH (Haas, 2007). Furthermore, the phagosom fuses with lysosomes, which enables the killing of the pathogen via lysosomal enzymes (Haas, 2007).

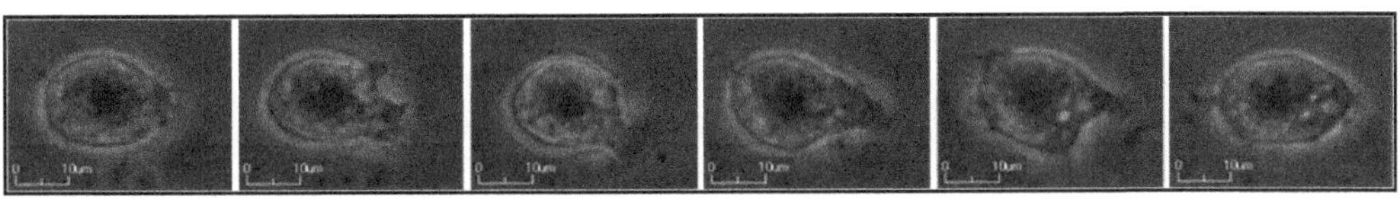

Fig. 2. Macrophage of the murine cell line RAW264.7 during phagocytosis (phase-contrast).

Macrophages produce a variety of toxic substances to kill engulfed microorganisms (figure 3). This includes antimicrobial peptides, nitric oxide (NO), the superoxide anion (O_2^-) and hydrogen peroxide (H_2O_2) (Pourova et al., 2010; Robinson, 2009). Nitric oxide is generated by the inducible nitric oxide synthase (iNOS) (Pourova et al., 2010; Robinson, 2009). Superoxide is synthesized by a multicomponent, membrane-associated NADPH oxidase in a process known as the respiratory burst, and further converted by the enzyme superoxide dismutase into H_2O_2 (Pourova et al., 2010; Robinson, 2009). Based on H_2O_2 a range of toxic chemicals, including the hydroxyl radical (˙OH), hypochlorite (OCl^-) and hypobromide (OBr^-) are produced by chemical and enzymatic reactions (Pourova et al., 2010; Robinson, 2009). Moreover, the activation of macrophages receptors promotes the expression of co-stimulating molecules as B7.1 and B7.2 (Glaros et al. 2009).

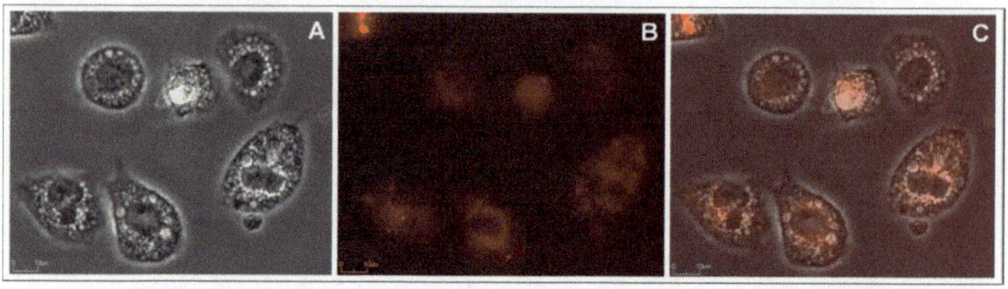

Fig. 3. Macrophages of the murine cell line RAW264.7 stimulated with phorbol-myristate-acetat (PMA). Intracellular respiratory burst is detected by the fluorogenic probe dihydrorhodamine 123.
A: Phase-contrast; B: Fluorescence channel Cy3; C: Overlay

2. Inflammation and bacterial resistance

2.1 Characteristics of an inflammation

An inflammation is defined as a local accumulation of fluid, plasma proteins and leucocytes caused by physical injuries, infections or locale immune reactions (Johnston et al., 2007). Characteristics of an inflammation are redness, swelling, heat and pain. During an acute inflammation the host actively fights invading microorganisms. This includes the inhibition of infection spread by means of physical barriers and the activation of the complement system (Johnston et al., 2007). The process is triggered by macrophage secreted cytokines (Johnston et al., 2007).

2.2 Bacterial resistance mechanisms

Several pathogens have evolved resistance mechanism to escape the immune defence (Johnston et al., 2007). Such persistent microorganisms are the cause of chronic infections. A chronic infection is a protracted process. Characteristics are an ongoing tissue damage accompanied with permanent proliferation processes (Germolec et al., 2010).
Bacterial resistance mechanisms are important factors of virulence, which have a significant impact on infection outcome. Via interaction with the immune system pathogens are able to modulate the defence mechanisms of the host thereby influencing the severity of disease (Veesenmeyer et al., 2009). Both the rate of pathogen elimination as well as the scale of tissue damage can be manipulated by the microorganisms. There is a multitude of bacterial resistance mechanisms. Typical examples are listed in table 1.
The impermeability of the membrane and the active transport of antimicrobial substances out of the cell impair the accumulation of antibiotics in the pathogens inside. Bacterial resistances against β-lactam antibiotics, fluoroquinolones, tetracyclines and aminoglycosides have been reported to be based on these mechanisms (Strateva & Yordanov, 2009).

Bacterial resistance mechanisms
Reduced permeability of the outer membrane
Constitutive (over-)expression of efflux channel proteins with broad substrate specifity
Biofilm formation
Quorum sensing

Table 1. Bacterial resistance mechanisms (Veesenmeyer et al., 2009; Strateva & Yordanov, 2009)

Via biofilm formation bacteria are able to colonise on all types of animal tissue, plants and inert surfaces (Boyen et al., 2009; Veesenmeyer et al., 2009). Furthermore, the resistance of the microorganisms against environmental conditions is improved. Biofilm formation hampers the killing of the pathogens by immune defence mechanisms or antimicrobial substances (Boyen et al., 2009; Veesenmeyer et al., 2009). As a consequence there are chronic infections, which are hard to treat by the means of antibiotics (Boyen et al., 2009; Veesenmeyer et al., 2009).

Quorum sensing is a communication mechanism, which is used by bacteria for collective coordination (Boyen et al., 2009). The microorganisms produce chemical signalling molecules as polypeptides (auto-inducing polypeptides. AIPs), N-acetyl-homoserine-lactone (auto inducer-1, AI-1) or furanosyl-borate-ester (auto inducer-2, AI-2) and secret them into the environment (Boyen et al., 2009). When exceeding a critical concentration the signal molecules modulate gene expression of the bacteria thus synchronising the behaviour of the whole population (Boyen et al., 2009). By this way quorum sensing promotes biofilm formation and manipulates virulence, mobility and sporulation of the microorganisms (Boyen et al., 2009).

2.3 Examples

2.3.1 *Rhodococcus equi*

Infections of immunocompetent humans with *R. equi* are rare. However, in case of immune-suppressing conditions as transplantations, cancer treatment and steroid medication pneumonia caused by *R. equi* have been observed (Kamboj, et al., 2005; Prescott, 1991). HIV positive people are particularly endangered. The mortality rate of infected AIDS patients is reported to be about 55% (Bell et al., 1998).

The facultative intracellular bacterium is known to survive extreme environmental conditions as low pH (Benoit, 2000) or oxidative stress (Benoit, 2002). In addition, *R. equi* blocks the process of phagosom maturation thus surviving and proliferating within macrophages (Fernandez-Mora et al., 2005). Internalised viable *R. equi* organisms prevent the fusion of their phagosom with lysosomes leading to an arrested phagosom neutral in pH and without lysosomal contents (Fernandez-Mora et al., 2005). The underlying mechanisms are not known, so far.

2.3.2 *Pseudomonas aeruginosa*

P. aeruginosa is one of the leading hospital bugs in the world. According to estimates the microorganism accounts for 10 to 15% of all nosocomial infections (Blanc et al., 1998). *P.*

aeruginosa colonises burns and wounds as well as the respiratory tract and the urinary tract of immunocompromised individuals (Trautmann et al., 2005). Due to the natural resistance of the opportunistic pathogen against numerous antibiotics *P. aeruginosa* infections are often hard to treat (Strateva & Yordanov, 2009). Moreover, the microorganism has a remarkably ability to acquire further resistance mechanisms against antimicrobial substances by the means of mutations (Strateva & Yordanov, 2009). Another notorious characteristic of *P. aeruginosa* is the biofilm formation (Boyen et al., 2009). The colonisation of surfaces of surgical implants, endotracheal tubes, catheters as well as the respiratory tract of individuals suffering from cystic fibrosis becomes an increasing medical problem. Further virulence factors of *P. aeruginosa* include the secretion of a number of toxins and the expression of flagella and type IV pili, which are of importance for surface attachment (Veesenmeyer et al., 2009). Two quorum sensing mechanisms of *P. aeruginosa* have been identified, so far: Las and Rhl (Veesenmeyer et al., 2009). A Pseudomonas quinolone signal (PQS) acts as mediator between the two systems (Pesci et al., 1999). Quorum sensing controls about 350 genes of *P. aeruginosa* (approximately 6% of the entire genome) modulating toxin synthesis and biofilm formation (Veesenmeyer et al., 2009).

3. Fatty acids and cellular membranes

3.1 Fatty acids

Fatty acids are composed of a hydrocarbon chain and a carboxyl group. Most naturally occurring fatty acids have a chain of an even number of carbon atoms. Fatty acids may be saturated or unsaturated depending on the existence of double bonds. In almost every unsaturated fatty acid the double bonds are in *cis* configuration (Löffler et al., 2007). This means that the adjacent hydrogen atoms are on the same side of the double bond resulting in a rigid binding, which restricts the conformational freedom of the fatty acid. The more *cis* double bonds a chain has, the less flexible it is. Thus, *cis* bonds limit the ability of a fatty acid to be closely packed (Stillwell & Wassall, 2003). Since fatty acids are parts of triglycerides in lipid droplets as well as of phospholipids in lipid bilayers the number of *cis* bonds of a fatty acid has an impact on basic physical properties of fat or biological membranes (Stillwell & Wassall, 2003).

Depending on the position of the double bonds unsaturated fatty acids are classified in several fatty acid families: n3, n6, n7 and n9. This terminology is based on the first double bond relative to the end of the hydrocarbon chain. For example, the term n3 signifies that the first unsaturation exist at the third carbon-carbon bond from the terminal methyl end of the chain. A transformation of a fatty acid from one family to another is not possible (Löffler et al., 2007). Animals and humans lack the ability to introduce double bonds in fatty acids beyond carbon 9. So, the fatty acids linoleic acid (C18:2n6) and linolenic acid (C18:3n3) are essential to the animal and human organisms (Löffler et al., 2007). Important examples of the n3, the n6, the n7 and the n9 family are listed in table 2.

Fatty acids are of great importance as membrane compound and in energy metabolism in the animal and human organisms. They can be found both as free fatty acids and as parts of acylglycerols, phospholipids, sphingolipids and cholesterol esters. Furthermore, some fatty acids serve as precursors of eicosanoid synthesis.

Non-scientific name	Chemical formula	Structural formula
N3 family		
Linolenic acid (LNA)	C18:3n3	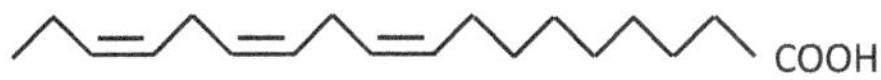
Eicosapentaenoic acid (EPA)	C20:5n3	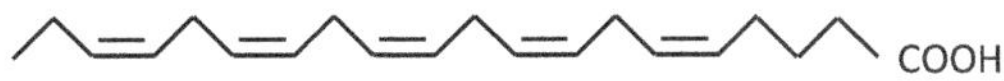
Docosahexaenoic acid (DHA)	C20:6n3	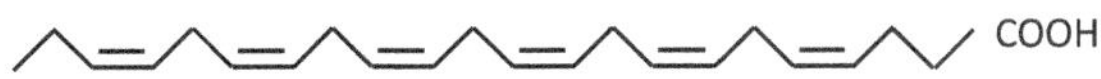
N6 family		
Linoleic acid (LA)	C18:2n6	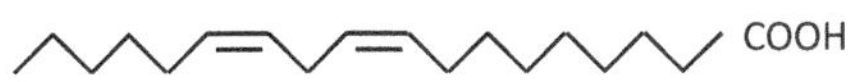
Gamma-linolenic acid (γ-LNA)	C18:3n6	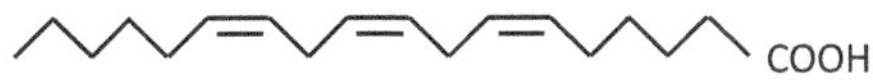
Arachidonic acid (AA)	C20:4n6	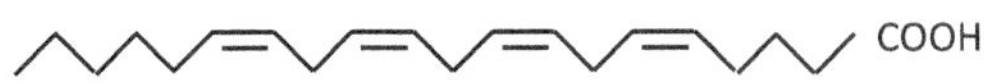
N7 family		
Palmitoleic acid	C17:1n7	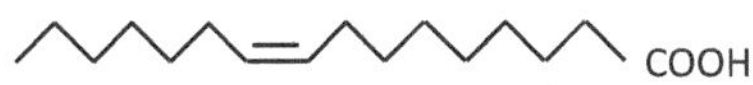
N9 family		
Oleic acid (OA)	C18:1n9	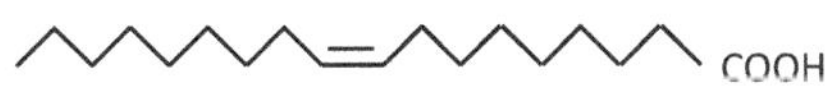

Table 2. Important examples of the n3, the n6, the n7 and the n9 fatty acid family

3.2 Cellular membranes

Cellular membranes are essential to life for all living beings. In prokaryotic organisms the plasma membrane separates the inner of the cell from the environment. In eukaryotic organisms beyond that there are additional intracellular membranes which encompass the cell organelles leading to a compartmentalisation of the cell. Furthermore, in eukaryotic organisms there are numerous membrane-enclosed vesicles, which ensure the directed exchange of materials and membrane components between the compartments of the cell as well as between the cell and the environment.

Membranes serve diverse functions in prokaryotic and eukaryotic cells. The plasma membrane is selectively-permeable to ions and organic molecules thus controlling the movement of substances in and out the cell. Biological membranes are involved in a variety of cellular processes as cell adhesion, ion conductivity and cell signalling. Moreover, membranes serve as an attachment surface both extracellular and intracellular.

The basic structure of biological membranes is a lipid bilayer, which is composed of phospholipids and sphingolipids. Further components of cellular membranes are cholesterol and proteins. Cholesterol crucially impacts the viscosity of the membrane. The hydrophobic interactions between the sterol scaffold of the cholesterol and the acyl chains of the phospholipids reduce the deformability of the lipid bilayer as well as the permeability of the membrane for small hydrophilic molecules (Quinn & Wolf, 2009). The proteins are the key to the overall functions of the membranes. They are either embedded into the membrane (integral proteins) or associated to it (peripheral and lipid-anchored proteins). Actions of membrane proteins include cell-cell contact, surface recognition, cytoskeleton contact, signalling, enzymatic activity and the transport of substances across the membrane.

Beside cholesterol the physical and chemical properties of biological membranes are determined by the fatty acid pattern. The packing density of saturated fatty acids differs widely from the packing density of unsaturated fatty acids (Stillwell & Wassall, 2003). An increase in the proportion of unsaturated fatty acids therefore results in a weakening in the intermolecular hydrophobic interactions (Stillwell & Wassall, 2003). In this way basal properties of biological membranes are modulated including the assembly of the acyl chains, the fluidity, permeability and compressibility of the membrane, melting and flip-flop mechanisms as well as the function of membrane proteins (Stillwell & Wassall, 2003; Wassall & Stillwell, 2008).

3.3 Lipid rafts

The phospholipids and sphingolipids are not distributed evenly in cellular membranes. Via lateral interactions among one another as well as with proteins specific micro domains are formed, the so called lipid rafts. Lipid rafts are structurally and functionally distinct domains that can be distinguished within the cell membrane due to their specific lipid compositions (Henderson et al., 2004; Lingwood & Simons, 2010; Pike, 2003; Tresset, 2009). Sphingolipids, cholesterol and saturated fatty acids predominate in the rafts (Pike, 2003). This allows for a tight packing of the acyl chains. The remaining liquid-ordered domain is characterized by a reduced fluidity compared to the surrounding plasma membrane.

Lipid rafts have been defined as "small (10-200 nm), heterogeneous, highly dynamic, sterol- and sphingolipid-enriched domains that compartmentalise cellular processes" (Pike, 2006). A variety of proteins has been shown to be enriched in membrane rafts such as GPI-anchored proteins, flotillin, receptor tyrosine kinases and G protein-coupled receptors (Pike, 2003). The spatial proximity of the proteins in the rafts enables a better coordination and an increased efficiency of proceeding reactions. Taking the dynamic nature of membrane domains into account the rafts have been supposed to scaffold certain molecules while excluding others thus function as a unique signalling platform (Ye et al., 2010). Further cellular processes lipid rafts have been implicated include membrane trafficking, molecular sorting, internalisation processes as well as membrane-cytoskeleton interactions (Simons & Toomre, 2000).

A number of macrophage functions have been shown to interrelate with membrane rafts. Examples include the endotoxin-mediated activation of macrophages, the MHCII-mediated presentation of antigens, phagocytosis as well as the production of pro-inflammatory cytokines (Gaus et al., 2005). Furthermore, lipid rafts have been shown to be used as target by a wide variety of pathogens to invade host cells (Hartlova et al., 2010). Bacterial toxins have been demonstrated to enter cells via certain toxin-associated receptors, which are known to be concentrated in membrane rafts (Van & Leo, 2002). Thus, the domains play an important role in infectious biology.

4. Fatty acid dependent modulation of the immune system

4.1 Fatty acids and the immune system

Fatty acids, in particular polyunsaturated fatty acids (PUFAs), possess immune modulating properties. PUFAs are shown to modulate the proliferative activity of neutrophil granulocytes (Prescott, 1984), macrophages (Hughes & Pinder, 2000), T cells (Anderson & Fritsche, 2004) and dendritic cells (Zeyda et al., 2005). Furthermore, impacts on the respiratory burst, the production of cytokines as well as the expression of adhesion

molecules have been described (Calder, 1998; Calder, 2006a). Of note, the effects triggered by the fatty acids depend on the fatty acid family. N3 fatty acids such as eicosapentaenoic acid (C20:5n3; table 2) and docosahexaenoic acid (C22:6n3; table 2) are thought to act anti-inflammatory (Calder, 2006a; Schmitz & Ecker, 2008). In contrast, fatty acids from the n6 family such as linoleic acid (C18:2n6; table 2) and arachidonic acid (C20:4n6; table 2) are described to act pro-inflammatory (Calder, 2006a; Schmitz & Ecker, 2008).
The interaction between fatty acids and the immune system is based on three known mechanisms (Benatti et al., 2004; Capkin et al, 2009): First, some fatty acids, e.g. eicosapentaenoic acid, docosahexaenoic acid and arachidonic acid, serve as precursors for the production of immune-modulating effectors. Second, fatty acids directly interact with intracellular receptors such as peroxisome proliferator-activated receptors (PPARs) or retinoid X receptors (RXRs) as well as G protein-coupled receptors (GPR120) (Oh et al., 2010). Third, the fatty acid composition of cell membranes modulates basic properties of the membrane thus influencing the activity of immune cells. A molecular model displaying the functional mechanisms, which underlay the interaction of fatty acids and the immune system, is shown in figure 4.

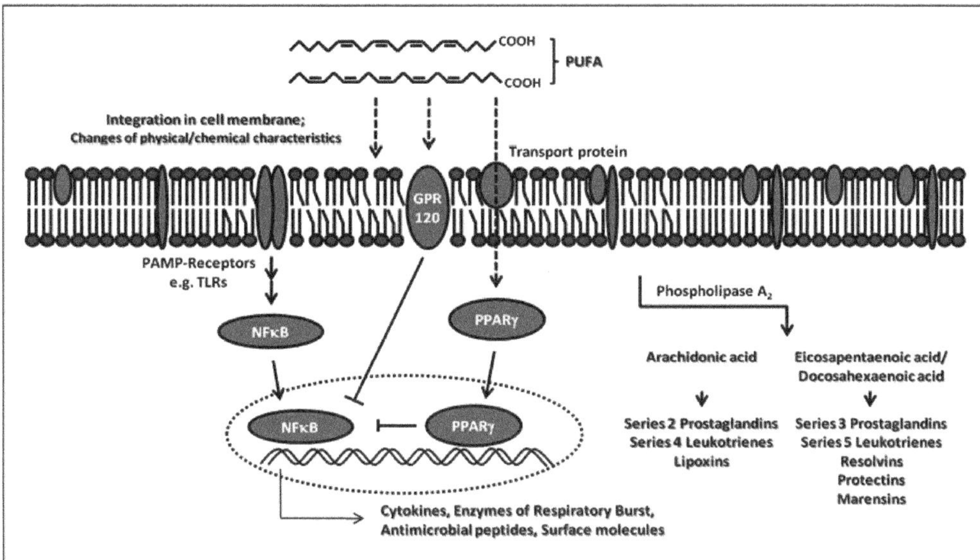

Fig. 4. Molecular model displaying the functional mechanisms, which underlay the interaction of fatty acids and the immune system

4.2 Eicosanoids, lipoxins, resolvins, protectins and marensins

Unsaturated fatty acids serve as precursors for the synthesis of several signal molecules and tissue hormones. These lipid mediators include the eicosanoids, the lipoxins, the resolvins, the protectins and the marensins.
There are four families of eicosanoids: prostaglandins, prostacyclins, thromboxanes and leukotrienes (Löffler et al., 2007). Each of these families can further be divided into separate series depending on the fatty acid family they derive from. The eicosanoid series differ widely in their biological activity. In general, n6 eicosanoids act pro-inflammatory, n3 eicosanoids are much less inflammatory (Lee, 1984; Lee, 1988).

Eicosanoids are synthesized in almost every animal and human tissue modulating numerous hormonal and other stimuli. The several physiological effects are triggered by specific membrane receptors of target cells and target tissues (Löffler et al., 2007). Acting as immune-modulators and neurotransmitters among others they influence the contraction of smooth muscle cells (vasoconstriction / vasodilatation), the experience of pain and the platelet aggregation (Löffler et al., 2007). Moreover, eicosanoids play an important role in hypersensitivity reactions and inflammatory processes (Benatti et al., 2004). An overview on the biological effects of major eicosanoids is shown in table 3.

Substance	Biological activity
Prostaglandin E_2	Bronchodilatation, Vasodilatation, Inducing of inflammation, fever and pain, Activation of osteoclasts, Inhibition of chloride secretion in the stomach and of lipolysis in fat tissue
Prostaglandin D_2	Bronchoconstriction, Promotion of sleep
Prostaglandin $F_{2\alpha}$	Bronchoconstriction, Vasoconstriction, Constriction of smooth muscle cells
Thromboxane A_2	Bronchoconstriction, Vasoconstriction, Platelet aggregation
Prostacyclin I_2	Vasodilatation, Increasing of vascular permeability, Inhibition of platelet aggregation, Inducing of inflammation

Table 3. Biological effects of major eicosanoids (Löffler et al., 2007)

The half-life of eicosanoids is about seconds to minutes. Thus, eicosanoids are considered as tissue hormones acting in an autocrine and paracrine manner (Löffler et al., 2007). The effect profile of eicosanoids therefore crucially depends on the type of eicosanoid receptors, which are expressed in close proximity to the eicosanoid-producing cell. In general, eicosanoid receptors are seven transmembrane receptors, which are also known as G protein-coupled receptors (Löffler et al., 2007). Subject to the type of receptor ligand binding results either in the modulation of the adenylate cyclase, which is followed by increased or decreased intracellular cAMP concentrations, or in an activation of the phosphatidylinositol cycle, which manipulates the concentration of cellular calcium (Löffler et al., 2007).

Depending on the fatty acid, which is used as precursor, eicosanoid synthesis results in discrete mediators. The n6 PUFA arachidonic acid is the substrate for production of series 2 prostaglandins and series 4 leukotrienes (Benatti et al., 2004). Starting from the n3 PUFA eicosapentaenoic acid series 3 prostaglandins and series 5 leukotrienes are formed (Benatti et al., 2004). In comparison to the arachidonic acid derivates series 3 prostaglandins and series 5 leukotrienes are notably less inflammatory. As an example: the leukotriene B_5 has been reported to have a 10 to 100 times reduced biological activity than the leukotriene B_4 (Lee et al., 1984; Lee et al., 1988).

Beside eicosanoids there is a genus of specialized pro-resolving mediators (SPM). The several families of these distinct local mediators include the lipoxins, the resolvins, the protectins and the marensins (Bannenberg & Serhan, 2010; Kohli & Levy, 2009; Norling & Serhan, 2010). SPM play a key role in the endogenous down-regulation of inflammation. For a long time inflammation resolution has been thought to occur passively by a dilution of pro-inflammatory signals and mediators. Only recently it has emerged, that instead it is an active process, which is orchestrated by a distinct set of chemical effectors (Serhan et al.,

2008). In resolving tissues an alteration in PUFA metabolism has been observed. A class switching in lipid mediator generation occurs, that leads to a change in enzymatic PUFA conversion from pro-inflammatory eicosanoids to pro-resolving mediators (Levy et al., 2001). SPM are derived from the n6 PUFA arachidonic acid and the n3 PUFAs eicosapentaenoic acid and docosahexaenoic acid as well (Bannenberg & Serhan, 2010; Kohli & Levy, 2009; Norling & Serhan, 2010). They exert influence at even picomolar to nanomolar concentrations (Serhan, 2005; Spite, 2009). Biological actions of SPM include the down-regulation of cell adhesion molecules, the reduction of chemotaxis, transendothelial migration and neutrophil activation, the stimulation non-phlogistic phagocytosis of apoptotic neutrophils and macrophages as well as the removal of inflammatory leukocytes (Bannenberg & Serhan, 2010). In table 4 there is an overview regarding the biological activities of major SPM.

The first SPM identified are the lipoxins (Serhan, 2005). Lipoxins are enzymatically generated by lipoxygenase from the n6 PUFA arachidonic acid, a process, which is triggerd by aspirin (Chiang, 2004). The potent anti-inflammatory effectors are special important in slowing down neutrophil-mediated tissue injury. They limit the recruitment and the adhesion of neutrophils to the site of inflammation. Furthermore, lipoxins force the phagocytosis of apoptotic neutrophils (Bannenberg & Serhan, 2010; Norling & Serhan, 2010). Major lipoxins are Lipoxin A_4 (LXA_4) and Lipoxin B_4 (LXB_4).

Resolvins are bioactive metabolites, which are synthesized from the enzymatic conversion of the n3 PUFA eicosapentaenoic acid and docosahexaenoic acid. The term resolvin is derived from 'resolution phase interaction products' (Serhan & Chiang, 2008). Depending on the fatty acid they are produced from resolvins are categorized as either E-series (from eicosapentaenoic acid) or D-series (from docosahexaenoic acid) (Serhan & Chiang, 2008). Aspirin-triggered forms have been described for each family (Serhan & Chiang). The E-series resolvins currently comprise Resolvin E1 (RvE1) and Resolvin E2 (RvE2). The D-series resolvins include Resolvin D1 (RvD1), Resolvin D2 (RvD2), Resolvin D3 (RvD3) and Resolvin D4 (RvD4). In general, resolvins efficiently block the synthesis of pro-inflammatory mediators, regulate the entry of neutrophils to inflammatory sites and help to clear neutrophils from mucosal surfaces (Norling & Serhan, 2010). At this, the bioactivity of the anti-inflammatory effectors has been shown to be highly stereoselective both *in vitro* and *in vivo* (Levy, 2010).

The n3 PUFA docosahexaenoic acid serves also as precursor for the synthesis of protectins. Protectins are characterized by their anti-inflammatory and protective actions, especially in neuronal tissues (Hong et al., 2003). As lipoxins and resolvins, protectins stop the infiltration of neutrophils and activate the resolution of inflammation (Hong et al., 2003; Serhan et al., 2006). The major protectin, Protectin D1 (PD1) has been shown to possess protective actions in the lung and in renal tissues thereby preserving them against injury and inflammation (Bannenberg & Serhan, 2010; Kohli & Levy, 2009; Levy, 2010; Norling & Serhan, 2010).

Recently, macrophages have been identified to synthesize anti-inflammatory and pro-resolving mediators from docosahexaenoic acid in a separate biosynthetic pathway (Norling & Serhan, 2010). These effectors have been termed maresins, for 'macrophage mediators in resolving inflammation' (Norling & Serhan, 2010). The production of marensins is triggered during phagocytosis (Bannenberg & Serhan, 2010). So far, Marensin 1 (MaR1), the major marensin, is known to reduce neutrophil migration and to stimulate phagocytosis by macrophages (Bannenberg & Serhan, 2010).

Substance	Biological activity
Resolvin E1	Decreasing of migration, pro-inflammatory signalling and infiltration of neutrophils; Stimulation of phagocytosis of apoptotic neutrophils by macrophages; Promotion of healing of diseased tissue
Resolvin E2	Decreasing of neutrophil infiltration
Resolvin D1	Decreasing of neutrophil infiltration; Protection from tissue damage and loss of function
Protectin D1	Decreasing of neutrophil infiltration and pro-inflammatory signalling; Stimulation of phagocytosis of apoptotic neutrophils by macrophages; Protection from tissue damage and loss of function

Table 4. Biological effects of major specialized pro-resolving mediators (SPM) (Kohli & Levy, 2009; Norling & Serhan, 2010)

The type of eicosanoids and specialized pro-resolving mediators produced depend on the fatty acid composition of the cell membrane. The main phospholipase, the phospholipas A2, preferably liberates the n6 PUFA arachidonic acid from membrane phospholipids, which acts as substrate for the synthesis of series 2 prostaglandin, series 4 leukotrienes and lipoxins (Löffler et al., 2007). Intake of n3 PUFA, such as eicosapentaenoic acid and docosahexaenoic acid, leads to increased levels of these fatty acids in the cell membrane. Products of eicosapentaenoic acid and docosahexaenoic acid are series 3 prostaglandins, series 5 leukotrienes, resolvins, protectins and marensins.

4.3 Interaction of fatty acids with nuclear receptors and G protein-coupled receptors

Fatty acids regulate gene expression via interaction with nuclear receptors and G protein-coupled receptors (GPCRs). Nuclear receptors are defined as intracellular ligand-inducible transcription factors, which modulate gene expression in response to hydrophobic endogenous and exogenous chemicals (Khan & Heuvel, 2003). Functions affected include the fatty acid metabolism, the reproductive development and the detoxification of substances (Khan & Heuvel, 2003). In general, nuclear receptors consist of distinct functional domains. The N-terminal A/B domain, has a weak transactivation activity (activation function 1 (AF-1)) (Bordoni et al., 2006; Khan & Heuvel, 2003). Adjacent there is the C domain, which is important for DNA binding (Bordoni et al., 2006; Khan & Heuvel, 2003). The DNA binding domain is the most conserved region of the nuclear receptor superfamily. It is composed of two zinc fingers, which bind to response elements (NREs) in their target promoters (Bordoni et al., 2006; Khan & Heuvel, 2003). The flanking D domain is a hinge region. This region may allow for conformational changes in the receptor structure following ligand binding (Bordoni et al., 2006; Khan & Heuvel, 2003). The C-terminal E/F domain contains the ligand binding site, which in every nuclear receptor is comprised of 10 to 13 α-helixes that form a hydrophobic binding cavity (Bordoni et al., 2006; Khan & Heuvel, 2003). At the extreme C-terminus there is the ligand-dependend transactivation function-2 (AF-2) (Bordoni et al., 2006; Khan & Heuvel, 2003). Furthermore, this region also contains nuclear localisation signals and protein interaction surfaces for dimerization with heat shock proteins, co-regulators and other transcription factors (Bordoni et al., 2006; Khan & Heuvel, 2003).

So far, five transcription factor families have been described to be modulated in their activity by fatty acids: peroxisome proliferator-activated receptors (PPARs), retinoid X receptors (RXRs), liver X receptors (LXRs), the hepatic nuclear factor 4 α (HNF-4α) and sterol regulatory element binding proteins (SREBPs) (Bordoni et al., 2006). The interaction between fatty acids and nuclear receptors is of importance in regulating lipid and glucose metabolism at this modulating the expression of specific enzymes as well as of fatty acid transporters (Bordoni et al., 2006). Beside, based on PPARs there is also a regulation of inflammation and immune response (Bishop-Bailey & Bystrom, 2009).

PPARs were identified 1990 as transcription factors (Issemann & Green, 1990). In 1992 linoleic acid (C18:2n6; table 2) and arachidonic acid were demonstrated to activate PPARs (Gottlicher et al., 1992). There are three PPAR family members: PPARα (NR1C1), PPARβ/δ (NR1C2; NUC1; FAAR fatty acid-activated receptor) and PPARγ (NR1C3). The isotypes are distinguished from each other by their tissue distribution and their differential activation (Grimaldi, 2001). PPARs are implicated in a number of biological processes, such as the regulation of lipid metabolism (uptake, activation, oxidation and esterification of fatty acids), development, cell proliferation and differentiation as well as inflammatory responses Escher & Wahli, 2000). PPARs exert their effects on gene expression as heterodimers with RXRs (Kliewer et al., 1992). The PPAR/RXR heterodimer binds to specific PPAR response elements (PPRE), which located in the promoter of target genes (Issemann et al., 1993). The consensus sequence consists of a direct repeat of the hexamer AGGTCA separated by single-nucleotide spacer, the so called direct repeat (DR-1) (Ijpenberg et al., 1997). The conformational change that occurs upon ligand binding leads to the dissociation of co-repressors as nuclear receptor co-repressor (NCoR) and silencing mediator for retinoid- and thyroid-hormone receptors (SMRT) (Feige et al., 2006). In addition, activated PPARs fascilitate the recruitment of co-activators, chromatin remodelling factors and of the transcription machinery (Bishop-Bailey & Bystrom, 2009). The activity of the PPARs can be modulated by phosporylation, nitration, ubiquitylation and sumoylation (Bordoni et al., 2006).

PPARα is mainly expressed in liver, intestinal tract, kidney, heart and brown adipose tissue (Bordoni et al., 2006). The receptor is of importance in fatty acid transport and oxidation, cell proliferation and inflammatory crosstalk (Bordoni et al., 2006). Synthetic ligands of PPARα have been shown to impair cytokine synthesis of phorbol ester stimulated monocytes (Jiang at el., 1998).

PPARβ/δ is almost ubiquitously expressed (Bishop-Bailey & Bystrom, 2009). It is implicated in the fatty acid oxidation of many tissues (Bishop-Bailey & Bystrom, 2009). Furthermore, PPARβ/δ has been reported to be involved in cell proliferation and development, wound healing, myelination of nerves as well as the adaptive response of skeletal muscle to exercise (Bordoni et al., 2006). In macrophages the receptor controls the inflammatory status at this diminishing the expression of pro-inflammatory cytokines and receptors as IL-1β, IL-6, TNF-α, macrophage inflammatory protein 1β, the MCP-1 receptor CC-chemokine receptor-2 and VCAM-1 (Bishop-Bailey & Bystrom, 2009).

PPARγ is expressed in various isoforms, which show tissue and differentiation specifity (Bishop-Bailey & Bystrom, 2009). The receptor plays a role in glucose homeostasis, lipid metabolism, cell proliferation and inflammation (Feige et al., 2006). PPARγ is the predominant PPAR receptor expressed by cells of the myeloid line (Stulnig, 2003). It is essential for differentiation of adipocytes and macrophages (Khan & Heuvel, 2003). Expression of PPARγ is upregulated during macrophage activation (Huang et al., 1999). Genes regulated include lipoprotein lipase, CD36 and scavenger receptors (Khan & Heuvel, 2003; Yaqoob, 2003). As with PPARα, synthetic ligands of PPARγ have been demonstrated to suppress production of IL-1β, IL-6, TNF-α as well as the inducible nitric oxide synthase (iNOS), matrix metalloprotease-9 and scavenger receptor A (Jiang at el., 1998; Ricote et al., 1998; Yang et al., 2000). PPARγ is activated by unsaturated fatty acids, the prostaglandin 15-deoxy PGJ_2 and non-steriodal anti-inflammatory drugs (NSAIDS) (Grimaldi, 2005; Khan & Heuvel, 2003; Stulnig, 2003).

Beside nuclear receptors recently five G protein-coupled receptors have been described, which can be activated by free fatty acids: GPR40 binding long-chain fatty acids, GPR41 binding short-chain fatty acids, GPR43 binding short-chain fatty acids, GPR84 binding medium-chain fatty acids and GPR120 binding long-chain fatty acids (Oh et al., 2010). From the perspective of immune modulation GPR120 emerges as a receptor of particular interest. In contrast to the other receptors of the family of fatty acid sensing GPCRs GPR120 is the only one, which is highly expressed in adipose tissue and macrophages (Oh et al., 2010). Moreover, ligand stimulation of GPR120 by the n3 PUFA DHA and EPA has been reported to result in potent anti-inflammatory effects, including inhibition of IL-6, TNF-α and MCP-1 mRNA expression and secretion (Oh et al., 2010). Activation of GPR120 by n3 fatty acids leads to a coupling of GPR120 to the adaptor protein β-arrestin2, which is followed by receptor and β-arrestin2 internalization (Oh et al., 2010). In the cytoplasm the GPR120/β-arrestin2 complex can associate with the TGF-beta activated kinase 1 binding protein 1 (TAB1) at this blocking the association of TAB1 with the TGF-beta activated kinase 1 (TAK1) (Oh et al., 2010). Thus, there is an inhibition of TAK1 activation and downstream signalling to the IKKβ/NFκB and JNK/AP1 system resulting in the inhibition of Toll-like receptor 2/3 and 4 as well as TNF-α action (Oh et al., 2010).

4.4 Fatty acid composition of cellular membranes

The lipid composition of cellular membranes is known to depend on the availability of fatty acids (Calder et al., 1994). Supplementation of cells with PUFAs results in an incorporation of the fatty acids into membrane phospholipids (Schmutzler et al., 2010; Schumann & Fuhrmann, 2010; Walloschke et al., 2010). Beyond that, the PUFAs were metabolized leading to an increase of the desaturation and elongation products of the fatty acids added (Schmutzler et al., 2010; Schumann & Fuhrmann, 2010; Walloschke et al., 2009). The enhanced proportion of unsaturated fatty acids in the cell membrane is accompanied by a heightening of the Methylene Bridge Index (MBI) of the lipid bilayer and an increasing of membrane fluidity (Schmutzler et al., 2010; Schumann & Fuhrmann, 2010; Walloschke et al., 2009). The MBI is calculated based on the ratio of a fatty acid (weight %) and the number of its bis-allyl-methylene positions (Kelley et al., 1995). The higher the MBI, the more fluid the membrane. Moreover, membranes with a heightened MBI are predicted to have an increased susceptibility against radical reactions (Kelley et al., 1995).

The modulation of membrane fluidity makes an impact on the activity of membrane-bound enzymes and also on the function of membrane receptors thus affecting signal transduction (Benatti et al., 2004; Calder et al., 1994). Many key proteins of signal transduction, as Toll-like receptors or Nod-like receptors, are localized in lipid rafts (Pike, 2003). After binding of the ligand, the activated receptor complexes are compartmentalized in the lipid rafts (Jury et al., 2007). At this, the lipid rafts facilitate the association of signal transduction molecules (Jury et al., 2007; Pike, 2003).

The membrane fluidity necessary for an optimal cell response is assumed to fall within particular boundaries (Calder et al., 1994). Changes in the lipid composition of the plasma membrane therefore directly affect cellular reactions on signals from the environmental.

Accordingly, there is a correlation between the activity of immune cells and the fatty acid pattern of their cell membrane.
Of note, the availability of fatty acids is modulated by the diet. The connection between the dietary intake of fatty acids and inflammation was first drawn in the late 1970s. Epidemiological observation showed that native Greenland Eskimos (Dyerberg & Bang, 1979) and Japanese (Hirai et al, 1980), which have a high intake of n3 PUFA from seafood, have a low incidence for myocardial infarction, chronic inflammation and autoimmune disorders. To date, there are numerous studies, which have investigated the effects of the amount and the type of fat in the diet on cellular physiology (Calder, 2006b; Galli & Calder, 2009). It is now well accepted that the fatty acid composition of body cells, including immune cells, is sensitive to alteration according to the fatty acid composition of the diet (Calder, 2001). In particular, proportions of PUFAs of the n3 and the n6 family are readily modified thus providing a link between dietary PUFA intake, inflammation and immunity (Calder, 2001). The findings from these studies led health care professionals to encourage the general population to consume more n3 fatty acids.

5. Conclusion

The importance of lipid bilayers for the overall processes of life is increasingly realized. Plasma membranes are just more than compartmentalization elements separating the inside of a cell from the surrounding environment. They have numerous functions in cell adhesion, ion conductivity and cell signalling acting as an attachment surface for intracellular and extracellular.
Infection processes and immune defence greatly depend on cellular membrane interactions. In an initial step of infection pathogens, as bacteria and viruses, as well as bacterial toxins, need to get inside the host cell (Murphy et al., 2008). The internalization enables the pathogens to proliferate and to poison the cell (Murphy et al., 2008). Thus, the attachment of pathogens to cellular surfaces and the binding to a cell-surface receptor are critical in the course of infection processes. Moreover, the mutual communication between immune cells crucially depends on signal molecules binding to cellular receptors as well as on direct membrane-membrane interactions. Stimulation of membrane receptors via cytokines and chemokines and direct cell-cell contacts are of importance in activating immune cells thus triggering immune defence (Murphy et al., 2008). Likewise, completion of the immune response after successful extinction of the pathogens is mediated by membrane-dependent signal transduction processes (Murphy et al., 2008). A further mechanism in immune defence, which involves the interaction between the plasma membranes of both pathogen and host, is the phagocytosis of pathogens by macrophages and dendritic cells.
Of note, membranes are very flexible in their overall composition. Depending on cell type and tissue the proportion of phospholipids and sphingolipids varies greatly. The same is the case with membrane proteins. There are numerous highly specialised mechanisms that allow for the particular allocation of membrane lipids and membrane proteins according to the requirements and functions of a cell. Beyond that, the lipid bilayer is characterized by an asymmetry in the distribution of phospholipids and sphingolipids between the inner and the outer leaflet (Löffler et al., 2007). This asymmetry is determined by the balance of specific transport proteins (Löffler et al., 2007). The disruption of the lipid asymmetry is a piece in the substrate recognition of macrophages (Löffler et al., 2007).

However, the lipid composition of cellular membranes, including immune cells, can be modulated depending on the availability of fatty acids, providing a link between the diet and the immune defence (Calder et al., 1994). In particular, highly unsaturated fatty acids are immediately incorporated into the lipid bilayer (Schumann & Fuhrmann, 2010). The physical properties of membranes are highly reliant on the fatty acid pattern. Features modulated include the fatty acid chain order, the phase behaviour, the elastic compressibility, the ion permeability, the fusion, the rapid flip-flop and several protein functions thus affecting cell signal transduction (Stillwell & Wassall, 2003; Wassall & Stillwell, 2008). Moreover, the unsaturated fatty acids of membrane phospholipids serve as substrate for the synthesis of lipid signal molecules, as eicosanoids, lipoxins, resolvins, protectins and marensins, which are known to efficiently modulate immune defence mechanisms (Bannenberg & Serhan, 2010; Kohli & Levy, 2009; Löffler et al., 2007; Norling & Serhan, 2010). Beside, the fatty acids also act as ligands for several nuclear receptors and G protein-coupled receptors thus directly influencing the immune system (Bordoni et al., 2006). This key position of fatty acids, in particular of PUFAs of the n3 and the n6 family, makes them particular promising in the supportive therapy of chronic diseases linked to persistent pathogens.

6. References

Anderson, M.J. & Fritsche, K.L. (2004). Dietary polyunsaturated fatty acids modulate in vivo, antigen-driven CD4+T-cell proliferation in mice. *Journal of Nutrition*, Vol.2004, No.8 (August 2004), pp. 1978-1983, ISSN 0022-3166

Bannenberg, G. & Serhan, C.N. (2010). Specialized pro-resolving mediators in the inflammatory resonse: An update. *Biochimica et Biophysica Acta*, Vol.1801, No.12 (December 2010), pp. 1260-1273, ISSN 1388-1981

Bell, K.S., Philp, J.C., Aw, D.W. & Christofi, N. (1998). The genus Rhodococcus. *Journal of Applied Microbiology*, Vol.85, No.2 (August 1998), pp. 195-210, ISSN 1364-5072

Benatti, P., Peluso G., Nicolai, R. & Calvani, M. (2004). Polyunsaturated fatty acids: niochemical, nutritional and epigenetic properties. *Journal of the American College of Nutrition*, Vol.23, No.4 (August 2004), pp. 281-302, ISSN 0731-5724

Benoit, S., Benachour, A., Taouji, S., Auffray, Y. & Hartke, A. (2002). H_2O_2, which causes macrophage-related stress, triggers induction of expression of virulence-associated plasmid determinants in Rhodococcus equi. *International Immunology*, Vol.70, No.7 (July 2002), pp. 3768-3776, ISSN 0019-9567

Benoit, S., Taouji, S., Benachour, A. & Hartke, A. (2000). Resistance of Rhodococcus equi to acid pH. *International Journal of Food Microbiology*, Vol.55, No.1-3 (April 2000), pp. 295-298, ISSN 0168-1605

Blanc, D.S., Petignat, C., Janin, B., Bille, J. & Francioli, P. (1998). Frequency and molecular diversity of Pseudomonas aeruginosa upon admission and during hospitalization: a prospective epidemiologic study. *Clinical Microbiological Infections*, Vol.4, No.5 (May 1998), pp. 242-247, ISSN 1469-0691

Bishop-Bailey, D. & Bystrom, J. (2009). Emerging role of peroxisome proliferator-activated receptor-β/δ in inflammation. *Pharmacology and Therapeutics*, Vol.124, No.2 (November 2009), pp. 141-150, ISSN 0163-7258

Bordoni, A., Di Nunzio, M., Danesi, F. & Biagi, P.L. (2006). Polyunsaturated fatty acids:From diet to binding to PPARs and other nuclear receptors. *Genes and Nutrition*, Vol.1, No.2 (June 2006), pp. 95-106, ISSN 1555-8932

Boyce, J.A., Broide, D., Matsumoto, K. & Bochner, B.S. (2009). Advances in mechanisms of asthma, allergy, and immunology in 2008. *Journal of Allergy and Clinical Immunology*, Vol.123, No.3 (March 2009), pp. 569-574, ISSN 0091-6749

Boyen, F., Eeckhaut, V., Van, I.F., Pasmans, F., Ducatelle, R. & Hasebrouck, F. (2009). Quorum sensing in veterinary pathogens: mechanisms, clinical importance and future perspectives. *Veterinary Microbiology*, Vol.135, No.3-4 (March 2009), pp. 187-195, ISSN 0378-1135

Bryant, C. & Fitzgerald, K.A. (2009). Molecular mechanisms involved in inflammasome activation. *Trends in Cell Biology*, Vol.19, No.9 (September 2009), pp. 455-464, ISSN 0962-8924

Calder, P.C. (2001). Polyunsaturated fatty acids, inflammation and immunity. *Lipids*, Vol.36, No.9 (September 2001), pp. 1007-1024, ISSN 0024-4201

Calder, P.C. (2006a). Polyunsaturated fatty acids and inflammation. *Prostaglandins, Leukotrienes and Essential Fatty Acids*, Vol.75, No.3 (September 2006), pp. 197-202, ISSN 0952-3278

Calder, P.C. (2006b). n-3 polyunsaturated fatty acids, inflammation, and inflammatory diseases. *American Journal of Clinical Nutrition*, Vol.83, No.6 (June 2006), pp. 1505S-1519S, ISSN 0002-9165

Calder, P.C., Yaqoob, P., Harvey, D.J., Watts, A. & Newsholme, E.A. (1994). Incorporation of fatty acids by concanavalin A-stimulated lymphocytes and the effect on fatty acid composition and membrane fluidity. *Biochemical Journal*, Vol.300, No.2 (June 1994), pp. 509-518, ISSN 0264-6021

Chapkin, R.S., Kim, W., Lupton, J.R. & McMurray, D.N. (2009). Dietary docosahexaenoic and eicosapentaenoic acid: emerging mediators of inflammation. *Prostaglandins, Leukotriens and Essential Fatty Acids*, Vol.81, No.2-3 (August-September 2009), pp. 187-191, ISSN 1532-2823

Chiang, N., Bermudez, E.A., Ridker, P.M., Hurwitz, S. & Serhan, C.N. (2004). Aspirin triggers anti-inflammatory 15-epi-lipoxin A_4 and inhibits thromboxane in a randomized human trial. *Proceedings of the National Academy of Science of the United States of America*, Vol.101, No.42 (October 2004), pp. 15178-15183, ISSN 0027-8424

Dyerberg, J. & Bang, H.O. (1979). Haemostatic function and platelet polyunsaturated fatty acids in Eskimos. *Lancet*, Vol.2, No.8140 (September 1979), pp. 433-435, ISSN 0140-6736

Escher, P. & Wahli, W. (2000). Peroxisome proliferator-activated receptors: insight into multiple cellular functions. *Mutation Research-Fundamental and Molecular Mechanisms of Mutagenesis*, Vol.448, No.2 (March 2000), pp. 121-138, ISSN 0027-5107

Feige, J.N., Gelman, L., Michalik, L., Desvergne, B. & Wahli, W. (2006). From molecular action to physiological outputs: peroxisome proliferator-activated receptors are nuclear receptors at the crossroads of key cellular functions. *Progress in Lipid Research*. Vol.45, No.2 (March 2006), pp. 120-159, ISSN 0163-7827

Fernandez-Mora, E., Polidori, M., Luhrmann, A., Schaible, U.E. & Haas, A. (2005). Maturation of Rhodococcus equi-containing vacuoles is arrested after completion of the early endosome stage. *Traffic*, Vol.6, No.8 (August 2005), pp. 635-653, ISSN 1398-9219

Galli, C. & Calder, P.C. (2009). Effects of fat and fatty acid intake on inflammatory and immune responses: a critical review. *Annals of Nutrition and Metabolism*, Vol.55, No.1-3 (September 2009), pp. 123-139, ISSN 0250-6807

Gaus, K., Rodriguez, M., Ruberu, K.R., Gelissen, I., Sloane, T.M., Kritharides, L. & Jessup, W. (2005). Domain-specific lipid distribution in macrophage plasma membranes. *Journal of Lipid Research*, Vol.46, No.7 (July 2005), pp. 1526-1538, ISSN 0022-2275

Germolec, D.R., Frawley, R.P. & Evans, E. (2010). Markers of inflammation. *Methods in Molecular Biology*, Vol.598 (February 2010), pp. 53-73, ISSN 1940-6029

Glaros, T. Larsen, M. & Li, L. (2009). Macrophaes and fibroblasts during inflammation, tissue damage and organ injury. *Frontiers in Biosciences*, Vol.12 (January 2009), pp. 3988-3993, ISSN 1093-9946

Gottlicher, M., Widmark, E., Li, Q. & Gustafsson, J.A. (1992). Fatty acids activate a chimera of the clofibric acid-activated receptor and the glucocorticoid receptor. *Proceedings of the national Academy of Sciences of the United States of America*, Vol.89, No.10 (May 1992), pp. 4653-4657, ISSN 0027-8424

Grimaldi, P.A. (2001). Fatty acid regulation of gene expression. *Current Opinion in Clinical Nutrition and Metabolic Care*, Vol.4, No.5 (September 2001), pp. 433-437, ISSN 1363-1950

Groves, E., Dart, A.E., Covarelli, V. & Caron, E. (2008). Molecular mechanisms of phagocytic uptake in mammalien cells. *Cellular and Molecular Life Sciences*, Vol. 65, No.13 (July 2008), pp. 1957-1976, ISSN 1420-682X

Haas, A. (2007). The phagosome: compartment with a license to kill. *Traffic*, Vol.8, No.4 (April 2007), pp. 311-330, ISSN 1398-9219

Hamilton, T.A., Ohmori, Y., Tebo, J.M. & Kishore, R. (1999). Regulation of macrophage gene expression by pro- and anti-inflammatory cytokines, *Pathobiology*, Vol.67, No.5-6 (1999), pp. 241-244, ISSN 1015-2008

Hartlova, A., Cerveny, L., Hubalek, M., Krocova, Z. & Stulnig, J. (2010). Membrane rafts: a potential gateway for bacterial entry into host cells. *Microbiology and Immunology*, Vol.54, No.4 (April 2010), pp. 237-245, ISSN 0385-5600

Henderson, R.M., Edwardson, J.M., Geisse, N.A. & Saslowsky, D.E. (2004). Lipid rafts: feeling is believing. *News in Physiological Sciences*, Vol.19 (April 2004), pp. 39-43, ISSN 0886-1714

Hirai, A., Hamazaki, T., Terano, T., Nishikawa, T., Tamura, Y., Kumagai, A. & Sajiki, J. (1980). Eicosapentaenoic acid and platelet function in Japanese. *Lancet*, Vol.2, No.8204 (November 1980), pp. 1132-1133, ISSN 0140-6736

Hong, S., Gronert, K., Devchand, P., Moussignac, R.-L. & Cerhan, C.N. (2003). Novel docosatrienes and 17S-resolvins generated from docosahexaenoic acid in murine brain, human blood and glial cells: autacoids in anti-inflammation. *Journal of Biologcal Chemistry*, Vol.278, No.17 (April 2003), pp. 14677-14687, ISSN 0021-9258

Huang, J.T., Welch, J.S., Ricote, M., Binder, C.J., Wilson, T.M., Kelly, C., Witztum, J.L., Funk, C.D., Conrad, D. & Glass, C.K. (1999). Interleukin-4-dependent production of PPAR-gamma ligands in macrophages by 12/15-lipoxygenase. *Nature*, Vol.400, No.6742 (July 1999), pp. 378-382, ISSN 0028-0836

Hughes, D.A. & Pinder, A.C. (2000). n-3 polyunsaturated fatty acids inhibit the antigen-presenting function of human monocytes. *American Journal of Clinical Nutrition*, Vol.71, No.1 (January 2000), pp. 357S-360S, ISSN 0002-9165

Ijpenberg, A., Jeannin, E., Wahli, W. & Desvergne, B. (1997). Polarity and specific sequence requirements of peroxisome proliferator-activated receptor (PPAR)/retinoid X receptor heterodimer binding to DNA. A functional analysis of the malic enzyme gene PPAR response element. *Journal of Biological Chemistry*, Vol.272, No.32 (August 1997), pp. 20108-20117, ISSN 0021-9258

Issemann, I. & Green, S. (1990). Activation of a member of the steroid hormone receptor superfamily by peroxisome proliferators. *Nature*, Vol.347, No.6294 (October 1990), pp. 645-650, ISSN 0028-0836

Issemann, I., Prince, R.A., Tugwood, J.D. & Green, S. (1993).The peroxisome proliferator-activated receptor:retinoid X receptor heterodimer is activated by fatty acids and fibrate hypolipidaemic drugs. *Journal of Molecular Endokrinology*, Vol.11, No.1 (August 1993), pp. 37-47, ISSN 0952-5041

Jiang, C., Ting, A.T. & Seed, B. (1998). PPAR-gamma agonists inhibit production of monocyte inflammatory cytokines. *Nature*, Vol.391, No.6662 (January 1998), pp. 82-86, ISSN 0028-0836

Johnston, J.B., Rahman, M.M. & McFadden, G. (2007). Strategies that modulate inflammasomes: insights from host-pathogen interactions. *Seminars in Immunopathology*, Vol.29, No.3 (September 2007), pp. 261-274, ISSN 1863-2297

Jury, E.C., Flores-Borja, F. & Kabouridis, P.S. (2007). Lipid rafts in T cell signaling and disease. *Seminars in cell & developmental biology*, Vol.18, No.5 (October 2007), pp. 608-615, ISSN 1084-9521

Kamboj, M., Kalra, A. & Kak, V. (2005). Rhodococcus brain abscess in a patient without HIV. *Journal of Clinical Pathology*, Vol.58, No.4 (April 2005), pp. 423-425, ISSN 0021-9746

Kelley, E.E., Buettner, G.R. & Burns, C.P. (1995). Relative alpha-tocopherol deficiency in cultured cells: free radical lipid peroxidation, lipid peroxidizability, and cellular polyunsaturated fatty acid content. *Archives of Biochemistry and Biophysics*, Vol.319, No.1 (May 1995), pp. 102-109, ISSN 0003-9861

Khan, S.A. & Heuvel, J.P.V. (2003). Reviews:Current Topics – Role of nuclear receptors in the regulation of gene expression by dietary fatty acids (Review). *Journal of Nutritional Biochemistry*, Vol.14, No.10 (October 2003), pp. 554-567, ISSN 0955-2863

Kliewer, S.A., Umesono, K., Noonan, D.J., Heyman, R.A. & Evans, R.M. (1992). Convergence of 9-cis retinoic acid and peroxisome proliferator signalling pathways through heterodimer formation of their receptors. *Nature*. Vol.358, No.6389, pp. 771-774, ISSN 0028-0836

Kohli, P. & Levy, B.D. (2009). Resolvins and protectins: mediating solutions to inflammation. *British Journal of Pharmacology*, Vol.158, No.4 (October 2009), pp. 960-971, ISSN 0007-1188

Lee, T.H., Menica-Huerta, J.M., Shih, C., Corey, E.J., Lewis, R.A. & Austen, K.F. (1984). Characterization and biologic properties of 5,12-dihydroxy derivates of eicosapentaenoic acid, including leukotriene B5 and the double lipoxygenase product. *Journal of Biology and Chemistry*, Vol.259, No.4 (February 1984), pp. 2383-2389, ISSN 0021-9258

Lee, T.H., Sethi, T., Crea, A.E., Peters, W., Arm, J.P. & Horton, C.E. (1988). Characterization of leukotriene B3: comparison of its biological activities with leukotriene B4 and leukotriene B5 in complement receptor enhancement, lysozyme release and chemotaxis of human neutrophils. *Clinical Science (London)*, Vol.74, No.5 (May 1988), pp. 467-475, ISSN 0143-5221

Levy, B.D. (2010). Resolvins and protectins: Natural pharmacophores for resolution biology. *Prostaglandins, Leukotrienes and Essential Fatty Acids*, Vol.82, No.4-6 (April-June 2010), pp. 327-332, ISSN 0952-3278

Levy, B.D., Clish, C.B., Schmidt, B., Gronert, K. & Serhan, C.N. (2001). Lipid mediator class switching during acute inflammation: signals in resolution. *Nature Immunology*, Vol.2, No.7 (July 2001), pp. 612-619, ISSN 1529-2908

Lingwood, D. & Simons, K. (2010). Lipid rafts as a membrane-organizing principle. *Science*, Vol.327, No.5961 (January 2010), pp. 46-50, ISSN 0036-8075

Löffler, G., Petrides, P.E. & Heinrich, P.C. (2007). *Biochemie & Pathobiochemie*, Springer Medizin Verlag, ISBN 3-540-32680-4, Heidelberg

Miles, E.A. & Calder, P.C. (1998). Modulation of immune function by dietary fatty acids. *Proceedings of the Nutrition Society*, Vol.57, No.2 (May 1998), pp. 277-292, ISSN 0029-6651

Milaud, T., Hammerling, G.J. & Garbi, N. (2010). Review of murine dendritic cells: types, location, and development. *Methods in Molecular Biology*, Vol.595, No.1 (February 2010), pp. 21-42, ISSN 1940-6029

Mogensen, T.H. (2009). Pathogen recognition and inflammatory signaling in innate immune defenses. *Clinical Microbiology Reviews*, Vol.22, No.2 (April 2009), pp. 240-273, ISSN 0893-8512

Murphy, K., Travers, P. & Walport, M. (2008). *Janeway`s Immunology*, Garland Science, Taylor and Francis Group, LLC, ISBN 0-8153-4123-7, New York

Norling, L.V. & Serhan, C.N. (2010). Profiling in resolving inflammatory exudates identifies novel anti-inflammatory and pro-resolving mediators and signals for termination. *Journal of Internal Medicine*, Vol.268, No.1 (July 2010), pp. 15-24, ISSN 0954-6820

Oh, D.Y., Talukdar, S., Bar, E.J., Imamura, T., Morinaga, H., Fan, W.Q., Li, P., Lu, W.J., Watkins, S.M. & Olefsky J.M. (2010). GPR120 is an omega-3 fatty acid receptor mediating potent anti-inflammatory and insulin-sensitizing effects. Cell, Vol.142, No.5 (September 2010), pp. 687-698, ISSN 0092-8674

Pesci, E.C., Milbank, J.B., Pearson, J.P., McKnight, S., Kende, A.S., Greenberg, E.P. & Iglewski, B.H. (1999). Quinolone signaling in the cell-to-cell communication system of Pseudomonas aeruginosa, *Proceedings of the National Academy of Science United States of America*, Vol.96, No.20 (September 1999), pp. 11229-11234, ISSN 0027-8424

Pike, L.J. (2003). Lipid rafts: bringing order to chaos. *Journal of Lipid Research*, Vol.44, No.4 (April 2003), pp. 655-667, ISSN 0022-2275

Pike, L.J. (2006). Rafts defined: a report on the Keystone symposium on lipid rafts and cell function. *Journal of Lipid Research*, Vol.47, No.7 (July 2006), pp. 1597-1598, ISSN 0022-2275

Pourova, J., Kottova, M., Voprsalova, M. & Pour, M. (2010). Reactive oxygen and nitrogen species in normal physiological processes. *Acta Physiologica*, Vol.198, No.1 (January 2010), pp. 15-35, ISSN 1748-1708

Prescott, J.F. (1991). Rhodococcus equi: an animal and human pathogen. *Clinical Microbiological Reviews*, Vol.4, No.1 (January 1991), pp. 20-34, ISSN 0893-8512

Prescott, S.M. (1984). The effect of eicosapentaenoic acid on leukotriene B production by human neutrophils. *Journal of Biological Chemistry*, Vol.259, No.12 (June 1984), pp. 7615-7621, ISSN 0021-9258

Quinn, P.J. & Wolf, C. (2009). The liquid-ordered phase in membranes. *Biochimica et Biophysica Acta*, Vol.1788, No.1 (January 2009), pp. 33-46, ISSN 0005-2736

Ricote, M., Li, A.C., Wilson, T.M., Kelly, C.J. & Glass, C.K. (1998). The peroxisome proliferator-activated receptor-gamma ia a negative regulator of macrophage activation. *Nature*, Vol.391, No.6662 (January 1998), pp. 79-82, ISSN 0028-0836

Robinson, J.M. (2009). Phagocytic leukocytes and reactive oxygen species. *Histochemistry and Cell Biology*, Vol.131, No.4 (April 2009), pp. 465-469, ISSN 0948-6143

Russell, D.G., Vanderven, B.C., Glennie, S., Mwandumba, H. & Heyderman, R.S. (2009). The macrophage marches on ist phagosome: dynamic assays of phagosome function. *Nature Reviews Immunology*, Vol.9, No.8 (August 2009), pp. 594-600, ISSN 1474-1733

Schmitz, G. & Ecker, J. (2008). The opposing effects of n-3 and n-6 fatty acids. *Progress in Lipid Research*, Vol.47, No.2 (March 2008), pp. 147-155, ISSN 0163-7827

Schmutzler, S., Bachmann, L., Fuhrmann, H. & Schumann, J. (2010). PUFA-dependent alteration of oxidative parameters of a canine mastocytoma cell line. *Acta Veterinaria Hungarica*, Vol.58, No.4 (June 2010), pp. 453-464, ISSN 0236-6290

Schumann, J. & Fuhrmann, H. (2010). Impairment of NFκB activity by unsaturated fatty acids. *International Immunopharmacology*, Vol.10, No.8 (August 2010), pp. 978-984, ISSN 1567-5769

Serhan, C.N., guest ed. (2005). Special issue on lipoxins and aspirin-triggered lipoxins. *Prostaglandins, Leukotrienes and Essential Fatty Acids*, Vol.73, No.3-4 (September-October 2005), pp. 139-321, ISSN 0952-3278

Serhan, C.N., Chiang, N., & Van Dyke, T.E. (2008). Resolving inflammation: dual anti-inflammatory and pro-resolution lipid mediators. *Nature Reviews Immunology*, Vol.8, No.5 (May 2008), pp. 349-361, ISSN 1474-1733

Serhan, C.N., Gotlinger, K., Hong, S., Lu, Y., Siegelman, J., Baer, T., Yang, R., Colgan, S.P. & Petasis, N.A. (2006). Anti-inflammatory actions of neuroprotectin D1/protectin D1 and its natural stereoisomers: assignements of dihydroxy-containing docosatrienes. *Journal of Immunology*, Vol.176, No.6 (March 2006), pp. 1848-1859, ISSN 0022-1767

Silva, M.T. (2010). When two is better than one: macrophages and neutrophils work in concert in innate immunity as complementary and cooperative partners of a myeloid phagocyte system. *Journal of Leukocyte Biology*, Vol.87, No.1 (January 2010), pp. 93-106, ISSN 0741-5400

Simons, K. & Toomre, D. (2000). Lipid rafts and signal transduction. *Nature Reviews Molecular Cell Biology*, Vol.1, No.1 (October 2000), pp. 31-39, ISSN 1471-0072

Spite, M., Norling, L.V., Summers, L., Yang, R., Cooper, D., Petasis, N.A., Flower, M., Perretti, C.N. & Serhan, C.N. (2009). Resolvin D2 is a potent regulator of leukocytes and controls microbial sepsis. *Nature*, Vol.461, No. 7268 (October 2009), pp. 1287-1291, ISSN 0028-0836

Stillwell, W. & Wassall, S.R. (2003). Docosahexaenoic acid: membrane properties of a unique fatty acid. *Chemistry and Physic of Lipids*, Vol.126, No.1 (November 2003), pp. 1-27, ISSN 0009-3084

Strateva, T. & Yordanov, D. (2009). Pseudomonas aeruginosa – a phenomenon of bacterial resistance. *Journal of Medical Microbiology*, Vol.58, No.9 (September 2009), pp. 1133-1148, ISSN 0022-2615

Stulnig, T.M. (2003). Immunomodulation by polyunsaturated fatty acids: Mechanisms and effects. *International Archives of Allergy and Immunology*, Vol.132, No.4 (December 2003), pp. 310-321, ISSN 1018-2438

Trautmann, M., Lepper, P.M. & Haller, M. (2005). Ecology of Pseudomonas aeruginosa in the intensive care unit and the evolving role of water outlets as a reservoir of the organism. *American Journal of Infection Control*, Vol.33, No.5 (June 2005), pp. S41-S49, ISSN 0196-6553

Tresset, G. (2009). The multiple faces of self-assembled lipidic systems. *PMC Biophysics*, Vol.2, No.1 (April 2009), pp.3, ISSN 1757-5036

Van, L.F. & Leo, O. (2002). Membrane lipid rafts: new targets for immunoregulation. *Current Molecular Medicine*, Vol.2, No.6 (September 2002), pp. 557-570, ISSN 1566-5240

Varol, C., Yona, S. & Jung, S. (2009). Origins and tissue-context-dependent fates of blood monocytes. *Immunology and Cell Biology*, Vol.87, No.1 (January 2009), pp. 30-38, ISSN 0818-9641

Veesenmeyer, J.L., Hauser, A.R., Lisboa, T. & Rello, J. (2009). Pseudomonas aeruginosa virulence and therapy: evolving translational strategies. *Critical Care Medicine*, Vol.37, No.5 (May 2009), pp. 1777-1786, ISSN 0090-3493

Walloschke, B., Fuhrmann, H. & Schumann, J. (2010). Enrichment of RAW264.7 macrophages with essential 18-carbon fatty acids affects both respiratory burst and production of immune modulating cytokines. *Journal of Nutritional Biochemistry*, Vol.21, No.6 (June 2010), pp. 556-560, ISSN 0955-2863

Wassall, S.R. & Stillwell, W. (2008). Docosahexaenoic acid domains: the ultimate non-raft membrane domain. *Chemistry and Physic of Lipids*, Vol.153, No.1 (May 2008), pp. 57-63, ISSN 0009-3084

Yang, X.Y., Wang, L.H., Chen, T., Hodge, D.R., Resau, J.H., DaSilva, L. & Farrar, W.L. (2000). Activation of human T lymphocytes is inhibited by peroxisome proliferator-activated receptor gamma (PPARgamma) agonists - PPARgamma co-association with transcription factor NFAT. *Journal of Biological Chemistry*, Vol.275, No.7 (February 2000), pp. 4541-4544, ISSN 0021-9258

Yaqoob, P. (2003). Lipids and the immune response: from molecular mechanisms to clinical applications. *Current Opinion in Clinical Nutrition and Metabolic Care*, Vol.6, No.2 (March 2003), pp. 133-150, ISSN 1363-1950

Ye, S., Tan, L., Ma, J., Shi, Q. & Li, J. (2010). Polyunsaturated docosahexaenoic acid suppresses oxidative stress induced endothelial cell calcium influx by altering lipid composition in membrane caveolar rafts. *Prostaglandins, Leukotrienes and essential fatty acids*, Vol.33, No.1 (July 2010), pp. 37-43, ISSN 0952-3278

Zeyda, M., Saemann, M.D., Stuhlmeier, K.M., Mascher, D.G., Nowotny, P.N. & Zlabinger, G.J. (2005). Polyunsaturated fatty acids block dendritic cell activation and function independently of NF-kappaB activation. *Journal of Biological Chemisry*, Vol.280, No.14 (April 2005), pp. 14293-14301, ISSN 0021-9258

4

Autoimmunity, Atherosclerosis and Apoptotic Cell Clearance

Tamar Aprahamian
Boston University School of Medicine
USA

1. Introduction

In recent years, it has been reported that there is an increased incidence of accelerated atherosclerosis among young women with systemic lupus erythematosus (SLE). Accelerated atherosclerosis has also been observed in other autoimmune diseases such as rheumatoid arthritis and systemic sclerosis. The end-organ damage most commonly observed in SLE patients is kidney failure. Recent advances in the treatment of kidney dysfunction, has led to the observation that many SLE patients also suffer from coronary heart disease and other endpoint cardiac events. As a result, studies have been designed and performed to better understand the basis for the accelerated disease progression in patients with autoimmune disease.

The development of atherosclerosis is driven, to a large extent, by inflammation. Initiation of atherosclerotic lesions can occur as a result of damage to the endothelium by a number of factors including oxidized low density lipoprotein (oxLDL), inflammatory cytokines, and immune complexes. The lesion progression involves inflammatory cell interactions with the endothelium and extravasation into the subendothelial space. Inflammation resulting from both atherosclerosis and autoimmunity is an essential, yet not well understood, factor in the initiation and progression of atherosclerosis associated with autoimmune diseases. Currently, one of the most widely studied areas among the genetic causes of SLE is decreased clearance of apoptotic bodies, which is thought to propagate the progression of the disease. There are numerous *in vivo* studies that support this hypothesis. For example, it has been shown that a long-term autoimmune response does not occur when there is efficient apoptotic body clearance. In cases where the machinery that is responsible for the clearance is disrupted in genetic mouse models, it has been shown that apoptotic bodies accumulate, resulting in lupus-like autoimmune diseases. This is evidenced by the variety of mouse models that develop autoimmunity in the absence of genes involved in apoptotic cell clearance. Apoptotic cell clearance also plays a role in atherosclerotic lesion development depending on the stage of the lesion. Our lab generated the first mouse model to study the interactions between SLE and atherosclerosis and subsequently, many new mouse models have been generated in order to further elucidate the mechanism by which the synergy between the two disease processes occurs.

The focus of this chapter will be to discuss the recognition and phagocytosis of an apoptotic cell, the machinery involved in apoptotic cell clearance, and the effects of alterations to various steps of this process. This will be demonstrated by including evidence of relevant genetic mouse models and examples of human disease resulting from impaired clearance. We will strive to illustrate the extent to which apoptotic cell clearance can affect the progression of not only autoimmune diseases such as lupus, but also extend to other pathological conditions including interactions with cardiovascular disease.

2. Systemic lupus erythematosus

Systemic lupus erythematosus (SLE) is a common autoimmune disease that affects an estimated 1.5 million Americans. Notably, the number of women of childbearing age that are affected versus men is increased 10-fold. It is also more common in the Afro-Caribbean and Asian populations (Lahita 1999). The mechanism(s) that leads to the breakdown of self-tolerance in SLE is not well understood. SLE is classified as a multi-systemic disease since the clinical presentations affect multiple organs. These signs can present with varying severity in skin, joints, kidneys, brain, heart and lungs (Lahita 1999). An abundance of autoantibody can be found in patients with SLE, and over 50 autoantibodies have been described. The major type of autoantibodies are primarily antinuclear and against DNA however, antibodies to components of RNA: anti-Sm or anti-ribonuclease, chromatin, nucleosomes, histones, and ribosomes are also commonly found (Lahita 1999).

One of the major clinical manifestations of SLE is glomerulonephritis in which blood and protein can accumulate in the urine as a result of disrupted function of the glomeruli. Decreased renal function can ultimately lead to renal failure. Most notably in SLE, autoantibody production leads to the formation of immune complexes with their specific antigens and these complexes can be deposited into the glomerular capillaries. Whether these immune complexes arise from deposition of circulating immune complexes or are formed in-situ, remains to be firmly established. Glomerulonephritis can lead to hypertension, contributing to interactions between autoimmune disease and other cardiovascular disorders. Thus, the accumulation and deposition of immune complexes made up of anti-DNA or antinuclear antibodies and their antigens are thought to spark the induction of the kidney dysfunction (Lahita 1999).

The end-organ damage most commonly observed in SLE patients is kidney failure. However, due to recent advances in the treatment of kidney dysfunction, it has been observed that there are an increased number of SLE patients with coronary heart disease (Manzi et al. 1997b; Petri et al. 1992; Urowitz et al. 1976). This has led to the study of atherosclerosis as a precursor to more advanced cardiovascular diseases in these patients. Atherosclerosis can eventually lead to major coronary heart disease and cardiovascular events, therefore it is prudent to monitor the progression of atherosclerosis in patients with SLE. In recent years, it has been reported that there is an increased incidence of accelerated atherosclerosis among young women with SLE (J.M. Esdaile et al. 2001b; Lockshin et al. 2001; Manzi 2000). These young women also have increased rates of coronary heart disease. More recently, this has also been shown to occur in other autoimmune diseases such as rheumatoid arthritis and systemic sclerosis (Lockshin et al. 2001; Riboldi et al. 2002; Van Doornum et al. 2002).

The cause of SLE remains unknown, although there are several genetic, environmental, and hormonal factors that can contribute to its initiation and progression. The presence of increased levels of autoantibodies is a hallmark of SLE, however, it is thought that simply having circulating auto-antibodies cannot cause autoimmune disease (Lahita 1999). There are environmental factors, such as ultraviolet light, that can cause an autoimmune disease like SLE to manifest itself. When taken into account that lupus occurs more frequently in women, it is thought that hormonal factors may also play a role in disease manifestation (Lahita 1999). Thus, the genetic factors may provide a predisposition to SLE, the flares of which could be triggered by environmental or hormonal factors.

Immune dysregulation can affect disease progression if there is T-cell dysfunction which presents via a shift in the cytokines produced by these helper T-cells. T-helper 1 (T_H1) pro-inflammatory cytokines such as tumor necrosis factor-alpha (TNFα), interferon-gamma (IFNγ), and IL-2 lead to B-cell growth, differentiation and activation that will in turn result in antibody production. In contrast, secretion of anti-inflammatory T_H2 cytokines such as IL-4, IL-5, and IL-10 functions to inhibit macrophage activation and downregulate T_H1 responses (Janeway et al. 2001). Therefore, modulation of cytokine production resulting in a shift towards a more pro-inflammatory response can affect lupus progression.

In SLE patients, accumulation of autoantibodies is characteristic and these autoantibodies can form immune complexes (Lahita 1999). During an SLE flare, these immune complexes can contribute to inflammation and injury to tissue. Immune complex injury and inflammatory response can occur in two ways. The first is when the antibody binds to its antigen, thus stimulating recruitment and activation of inflammatory cells such as macrophages via complement and Fc receptors. This occurs in cells or extracellular tissues and will lead to tissue injury. Second, immune complexes that form in the circulation can deposit on the vessel wall and cause an inflammatory response on the endothelium by recruitment of inflammatory cells (Abbas and Lichtman 2003). This may be of particular interest concerning the association of accelerated atherosclerosis with SLE. Aggravation of the endothelial lining by autoantibodies and immune complexes will be discussed later in more detail with relation to promoting atherosclerotic lesion formation.

Currently, one of the most widely studied areas among the genetic causes of SLE is in decreased clearance of apoptotic bodies that are thought to propagate the progression of the disease. There are numerous studies of different genetic mouse models that support this hypothesis (Bickerstaff et al. 1999; Botto et al. 1998; Clynes et al. 1998; Cohen et al. 2002; Hanayama et al. 2004; Korb and Ahearn 1997; Napirei et al. 2000; Taylor et al. 2000). It has been demonstrated that short-term autoimmunity, i.e. production of autoantibodies, can be achieved by immunization with apoptotic cells. However, a long-term autoimmune response does not occur when there is efficient apoptotic body clearance (Qian et al. 2004). In cases where the machinery that is responsible for the clearance is disrupted, it has been shown that apoptotic bodies accumulate, resulting in lupus-like diseases. These studies will be discussed later in the chapter.

3. Apoptosis

Apoptosis is programmed cell death that is necessary for tissue remodeling during development. It also occurs when a cell may pose a threat to the organism. For example, cells with DNA damage that could become cancerous, or cells infected by a virus, will be recognized by cytotoxic T-cells and, in almost all cases, removed. Therefore, the role of apoptosis is not limited to development but plays a role in maintaining cellular homeostasis throughout an organism's life.

A main feature of apoptosis is its well-defined sequence of morphological changes. The cell begins by condensing both chromatin and cytoplasm resulting in nuclear blebbing and a change in cell appearance. Chromosomal DNA is digested into 200bp fragments by endogenous nucleases that cleave at the inter-nucleosomal linker regions. This is important to note since SLE patients develop antibodies to nucleosomes that are found prior to anti-DNA antibodies. The genes involved in the digestion of DNA and chromatin from cells undergoing apoptosis are DNaseI and serum amyloid P (SAP). Deoxyribonuclease I (DNaseI) is responsible for digesting extracellular chromatin and the lack of this enzyme results in an autoimmune phenotype in mice, which develop auto-antibodies to chromatin as well as glomerulonephritis caused by immune complex deposition (Napirei et al. 2000). SAP is known to bind chromatin and perhaps act as a cover to prevent an inflammatory immune response and assist in its clearance. The absence of SAP results in auto-antibodies to chromatin which can deposit in the kidney and cause glomerulonephritis (Bickerstaff et al. 1999). The next step of apoptosis involves further shrinking of the cell and blebbing off of small membrane bound vesicles, apoptotic bodies, which will then be phagocytosed.

Apoptosis is not limited to organism development. For example, each day there are more than 10^{11} senescent red blood cells that must be eliminated, (Alberts et al. 2002) and the bone marrow produces millions of new red blood cells, monocytes, neutrophils, and lymphocytes. Regulated loss of all these blood cells occurs by apoptosis, and the dying cells are finally phagocytosed by specialized macrophages in the liver and spleen. Macrophages and dendritic cells are phagocytic cells deriving from hematopoietic stem cells. They are major players in the body's defense against infection, in addition to T-cells, B-cells, and neutrophils. The phagocytic properties which they possess are also critical to removal of dead cells. Apoptosis plays an important role in development, homeostasis, and disease. Apoptotic cell debris is efficiently removed by phagocytic cells through a process that requires a complex system of signals and receptors. Many studies show that a breakdown in the removal of apoptotic cell corpses will promote inflammation and, at its extreme, autoimmunity.

Therefore, this process is very important since the production of new cells must be balanced by an equal loss of these cells. Related to this idea, it has been suggested that the balance is maintained in a 'Yin' and 'Yang' process involving apoptosis and wound healing, respectively (Khatami 2008, 2011). With regard to inflammation, apoptotic events ('Yin') stimulate the initial responses of immune cells for the recognition and clearance of the offender. The post-inflammatory events involved in wound healing ('Yang') are important in reconstruction and repair, thereby contributing to the resolution of inflammation (Khatami 2008, 2011). In the following sections, the recognition of the apoptotic cells and their various receptors or opsonizers will be discussed.

3.1 Recognition of the apoptotic cell

Proper maintenance within the body must occur to clear the apoptotic bodies in a non-inflammatory manner. Phagocytosis is an action of engulfment that requires activation of receptors in order to initiate the process of ingestion and degradation. The final steps in the process of apoptosis occur in concert with the phagocytes. Recognition of the apoptotic cell involves a complex system of signals and receptors. This system has been the focus of intense research and has yielded evidence towards recruitment signals, including chemokines and cell surface changes, as well as the receptors responsible for physical contact with the apoptotic cells. This section will categorize and discuss phagocytic clearance, the various stages of apoptosis from initial breakdown of the cells and nucleosomes, to the eventual clearance of the apoptotic debris, and the relevant mouse models that have been useful in studying the development of SLE.

A chemoattractant that signals recruitment of macrophages to the sites of apoptotic cell death has recently been described. The apoptotic cell will release a chemokine called lysophosphatidylcholine (LPC) that signals to macrophages to engulf and digest the apoptotic body (Lauber et al. 2003). LPC is produced as a result of hydrolysis of phosphatidylcholine in LDL and cell membranes, and can be produced by phospholipase-A2 (PLA_2) or by oxidation. LPC was previously known as a chemoattractant for monocytes (Hoffman et al. 1982), however, the role in apoptotic cell clearance was not known until recently. In terms of cardiovascular disease, LPC has been shown to be a component of atherosclerotic plaques, and expression of PLA_2 is observed in the arterial wall. PLA_2 is known to be induced by proinflammatory cytokines, such as TNFα and IL-6. Since these cytokines are known to promote inflammation in both cardiovascular and autoimmune diseases, this has potential consequences not only to atherosclerosis, but also towards SLE.

A relationship between LPC and SLE has been described in several studies. First, levels of anti-LPC antibodies are elevated in patients with SLE compared to their healthy counterparts (Wu et al. 1999). Although the levels of LPC have not been analyzed in the sera of patients with SLE, it has been determined that they have increased PLA_2 activity (Pruzanski et al. 1994). Therefore it is possible that they may also have increased levels of LPC. Similar antigenic epitopes among phospholipids such as oxLDL and LPC have been identified, and these were also found to be similar to those found in endothelial cells. Further studies have demonstrated that anti-LPC antibody levels are decreased in male patients with borderline hypertension compared to normotensive controls (Wu et al. 2001). This provides evidence further linking inflammation to cardiovascular disease. Thus, the significance of LPC involvement in SLE has potential benefits to understanding the links between SLE and cardiovascular disease.

To date, the most well understood recognition signal to trigger phagocytosis is the expression of PS on the surface of the apoptotic cell membrane. When a cell undergoes apoptosis, the distribution of lipids in the plasma membrane is disrupted. Negatively charged PS will be flipped in the lipid bilayer to be exposed on the outside layer. As a consequence, this is recognized as an "eat me" signal by phagocytes (Fadok et al. 1992; Fadok et al. 2001). This is the one of the first steps that will allow recognition of the cell as apoptotic, and eventual uptake by the phagocyte. Apoptotic cells that are not cleared can undergo secondary necrosis, and this leads to the release of the intracellular components, promoting a pro-inflammatory response. Therefore, it is crucial that cells are recognized as apoptotic and cleared in a timely manner.

Phosphatidylserine content has been used as a measurement for circulating levels of microparticles, which are vesicles released from plasma membranes after injury or apoptosis. Increased levels of endothelial microparticles have been found in human plasma under a variety of pathological conditions and are thought to play a role in systemic cell activation. Endothelial microparticles are present in atherosclerotic plaque (Mallat et al. 1999; Nomura et al. 2000), and there is a relationship between circulating microparticles and arterial stiffness in patients with end-stage renal failure (Amabile et al. 2005). In addition, increases in endothelial microparticles have been documented in patients with severe hypertension compared to healthy controls (Preston et al. 2003). Recent work has shown a correlation between microparticles and disease activity in patients with SLE, primary Sjorgren's syndrome and rheumatoid arthritis (Pereira et al. 2006; Sellam et al. 2009).

After successful localization to the site of the apoptotic cell, further recognition signals facilitate initial attachment of the macrophage via a variety of specialized surface receptors.

Several receptors have been linked to recognizing apoptotic cells, a majority of which are known to distinguish various forms of phospholipids, including phosphatidylserine (PS). There are three types of receptors that will be discussed: those that respond to PS on the cell surface of the apoptotic cell, both directly and indirectly, and those that recognize and bind to various molecules that opsonize the apoptotic cell for ingestion.

3.2 Direct binding to PS

The presence of PS on the cell surface is known to stimulate various receptors on the macrophage in order to facilitate clearance and promote an anti-inflammatory response (Fig. 1). A macrophage receptor with a direct interaction with PS, a PS-specific receptor appears to exist (Fadok et al. 2000). Data shows macrophage binding of apoptotic cells can be mediated by a specific PS receptor (PSR). This action is associated with the production of TGF-β and the downregulation of inflammatory cytokines (Fadok et al. 1998). Another study corroborating the notion that apoptotic clearance is normally anti-inflammatory observed that tumor necrosis factor-alpha (TNF-α), a cytokine released by macrophages during a pro-inflammatory response, is downregulated by PS-liposomes (Aramaki et al. 1997). Therefore, PS is important not only for recognition by phagocytes, but also for controlling the immune response and maintaining an anti-inflammatory setting.

3.3 Bridging molecules

Other receptors exist that are linked to PS via bridging molecules (Fig. 1). These receptors include β2-Glycoprotein I (β2GPI), and Mer (Balasubramanian et al. 1997; Balasubramanian and Schroit 1998; Scott et al. 2001). β2GPI is a plasma protein that binds phospholipids, in particular, it has been found to bind directly to PS. Several studies suggest that β2GPI bound to PS on apoptotic cells contributes to clearance by then binding to its receptor (β2GPI-R) found on macrophages. Therefore, β2GPI is a candidate protein that could contribute to autoimmune disease if altered. Mer, a member of the receptor tyrosine kinase family, binds to the growth arrest-specific protein 6 (Gas-6). The function of Gas-6 in apoptotic clearance is to bind the exposed PS on apoptotic cells, then bind to mer on macrophages (K. Nagata et al. 1996). This action leads to phagocytosis of the apoptotic cell and, at the same time, TNFα levels decrease though the reason for this effect remains to be elucidated (Camenisch et al. 1999). This suggests that mer involvement in apoptotic cell removal may contribute to the anti-inflammatory response seen in normal clearance. Evidence of this is provided by a mouse model whereby the absence of mer results in the manifestation of autoimmunity resembling SLE (Cohen et al. 2002). Apoptotic material accumulates in lymphoid tissue, evidenced by the enlarged spleen. The autoimmunity observed in these mice is characterized by autoantibody production including anti-DNA, ANAs, and anti-phospholipid. A mild form of glomerulonephritis also occurs (Cohen et al. 2002). In addition, the liver X receptor transcription factors have been shown to be necessary for proper clearance of apoptotic bodies, by the induction of mer expression (A-Gonzalez et al. 2009). Liver X receptor-deficient mice are impaired in their ability to respond to apoptotic clearance, have dysregulated inflammatory pathway signalling, and develop lupus like disease. Taken together, these mouse models deficient in machinery necessary for apoptotic cell clearance provide further evidence to implicate impaired apoptotic cell clearance in autoimmunity.

3.4 Scavenger receptors

There are several scavenger receptors that have been implicated in apoptotic clearance: CD-36, scavenger receptor A and B1 (SR-A, SR-B), LOX -1, and CD68 (Gillotte-Taylor et al. 2001; Imachi et al. 2000; Rigotti et al. 1995; Shiratsuchi et al. 1999) (Fig. 1). Of all these receptors, CD-36 is the only one to have a known ligand. CD-36 is linked to the apoptotic body via a thrombospondin bridge. Since, these receptors also recognize and uptake oxLDL as part of macrophage foam cell formation, they are thought to function by recognizing oxidized sites on apoptotic cells.

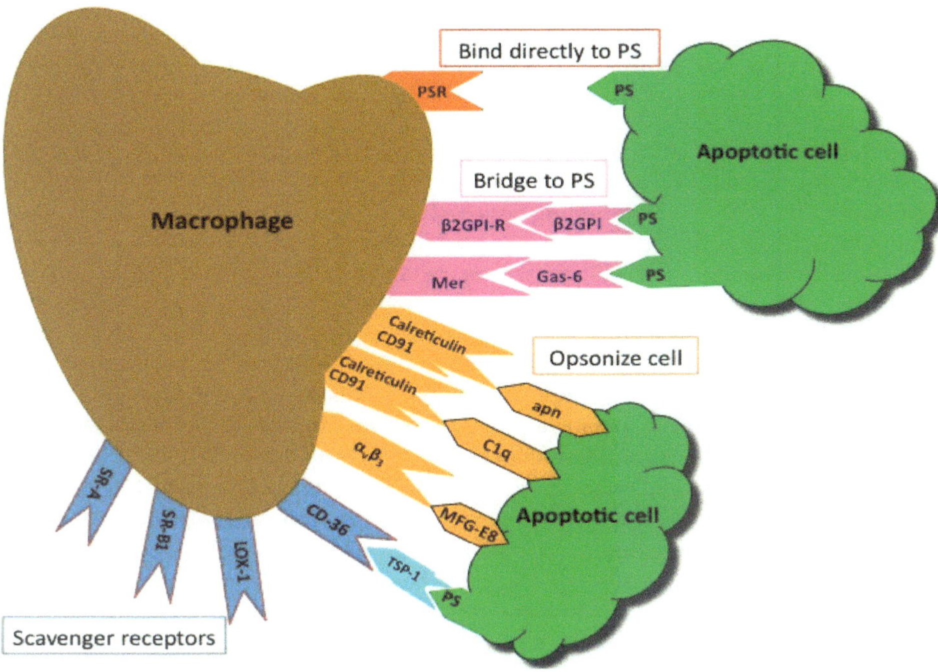

Fig. 1. Receptors associated with apoptotic cell clearance. Four types of receptors exist on macrophages to promote attachment and phagocytosis of apoptotic cells. Phosphatidylserine receptor (PSR) binds directly to phosphatidylserine (PS). Two receptors, β2-Glycoprotein I receptor (β2GPI-R) and Mer, bind to β2-Glycoprotein I (β2-GPI) and growth arrest-specific protein 6 (Gas-6) respectively; β2GPI and Gas-6 bind PS and act as a bridge between the macrophage and the apoptotic cell. Adiponectin, complement protein C1q and milk fat globule epidermal growth factor 8 (MFG-E8) opsonize the apoptotic cell and bridge to the macrophage via calreticulin/CD91 and $\alpha_v\beta_3$ receptors, respectively. The final group includes scavenger receptor A (SR-A), scavenger receptor B1 (SR-B1), LOX1, and CD-36. CD-36 joins thrombospondin-1 (TSP-1) bound to PS on the apoptotic cell.

3.5 Opsonization of the apoptotic body

Among the genetic factors that have been implicated in the progression of SLE, is a third group that helps to regulate clearance by opsonizing the apoptotic body and facilitating antigen clearing mechanisms (Fig. 1). Opsonization is the process of making bacteria or other cells more attractive to phagocytes; therefore, this can play a large role in the recognition and removal of apoptotic cells. Further evidence involving an opsonization mechanism is observed by a protein that is secreted by activated macrophages and dendritic cells: milk fat globule-EGF-factor 8 (MFG-E8). MFG-E8 facilitates phagocytosis of apoptotic cells by linking the apoptotic cell to the phagocyte. It binds specifically to the phosphotidylserine that is exposed on the apoptotic cells, and then binds to the $\alpha_v\beta_3$ integrin expressed on the phagocyte (Hanayama et al. 2002). Co-culture of peritoneal macrophages with a mutant MFG-E8 protein results in inhibited phagocytosis. In addition, the levels of the anti-inflammatory cytokine IL-10 are suppressed. Under normal conditions, expression of IL-10 is upregulated by macrophages that are actively engulfing apoptotic cells. This study also showed that intravenous injection of mutant MFG-E8 protein stimulated the production of autoantibodies (Asano et al. 2004). A mouse model lacking MFG-E8 revealed an autoimmune phenotype showing autoantibody production, splenomegaly, and glomerulonephritis. In addition, macrophages from MFG-E8$^{-/-}$ mice engulfed fewer apoptotic cells than wild type macrophages which could be corrected with the addition of recombinant MFG-E8. A similar finding occurred *in vivo* where there was less co-localization of apoptotic cells with the macrophages located in the spleen (Hanayama et al. 2004). This study suggests that apoptotic cell clearance is impaired in the absence of MFG-E8, and this contributes to the propagation of autoimmune disease.

Another molecule, Complement C1q, is part of the complement system which is a major effector of the humoral immune response, but also contributes to the opsonization of apoptotic cells. The removal of apoptotic cells is facilitated by binding a portion of the globular head of C1q (independent of antibody) to the apoptotic cell (Korb and Ahearn 1997). The collagenous domain of C1q then binds to the receptor calreticulin, which is found on the macrophage (Ogden et al. 2001). In both cases, the end result is ingestion and degradation in an anti-inflammatory manner. In a mouse model, the absence of C1q results in antinuclear antibody accumulation and immune complex renal disease. In addition, disease severity related to the absence of complement decreases in relation to the placement in the pathway. C1q$^{-/-}$ mice demonstrate a severe form of SLE compared to C4-/- mice (Botto et al. 1998; Taylor et al. 2000). Complement deficiency has also been linked to SLE pathogenesis in humans. This implicates apoptotic body clearance via the complement pathway as a major factor in SLE initiation and progression.

Adiponectin is an adipose-derived cytokine known to be cardio-protective, but also opsonizes apoptotic bodies and facilitates an efficient clearance in order to promote phagocytosis that is non-inflammatory. Adiponectin has a similar structure to C1q and facilitates clearance by opsonization of the apoptotic cell body and uptake through one of its receptors, calreticulin-CD91, which is expressed on the surface of the macrophage. In vitro treatment of macrophages with adiponectin results in increased apoptotic body clearance. In addition, lupus-prone mice on a C57 background, deficient in adiponectin have a defect in clearance of apoptotic bodies and a worsened lupus disease phenotype (Takemura et al. 2007). Another mouse model, combining a lupus phenotype with adiponectin deficiency, on the MRL background which is in itself permissive to autoimmunity, results in exacerbated kidney morphology including crescent formation, mesangial expansion, and increased IgG and complement C3 deposits (Parker et al. 2011). Paradoxically, SLE patients with renal dysfunction have been reported to have increased adiponectin levels compared to SLE patients with normal renal function, and adiponectin levels are also increased in the urine of SLE patients having an active renal flare (Rovin et al. 2005). This finding was one of the first that lead to the finding that many chronic inflammatory diseases have increased levels of adiponectin, however this is an area of research currently being investigated.

More recently, the nuclear receptor, peroxisome-proliferator activated receptor-δ (PPARδ) has been shown to act as an enhancer of opsonization molecules. Mouse models with ubiquitous or macrophage-specific deletion of PPARδ have impaired clearance of apoptotic cells, resulting in increased auto-antibody production and a lupus-like phenotype. The opsonins controlled by PPARδ in this study are C1q and MFG-E8 (Mukundan et al. 2009). Similarly, macrophage-specific deletion of other members of the nuclear receptor family, PPARγ or retinoid X receptor-α results in autoantibody accumulation and glomerular injury (Roszer et al. 2011). In addition to the lupus phenotype, mice deficient in PPARγ or retinoid X receptor-α are unable to efficiently clear apoptotic cells, again providing evidence that impaired clearance is important to the pathogenesis of SLE. Taken together, it would be interesting to speculate if adiponectin expression and opsonization is also maximized, since PPARγ is known to upregulate adiponectin.

The above are genes that are involved in both the binding and clearance of apoptotic debris and immune complexes, as well as in the digestion of DNA and chromatin. These are especially interesting because they support the hypothesis, using both human and murine data, that impaired clearance of apoptotic bodies will lead to synergistic effects between atherosclerosis and autoimmune disease.

3.6 Non-inflammatory vs. pro-inflammatory phagocytosis

Macrophages have various receptors that are responsible for the uptake of apoptotic debris which typically results in an anti-inflammatory response. However, various instances of phagocytic uptake, or the inhibition of it, can cause a pro-inflammatory response. In addition, evidence exists of complications and consequential pro-inflammatory cytokine release from immune complexes and autoantibodies observed in SLE.

In general, upon ingestion of an apoptotic cell by a phagocyte, normal clearance will occur by filtration through the lymph nodes and normal degradation and digestion of the apoptotic body by the macrophage. Usually this occurs in a non-inflammatory manner (Fig. 2a) (Fadok et al. 1998). In the instance where the macrophage does not, or is unable to phagocytose the apoptotic body, other phagocytic cells called dendritic cells will proceed to take up the apoptotic body. In this case, follicular dendritic cells which reside with B-cells in the germinal center of the lymph nodes, present the apoptotic bodies as antigens to the B-cells, which will stimulate the release of antibodies. This has consequences for autoimmune diseases such as SLE by further propagating and increasing the amount of antibodies and autoantibodies being produced in the body.

Uptake and degradation of apoptotic cells through scavenger receptors does not normally stimulate an inflammatory response, however, there are instances where pro-inflammatory signaling does occur. Scavenger receptors that recognize oxidized or otherwise modified low-density lipoprotein (LDL) are also capable for the removal of apoptotic cells. Competition for binding can occur for example, in a hyperlipidemic state, with oxidized LDL (oxLDL) and inhibit uptake of the apoptotic cell (Fig. 2b). This will result in increased circulating apoptotic cells which can further degrade and go into secondary necrosis, releasing pro-inflammatory cytokines. Therefore, it is reasonable to suggest that in hyperlipidemic environments such as those found in cardiovascular disease, there will be propagation of inflammation when apoptotic cells are not cleared from the circulation.

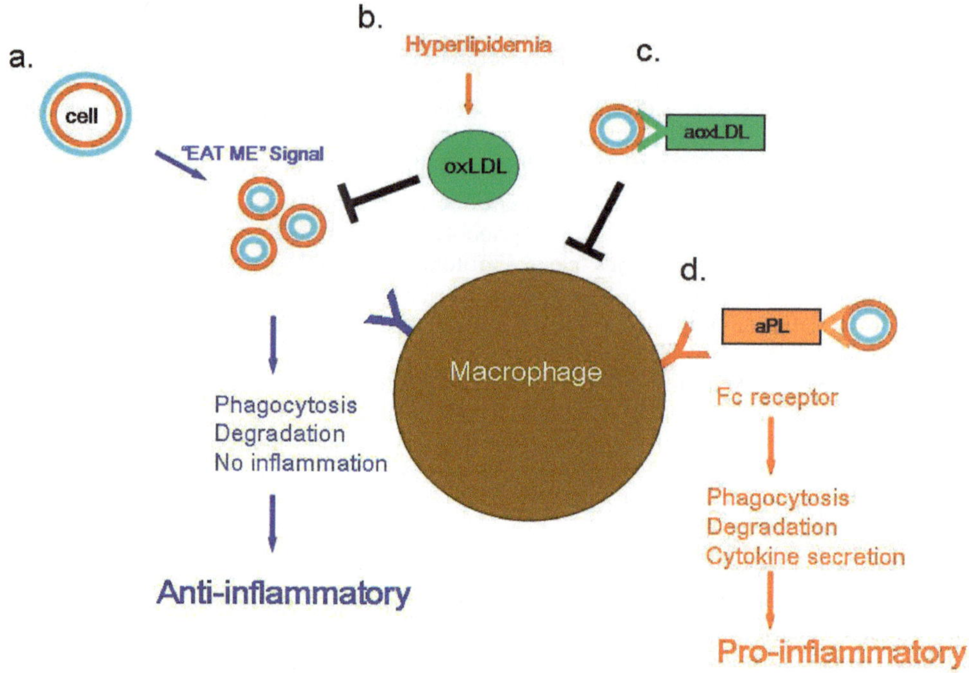

Fig. 2. Normal vs. impaired clearance of apoptotic cells. a) Apoptotic cell clearance does not promote inflammation. b) Elevated circulating lipids may contribute to increased oxidized LDL which can compete with apoptotic cells for receptor uptake. c) Apoptotic cell clearance can be inhibited by binding of anti-oxLDL. d) Opsonization of an apoptotic cell by anti-phospholipids results in uptake by macrophage Fc receptor and pro-inflammatory cytokine signaling.

Relevant to autoimmune diseases, an abundance of circulating autoantibodies to oxidized LDL for example, provides an environment suitable to a pro-inflammtory response with regard to apoptotic clearance. Anti-oxLDL can bind the apoptotic cells by forming an immune complex which inhibits phagocytosis by macrophages and has the potential to further damage tissue (Fig. 2c). In addition, antibodies such as antiphospholipid and anti-β2GPI have been shown to bind to apoptotic cells and opsonize them for recognition by the macrophage Fc receptor (Manfredi et al. 1998b; Manfredi et al. 1998a) (Fig 2d). Apoptotic cell opsonization by β2GPI results in dendritic cell stimulation and presentation to T-cells. Activation of B-cells occurs as a result of T-cell signaling, and subsequent autoantibody production ensues (Manfredi et al. 2005). Cross-linking of Fc receptors by IgG immune complex opsonized molecules results in pro-inflammatory cytokine secretion (Fig. 2d). Specifically, FcγIIA on apoptotic neutrophils is bound by immune complexes, and this increases phagocytosis of the apoptotic cell by macrophages. However, phagocytosis by the macrophage in this context results in secretion of TNFα and IL-6, both of which are known to promote inflammation (Hart et al. 2004). Therefore, in an environment where autoantibodies are produced, such as in SLE, this can serve to exacerbate the disease.

4. Apoptotic clearance in autoimmune disease

Currently, one of the most widely studied areas among the genetic causes of SLE is in decreased clearance of apoptotic bodies which are thought to propagate the progression of the disease. It is thought that immune complexes play a role in the pathogenesis of SLE. Evidence to support this idea is provided in a study investigating cytokine production in SLE patients. Both *in vitro* and *in vivo* data has demonstrated that material released from necrotic and apoptotic cells will combine with IgG found in serum from SLE patients. This results in production of IFNα, a pro-inflammatory cytokine that is elevated in SLE patients (Lovgren et al. 2004). This study suggests that the autoantibodies present in serum from SLE patients can form immune complexes with nucleic acids released by apoptotic cells. This will stimulate IFNα production, thus contributing to disease pathogenesis. In addition, administration of IFNα to patients for diseases unrelated to SLE revealed that about 25% of these subjects developed serum anti-nuclear antibodies (ANAs), and a small number if these then went on to develop subsequent autoimmunity (Baechler et al. 2004). From these studies, it is reasonable to suggest that increased IFNα production is, in part, a result of impaired clearance of apoptotic cells.

Evidence exists of autoimmune disease in humans with gene defects of key players in apoptotic clearance machinery. For example, recent evidence has shown that circulating levels of Gas6 and soluble Axl, involved in the bridging of apoptotic cells to the macrophage, correlate to disease activity in SLE especially with the involvement of lupus nephritis (Ekman et al. 2011). In addition, complement deficiency has been noted to occur and result in SLE. In a healthy individual, complement C1q opsonizes antigen-antibody complexes for ingestion and degradation in an anti-inflammatory manner. In addition, a second function of C1q is its ability to bind apoptotic debris through a portion of its globular head independent of antibody (Korb and Ahearn 1997). This is made more efficient if it occurs in conjunction with simultaneous activation of the Fcγ receptors by IgG molecules that have also bound to the antigen or immune complex (Abbas and Lichtman 2003). Adding complement proteins *in vitro* to a phagocytosis assay using human monocyte-derived macrophages from C1q deficient humans resulted in a three-fold increase in phagocytosis of apoptotic cells (Mevorach et al. 1998a). Complement deficient humans follow similar patterns in terms of what is observed in experimental mice: the more upstream in the pathway, the more severe SLE that will develop (Botto and Walport 1993; Botto et al. 1998). The most common deficiencies and also the ones that present the most severe signs of SLE occur with proteins in C1 and C4. In contrast, deficiencies in C2 and C3 have lower occurrences in humans and are also less associated with the development of SLE. Thus, a trend leading towards varying flares of SLE is observed in humans and related to decreased apoptotic cell clearance (Walport 2002). Therefore, it is reasonable to suggest that a hierarchy exists among the proteins of the complement pathway with regard to anti-inflammatory phagocytic clearance.

Another group of defects implicated in autoimmunity involves genes that normally bind immune complexes and aid in their removal. Polymorphisms predisposing people to SLE are known to occur in the receptors FcγRIIA and FcγRIII, also known as CD32 and CD16, respectively. These genes are part of a family of receptors that bind to the Fc domains of many IgG isotypes. FcγRIIA and FcγRIII are low-affinity receptors, so IgG monomers are unable to bind and activate the receptors. These receptors are found on macrophages as well as dendritic cells and neutrophils and mediate the phagocytosis of opsonized particles, and stimulate other leukocytes to degrade the phagocytosed particles. In a lupus mouse model where the Fcγ receptor is disrupted, immune complexes still deposit in the glomeruli but do not contribute to mortality of the animal (Clynes et al. 1998). Therefore, Fcγ receptors play a role in inflammatory cytokine signaling that can contribute to autoimmunity.
An *in vitro* study utilizing monocyte-derived macrophages from SLE patients revealed a significantly lower ability of these macrophages to phagocytose apoptotic cells, compared to healthy controls (Herrmann et al. 1998). In addition, Baumann and colleagues have provided *in vivo* clinical evidence that human patients with SLE have impaired clearance of their apoptotic debris. They showed that apoptotic cells accumulated within the germinal centers of the lymph nodes of SLE patients. They studied macrophages within the lymph nodes and found that they not only have an abnormal morphology, but also that there is a decreased amount of apoptotic body co-localization, suggesting that macrophage phagocytosis is disrupted in these patients. Further, the apoptotic bodies were found to colocalize more frequently with follicular dendritic cells (DCs). This association could lead to presentation by the DCs of the apoptotic body as an antigen, and promote auto-antibody production by the B-cells (Baumann et al. 2002). Thus, there are several lines of evidence that implicate impaired apoptotic body clearance in the progression of autoimmune diseases such as SLE.

5. Cardiovascular disease- conventional vs. SLE-specific risk factors

Clinical studies have largely examined the relationship between SLE and endpoint cardiac events including myocardial infarction and stroke. More recently, attention has shifted towards the *causes* of advanced cardiovascular diseases; the focus now being on the contribution of accelerated atherosclerosis in SLE patients (J.M. Esdaile et al. 2001b; Lockshin et al. 2001; Manzi 2000). Conventional risk factors for development of atherosclerotic vascular and coronary artery disease include age, circulating levels of high-density lipoprotein (HDL) and total cholesterol, blood pressure, smoking, and diabetes mellitus. This list of risk factors continues to expand since further study has revealed that systolic and diastolic blood pressure levels can be considered separate risk factors; independent roles for obesity and specific adipose tissue distribution has stemmed from studies of diabetes mellitus associated with coronary artery disease. Additions that are actively being researched include C-reactive protein, lipoprotein(a), fibrinogen, and homocysteine (Hackam and Anand 2003). The list of risk factors is constantly being updated as studies continue to search for new markers to predict disease.
Risk factors have also been identified specifically for SLE patients with cardiovascular disease (CVD), in addition to the conventional risk factors discussed above. These are a distinct set of risk factors that separate these patients from SLE patients without CVD as well as their healthy counterparts (Svenungsson et al. 2001). Using the risk factors defined by the Framingham study, a significant proportion of CVD associated with SLE was shown

to occur based on other unknown risk factors. In this study, when traditional Framingham risk factors were accounted for, it was observed that there was an 8- to 17-fold increase in nonfatal myocardial infarction, stroke, death from CHD and overall occurrences of CHD, in patients with SLE (J. M. Esdaile et al. 2001a). In young, pre-menopausal women, this increase was as high as 50-fold. In another study, women with SLE and no evidence of CVD were studied with regards to carotid plaque, intima-media wall thickness (IMT), and aortic stiffness. It was determined that the risk factors for carotid plaque and IMT were the same for cardiovascular disease in the absence of SLE. However, other risk factors with respect to aortic stiffness were found to be specific to SLE patients. For example increased C3 complement levels were observed in SLE patients with higher vascular stiffness. This suggests that immune dysregulation and complement metabolism play a role in the interactions between these two disease processes (Selzer et al. 2004). It has also been shown that patients with SLE have significant endothelial dysfunction that occurs at rates higher than those predicted after taking traditional CHD risk factors into account (El-Magadmi et al. 2004). Several other studies evaluating the role of traditional CVD risk factors in patients with SLE have been performed, but have excluded SLE patients with various existing risk factors.

5.1 Atherosclerosis

Atherosclerosis is the underlying cause of most cardiovascular disease accounting for the majority of death in the Western world. It is a disorder in which intimal thickening and lipid deposition occur in the elastic arteries such as the aorta, and places of turbid flow, as well as in the larger arteries such as the coronary arteries. There are six levels of atherosclerotic lesion progression; the last three are considered complex and occlusive, having a thinner cap and a very cholesterol-rich core, making it more susceptible to rupture. Plaque deposition and rupture can lead to a cardiovascular event such as a myocardial infarction or stroke. Initial events that lead to lesion development occur when LDL is allowed to migrate into the vessel wall. This can occur in one of two ways: a diffusion like-mechanism if the serum LDL level is extremely high; or injury to the endothelial lining, occuring from hypertension, toxins, bacteria, viruses, or immune complexes (Ross 1993).

About half of all the circulating LDL within the body is cleared daily. Although two-thirds of LDL particles are taken up through the LDL receptors during normal clearance of lipids from the body, the remaining LDL is cleared by other mechanisms. For example, within the interstitium, LDL can become modified to various oxidized forms. This allows the LDL to be engulfed by type A scavenger receptors on macrophages and/or smooth muscle cells which are then termed "foam cells." These foam cells contribute to the initiation and progression of atherogenesis.

Accelerated atherosclerosis is believed to be a critical factor contributing to stroke and coronary heart disease (CHD), which is one of the leading causes of death among young women with SLE (Manzi et al. 1997a; Petri et al. 1992; Urowitz et al. 1976). Clinical studies have largely examined the relation between SLE and endpoint cardiac events including myocardial infarction and stroke. Attention has shifted towards the causes of advanced cardiovascular diseases; the focus now being on the contribution of accelerated atherosclerosis in SLE patients (J. M. Esdaile et al. 2001a; Lockshin et al. 2001; Manzi 2000).

As mentioned earlier, progress in elucidating the feedback interactions between atherosclerosis and autoimmune disease has been impaired by the lack of appropriate animal models, and further research is necessary to determine the mechanisms in order to provide more beneficial treatment to patients. A mouse model developed by our lab has demonstrated a synergy between atherosclerosis and SLE (Aprahamian et al. 2004). This model combined an autoimmune phenotype, *gld*, (due to FasL deficiency) with an atherosclerotic background, apoE-/-, (due to apoE deficiency). Fas ligand (FasL) is a type II membrane protein that induces apoptotic cell death in cells that bear the Fas (CD95/Apo-1) receptor (S. Nagata and Golstein 1995). Mice lacking Fas or FasL have a marked deficiency in apoptosis, leading to the accumulation of lymphocytes. The *gld*.apoE-/- double mutant mouse was subjected to a high cholesterol Western-type diet and compared to the wild type, *gld*, and apoE-/- mice controls. Through analysis of cholesterol levels and atherosclerotic lesion area, it was found that the atherogenic phenotypes were exacerbated in the presence of inflammatory autoimmune disease. In addition, analysis of autoantibody levels, splenomegaly, and lymphadenopathy revealed that the autoimmune phenotypes were exacerbated when subjected to an atherogenic background. Although to a lesser extent, these results were also significant when mice were maintained on normal diet. Next, the mechanism by which this observed synergy occurred was dissected by first examining the number of apopotic cells within the lymph nodes of *gld* and *gld*.apoE-/- mice. A significant number of TUNEL positive stained cells in *gld* mice compared to wild type and apoE-/- mice was observed, and this number was further increased in *gld*.apoE-/- mice. In addition, examination of apoptotic bodies within the circulation corroborates this finding. Histological analysis in lymph nodes revealed that fewer macrophages colocalized with TUNEL positive material in the *gld*.apoE-/- mice, indicating impaired uptake of the apoptotic bodies by macrophages. Disruption of the chemoattractant gradient for macrophage clearance in *gld* mice resulted in an increase in apoptotic bodies within the lymph nodes. Taken together, these data suggest that the synergy between the two disease processes observed in the *gld*.apoE-/- mouse may occur in part from impaired clearance of apoptotic bodies.

Other studies followed, utilizing mouse models to further elucidate the interaction between atherosclerosis and lupus. Using the lupus-susceptible *Sle*1.2.3 mouse model and creating LDLr bone marrow chimeras resulted in accelerated atherosclerosis associated with increased T and B cell activation when maintained on a high cholesterol Western diet (Stanic et al. 2006). In addition, the same group has shown that high fat fed LDLr.SLE chimeras have increased mortality and are significantly more hypertensive, indicating a synergy between the lupus disease and vascular complications (Braun et al. 2008). Another bone marrow chimera experiment transplant using *gld* bone marrow to LDLr-/- mice was shown to accelerate plaque progression (Gautier et al. 2007). Ma et al., has demonstrated that induction of cGVH in B6.*ApoE-/-* mice, breeding a Fas null gene onto these B6/*lpr.ApoE-/-* mice, and breeding the ApoE-/- defect onto MRL/*lpr* mice all caused a modest increase of atherosclerosis at 24 weeks of age compared to B6.*ApoE-/-* controls, as well as increased lupus like symptoms (Ma et al. 2008). The involvement of adiponectin has not been examined in these models, however given the importance of this adipokine in regulating SLE as well as inflammatory processes involved in atherosclerosis, it would be of great interest to study not only the levels of adiponectin, but also to administer exogenous adiponectin to determine if the phenotypes could be rescued. The paradox of low levels of adiponectin during flares of SLE is an interesting area that requires further exploration.

In addition, it is known that chronic inflammation can affect bone metabolism and that the pro-inflammatory cytokines TNF, IL-1beta, and IL-6 may play a major role. To this end, *lpr* mice, which have a mutation in the fas receptor, were crossed to apoE-/- mice and this double mutant was reported to develop lupus nephritis, atherosclerosis and decreased bone mineral and volume density, which may be helpful to study the role of osteopenia in lupus (Feng et al. 2007). In a further study, these mice were treated with pravastatin and an apo1 mimetic, and results showed beneficial effects. This is particularly interesting since pravastatin has been shown to increase adiponectin expression at both the mRNA and protein level, as well as enhance insulin sensitivity (Sugiyama et al. 2007). Although there is little data about the role of adipokines in degenerative bone disease, decreased adiponectin levels have been observed in the bone marrow supernatant fluid of women with osteroporosis when compared to non-osteoporotic (Pino et al. 2010). In addition, Oshima et al demonstrated that exogenous overexpression of adiponectin in wild type mice resulted in increased bone mass and decreased number of osteoclasts. Further study in vitro showed that adiponectin can prevent development of osteoclasts by inhibiting differentiation of mouse bone marrow macrophages as well as human mononuclear cells (Oshima et al. 2005). In addition to facilitating apoptotic clearance, adiponectin inhibits the expression of TNFalpha, and there is a feedback loop whereby both TNFalpha and IL-6 inhibit the production of adiponectin in adipocytes It is therefore interesting to speculate that varying levels of adiponectin can affect inflammatory processes that could result in degenerative bone disorders found in some inflammatory conditions such as obesity, inflammatory bowel disease, and diabetes.

Based on these data, it is reasonable to suggest that the presence of two disease states involving inflammation promotes impaired apoptotic cell clearance and thus provides a positive feedback mechanism which drives the progression of the two diseases. Therefore, the two disease processes result in a vicious cycle that catalyzes the progression of atherosclerotic lesion formation and autoimmune disease.

5.2 Hypercholesterolemia and impaired clearance

Apoptotic cell ingestion by macrophages normally induces a non-inflammatory response. Conversely, phagocytosis of many bacteria and foreign antigens normally results in a pro-inflammatory response by macrophages which could include the generation of reactive oxygen species, proteolytic enzyme release, and the production of numerous inflammatory cytokines and growth factors (Fadok et al. 1998). If the immune system is disrupted, apoptotic cell phagocytosis may result in a pro-inflammatory response. This is not limited to conventional immune disorders since there is evidence that hyperlipidemia can disrupt proper phagocytosis of apoptotic cells.

Aggravated autoimmune disease may result from interference with the signal gradients that are required for the normal recruitment of phagocytes to dying cells. As discussed earlier, apoptotic bodies release LPC, facilitating macrophage recruitment to the dying cell. LPC is a major component of oxLDL, which is a proatherogenic form of LDL cholesterol (Lauber et al. 2003). Thus, hyperlipidemic conditions may provide elevated levels of oxLDL, thereby disrupting the LPC chemoattractant gradient. This would render the apoptotic cell "lost" as far as macrophage recognition. It has previously been shown that increased levels of LPC disrupts phagocytic uptake of apoptotic bodies, which is further exacerbated in mice on an atherogenic background (Aprahamian et al. 2004). Therefore, atherosclerosis may compound the impaired clearance of apoptotic cells in patients with SLE.

Similarly, it has been shown that apoptotic bodies are recognized and taken up through many of the same receptors that bind oxLDL, a modified form of LDL that has been shown to be proatherogenic (Oka et al. 1998; Platt et al. 1996; Sambrano and Steinberg 1995). Therefore, an atherogenic environment may provide an increased amount of oxLDL that can compete with the apoptotic cell for binding to the scavenger receptor. This would interfere with the recognition of apoptotic bodies by macrophages and contribute to further inflammation. Increased levels of both oxLDL and anti-oxLDL have been proposed as risk factors for cardiovascular disease in female patients with SLE (Wu et al. 1999). In addition, antibodies to other phospholipids are risk factors that are involved in the progression of atherosclerosis and advanced cardiovascular outcomes such as myocardial infarction (Puurunen et al. 1994; Salonen et al. 1992; Wu et al. 1997). Anti-oxLDL antibodies are capable of binding to apoptotic cells and this inhibits phagocytosis by macrophages (Chang et al. 1999). Therefore, a number of reasons suggest that hypercholesterolemia may contribute to macrophage disruption and the impaired clearance of apoptotic cells leading to a more severe manifestation of SLE outbreak.

It is interesting to note that another phospholipid, cardiolipin, and its autoantibodies, are found at increased levels in patients with SLE, and also in patients with cardiovascular disease (Vaarala 2000). It has been shown that antinuclear antibodies and anti-cardiolipin antibodies can arise after *in vivo* administration of apoptotic cells to healthy wild-type mice (Mevorach et al. 1998b). Of note, antibodies to cardiolipin cross-react with oxLDL in patients with SLE (Vaarala et al. 1993). Another interesting feature of anti-phospholipids is that they also cross react with anti-endothelial cell antibodies (Hasselaar et al. 1990). Since antibodies directed towards negatively charged phospholipids can bind to endothelial cells, they could therefore be a driving force in the initiation of endothelial activation and dysfunction, ultimately leading to atherosclerosis.

Activated endothelial cells are characterized by changes in the vascular integrity and expression levels of adhesion molecules and cytokines (Hunt 2000). Human anti-cardiolipin antibodies have been implicated in the activation of endothelial cells, resulting in expression of E-selectin, vascular cell adhesion molecule-1, and intracellular adhesion molecule-1, all of which facilitate monocyte adhesion to the vessel wall (Simantov et al. 1995; Simantov et al. 1996). This suggests that anti-cardiolipin may facilitate extravasation of these monocytes and contribute to inflammation within the vessel wall, whether in atherogenesis, or autoimmune disease. In addition, patients with SLE and in particular, those with cardiovascular disease, have enhanced levels of lipid peroxidation (Frostegard et al. 2005). It is likely that hyperlipidemic conditions contribute to the severity of autoimmune disease by promoting the accumulation of apoptotic debris.

6. Conclusion

Published data provides mounting evidence that accelerated atherosclerosis and cardiovascular disease is a growing problem in patients with SLE and other autoimmune diseases. This chapter has focused on the role that clearance of apoptotic bodies plays in the progression of both the autoimmune and cardiovascular components of disease. Specifically, in vitro and in vivo data have been presented to demonstrate the roles of the various individual molecules involved in the machinery of the apoptotic and phagocytic processes. These studies clearly show an intricate connection between impaired apoptotic clearance and the development or progression of autoimmune disease. Further, the role of inflammation in atherosclerosis, accelerated in the presence of autoimmune disease, has been shown to be important to the progression of both diseases. The driving mechanisms of impaired clearance of apoptotic cells and precise etiology of these results in driving disease development are currently an intense area of research.

7. References

A-Gonzalez, N, et al. (2009), 'Apoptotic cells promote their own clearance and immune tolerance through activation of the nuclear receptor LXR', *Immunity,* 31 (2), 245-58.

Abbas, AK and Lichtman, AH (2003), *Cellular and Molecular Immunology* (Saunders, Elsevier Science USA) Chapter 18.

Alberts, B., et al. (2002), 'Chapter 13', *Molecular biology of the cell.* (New York, N.Y.: Garland Publishing, Inc.).

Amabile, N., et al. (2005), 'Circulating endothelial microparticles are associated with vascular dysfunction in patients with end-stage renal failure', *J Am Soc Nephrol,* 16 (11), 3381-8.

Aprahamian, T., et al. (2004), 'Impaired clearance of apoptotic cells promotes synergy between atherogenesis and autoimmune disease', *J Exp Med,* 199 (8), 1121-31.

Aramaki, Y., et al. (1997), 'Negatively charged liposomes inhibit tyrosine phosphorylation of 41-kDa protein in murine macrophages stimulated with LPS', *Biochem Biophys Res Commun,* 231 (3), 827-30.

Asano, K., et al. (2004), 'Masking of phosphatidylserine inhibits apoptotic cell engulfment and induces autoantibody production in mice', *J Exp Med,* 200 (4), 459-67.

Baechler, E. C., Gregersen, P. K., and Behrens, T. W. (2004), 'The emerging role of interferon in human systemic lupus erythematosus', *Curr Opin Immunol,* 16 (6), 801-7.

Balasubramanian, K. and Schroit, A. J. (1998), 'Characterization of phosphatidylserine-dependent beta2-glycoprotein I macrophage interactions. Implications for apoptotic cell clearance by phagocytes', *J Biol Chem,* 273 (44), 29272-7.

Balasubramanian, K., Chandra, J., and Schroit, A. J. (1997), 'Immune clearance of phosphatidylserine-expressing cells by phagocytes. The role of beta2-glycoprotein I in macrophage recognition', *J Biol Chem,* 272 (49), 31113-7.

Baumann, I., et al. (2002), 'Impaired uptake of apoptotic cells into tingible body macrophages in germinal centers of patients with systemic lupus erythematosus', *Arthritis Rheum,* 46, 191-201.

Bickerstaff, M. C., et al. (1999), 'Serum amyloid P component controls chromatin degradation and prevents antinuclear autoimmunity', *Nat Med,* 5 (6), 694-7.

Botto, M. and Walport, M. J. (1993), 'Hereditary deficiency of C3 in animals and humans', *Int Rev Immunol,* 10 (1), 37-50.

Botto, M., et al. (1998), 'Homozygous C1q deficiency causes glomerulonephritis associated with multiple apoptotic bodies.', *Nat Genet,* 19, 56-9.

Braun, N., et al. (2008), 'Accelerated atherosclerosis is independent of feeding high fat diet in systemic lupus erythematosus-susceptible LDLr(-/-) mice', *Lupus,* 17 (12), 1070-8.

Camenisch, T. D., et al. (1999), 'A novel receptor tyrosine kinase, Mer, inhibits TNF-alpha production and lipopolysaccharide-induced endotoxic shock', *J Immunol,* 162 (6), 3498-503.

Chang, M. K., et al. (1999), 'Monoclonal antibodies against oxidized low-density lipoprotein bind to apoptotic cells and inhibit their phagocytosis by elicited macrophages:

evidence that oxidation-specific epitopes mediate macrophage recognition', *Proc Natl Acad Sci U S A*, 96, 6353-58.

Clynes, R., Dumitru, C., and Ravetch, J. V. (1998), 'Uncoupling of immune complex formation and kidney damage in autoimmune glomerulonephritis', *Science*, 279 (5353), 1052-4.

Cohen, P. L., et al. (2002), 'Delayed apoptotic cell clearance and lupus-like autoimmunity in mice lacking the c-mer membrane tyrosine kinase', *J Exp Med*, 196 (1), 135-40.

Ekman, C., et al. (2011), 'Plasma concentrations of Gas6 and sAxl correlate with disease activity in systemic lupus erythematosus', *Rheumatology (Oxford)*, 50 (6), 1064-9.

El-Magadmi, M., et al. (2004), 'Systemic lupus erythematosus: an independent risk factor for endothelial dysfunction in women', *Circulation*, 110 (4), 399-404.

Esdaile, J. M., et al. (2001a), 'Traditional Framingham risk factors fail to fully account for accelerated atherosclerosis in systemic lupus erythematosus', *Arthritis Rheum*, 44 (10), 2331-7.

Esdaile, J.M., et al. (2001b), 'Traditional Framingham risk factors fail to fully account for accelerated atherosclerosis in systemic lupus erythematosus.', *Arthritis Rheum.*, 44, 2331-37.

Fadok, V. A., et al. (2001), 'Loss of phospholipid asymmetry and surface exposure of phosphatidylserine is required for phagocytosis of apoptotic cells by macrophages and fibroblasts', *J Biol Chem*, 276 (2), 1071-7.

Fadok, V.A., et al. (1992), 'Exposure of phosphatidylserine on the surface of apoptotic lymphocytes triggers specific recognition and removal by macrophages', *J Immunol*, 148 (7), 2207-16.

Fadok, V.A., et al. (1998), 'Macrophages that have ingested apoptotic cells in vitro inhibit proinflammatory cytokine production through autocrine/paracrine mechanisms involving TGF-beta, PGE2, and PAF', *J Clin Invest*, 101 (4), 890-8.

Fadok, V.A., et al. (2000), 'A receptor for phosphatidylserine-specific clearance of apoptotic cells', *Nature*, 405 (6782), 85-90.

Feng, X., et al. (2007), 'ApoE-/-Fas-/- C57BL/6 mice: a novel murine model simultaneously exhibits lupus nephritis, atherosclerosis, and osteopenia', *J Lipid Res*, 48 (4), 794-805.

Frostegard, J., et al. (2005), 'Lipid peroxidation is enhanced in patients with systemic lupus erythematosus and is associated with arterial and renal disease manifestations', *Arthritis Rheum*, 52 (1), 192-200.

Gautier, E. L., et al. (2007), 'Enhanced immune system activation and arterial inflammation accelerates atherosclerosis in lupus-prone mice', *Arterioscler Thromb Vasc Biol*, 27 (7), 1625-31.

Gillotte-Taylor, K., et al. (2001), 'Scavenger receptor class B type I as a receptor for oxidized low density lipoprotein', *J Lipid Res*, 42 (9), 1474-82.

Hackam, D. G. and Anand, S. S. (2003), 'Emerging risk factors for atherosclerotic vascular disease: a critical review of the evidence', *Jama*, 290 (7), 932-40.

Hanayama, R., et al. (2002), 'Identification of a factor that links apoptotic cells to phagocytes', *Nature*, 417 (6885), 182-7.

--- (2004), 'Autoimmune disease and impaired uptake of apoptotic cells in MFG-E8-deficient mice', *Science*, 304 (5674), 1147-50.

Hart, S. P., Alexander, K. M., and Dransfield, I. (2004), 'Immune complexes bind preferentially to Fc gamma RIIA (CD32) on apoptotic neutrophils, leading to augmented phagocytosis by macrophages and release of proinflammatory cytokines', *J Immunol,* 172 (3), 1882-7.

Hasselaar, P., et al. (1990), 'Crossreactivity of antibodies directed against cardiolipin, DNA, endothelial cells and blood platelets', *Thromb Haemost,* 63 (2), 169-73.

Herrmann, M., et al. (1998), 'Impaired phagocytosis of apoptotic cell material by monocyte-derived macrophages from patients with systemic lupus erythematosus', *Arthritis Rheum,* 41 (7), 1241-50.

Hoffman, R. D., et al. (1982), 'Stereospecific chemoattraction of lymphoblastic cells by gradients of lysophosphatidylcholine', *Proc Natl Acad Sci U S A,* 79 (10), 3285-9.

Hunt, B. J. (2000), 'The endothelium in atherogenesis', *Lupus,* 9 (3), 189-93.

Imachi, H., et al. (2000), 'Human scavenger receptor B1 is involved in recognition of apoptotic thymocytes by thymic nurse cells', *Lab Invest,* 80 (2), 263-70.

Janeway, CA, et al. (2001), *Immunobiology 5* (Fifth edn.: Garland Publishing).

Khatami, M. (2008), ''Yin and Yang' in inflammation: duality in innate immune cell function and tumorigenesis', *Expert Opin Biol Ther,* 8 (10), 1461-72.

Khatami, M. (2011), 'Unresolved inflammation: 'immune tsunami' or erosion of integrity in immune-privileged and immune-responsive tissues and acute and chronic inflammatory diseases or cancer', *Expert Opin Biol Ther.*

Korb, LC and Ahearn, JM (1997), 'C1q binds directly and specifically to surface blebs of apoptotic human keratinocytes: complement deficiency and systemic lupus erythematosus revisited.', *J. Immunol,* 158, 4525-8.

Lahita, RG (1999), *Systemic Lupus Erythematosus* (Third edn.: Academic Press).

Lauber, K., et al. (2003), 'Apoptotic cells induce migration of phagocytes via caspase-3-mediated release of a lipid attraction signal', *Cell,* 113, 717-30.

Lockshin, M.D., Salmon, J.E., and Roman, M.J. (2001), 'Atherosclerosis and lupus: a work in progress.', *Arthritis Rheum.,* 44, 2215-17.

Lovgren, T., et al. (2004), 'Induction of interferon-alpha production in plasmacytoid dendritic cells by immune complexes containing nucleic acid released by necrotic or late apoptotic cells and lupus IgG', *Arthritis Rheum,* 50 (6), 1861-72.

Ma, Z., et al. (2008), 'Accelerated atherosclerosis in ApoE deficient lupus mouse models', *Clin Immunol,* 127 (2), 168-75.

Mallat, Z., et al. (1999), 'Shed membrane microparticles with procoagulant potential in human atherosclerotic plaques: a role for apoptosis in plaque thrombogenicity', *Circulation,* 99, 348-53.

Manfredi, A. A., Sabbadini, M. G., and Rovere-Querini, P. (2005), 'Dendritic cells and the shadow line between autoimmunity and disease', *Arthritis Rheum,* 52 (1), 11-5.

Manfredi, A. A., et al. (1998a), 'Apoptotic cell clearance in systemic lupus erythematosus. II. Role of beta2-glycoprotein I', *Arthritis Rheum,* 41 (2), 215-23.

Manfredi, A.A., et al. (1998b), 'Apoptotic cell clearance in systemic lupus erythematosus. I. Opsonization by antiphospholipid antibodies', *Arthritis Rheum,* 41, 205-14.

Manzi, S. (2000), 'Systemic lupus erythematosus: a model for atherogenesis?', *Rheumatology (Oxford),* 39, 353-59.

Manzi, S., et al. (1997a), 'Age-specific incidence rates of myocardial infarction and angina in women with systemic lupus erythematosus: comparison with the Framingham Study', *Am J Epidemiol,* 145 (5), 408-15.

Manzi, S., et al. (1997b), 'Age-specific incidence rates of myocardial infarction and angina in women with systemic lupus erythematosus: comparison with the Framingham Study.', *Am. J. Epidemiol.*, 145, 408-15.

Mevorach, D., et al. (1998a), 'Complement-dependent clearance of apoptotic cells by human macrophages', *J Exp Med*, 188 (12), 2313-20.

Mevorach, D., et al. (1998b), 'Systemic exposure to irradiated apoptotic cells induces autoantibody production', *J Exp Med*, 188 (2), 387-92.

Mukundan, L., et al. (2009), 'PPAR-delta senses and orchestrates clearance of apoptotic cells to promote tolerance', *Nat Med*, 15 (11), 1266-72.

Nagata, K., et al. (1996), 'Identification of the product of growth arrest-specific gene 6 as a common ligand for Axl, Sky, and Mer receptor tyrosine kinases', *J Biol Chem*, 271 (47), 30022-7.

Nagata, S. and Golstein, P. (1995), 'The Fas death factor.', *Science*, 267, 1449-56.

Napirei, M., et al. (2000), 'Features of systemic lupus erythematosus in Dnase1-deficient mice', *Nat Genet*, 25 (2), 177-81.

Nomura, S., et al. (2000), 'Platelet-derived microparticles in patients with arteriosclerosis obliterans: enhancement of high shear-induced microparticle generation by cytokines', *Thromb Res*, 98 (4), 257-68.

Ogden, C. A., et al. (2001), 'C1q and mannose binding lectin engagement of cell surface calreticulin and CD91 initiates macropinocytosis and uptake of apoptotic cells', *J Exp Med*, 194 (6), 781-95.

Oka, K., et al. (1998), 'Lectin-like oxidized low-density lipoprotein receptor 1 mediates phagocytosis of aged/apoptotic cells in endothelial cells', *Proc Natl Acad Sci U S A*, 95 (16), 9535-40.

Oshima, K., et al. (2005), 'Adiponectin increases bone mass by suppressing osteoclast and activating osteoblast', *Biochem Biophys Res Commun*, 331 (2), 520-6.

Parker, J., et al. (2011), 'Modulation of lupus phenotype by adiponectin deficiency in autoimmune mouse models', *J Clin Immunol*, 31 (2), 167-73.

Pereira, J., et al. (2006), 'Circulating platelet-derived microparticles in systemic lupus erythematosus. Association with increased thrombin generation and procoagulant state', *Thromb Haemost*, 95 (1), 94-9.

Petri, M., et al. (1992), 'Risk factors for coronary artery disease in patients with systemic lupus erythematosus.', *Am. J. Med.*, 93, 513-19.

Pino, A. M., et al. (2010), 'Concentration of adipogenic and proinflammatory cytokines in the bone marrow supernatant fluid of osteoporotic women', *J Bone Miner Res*, 25 (3), 492-8.

Platt, N., et al. (1996), 'Role for the class A macrophage scavenger receptor in the phagocytosis of apoptotic thymocytes in vitro', *Proc Natl Acad Sci U S A*, 93 (22), 12456-60.

Preston, R. A., et al. (2003), 'Effects of severe hypertension on endothelial and platelet microparticles', *Hypertension*, 41 (2), 211-7.

Pruzanski, W., et al. (1994), 'Circulating group II phospholipase A2 activity and antilipocortin antibodies in systemic lupus erythematosus. Correlative study with disease activity', *J Rheumatol*, 21 (2), 252-7.

Puurunen, M., et al. (1994), 'Antibody against oxidized low-density lipoprotein predicting myocardial infarction', *Arch Intern Med*, 154 (22), 2605-9.

Qian, Y, Wang, H., and Clarke, SH (2004), 'Impaired clearance of apoptotic cells induces the activation of autoreactive anti-Sm marginal zone and B-1 B cells.', *J. Immunol*, 172, 625-35.

Riboldi, P., et al. (2002), 'Cardiac involvement in systemic autoimmune diseases', *Clin Rev Allergy Immunol*, 23, 247-61.

Rigotti, A., Acton, S. L., and Krieger, M. (1995), 'The class B scavenger receptors SR-BI and CD36 are receptors for anionic phospholipids', *J Biol Chem*, 270 (27), 16221-4.

Ross, R. (1993), 'The pathogenesis of atherosclerosis: a perspective for the 1990s.', *Nature (London)*, 362, 801-09.

Roszer, T., et al. (2011), 'Autoimmune kidney disease and impaired engulfment of apoptotic cells in mice with macrophage peroxisome proliferator-activated receptor gamma or retinoid X receptor alpha deficiency', *J Immunol*, 186 (1), 621-31.

Rovin, B. H., et al. (2005), 'Plasma, urine, and renal expression of adiponectin in human systemic lupus erythematosus', *Kidney Int*, 68 (4), 1825-33.

Salonen, J. T., et al. (1992), 'Autoantibody against oxidised LDL and progression of carotid atherosclerosis', *Lancet*, 339 (8798), 883-7.

Sambrano, G. R. and Steinberg, D. (1995), 'Recognition of oxidatively damaged and apoptotic cells by an oxidized low density lipoprotein receptor on mouse peritoneal macrophages: role of membrane phosphatidylserine', *Proc Natl Acad Sci U S A*, 92, 1396-400.

Scott, R. S., et al. (2001), 'Phagocytosis and clearance of apoptotic cells is mediated by MER', *Nature*, 411 (6834), 207-11.

Sellam, J., et al. (2009), 'Increased levels of circulating microparticles in primary Sjogren's syndrome, systemic lupus erythematosus and rheumatoid arthritis and relation with disease activity', *Arthritis Res Ther*, 11 (5), R156.

Selzer, F., et al. (2004), 'Comparison of risk factors for vascular disease in the carotid artery and aorta in women with systemic lupus erythematosus', *Arthritis Rheum*, 50 (1), 151-9.

Shiratsuchi, A., et al. (1999), 'Role of class B scavenger receptor type I in phagocytosis of apoptotic rat spermatogenic cells by Sertoli cells', *J Biol Chem*, 274 (9), 5901-8.

Simantov, R., et al. (1996), 'Antiphospholipid antibodies activate vascular endothelial cells', *Lupus*, 5 (5), 440-1.

Simantov, R., et al. (1995), 'Activation of cultured vascular endothelial cells by antiphospholipid antibodies', *J Clin Invest*, 96 (5), 2211-9.

Stanic, A. K., et al. (2006), 'Immune dysregulation accelerates atherosclerosis and modulates plaque composition in systemic lupus erythematosus', *Proc Natl Acad Sci U S A*, 103 (18), 7018-23.

Sugiyama, S., et al. (2007), 'Pravastatin improved glucose metabolism associated with increasing plasma adiponectin in patients with impaired glucose tolerance and coronary artery disease', *Atherosclerosis*, 194 (2), e43-51.

Svenungsson, E., et al. (2001), 'Risk factors for cardiovascular disease in systemic lupus erythematosus', *Circulation*, 104 (16), 1887-93.

Takemura, Y., et al. (2007), 'Adiponectin modulates inflammatory reactions via calreticulin receptor-dependent clearance of early apoptotic bodies', *J Clin Invest*, 117 (2), 375-86.

Taylor, P. R., et al. (2000), 'A hierarchical role for classical pathway complement proteins in the clearance of apoptotic cells in vivo', *J Exp Med,* 192, 359-66.

Urowitz, M.B., et al. (1976), 'The bimodal mortality pattern of systemic lupus erythematosus.', *Am. J. Med.,* 60, 221-25.

Vaarala, O. (2000), 'Autoantibodies to modified LDLs and other phospholipid-protein complexes as markers of cardiovascular diseases', *J Intern Med,* 247, 381-84.

Vaarala, O., et al. (1993), 'Crossreaction between antibodies to oxidised low-density lipoprotein and to cardiolipin in systemic lupus erythematosus', *Lancet,* 341 (8850), 923-5.

Van Doornum, S., McColl, G., and Wicks, I. P. (2002), 'Accelerated atherosclerosis: an extraarticular feature of rheumatoid arthritis?', *Arthritis Rheum,* 46, 862-73.

Walport, M. J. (2002), 'Complement and systemic lupus erythematosus', *Arthritis Res,* 4 Suppl 3, S279-93.

Wu, R., et al. (2001), 'Antibodies to Lysophosphatidylcholine Are Decreased in Borderline Hypertension', *Hypertension,* 37 (1), 154-59.

Wu, R., et al. (1997), 'Antibodies against cardiolipin and oxidatively modified LDL in 50-year-old men predict myocardial infarction', *Arterioscler Thromb Vasc Biol,* 17 (11), 3159-63.

Wu, R., et al. (1999), 'Antibodies against lysophosphatidylcholine and oxidized LDL in patients with SLE', *Lupus,* 8 (2), 142-50.

5

The Platelet as an Immunomodulator: The Old Thespian with New Roles in Atherosclerosis, Sepsis and Autoimmune Disease

Omar L. Esponda[1], Yaliz Loperena[2],
Gladiany Ramos[2] and A. Valance Washington[2]
[1]*Internal Medicine Department, University Hospital Dr. Ramón Ruiz Arnaú*
[2]*Laboratory of Anatomy and Cell Biology, Universidad Central del Caribe*
Bayamón, Puerto Rico,
USA

1. Introduction

Models of the inflammatory process depict scenes of a drama that has being studied for millenniums. A drama that began at the macroscopic level, with Celsus and the aphoristic comment "*Vero notae inflammationis sunt quatuor: rubor et tumor cum calore et dolore*"[1] ; with the four cardinal signs of inflammation, followed by Virchow at the microscopic level by proposing a response to insult model, and one that continues to unfold as we develop molecular representations of this process, in an attempt to complete the story of a drama.

> *"If therefore we speak of an irritament[2], we cannot properly intend to attach any other meaning to it, than that, in consequence of some cause or other external to the part which falls into a state of irritation, and acting upon it either directly or through the medium of the blood the composition and constitution of this part undergo alterations which at the same time alter its relations to the neighboring parts (whether they be blood-vessels or other structures) and enable it to attract to itself and absorb from them a larger quantity of matter than usual, and to transform it according to circumstances. Every form of inflammation with which we are acquainted, may be naturally explained in this way".*
>
> Rudolf Virchow 1858

It's an open secret, and we continue to publish it as if it is a surprise or new knowledge even. Whether we realize it or not we have evolved a new field; a field that is defined by the intersection of immunology and hemostasis. Platelets whose main purpose has traditionally been considered as a plug forming device, is currently participating in new paradigms of disease, as a sophisticated mediator in a milieu of chemokines and adhesion molecules which modulate the immune response and consequently inflammation. Studies from

---

[1] *"But the signs of inflammation are four; redness, and swelling, with heat & pain"*
[2] Inflammatory stimulus

inflammatory diseases such as sepsis, rheumatoid arthritis, and acute lung injury set the stage for modification of the thespian paradigm. One that helps us complete the continuum from coagulation to inflammation and back to coagulation again. Here we propose to name this field of study "Immunohemostasis". No better model to appreciate the crosstalk between coagulation and inflammation than atherosclerosis.

2. Platelets have a role early in the development of atherosclerosis

Although platelets are not solely responsible for the development of atherosclerosis, their contribution to the inception of the vascular lesion, up until to atherothrombosis - its most critical consequence - is conceptually best understood as a model of inflammation. This is somewhat amusingly explained by Rudolf Virchow on a footnote in, *Cellular Pathology* (1865), "Suppose three people were sitting quietly on a bench, and suddenly a stone came and injured one of them, the others would be excited, not only by the sudden appearance of the stone, but also by the injury done to their companion, to whose help they would feel bound to hasten. Here the stone would be the irritant, the injury the irritament, the help an expression of the irritation called forth in the bystanders". Following Dr. Virchow's thought process, modern science not only has documented many different stones but also acknowledges that at times, these bystanders can hasten the *irritament* (inflammatory stimulus), therefore as we will understand an overzealous and excited bystander could prove to be, vessel hardening.

If we look at atherosclerosis as a model of inflammatory disease, platelet adhesion could similarly be regarded as a model of platelet induced disease (Langer & Gawaz, 2008). Atherogenesis is influenced by platelets that adhere to activated vascular endothelial cells and feed chemotactic mediators to adjoining cells. Although the underlying mechanism of atherosclerosis is attributed to endothelial impairment due to insults from genetic and environmental factors (Lusis, 2000), it needs platelet firm adhesion to the endothelium for inception of the atheromatous plaque (Spagnoli et al., 2007). Genetic and environmental factors that trigger injurious events, which include the formation of reactive oxygen species, reduce the bioavailability of nitric oxide (Lowenstein et al., 2005). Then the non-denuded, but aggravated endothelium fails to inhibit control over Weibel-Palade body exocytosis translocating P-selectin and von Willebrand Factor (vWF) from within the granules to the outer cellular surface (Wagner & Frenette, 2008). These two proteins allow the adhesion of platelets to the vascular endothelium in a multistep process. First platelets are tethered to the vascular wall with assistance by endothelial selectins. Platelets then roll on the vascular endothelial cells (Polgar et al., 2005). Depending on further activation of the endothelial cell and expression of endothelial integrins, the platelet adheres firmly to the vascular wall (May et al., 2008), or in the absence of further endothelial activation, the platelet, disengages from the vessel wall and returns to circulation (White, 2007). Remarkably this can occur due to the fact that platelet activation is not required for platelet rolling (Harrison, 2005). In contrast, experimental models of mice infused with activated platelets also stimulate Weibel-Palade body exocytosis, promoting the development of atherosclerosis which is attributed to platelet P-selectin – mediated delivery of platelet-derived proinflammatory factors to monocytes/leukocytes and the vessel wall (Delvaeye & Conway, 2009).

Molecule	Tissue Distribution	Function	Ligand
Selectins			
P-selectin	Endothelium & platelets	Rolling of leukocytes on endothelium and platelets & of platelets on endothelium	PSGL-1
E-selectin	Endothelium	Rolling of leukocytes on endothelium	PSGL-1 ESL-1 CD44
Immunoglobulins			
ICAM-1	Endothelium	Firm adhesion and transmigration of leukocytes	β2-integrins
ICAM-2	Endothelium, dendritic cells	Firm adhesion & transmigration of leukocytes; platelet adhesion to leukocytes	β2-integrins
VCAM-1	Endothelium	Firm adhesion & transmigration of leukocytes	α4-integrins
PECAM-1	Leukocytes, endothelial cell-cell junctions	Transmigration	PECAM-1
Glycoprotein			
von Willebrand Factor	Endothelium, α-granules of platelets, & subendothelial connective tissue	Binding to other proteins, most efficient under high shear stress	Factor VIII, Collagen, Platelet GPIb
Glycoprotein IV	Platelets & monocytes	Scavenger receptor, implicated in hemostasis, thrombosis, inflammation, lipid metabolism & atherogenesis	Collagen, thrombospondin, platelet-agglutinating protein p37, oxLDL & long-chain fatty acids
Integrins			
β2-integrins	Leukocytes	Firm adhesion to endothelium & platelets	ICAMs VCAM fibrinogen
MAC-1	Polymorphonuclear leukocytes, NK cells, & mononuclear phagocytes	Pattern recognition receptor causes phagocytosis	various
β3-integrins	Platelets & neutrophils/endothelium	Firm cell adhesion	Fibrinogen; ECM
IIβIIIα	Platelets	Aids in platelet activation	Fibrinogen, vWF and fibronectin
Tumor necrosis factor family			
CD40 **CD40L**	endothelium, leukocyte & platelet	Activates different endothelium, leukocyte & platelet function	CD40L CD40; αIIbβ3 on platelets

Table 1. Major Receptor molecules in endothelium, platelet, and leukocyte interactions (Modified from Harrison, 2005)

Activated platelets propel inflammation, by forming platelet-leukocyte complexes which facilitate leukocyte migration into the arterial wall. Since the density of P-selectin on platelets after activation is much higher than on endothelium, leukocytes are easily recruited to the adherent activated platelets (White, 2007). In these dynamics, the balance between homeostasis and inflammation is easily shifted to inflammation in a vicious cycle as soluble P-selectin, shed from activated platelets and endothelium, stimulate leukocytes to produce tissue factor which subsequently activates more platelets (Vicic & Weiss, 1983). In further interaction with leukocytes; polymorphonuclear cells adhere to platelets in a Mac-1–dependent manner, inducing complex activation cascades in monocytes that promote monocyte or neutrophil adhesion, thrombosis, monocytic chemokine and cytokine release, or the oxidative burst of neutrophils (Rivera et al., 2009). See table 1. Among the many receptor pairs, that contribute to neutrophil activation in platelet-neutrophil interactions, there is neutrophil surface triggering receptor expressed on myeloid cells 1 (TREM-1) and platelet surface TREM-1 ligand, although not required for platelet-neutrophil aggregate formation, cellular interactions involving this receptor pair induce respiratory burst activity and IL-8 secretion in neutrophils which attract leukocytes and further activate other platelets (Minors, 2007).

By no means are platelets, endothelial cells and leukocytes innocent bystanders; through years of evolution these eager to protect cells fight infection, hemorrhage and constant insults. In the theater of inflammation, as it often happens, we undergo friendly fire, which make our vessels harder but not tougher. Without regard to its etiology, the interactions between platelets, endothelial cells, and leukocytes as a result of platelet activation, endothelial dysfunction and leukocyte adhesion, causes inflammatory responses which lead to the origin and establishment of atherosclerosis.

3. Platelets resourceful machinery in function

Platelets are the smallest of the many types of cells in circulating blood, with an average size of only 2.0 to 5.0 μm in diameter, 0.5 μm in thickness, with a mean cell volume of 6 to 10 femtoliters (Riddel, Jr. et al., 2007). Platelets are anucleate, discoid shaped blood cells that partake in pathophysiological roles like: hemostasis, thrombosis, clot retraction, vessel constriction/repair, inflammation and other aspects of host defense (Austin S.K., 2008). They are critical players in immune oversight and an important key to cellular interactions during the coagulation and inflammation process (Brass, 2010). Their sheer number, shape and small size make possible for platelets to localize to the vessel wall under flow, making possible a constant survey of the wall integrity (Coughlin, 2000). Platelets contain scarce functional mitochondria, glycogen, an intricate membranous system, and three major morphologically different, secretory organelles which are: α-granules, dense core granules & lysosomes (Coughlin, 2005). Inside the α-granules can be found a wide variety of coagulation/adhesive proteins, growth factors and protease inhibitors involved in both primary and secondary hemostatic mechanisms (Kahn et al., 1999). The platelet membrane is covered by a wide variety of mobile transmembrane receptors, including integrins (e.g., αIIbβ3: IIβ IIIα), leucine-rich repeated receptors (e.g., GPIb/IX/V), G-protein coupled seven transmembrane receptors (e.g., PAR-1 and PAR-4 thrombin receptors) and C-type lectin receptors (e.g., P-selectin) (Coughlin, 2000).

Under normal conditions, hemostasis occurs by two independent, but related processes: the platelet activation pathway and the coagulation cascade (Sivaraman & Latour, 2011).

The primary role of platelets in hemostasis is the formation of an initial plug at the site of the vascular injury or as commonly known, primary hemostasis. The formation of a stable plug consists of three principal events: adhesion, activation and aggregation. When the vessel wall is damaged, it exposes the blood to subendothelial collagen and microfibrilis, which stimulate the initial step that allows platelet adhesion (Delvaeye & Conway, 2009). Adhesion is also mediated via von Willebrand Factor (vWF), a multimeric protein synthesized by endothelial cells that serves as a bridge between the tissue and platelets. vWF binds to both exposed collagen at sites of vascular injury and the platelet membrane glycoprotein Ib-V-IX (GPIb-V-IX) receptor complex (Romney & Glick, 2009). Platelet activation is caused by exposure of various agonists, such as thrombin, thromboxane A2 (TxA_2), adenosine diphosphate (ADP), collagen, and arachidonic acid to their particular receptors (Perez-Gomez & Bover, 2007). One example is the G protein-coupled receptors on the platelet surface whose ligand are TxA_2 , ADP, and thrombin (Satran & Almog, 2003).
The PARs are G-protein-coupled receptors that use a unique mechanism to convert an extracellular proteolytic cleavage of the receptor into a transmembrane signal (Eyre L. & Gamlin F., 2010), hence the derivation of the thrombin receptor activating peptide (TRAP). Human platelets express two different G-coupled protease activated receptors, PAR-1 and PAR-4, while mouse platelets express PAR-3 and PAR-4 (Brass, 2010). In human platelets, PAR-1 is a high-affinity receptor that is activated at low concentrations of thrombin, PAR-4 is the lower-affinity receptor that mediates thrombin signaling at higher concentrations of thrombin than PAR-1 (Johns, 2004), but it initiates signaling for a more extended duration that its PAR-1 counterpart. The activation of both PAR-1 and PAR-4 is enough to trigger platelet secretion and aggregation (Cambien & Wagner, 2004).
Activation of platelets results in a conformational change from normal disc shape to a compact sphere with long dendritic extensions called pseudopods, which facilitate platelet-platelet interaction. This process alters the membrane permeability and allows the entry of calcium into the platelet cytosol, leading to integrin activation. Following platelet activation, the membrane receptor glycoprotein IIβ/IIIα (IIβ IIIα) undergoes a conformational change, which takes us to the adhesion phase mediated by platelet IIβ IIIα binding to fibrin(ogen), allowing the formation of multiple stable crosslinks between adjacent platelets. The GPIb-IX-V receptor complex and IIβ IIIα are two unique platelets receptors responsible of platelet adhesion and thrombus formation to regulate hemostasis (Furie & Furie, 2004).
A revised model of hemostasis described by Satran & Almog (Satran & Almog, 2003), emphasizes the role of different cell surfaces in the localization and control of the coagulation processes, this includes three overlapping phases: initiation, amplification, and propagation. Tissue Factor (TF) is the key initiator of coagulation and is expressed primarily by subendothelial mural cells and adventitial fibroblast in and around the vessel wall (Filice & Niewoehner, 1987). The initiation phase starts when exposed collagen causes accumulation and activation of platelets, while exposed TF initiates the process of generating thrombin through binding to factor VII, creating the tissue factor-factor VIIa complex (TF/FVIIa) (Spitznagel & Shafer, 1985). TF/FVIIa complex activates factor X, either directly or indirectly via factor IX, and transforms prothrombin into thrombin in small amounts that are insufficient to complete the process of fibrin formation. The amplification phase occurs after platelet adhesion to the initiation site while in a state of partial activation. At that point thrombin, generated in the initiation phase and responsible for activating coagulation factors V, VIII, and IX, binds to platelets enhancing both their binding to the

vessel injury and activation. In the propagation phase the generation of thrombin is continuous. Factor X_a production is maintained by intrinsic tenase complex which, consist of factor VIII_a the cofactor for factor IX_a (Spitznagel & Shafer, 1985). These three overlapping phases allow a fibrin platelet clot to form over an area of injury; this clotting process is limited by negative feedback by activated protein C which inactivates factors V_a and VIII_a to avoid thrombotic occlusion in surrounding normal areas of the vasculature. The formation of a stable hemostatic plug is possible by important platelets properties which include their shape, the secretory granules, high density regulatory and adhesion receptors, and the ability to promote thrombin generation (Goncalves et al., 2011). The coagulation cascade, although important to platelet activation, is outside of the scope of this review

Platelet disorders can be divided into two categories: quantitative and qualitative. Quantitative defects are abnormalities in platelet number, whereas qualitative defects are abnormalities in platelet function (Siljander, 2011). This classification is somewhat random as some platelet disorders are characterized by both decreased number and function (Heijnen et al., 1999). Platelet defects such as storage granule diseases like Hermansky-Pudlak & Grey platelet syndromes or Glansmann thrombasthenia in which the platelets lack IIβIIIα are rare qualitative diseases.

An important receptor in platelet interactions which has being studied in models of qualitative platelets defects is P-selectin (CD62P), formerly known as PADGEM or GMP-140, is a member of the selectin family of cell adhesion receptors, and as its name implies, it is a lectin that binds various sugar moieties (Castaman et al., 1996). P-selectin , is stored premade in the Weibel-Palade bodies of endothelial cells and the platelet α-granules (Berckmans et al., 2001) and remains inaccessible when these cells are in the resting state (Wolf et al., 1999).

Activation of either/or both platelets and endothelial cells brings P-selectin to the cell surface. Thus control of P-selection dependant interactions is conditional of the presence of P-selectin on the cell that is in the active state. Upon cell activation, P-selectin is translocated to the plasma membrane, mediating the interaction of stimulated platelets and endothelial cells with leukocytes though its interaction with P-selectin glycosylated ligand (PSGL-1). PSGL-1 is a constitutively expressed receptor on platelets, leukocytes, and a subset of lymphocytes (Heemskerk et al., 2002) (psgl-1 does bind E- and L selectin as well). P-selectin mediates the formation of preliminary platelet-leukocyte aggregates (Yang & Wilson, 1996). Early studies on P-selectin demonstrated that P-selectin mediated *in vitro* platelet-leukocyte interactions and induced leukocyte rolling in a flow chamber system (Elzey et al., 2003). These studies were confirmed in the P-selectin null mouse where leukocyte rolling was attenuated and neutrophil migration to the peritoneum was delayed (Amabile et al., 2010). The implications of these findings have been profound and have set the stage for us to discern the relationship between hemostasis and inflammation.

4. Platelets as dedicated players in immune function

The inflammatory process in the classical sense has been defined by the innate and adaptive systems where early contact to foreign invaders is mediated by the innate compartment and if the danger persists the adaptive compartment will assist. There is an intricate series of communication behaviors within and between these compartments that include physical interaction and a series of chemical signals which regulate the migration of the white blood cell population. Although we understand many of the individual parts, the system as a whole gets very complicated. The innate immune response is designed as our first response by identifying pieces of our puzzle that just don't fit. Using a series of basic pattern recognition receptors, the innate immune system identifies foreign substances and seeks to destroy or remove them from our body. The cells of the innate immune system have a complicated system of chemical communications that act as sentinels attractants or differentiation agents that push the limits of the innate immune system to adapt to the problem at hand. Traditionally, natural killer cells, monocytes, monocyte derived cells and polymorphonuclear cells (a vast majority of which are neutrophils) form the major portion of our innate immune system. Complement is a series of soluble factors that form a cascade, similar to the serine proteases of the coagulation cascade, that results in lysis of microbial and apoptotic cells. Platelets not having the ability to rearrange receptors to acquire antigen specificity and having the ability to respond quickly to insult would be considered a member of the innate immune system.

4.1 Platelet regulation of neutrophil function

Foreign invaders are recognized by neutrophils and neutrophils are considered to form our first line of defense (Puddu et al., 2010). Next to platelets, neutrophils are the most numerous white blood cells in our body and they are innate immune effectors. Neutrophils are dangerous to foreign substances as well as to ourselves if left unchecked. When they identify foreign invaders they use one of several killing mechanisms to dispose of the identified threat. Neutrophils will phagocytose bacteria or when the conditions are right they will release their granule contents causing non-specific damage to the quarry as well as the host (Chen et al., 1995). Here we will argue that even though neutrophils MAY be our first line of defense, they need platelets to regulate their decision making at point of endothelial contact (figure 1). Platelet regulation of neutrophil function is best introduced by evaluation of platelet depletion studies.

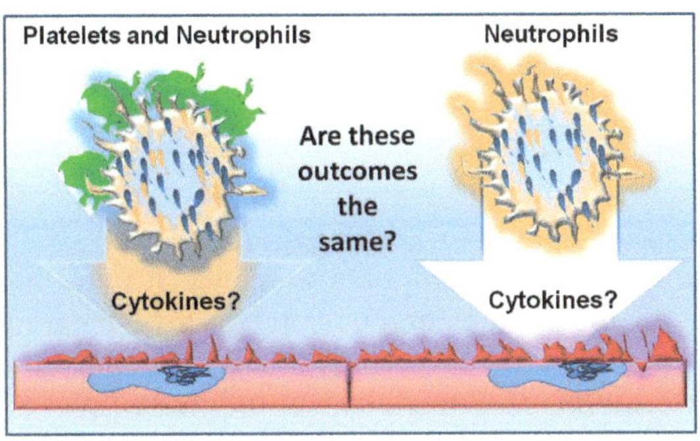

Fig. 1. Do platelets maintain vascular integrity preemptively by regulating neutrophil function?

Over the past five years, a wealth of investigators has used platelet depletion in mouse based disease models to better understand the platelet's role in inflammation. These studies have begun to show that the depletion of platelets leads to abbreviated neutrophil derived inflammation and neutrophil transendothelial migration. For example, using a corneal epithelium abrasion model, (Lam et al., 2011) demonstrated that platelet depletion lowers neutrophil transmigration across corneal endothelium at six and twelve hours. Using P-selectin glycosylated ligand (psgl)-1 null mice Zarbock et al. implicate the psgl-1/P-selectin ligand pair as a key regulator in the connection between platelets and neutrophils. In models of acute lung injury, platelet depletion reduced neutrophil influx (Zarbock et al., 2006). Zarbock and colleagues show that platelets recruit neutrophils to the lungs and use P-selectin and TxA_2 dependant mechanisms to mediate damage. TxA_2 is an arachadonic acid derived inflammatory mediator librated from activated platelets (Zarbock et al., 2006). Using a two hit lung injury model Looney et al., demonstrated that platelet depletion actually seemed to improve survival outcomes (Looney et al., 2009). The two hit model was shown to be P-selectin independent, but the investigator's use of aspirin, which lowered lung injury and improved survivorship supports a role for TxA_2. Aspirin inhibits TxA_2 production from platelets. Kornerup et al., used two different models (LPS inhalation and xymosan induced peritonitis) to show that platelet depletion reduces neutrophil recruitment to the inflammatory site in the lungs and the liver (Kornerup et al., 2010). Their data suggests that platelets activate the neutrophils forming platelet/neutrophil complexes which aid in neutrophil transmigration. Depletion of platelets was also shown to lower recruitment of eosinophils and lymphocytes in allergic inflammation (Pitchford et al., 2005), and apparently increases the efficacy of breast cancer chemotherapy (Demers et al., 2011). Taken together, therapeutic targeting of inflammation may need to focus on platelet function in addition, if not totally, to control the immune response.

A recent platelet derived mechanism that was identified is the neutrophil extracellular traps (NETs: (Clark et al., 2007), in which the toll like receptor on platelets recognizes its ligand and mediates platelets to influence to neutrophils to release their DNA. The DNA is used to ensnare bacteria in the lungs and liver sinusoids. Neutrophils are born to die protecting their host, in many ways they are like larger nucleated platelets performing many of the same functions including: aggregation, microparticle release, and phagocytosis, with the addition of the ability to extravate into the tissue. There are two points to be made here: first, in the neutrophil NET study, they demonstrate that platelet recruitment to the lungs during sepsis is neutrophil dependent, a finding that is in stark contrast to the work by Zarbock, where they show the opposite. Secondly, they clearly show a different outcome as a result of platelet-neutrophil interactions. Why were these outcomes so very different, although they used similar stimulants (LPS)?

4.2 Monocytes and platelets line up to work against infection

The second part of the innate immune system is monocytes and monocyte derived cells (macrophages). Monocytes are innate immune regulators with the responsibility to clean up the debris left from dying and apoptotic neutrophils that have engaged in battle. Monocytes usually arrive to scenes of inflammation after neutrophils and platelets and will persist in the inflamed tissue until the infection subsides. The expression of tissue factor by monocytes will attract the coagulation factor VII_a and is believed to be a primary cause for the initiation of the coagulation cascade and subsequent deregulation of hemostasis during sepsis. Monocytes, however, are also the primary link between the innate and the adaptive immune system (Ziegler-Heitbrock, 2007). Monocytes maintain the ability to differentiate into tissue macrophages or dendritic cells which present antigen to lymphocytes and prime the adaptive immune system. Once in the tissue, monocytes quickly mature into tissue macrophages and they are often referred to by a different name, dependant on the tissue.

For example the resident macrophage of the liver is called the Kupffer cell. Tissue macrophages release a battery of cytokines and chemokines that gage the enormity of the task at hand using chemoattractants to call in neutrophils, platelets, or more macrophages if deemed necessary. In a model of sepsis, where LPS from *Klebsiella* was given intravenously, Kupffer cells were shown to be responsible for the recruitment of platelets to the liver (Yamaguchi et al., 2006). However, in a model of *Leishmaina major*, platelets were demonstrated to recruit monocytes indirectly through the release of platelet derived growth factor (PDGF) (Goncalves et al., 2011). The model that the Goncalves et al., puts forth suggests that the release of PDGF from activated platelets cause a release of the cytokine CCL2 from a multitude of cell types which in turn attracts monocytes. Platelet depletion reduced the accumulation of effector monocytes and reduced clearance of *Leishmanina*, therefore demonstrating the importance of platelets in the removal of parasitic infections. Interestingly, platelet activation was dependent on complement factor 3 (C3), allowing us to address in the next scene in our drama, platelet interaction with complement.

4.3 Complement and new pathways in platelet function

Complement is a major immune regulation pathway. The complement system is ancient, abundant, and redundant (Ricklin et al., 2010). Not only is the system ancient, so has been our understanding of complement until recently. The biochemical origin of our understanding of complement is revealed by the terminology used with complement components, which are called factors. Much like the coagulation system where fractions of blood components with activity were isolated and its activity was given a number; our understanding of the complement system has grown from these obscure beginnings. Molecular genetics has breathed new life into our understanding this, one of our oldest and most conserved systems. In immunity, complement is a major component in the control of bacterial infection. In a process called, opsonization, a cascade involving a series serine proteases and proteins result in a membrane attack complex or MAC that forms pores on foreign cells such as bacteria and apoptotic cells and is chemoattractant to white blood cells.

Complement in its most basic sense is focused around factor C3 (Lambris et al., 2008). There are three major pathways that lead to the formation of C3 activators or convertases. These pathways are the lectin, classical, and alternative pathways. The lectin pathway is activated by the mannose binding protein leading to the formation of the C3 convertase 4b2b. However, to date not much information in regards to the lectin pathway and platelets is published and we will focus this portion of the review on the classical and alternative pathways of complement activation.

The classical pathway is most commonly activated when complement factor C1q interacts with IgG or IgM (MacKenzie et al., 1971). The binding of C1q to immunoglobulin allows the complement/Ig complex to activate components C1r and C1s, leading to the cleavage of C4 and C2. C4 is cleaved into C4a and C4b. While C4a diffuses away, C4b is momentarily enzymatically active and may form covalent bonds with the complement/Ig complex or bind to endothelial cells. In the event that neither of these options happen, the interaction of C4b with the surrounding water converts C4b into a ligand for C2 allowing C2's conversion into C2a and C2b by C1s. C2b bound to C4b forms the C3 convertase C4b2b cleaving the central complement factor C3 into C3a and C3b. (there is controversy in the literature to nomenclature of the C4b2b convertase, in some references it is called C4b2a). Platelets contain C1q and have demonstrated activity of the classical pathway (Nayak et al., 2010; Yin et al., 2007). Platelet activation of the classical pathway is associated with anti-phospholipid syndrome and immune thrombocytopenia purpura (Peerschke et al., 2010).

The alternative pathway is responsible for up to 95% of the activated C3b (Bexborn et al., 2008). The tick over theory provides a model for the activation of the alternative pathway. C3 is relatively dormant in circulation; however a small amount is spontaneously activated to $C3_{H2O}$, and provides windows of opportunity for C3 to behave essentially as a pattern receptor recognizing potentially harmful substances. $C3_{H2O}$ is primed to bind factor B and subsequently cleaved by factor D into C3a which is chemoattractive and the C3 convertase, C3b (Fearon et al., 1973; Fearon & Austen, 1975). Under the correct circumstances C3b will insert into cells causing an increase in deposition of C3b eventually tipping the scales toward complement opsonization of cells and initiation of the complement cascade (Bexborn et al., 2008). Increased C3b activates C5 leading to the deposition of the C5-9 membrane attack complex (MAC), which functions to produce pores in cells eventually leading to cell destruction.

Opsonization of cells by C1, C3b and C5b can also lead to phagocytosis when complement bound cells are recognized by their corresponding receptors (Ricklin et al., 2010). CD35 (CR1), which is found on many white blood cells and in the granules of neutrophils, recognizes C3b and C4b deposited on cells mediating phagocytosis. The integrins CD11b (CR3) and CD11c (CR4: both of these integrins are complexed with CD18 (Gahmberg, 1997)) mediate binding to complement iC3b which is the inactivated form of C3b, and mediates phagocytosis as well (Arnaout, 1990; Ross, 2000). Although CD11c is constitutively expressed on neutrophils both CD11b/CD18 complexes and CD35 are stored in neutrophil granules and are upregulated on activated neutrophils. When deposition of complement is in the endothelium, neutrophils are prompted to release their granules and phagocytize opsonized cells (Yin et al., 2007). It is suspected that complement deposition is a major cause of loss of vascular integrity, edema, and bleeding associated with inflammation.

Tight regulation is maintained on complement. An overzealous complement system will lead to self-attack of endothelium and may be an initiation factor of pathways leading to hemorrhage. Factor I (fI) is a major inhibitor of C3b and in conjunction with Factor H (fH) mediate the deceleration of the MAC formation. Factor H is a cofactor in fI binding and deactivating C3b that has bound the cell surface (Paixao-Cavalcante et al., 2009). Once bound, active C3b is transformed to iC3b which stops further opsonization, iC3b becomes the ligand of neutrophils and monocytes expressing CD11b or CD11c. Oddly enough, CD35 while initiating phagocytosis also mediates inactivation by fI (Ricklin et al., 2010).

Mutations in factor H are associated with hemolytic uremic sysdrome (HUS) (Licht et al., 2009; Stahl et al., 2008). Studies in fH deficient mice show that platelets are in large part responsible for this association. Platelets are a sink for fH (Vaziri-Sani et al., 2005). Platelets uptake fH from the plasma and store fH in various locations including the α-granules (Devine & Rosse, 1987; Licht et al., 2009). Mutations in fH lead to increased complement deposition on platelets and increased platelet activation (Stahl et al., 2008). These findings are consistent with the thrombocytopenia and thrombus formation seen in the kidneys of HUS patients.

Platelets are not immune to opsonization and there are numerous reports of complement binding to platelets, but these waters remain murky. Upon platelet activation there is a drastic increase in the binding of each of the anaphalaxins (C3b, C4b and C5 - 9) as well as C1q (Peerschke & Ghebrehiwet, 1997). Furthermore, P-selectin has recently been shown to propagate C3 activation opening a point of possible crosstalk between the hemostatic and innate immune systems (Del Conde et al., 2005). Subsequent studies, however, suggest that even though C3 binds to activated platelets it doesn't necessitate proteolytic activation. The C3 associated with platelets was estimated to be $C3_{H2O}$ containing an exposed thioester, which in the presence of fH and fI is inactivated rapidly (Martel et al., 2011). Coincidently, the C3 associated with the platelets facilitated binding of a soluble CR1, consistent with the idea that platelets facilitate the inactivation of the $C3_{H2O}$. In fact, in support of this idea, Martel et al. demonstrate that the C5-9 complex will form on less than 15% of platelets indicating that the MAC pathway is not a major form of platelet destruction or mechanism of platelet immune crosstalk (Martel et al., 2011). They suggest that the binding of the C5-9 complex may contribute to micropartical formation. Thus the binding and activation of C3b by P-selectin may need additional triggers such as sheer to induce C3 activation.

The studies in patients with aHUS strongly suggest that the regulation of C3b is a major mechanistic contact point between the immune and hemostatic systems. Platelets from patients lacking a functional fH, have increased deposits of C3 and C5-9 and are subject to complement mediated activation. As mentioned above, aHUS patients have the tendency to develop microthrombi in their kidneys that lead to kidney damage and accordingly they suffer from thrombocytopenia (Hirahashi et al., 2009; Stave & Croker, 1984). Thus, the ratio between C3 and fH represent the delicate balance that has to be overcome for complement to involve platelet participation. Early sepsis studies demonstrated that C3 depletion alleviated the thrombocytopenia associated with the sepsis response (Ulevitch & Cochrane, 1978), supporting the notion that from the immune system, it is C3 that initiates the participation of platelets. Here we submit that the complement cascade is the immunological system's major pathway to platelet participation (see figure 2). Complement activates platelets in a manner similar to the coagulation system, but with less of a robust reaction. A complement derived platelet activation cascade would not be to form an occlusive clot but localized thrombi, such as that to contain bacterial infection. Complement activation may lead to differential release of specific subsets of platelet α-granules (Italiano, Jr. et al., 2008). When platelets are depleted, complement activation leads to hemorrhage (Goerge et al., 2008).

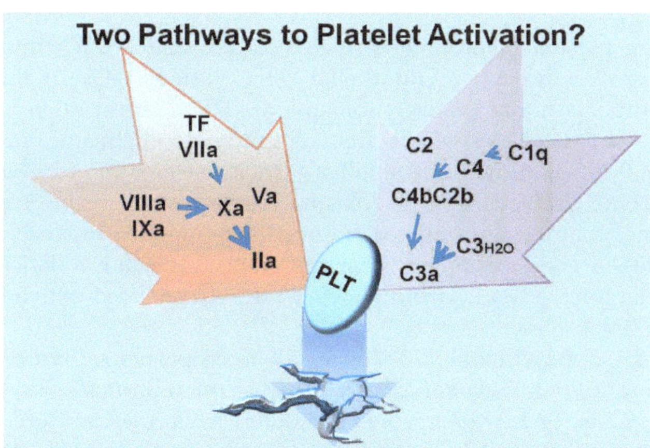

Fig. 2. Platelets are activated by both coagulation and complement cascades. The complement cascade represents the immune systems access to platelet function.

4.4 Adaptive immunity

Although we will not focus on adaptive immunity in this review, we will mention that lymphocytes comprise our adaptive immune system. Lymphocytes produce molecules that are derived to specifically recognize foreign potentially dangerous substances. Humoral immunity, mediated by B-cells, involves the production of antibodies. B-Cells will produce classes of antibodies that specifically recognize regional markers on foreign substances and cause clustering of the identified antigen into immune complexes (ICs). ICs can be bound by complement and targeted for destruction, or are directly removed by the cells of our innate immune system which include neutrophils and monocytes.

Oddly enough, the antibodies produced by B-cells are made in a sequential manner. For example, the pentametric IgM class is made first. IgM is subsequently changed to dimeric IgG in a process called class switching. Class switching is regulated by the CD40-CD40 ligand (CD40L) interaction. Mice lacking CD40L develop a hyper IgM syndrome, where the B-cells fail to change from production of IgM to IgG. CD40L is expressed on platelets and is believed to be a major source of CD40L. Transfer of wild type platelets to CD40L null mice rescues this syndrome, demonstrating an important regulatory role for platelets in the adaptive immune system (Elzey et al., 2003).

T-lymphocytes or T-cells mediate cellular immunity through a T-cell receptor that is made to specifically recognize one antigen. The T-cell receptor directs the T-cell to its antigen where it mediates a supportive function (T-helper cells) or can mediate cytotoxicity (cytotoxic T-cells). Cytotoxic T-cells recognize cells in distress such as cancer or virally infected cells. Using two different models of hepatic viral infection Iannacone et al. demonstrated that platelet depletion during a hepatic viral infection lowered the amount of cytotoxic T-cells that entered the liver and lowering hepatic cell damage. However, even though there was reduced liver damage, viral clearance was also reduced. Reintroduction of activated platelets restored the hepatic damage, but also allowed the viral load to be removed (Iannacone et al., 2005). In the theatrical setting of adaptive immunity, platelets demonstrate an indispensible role.

5. Platelet derived microparticles fuel the inflammatory response

Microparticles are plasma membrane-derived vesicles shed from stimulated cells which include leukocytes, erythrocytes, endothelial cells, various cells in the central nervous system (CNS), adipocytes and platelets (Siljander, 2011). Platelet microparticles (PMP) are small membrane-coated vesicles which circulate in the blood stream. PMP are estimated to vary in size from 0.1–1.0 μm with the smaller particles originating from α-granules and the larger particles being derived from the plasma membrane (Heijnen et al., 1999). There is increasing evidence that these submicron fragments, termed microparticles, have important physiological roles. A good example is Castaman defect, which is a deficiency in the ability to generate platelet microparticles from platelets that is associated with a bleeding tendency (Castaman et al., 1996).

PMP constitute for approximately 70-90% of all microparticles (Berckmans et al., 2001). Recently it was found, that megakaryocytes generate microparticles. Using a system where particles bearing CD62 or LAMP-1 were considered to be platelet derived and those that expressed filamin A were megakaryocyte derived. Flaumenhaft et al., determined that the microparticles circulating in healthy individuals are surprisingly predominantly megakaryocyte derived (Flaumenhaft et al., 2009). Characterization of microparticles, using proteomics and functional approaches, has shown that PMP can be separated into different size classes. Each of these size classes can differ in protein components, protein/lipid ratio, and functional effects on neighboring platelets and endothelial cells. When separated by centrifugation, PMP can be separated into four fractions: two of which (fractions 2 and 3) the phospholipid/protein ratios are typical of the plasma membranes, while the composition of fractions 1 and 4 indicate a greater proportion of lipid (Dean et al., 2009). The study of PMP has evolved rapidly, putting them as central mediators of many physiological processes such as inflammation. This part of the chapter will describe the origin of PMP and discuss their role in the inflammatory process under different conditions.

PMP are mainly released by the α-granules and multivesicular bodies of activated platelets, having exposed phosphatidylserine (PS), and resembling apoptotic cells. In a cell, aminophospholipids such as PS and phosphatidylethanolamine (PEA) are specifically segregated on the internal leaflet of the plasma membrane, whereas phosphatidylcholine and sphingomyelin are enriched on the external one. The greater proportion of PS exposed on the surface of activated platelets is reflected in PMP derived from the platelet membrane. A significant and sustained increase of cytosolic $Ca2^{+}$ accompanying cell stimulation may lead to the collapse of the membrane asymmetry by stimulating scramblase and floppase enzymatic activities and concomitantly inhibiting the flippase. The mechanisms involved in PMP release include platelet activation, which is calcium-dependant and Bak/Bax/caspase mediated release, which is independent of platelet activation (Schoenwaelder et al., 2009). The calcium dependant mechanisms involve membrane fragmentation or blebbing, loss of membrane integrity, microvesiculation, and the exposure of PS on the platelet surface followed by release of the PMP caused by cytoskeleton degradation of filamin 1A and gelsolin by Ca2+-dependent calpalin (Wolf et al., 1999). Bak/Bax mechanisms described by Schoenwaelder *et al.*, showed that prosurvival Bcl-xL maintains platelet viability, primarily by restraining the pro-apoptotic function of Bak (Schoenwaelder et al., 2009). It has been reported that Bcl-xL levels decline in stored platelets. This is consistent with an increase of PS exposure seen in platelets, a process which requires the Bak/Bax proteins, which play a central role in apoptosis. The release of PS expressing PMPs increases platelet procoagulant activity. Accordingly, the mechanisms of PMP release affect the size, constituents and function of the PMP.

5.1 Functional importance of platelet microparticles

PMP function is largely defined by the receptors and any molecules trapped in and on the vesicle at the time of release. PMP reflects a subset of the total receptors on the platelet surface or from the platelet α-granules at any given time. The major functional significance of these bioactive vesicles is associated with its procoagulant activity. For example, PMPs are enriched with membrane receptors for coagulation factor V_a and the fibrinogen receptor IIβ IIIα. When PS is exposed on the surface of activated platelets, membrane assembly of coagulation factor complexes occurs (Heemskerk et al., 2002). The presence of factor Va and PS form the foundation of the tenase complex and facilitate the assembly of the prothombinase complex. PMPs with IIβ IIIα facilitate polymerization though the binding of fibrin forming mini scaffolding stations that support the generation of thrombin. Together these molecules provide a catalytic surface for the prothrombinase reaction, thus contributing to the acceleration of thrombin generation (Ando et al., 2002). PMPs can also become membrane templates for fibrinolytic and proteolytic factors as well.

5.2 PMP and disease

CD40 is a receptor expressed on a wide range of cells such as B cells, neutrophils, monocytes, macrophages, platelets, dendritic cells, endothelial cells, fibroblast, keratinocytes and smooth muscle cells; modulating humoral and cellular immunity. As a member of the tumor necrosis factor (TNF) superfamily, the activation of CD40 by CD40L (CD40L/CD154) plays a crucial role for the development and progression of a variety of inflammatory processes including T-cell priming, enhanced T-cell cytotoxicity, and T-cell depended B-cell responses (Yang & Wilson, 1996). As mentioned above, platelets express CD40L. Matrix metalloproteinase-2 (MMP-2) releases CD40L from the platelet membrane creating the bioactive soluble fragment, sCD40L. Platelets are responsible for the production of approximately 95% of sCD40L in the peripheral blood (Elzey et al., 2003). Furthermore, CD40L is found on PMP which implicates PMPs in several diseases. Multiple sclerosis (MS), for example, is characterized by the formation sclerotic plaques in the central nervous system. During MS, the cells responsible for the production of myelin sheaths, oligodendrocytes, are destroyed. Auto reactive T cells attack the sheaths, causing neuronal destruction. In the case of MS, chronic platelet activation leads to the release of CD40L, implicating PMP as a potential effector in the development of MS.

The autoimmune disease, rheumatoid arthritis (RA), manifests as a chronic inflammation of the synovial lining in the joints, which results in pain, swelling and in the most severe cases a destruction of the bone and cartilage. In an elegant study, Boilard et al., implicate PMPs in the pathology of RA. They were investigating the presence of platelets in the synovial fluid of RA patients. Using flow cytometry and the platelet specific marker, CD41 to detect the platelet specific integrin IIβ IIIα, they demonstrated an average of $2x10^5$ PMP/µl in RA patients compared to non-detectable levels in patients with osteoarthritis. Interestingly enough there were a subset of platelets that rosetted the leukocytes that were present in the synovial fluid (Boilard et al., 2010). RA can be induced in mice by the passive transfer of immunoglobulin G (IgG) auto-antibodies from K/BxN mice to wild type. Using the K/BxN system, the authors demonstrated that platelet depletion greatly reduced arthritic symptoms, supporting a role for platelets in the progression of RA. They subsequently determined using glycoprotein VI (GPVI) deficient mice that the microparticles were generated by activation by collagen and that these PMPs contained the ability to release IL-1. IL-1 subsequently induced proinflammatory cytokines IL-6 and neutrophil chemoattractant IL-8 production leading to the recruitment of neutrophils. Thus, PMP are major regulators of RA. The finding answered several nuances found in patients with RA. For instance how come patients with RA have platelet proteins in their synovial fluid but no platelets? Here the aerosolized platelets in the form of PMP delivered discrete packets of platelet function resulting in bone damage and the recruitment of neutrophils by an indirect method.

Therefore, aerosolized PMPs allow the delivery of skewed platelet function as opposed to the complete regulatory balance of platelet function. The recruitment of inflammatory cells at the sites of vessels injury can drive the development of arthrosclerosis, in which the participation of PMP is mostly the formation of the plaque and its progression (Amabile et al., 2010). PMP participate by amplifying and sustaining coagulation and inflammatory response after the rupture of the plaque (Puddu et al., 2010). β-amyloid, for example, is found in PMP and is implicated in the progression of Alzheimer disease. Platelets are the major source of β-amyloid in the peripheral blood (Chen et al., 1995). In fact, it was shown that β-amyloid secretion supersedes that of all other proteins shed from the platelet surface upon activation (Fong et al., 2011). Accordingly, PMPs have been cited as carriers of soluble Alzheimer's beta amyloid (Matsubara et al., 2002). In the case of cancer PMP contributes to the metastasis by producing MMP and VEGF (vascular endothelial growth factor) among other important factors. Following a paradigm where platelets are strictly hemostatic vessels, the delivery of PMP would strictly cause coagulatory disarray. However, here we show that while PMP does play a coagulatory role in situations like atherosclerosis, they also play diverse role like those seen with activation of T-cells or exacerbation or RA in the synovial fluid of joints. PMPs may be important force working toward unresolved inflammation as described by Khatami, where two opposing inflammatory forces (wound healing and apoptotic) are shifted leading to a chronic inflammatory state (Khatami, 2011).

6. Immunohemostasis

Our laboratory's interest in the intersection of inflammation and hemostasis is derived from the study of a platelet specific gene that mediates platelet involvement in inflammation called TREM-Like transcript (TLT)-1 (Washington et al., 2002). TLT-1 is a single Ig domain receptor found on platelets and megakaryocytes (Barrow et al., 2004; Washington et al., 2004). Like the adhesion molecule p-selectin, TLT-1 is stored in the platelet α-granules until activation when it is quickly bought to the surface (Washington et al., 2004).

6.1 TLT-1

The TLT-1 gene (*treml-1*) is situated in the TREM cluster, amongst a group of immunoregulatory receptors that are found on leukocytes and endothelial cells (Allcock et al., 2003). TLT-1 is the first member of the cluster found on platelets giving it a unique role among the TREM family of genes (note; TLT-2 has recently been found in platelet releasates suggesting it is present on platelets; (Fong et al., 2011)). There are two published forms of TLT-1 which include a long form that has several interesting motifs in the cytoplasmic domain and a splice variant form that only has a 16 amino acid tail (Allcock et al., 2003; Washington et al., 2002). Interactions with the phosphatases SHP-1, -2 and moesin have been described but the significance of these interactions have not been uncovered (Barrow et al., 2004; Washington et al., 2002). Nevertheless, an activation role for TLT-1 was supported when single chain antibodies specific to TLT-1 were shown to inhibit platelet aggregation in the presence of low levels of agonist in vitro (Giomarelli et al., 2007). These results support an enhancing role for TLT-1 and suggest that TLT-1 may play an important role in maintaining platelet activation.

To better understand TLT-1's potential in vivo, a null mouse model was developed (Washington et al., 2009). The TLT-1 mouse is viable with negligible differences seen in platelet counts. During platelet aggregation assays we found that the null platelets show reduced capacity for aggregation with the secondary platelet agonists ADP and the TxA_2 mimetic U46619 compared to wild type *(wt)*. Consistent with these results, tail bleeding assays demonstrate and overall increase in time to secession of bleeding compared to wild type mice, however the difference between null and wt mice were not as substantial as a PAR1 or GPVI null mouse suggesting that TLT-1's role in hemostasis was not of primary hemostasis, but one that was "unique".

To gain a clearer picture of TLT-1 function we used an acute sepsis model where we inject LPS intraperitoneally and monitored hemostatic and immunological parameters as well as survival (Washington et al., 2009). Sepsis is an interesting model because it starts with a strictly immunological challenge and mortality is a direct response to rife platelet activation and microthrombi. Platelets play an indispensible role during hemostasis and an often unappreciated role during inflammation (Levi & van der Poll, 2004). The involvement of platelets in the immune response and sepsis is undeniable, but never the less not completely understood.

Treatment of null and wt mice with LPS causes the TLT-1$^{-/-}$ mice to succumb faster and in greater numbers to the immunological challenge. Null mice display a distortion of both hemostatic and immunological parameters. Plasma levels of one of the major inflammatory mediators, tissue necrosis factor- α (TNF- α), is also elevated in the null mouse, demonstrating TLT-1 either directly or indirectly modulates immune function. Platelet counts in the null mouse are significantly lower, while the levels of d-dimers are elevated. These two important markers of sepsis, platelet count and d-dimers, suggest the presence of a more severe DIC in the null mouse than *wt* (Washington et al., 2009).

The severity of DIC in the null mouse compared to the wild type mouse was further supported in the localized Shwartzman model of vasculitis. The localized Shwartzman reaction, which correlates well with the presence of DIC in humans, challenges the animal subcutaneously with the inflammatory mediators LPS and TNF-α and subsequently the lesion is evaluated for hemorrhage, clotting, and leukocyte infiltration. Null mice showed slightly increased amounts of microclots, and neutrophil infiltration, however the quantity of hemorrhage was twofold and the area of the lesion was almost three fold greater than in *wt* mice (Washington et al., 2009). These results are indicative of a role in the integration of inflammation with hemostasis; however at the time, this idea, although reported in numerous publications, was not quite accepted.

6.2 Immune – Hemostasis

It was in a series of articles originating from the Wagner laboratory that light was shed on the connection between inflammation and hemorrhage. In essence they asked, "When you are thrombocytopenic, where do you bleed?" A surprising answer was in inflamed tissue (Goerge et al., 2008). In a series of eloquent experiments they provide convincing evidence that platelets are necessary to control immune derived bleeding, and what's more they (platelets) use other than the classical hemostatic mechanisms involved in plug formation. Using the reverse arthus model significant hemorrhage is witnessed only in the group of mice that are thrombocytopenic, confirming the importance of platelets to **immune-hemostasis**. The authors go on to show that deletion mutants for IIβ IIIα, GPIV, GP1b, or p-selectin, like *wt* mice, maintained their ability to control hemorrhage, demonstrating that the members of the classical pathways of platelet function are not necessary to mandate an **immune-hemostasis**; signifying that there are alternate pathways to hemostasis. They also used a LPS inhalation model to show that mice that are thrombocytopenic bleed in the lungs demonstrating the hemostatic effect at the organ level (Goerge et al., 2008). Both of these models induce complement deposition, neutrophil activation, and endothelial damage that ultimately recruit platelet involvement. It is easy to imagine that the bleeding diathesis could be reproduced by the inhibition of only a handful of specific molecules important to the cause, which in essence is what they were testing with the deficient mice in the reverse arthus model.

The mechanisms that regulate the hemorrhage seen at sites of inflammation and in cancer seem to be similar. In a cancer model, it was shown that the addition of resting platelets, but not activated platelets, rescues the hemorrhage seen during inflammation in cancer. One of the major differences between resting and activated platelets is that resting platelets maintain the contents of their α-granules and accordingly, they go on to show that supernatants from activated platelets will rescue the bleeding seen at a tumor. These results indicate that platelet α-granules contain a soluble factor or factors that have the ability to maintain vascular integrity at sites of hemorrhage induced by inflammation. Although they were able to show distinct changes of various culprit α-granule proteins, their work did not reveal the protein or proteins responsible for the control of hemorrhage (Ho-Tin-Noe et al., 2008). Their conclusion is that platelets continually maintain hemostasis in the face of inflammation using mechanisms other than those well described during plug formation. This opens the idea that platelets may work preemptively to stop hemorrhage by regulating leukocyte activity at the vessel wall. So the question remains, is there a molecule or a hand full of molecules responsible for maintaining hemostasis in the face of inflammation?

These series of experiments clearly define what we have known since the time of Celsius, but have ignored. In light of these experiments, our interpretation of TLT-1's "unique" role becomes plausible. TLT-1's purpose on platelets appears to be that of transition. In conjunction with molecules like p-selectin, GpIb, and TREM-1, TLT-1 mediates the integration of inflammatory signals with platelet function, mediating coagulation when only secondary agonists like TxA_2 or low levels of thrombin are present. TLT-1 may be one of a handful of molecules regulating immuno-hemostasis. These eloquent experiments (Goerge et al., 2008; Ho-Tin-Noe et al., 2008; Ho-Tin-Noe et al., 2009) also call for an official beginning of a new field that defines the intersection between immunology and hemostasis, one that we refer to as Immunohemostasis.

It is no longer adequate to state that platelets are linked to the inflammatory response. Here we have outlined numerous publications that demonstrate: how platelets influence neutrophil function (Clark et al., 2007; Looney et al., 2009; Zarbock et al., 2006), monocyte function (Goncalves et al., 2011), both T and B cell function (Elzey et al., 2003; Iannacone et al., 2005), the interrelation with complement and the effect of microparticles on the immune system (Boilard et al., 2010). These studies clearly demonstrate that platelets play an important role in inflammation. What is called for now is the kinetics of interactions and outcomes from studies using enhanced or decreased platelet count in immune reactions.

While all of the studies mentioned point out that platelets influence immune function, very few point out the outcomes from having increased or decreased platelet involvement. We pointed out earlier in this discussion, seemingly conflicting results between studies with similar stimuli but that had with different outcomes. Using LPS, Zarbock *et al.*, show that platelet depletion decreases inflammation. Clark et al., uses LPS and show that platelets are critical for NET formation. Why are they different and do they connect? Zarbock *et al.*, looks at a 2 hour time point (Zarbock et al., 2006) where Clark *et al.*, uses longer time points (Clark et al., 2007). NETS are notoriously slow in formation (Massberg et al., 2010); therefore these two results could be different stages of the same continuum. Neither of the articles describes outcomes, but leave open for debate which comes first, the platelet or the neutrophil. Looney *et al.*, (Looney et al., 2009) show an acute lung injury model where platelet depletion decreases mortality, but they used a two hit model where LPS was followed by antibodies to MHC. It is easy to see how platelet depletion could be life preserving. Their studies however, suggest that it is the neutrophils that recruit the platelets.

In reports that do report outcome, they show that even though platelet depletion reduces inflammation, they also point out that without the platelets, the immune response was inadequate. In the *Leishmania* study for example, platelet depletion lowered monocyte recruitment and inflammation, but at the same time the *Leishmania* infection was not cleared (Goncalves et al., 2011). In the thrombotic glomerular nephritis model, platelet depletion increased lethality of the treatment suggesting that platelets play a protective role. Similar outcomes were seen with viral models, where platelets caused hepatic damage and removal of platelets reduced the damage. Iannacone *et al.*, demonstrated that although there was less damage without platelets, the T-cells were unable to remove the viral infection, demonstrating that platelets are a critical part of the inflammatory response (Iannacone et al., 2005).

In a final note, it was shown that coagulation was important in bacterial immune response to help contain the infection (Massberg et al., 2010). It was ascertained that neutrophils release nucleosomes containing serine proteases. These nucleosomes function to make NETs and also that degrade platelet derived tissue factor pathway inhibitor, thus shifting the hemostatic balance at the platelet neutrophil interface toward coagulation. The authors point out the conserved nature of coagulation's role in controlling infection in stating that insects don't have an adaptive immune system and use coagulation as a mechanism to control infection in the hemolymph. Therefore they maintain that coagulation is an evolutionally efficient mechanism to control infection. Thus coagulation and platelets play a critical role in maintaining disease during process of **immuno-hemostasis**.

In conclusion, platelets are key regulators of the immune system and immune function cannot be considered complete without considering platelet function. It may be hard for those who prescribe to the self non-self theory of immune function to swallow platelets as playing more than a bystander a role in immune function. If we look at platelets as derived from megakaryocytes, recent studies show that bacterial infection changes the profile of what transcripts platelets store and therefore produce after activation (Freishtat et al., 2009). Thus, maybe it is not the platelets that are in control, but feedback to and from the megakaryocyte. Alternatively, if we subscribe to the newly derived Danger theory of immune function (Matzinger, 2001; Matzinger, 2002), platelets as well as neutrophils fit the bill as perfect detectors of danger and mediators of immune response. We can easily see how over activation of platelets and neutrophils could signal danger and elicit a more robust immune response. Either way, platelets play an indispensible role in the immune system and the hemostatic response to immune challenges and we propose the beginning of a new scene in our studies, a scene where the platelet is the immunomodulator; in a scene called **Immunohemostasis**.

6.3 Acknowledgements

This publication was possible by Grant Number 1U54RR026139-01A1 and G12RR-03035 from the National Center for Research Resources (NCRR), a component of the National Institutes of Health (NIH) and grant number SC2GM081237 from the National Heart Lung and Blood Institute

7. References

Allcock, Barrow, Forbes, Beck, & Trowsdale (2003). The human TREM gene cluster at 6p21.1 encodes both activating and inhibitory single IgV domain receptors and includes NKp44, *Eur J Immunol* Vol.33(No. 2): 567-577.

Amabile, Rautou, Tedgui, & Boulanger (2010). Microparticles: key protagonists in cardiovascular disorders, *Semin Thromb Hemost* Vol.36(No. 8): 907-916.

Ando, Iwata, Ozeki, Tsuchiya, Akiba, & Nihei (2002). Circulating platelet-derived microparticles with procoagulant activity may be a potential cause of thrombosis in uremic patients, *Kidney Int* Vol.62(No. 5): 1757-1763.

Arnaout (1990). Structure and function of the leukocyte adhesion molecules CD11/CD18, *Blood* Vol.75(No. 5): 1037-1050.

Austin S.K. (2008). Haemostasis, *Medicine* Vol.37(No. 3): 133-136.

Barrow, Astoul, Floto, Brooke, Relou, Jennings, Smith, Ouwehand, Farndale, Alexander, & Trowsdale (2004). Cutting edge: TREM-like transcript-1, a platelet immunoreceptor tyrosine-based inhibition motif encoding costimulatory immunoreceptor that enhances, rather than inhibits, calcium signaling via SHP-2, *J Immunol* Vol.172(No. 10): 5838-5842.

Berckmans, Nieuwland, Boing, Romijn, Hack, & Sturk (2001). Cell-derived microparticles circulate in healthy humans and support low grade thrombin generation, *Thromb Haemost* Vol.85(No. 4): 639-646.

Bexborn, Andersson, Chen, Nilsson, & Ekdahl (2008). The tick-over theory revisited: formation and regulation of the soluble alternative complement C3 convertase (C3(H2O)Bb), *Mol Immunol* Vol.45(No. 8): 2370-2379.

Boilard, Nigrovic, Larabee, Watts, Coblyn, Weinblatt, Massarotti, Remold-O'Donnell, Farndale, Ware, & Lee (2010). Platelets amplify inflammation in arthritis via collagen-dependent microparticle production, *Science* Vol.327(No. 5965): 580-583.

Brass (2010). Understanding and evaluating platelet function, *Hematology Am Soc Hematol Educ Program* Vol.2010: 387-396.

Cambien & Wagner (2004). A new role in hemostasis for the adhesion receptor P-selectin, *Trends Mol Med* Vol.10(No. 4): 179-186.

Castaman, Yu-Feng, & Rodeghiero (1996). A bleeding disorder characterised by isolated deficiency of platelet microvesicle generation, *Lancet* Vol.347(No. 9002): 700-701.

Chen, Inestrosa, Ross, & Fernandez (1995). Platelets are the primary source of amyloid beta-peptide in human blood, *Biochem Biophys Res Commun* Vol.213(No. 1): 96-103.

Clark, Ma, Tavener, McDonald, Goodarzi, Kelly, Patel, Chakrabarti, McAvoy, Sinclair, Keys, Allen-Vercoe, Devinney, Doig, Green, & Kubes (2007). Platelet TLR4 activates neutrophil extracellular traps to ensnare bacteria in septic blood, *Nat Med* Vol.13(No. 4): 463-469.

Coughlin (2000). Thrombin signalling and protease-activated receptors, *Nature* Vol.407(No. 6801): 258-264.

Coughlin (2005). Protease-activated receptors in hemostasis, thrombosis and vascular biology, *J Thromb Haemost* Vol.3(No. 8): 1800-1814.

Dean, Lee, Cummins, Schultz, & Powell (2009). Proteomic and functional characterisation of platelet microparticle size classes, *Thromb Haemost* Vol.102(No. 4): 711-718.

Del Conde, Cruz, Zhang, Lopez, & fshar-Kharghan (2005). Platelet activation leads to activation and propagation of the complement system, *J Exp Med* Vol.201(No. 6): 871-879.

Delvaeye & Conway (2009). Coagulation and innate immune responses: can we view them separately?, *Blood* Vol.114(No. 12): 2367-2374.

Demers, Ho-Tin-Noe, Schatzberg, Yang, & Wagner (2011). Increased efficacy of breast cancer chemotherapy in thrombocytopenic mice, *Cancer Res* Vol.71(No. 5): 1540-1549.

Devine & Rosse (1987). Regulation of the activity of platelet-bound C3 convertase of the alternative pathway of complement by platelet factor H, *Proc Natl Acad Sci U S A* Vol.84(No. 16): 5873-5877.

Elzey, Tian, Jensen, Swanson, Lees, Lentz, Stein, Nieswandt, Wang, Davidson, & Ratliff (2003). Platelet-mediated modulation of adaptive immunity. A communication link between innate and adaptive immune compartments, *Immunity* Vol.19(No. 1): 9-19.

Eyre L. & Gamlin F. (2010). Haemostasis, blood platelets and coagulation, *Anaesthesia & Intensive Care Medicine* Vol.11(No. 6): 244-246.

Fearon & Austen (1975). Properdin: binding to C3b and stabilization of the C3b-dependent C3 convertase, *J Exp Med* Vol.142(No. 4): 856-863.

Fearon, Austen, & Ruddy (1973). Formation of a hemolytically active cellular intermediate by the interaction between properdin factors B and D and the activated third component of complement, *J Exp Med* Vol.138(No. 6): 1305-1313.

Filice & Niewoehner (1987). Contribution of neutrophils and cell-mediated immunity to control of Nocardia asteroides in murine lungs, *J Infect Dis* Vol.156(No. 1): 113-121.

Flaumenhaft, Dilks, Richardson, Alden, Patel-Hett, Battinelli, Klement, Sola-Visner, & Italiano, Jr. (2009). Megakaryocyte-derived microparticles: direct visualization and distinction from platelet-derived microparticles, *Blood* Vol.113(No. 5): 1112-1121.

Fong, Barry, Tran, Traxler, Wannemacher, Tang, Speicher, Blair, Speicher, Grosser, & Brass (2011). Deciphering the human platelet sheddome, *Blood* Vol.117(No. 1): e15-e26.

Freishtat, Natale, Benton, Cohen, Sharron, Wiles, Ngor, Mojgani, Bradbury, Degnan, Sachdeva, Debiase, Ghimbovschi, Chow, Bunag, Kristosturyan, & Hoffman (2009). Sepsis alters the megakaryocyte-platelet transcriptional axis resulting in granzyme B-mediated lymphotoxicity, *Am J Respir Crit Care Med* Vol.179(No. 6): 467-473.

Furie & Furie (2004). Role of platelet P-selectin and microparticle PSGL-1 in thrombus formation, *Trends Mol Med* Vol.10(No. 4): 171-178.

Gahmberg (1997). Leukocyte adhesion: CD11/CD18 integrins and intercellular adhesion molecules, *Curr Opin Cell Biol* Vol.9(No. 5): 643-650.

Giomarelli, Washington, Chisholm, Quigley, McMahon, Mori, & McVicar (2007). Inhibition of thrombin-induced platelet aggregation using human single-chain Fv antibodies specific for TREM-like transcript-1, *Thromb Haemost* Vol.97(No. 6): 955-963.

Goerge, Ho-Tin-Noe, Carbo, Benarafa, Remold-O'Donnell, Zhao, Cifuni, & Wagner (2008). Inflammation induces hemorrhage in thrombocytopenia, *Blood* Vol.111(No. 10): 4958-4964.

Goncalves, Zhang, Cohen, Debrabant, & Mosser (2011). Platelet activation attracts a subpopulation of effector monocytes to sites of Leishmania major infection, *J Exp Med* Vol.208(No. 6): 1253-1265.

Harrison (2005). Platelet function analysis, *Blood Rev* Vol.19(No. 2): 111-123.

Heemskerk, Bevers, & Lindhout (2002). Platelet activation and blood coagulation, *Thromb Haemost* Vol.88(No. 2): 186-193.

Heijnen, Schiel, Fijnheer, Geuze, & Sixma (1999). Activated platelets release two types of membrane vesicles: microvesicles by surface shedding and exosomes derived from exocytosis of multivesicular bodies and alpha-granules, *Blood* Vol.94(No. 11): 3791-3799.

Hirahashi, Hishikawa, Kaname, Tsuboi, Wang, Simon, Stavrakis, Shimosawa, Xiao, Nagahama, Suzuki, Fujita, & Mayadas (2009). Mac-1 (CD11b/CD18) links inflammation and thrombosis after glomerular injury, *Circulation* Vol.120(No. 13): 1255-1265.

Ho-Tin-Noe, Goerge, Cifuni, Duerschmied, & Wagner (2008). Platelet granule secretion continuously prevents intratumor hemorrhage, *Cancer Res* Vol.68(No. 16): 6851-6858.

Ho-Tin-Noe, Goerge, & Wagner (2009). Platelets: guardians of tumor vasculature, *Cancer Res* Vol.69(No. 14): 5623-5626.

Iannacone, Sitia, Isogawa, Marchese, Castro, Lowenstein, Chisari, Ruggeri, & Guidotti (2005). Platelets mediate cytotoxic T lymphocyte-induced liver damage, *Nat Med* Vol.11(No. 11): 1167-1169.

Italiano, Jr., Richardson, Patel-Hett, Battinelli, Zaslavsky, Short, Ryeom, Folkman, & Klement (2008). Angiogenesis is regulated by a novel mechanism: pro- and antiangiogenic proteins are organized into separate platelet alpha granules and differentially released, *Blood* Vol.111(No. 3): 1227-1233.

Johns (2004). Platelet Function Testing, *Clinical Hemostasis Review* Vol.18(No. 4): 1-9.

Kahn, Nakanishi-Matsui, Shapiro, Ishihara, & Coughlin (1999). Protease-activated receptors 1 and 4 mediate activation of human platelets by thrombin, *J Clin Invest* Vol.103(No. 6): 879-887.

Khatami (2011). Unresolved inflammation: 'immune tsunami' or erosion of integrity in immune-privileged and immune-responsive tissues and acute and chronic inflammatory diseases or cancer, *Expert Opin Biol Ther*

Kornerup, Salmon, Pitchford, Liu, & Page (2010). Circulating platelet-neutrophil complexes are important for subsequent neutrophil activation and migration, *J Appl Physiol* Vol.109(No. 3): 758-767.

Lam, Burns, Smith, & Rumbaut (2011). Platelets enhance neutrophil transendothelial migration via P-selectin glycoprotein ligand-1, *Am J Physiol Heart Circ Physiol* Vol.300(No. 2): H468-H475.

Lambris, Ricklin, & Geisbrecht (2008). Complement evasion by human pathogens, *Nat Rev Microbiol* Vol.6(No. 2): 132-142.

Langer & Gawaz (2008). Platelet-vessel wall interactions in atherosclerotic disease, *Thromb Haemost* Vol.99(No. 3): 480-486.

Levi & van der Poll (2004). Coagulation in sepsis: all bugs bite equally, *Crit Care* Vol.8(No. 2): 99-100.

Licht, Pluthero, Li, Christensen, Habbig, Hoppe, Geary, Zipfel, & Kahr (2009). Platelet-associated complement factor H in healthy persons and patients with atypical HUS, *Blood* Vol.114(No. 20): 4538-4545.

Looney, Nguyen, Hu, Van Ziffle, Lowell, & Matthay (2009). Platelet depletion and aspirin treatment protect mice in a two-event model of transfusion-related acute lung injury, *J Clin Invest* Vol.119(No. 11): 3450-3461.

Lowenstein, Morrell, & Yamakuchi (2005). Regulation of Weibel-Palade body exocytosis, *Trends Cardiovasc Med* Vol.15(No. 8): 302-308.

Lusis (2000). Atherosclerosis, *Nature* Vol.407(No. 6801): 233-241.

MacKenzie, Creevy, & Heh (1971). The interaction of human IgM and C1q, *J Immunol* Vol.106(No. 1): 65-68.

Martel, Cointe, Maurice, Matar, Ghitescu, Theroux, & Bonnefoy (2011). Requirements for membrane attack complex formation and anaphylatoxins binding to collagen-activated platelets, *PLoS One* Vol.6(No. 4): e18812-

Massberg, Grahl, von Bruehl, Manukyan, Pfeiler, Goosmann, Brinkmann, Lorenz, Bidzhekov, Khandagale, Konrad, Kennerknecht, Reges, Holdenrieder, Braun, Reinhardt, Spannagl, Preissner, & Engelmann (2010). Reciprocal coupling of coagulation and innate immunity via neutrophil serine proteases, *Nat Med* Vol.16(No. 8): 887-896.

Matsubara, Shoji, Murakami, Abe, Frangione, & Ghiso (2002). Platelet microparticles as carriers of soluble Alzheimer's amyloid beta (sAbeta), *Ann N Y Acad Sci* Vol.977: 340-348.

Matzinger (2001). Essay 1: the Danger model in its historical context, *Scand J Immunol* Vol.54(No. 1-2): 4-9.

Matzinger (2002). The danger model: a renewed sense of self, *Science* Vol.296(No. 5566): 301-305.

May, Seizer, & Gawaz (2008). Platelets: inflammatory firebugs of vascular walls, *Arterioscler Thromb Vasc Biol* Vol.28(No. 3): s5-10.

Minors (2007). Haemostasis, blood platelets and coagulation, *Anaesthesia & Intensive Care Medicine* Vol.8(No. 5): 214-216.

Nayak, Ferluga, Tsolaki, & Kishore (2010). The non-classical functions of the classical complement pathway recognition subcomponent C1q, *Immunol Lett* Vol.131(No. 2): 139-150.

Paixao-Cavalcante, Hanson, Botto, Cook, & Pickering (2009). Factor H facilitates the clearance of GBM bound iC3b by controlling C3 activation in fluid phase, *Mol Immunol* Vol.46(No. 10): 1942-1950.

Peerschke & Ghebrehiwet (1997). C1q augments platelet activation in response to aggregated Ig, *J Immunol* Vol.159(No. 11): 5594-5598.

Peerschke, Yin, & Ghebrehiwet (2010). Complement activation on platelets: implications for vascular inflammation and thrombosis, *Mol Immunol* Vol.47(No. 13): 2170-2175.

Perez-Gomez & Bover (2007). [The new coagulation cascade and its possible influence on the delicate balance between thrombosis and hemorrhage], *Rev Esp Cardiol* Vol.60(No. 12): 1217-1219.

Pitchford, Momi, Giannini, Casali, Spina, Page, & Gresele (2005). Platelet P-selectin is required for pulmonary eosinophil and lymphocyte recruitment in a murine model of allergic inflammation, *Blood* Vol.105(No. 5): 2074-2081.

Polgar, Matuskova, & Wagner (2005). The P-selectin, tissue factor, coagulation triad, *J Thromb Haemost* Vol.3(No. 8): 1590-1596.

Puddu, Puddu, Cravero, Muscari, & Muscari (2010). The involvement of circulating microparticles in inflammation, coagulation and cardiovascular diseases, *Can J Cardiol* Vol.26(No. 4): 140-145.

Ricklin, Hajishengallis, Yang, & Lambris (2010). Complement: a key system for immune surveillance and homeostasis, *Nat Immunol* Vol.11(No. 9): 785-797.

Riddel, Jr., Aouizerat, Miaskowski, & Lillicrap (2007). Theories of blood coagulation, *J Pediatr Oncol Nurs* Vol.24(No. 3): 123-131.

Rivera, Lozano, Navarro-Nunez, & Vicente (2009). Platelet receptors and signaling in the dynamics of thrombus formation, *Haematologica* Vol.94(No. 5): 700-711.

Romney & Glick (2009). An updated concept of coagulation with clinical implications, *J Am Dent Assoc* Vol.140(No. 5): 567-574.

Ross (2000). Regulation of the adhesion versus cytotoxic functions of the Mac-1/CR3/alphaMbeta2-integrin glycoprotein, *Crit Rev Immunol* Vol.20(No. 3): 197-222.

Satran & Almog (2003). The coagulopathy of sepsis: pathophysiology and management, *Isr Med Assoc J* Vol.5(No. 7): 516-520.

Schoenwaelder, Yuan, Josefsson, White, Yao, Mason, O'Reilly, Henley, Ono, Hsiao, Willcox, Roberts, Huang, Salem, Kile, & Jackson (2009). Two distinct pathways regulate platelet phosphatidylserine exposure and procoagulant function, *Blood* Vol.114(No. 3): 663-666.

Siljander (2011). Platelet-derived microparticles - an updated perspective, *Thromb Res* Vol.127 Suppl 2: S30-S33.

Sivaraman & Latour (2011). Delineating the roles of the GPIIb/IIIa and GP-Ib-IX-V platelet receptors in mediating platelet adhesion to adsorbed fibrinogen and albumin, *Biomaterials* Vol.32(No. 23): 5365-5370.

Spagnoli, Bonanno, Sangiorgi, & Mauriello (2007). Role of inflammation in atherosclerosis, *J Nucl Med* Vol.48(No. 11): 1800-1815.

Spitznagel & Shafer (1985). Neutrophil killing of bacteria by oxygen-independent mechanisms: a historical summary, *Rev Infect Dis* Vol.7(No. 3): 398-403.

Stahl, Vaziri-Sani, Heinen, Kristoffersson, Gydell, Raafat, Gutierrez, Beringer, Zipfel, & Karpman (2008). Factor H dysfunction in patients with atypical hemolytic uremic syndrome contributes to complement deposition on platelets and their activation, *Blood* Vol.111(No. 11): 5307-5315.

Stave & Croker (1984). Thrombotic microangiopathy in anti-glomerular basement membrane glomerulonephritis, *Arch Pathol Lab Med* Vol.108(No. 9): 747-751.

Ulevitch & Cochrane (1978). Role of complement in lethal bacterial lipopolysaccharide-induced hypotensive and coagulative changes, *Infect Immun* Vol.19(No. 1): 204-211.

Vaziri-Sani, Hellwage, Zipfel, Sjoholm, Iancu, & Karpman (2005). Factor H binds to washed human platelets, *J Thromb Haemost* Vol.3(No. 1): 154-162.

Vicic & Weiss (1983). Evidence that platelet alpha-granules are a major determinant of platelet density: studies in storage pool deficiency, *Thromb Haemost* Vol.50(No. 4): 878-880.

Wagner & Frenette (2008). The vessel wall and its interactions, *Blood* Vol.111(No. 11): 5271-5281.

Washington, Gibot, Acevedo, Gattis, Quigley, Feltz, De La Mota, Schubert, Gomez-Rodriguez, Cheng, Dutra, Pak, Chertov, Rivera, Morales, Lubkowski, Hunter, Schwartzberg, & McVicar (2009). TREM-like transcript-1 protects against inflammation-associated hemorrhage by facilitating platelet aggregation in mice and humans, *J Clin Invest* Vol.119(No. 6): 1489-1501.

Washington, Quigley, & McVicar (2002). Initial characterization of TREM-like transcript (TLT)-1: a putative inhibitory receptor within the TREM cluster, *Blood* Vol.100(No. 10): 3822-3824.

Washington, Schubert, Quigley, Disipio, Feltz, Cho, & McVicar (2004). A TREM family member, TLT-1, is found exclusively in the alpha-granules of megakaryocytes and platelets, *Blood* Vol.104(No. 4): 1042-1047.

White (2007). Chapter 3: Platelet Structure, Vol.2nd(No. 3): 45-73.

Wolf, Goldstein, Stennicke, Beere, Amarante-Mendes, Salvesen, & Green (1999). Calpain functions in a caspase-independent manner to promote apoptosis-like events during platelet activation, *Blood* Vol.94(No. 5): 1683-1692.

Yamaguchi, Yu, Kumamoto, Sugawara, Kawamura, Takada, Yokochi, Sugawara, & Endo (2006). Involvement of Kupffer cells in lipopolysaccharide-induced rapid accumulation of platelets in the liver and the ensuing anaphylaxis-like shock in mice, *Biochim Biophys Acta* Vol.1762(No. 3): 269-275.

Yang & Wilson (1996). CD40 ligand-dependent T cell activation: requirement of B7-CD28 signaling through CD40, *Science* Vol.273(No. 5283): 1862-1864.

Yin, Ghebrehiwet, Weksler, & Peerschke (2007). Classical pathway complement activation on human endothelial cells, *Mol Immunol* Vol.44(No. 9): 2228-2234.

Zarbock, Singbartl, & Ley (2006). Complete reversal of acid-induced acute lung injury by blocking of platelet-neutrophil aggregation, *J Clin Invest* Vol.116(No. 12): 3211-3219.

Ziegler-Heitbrock (2007). The CD14+ CD16+ blood monocytes: their role in infection and inflammation, *J Leukoc Biol* Vol.81(No. 3): 584-592.

6

Inflammation, Immunity and Redox Signaling

Joshua Jabaut and Karina Ckless
State University of New York at Plattsburgh (SUNY Plattsburgh), Chemistry Department
USA

1. Introduction

It has long been known that several types of antioxidants also possess anti-inflammatory properties indicating a strong relationship between inflammation and oxidative stress. Reactive oxygen species (ROS) generated by inflammatory cells not only help to kill pathogens but also act on the inflammatory cells themselves, altering the intracellular redox balance and functioning as signaling molecules involved with the regulation of inflammatory and immunomodulatory genes. Indeed, at the transcriptional level, ROS play a key role in the control of nuclear factor kappa B (NF-κB), activator protein-1 (AP-1), and other transcription factors involved in gene expression of both inflammatory and immune mediators. More interestingly, ROS and also reactive nitrogen species (RNS) can either activate or inactivate these transcription factors by chemically modifying critical amino acid residues within these proteins or on residues of accessory proteins of the respective signaling pathways. The interest in the molecular mechanisms involved in redox regulation of inflammatory and immune responses has gone beyond the transcription factors as target proteins. Proteins involved in signaling cascades that ultimately culminate in the production of inflammatory and immune mediators have been investigated as redox sensors and therefore targets for ROS and or RNS modulation. For instance, NLRP3 inflammasome is a cysteine-rich multidimeric protein that participates in the formation of a molecular platform for caspase1-dependent IL-1β secretion. It has been suggested that IL-1β production and secretion in monocytes is a redox regulated event. However, the mechanisms of production and the nature of ROS involved in inflammasome activation are still unknown. This chapter will discuss some of the latest concepts on how ROS and RNS can modulate the inflammatory and immune responses at the molecular level, from redox regulated transcription factors to redox sensitive proteins involved in inflammatory and immune signaling pathways.

2. Chemistry, source and biological activity of reactive oxygen and nitrogen species

By definition, free radicals are reactive molecules that can exist independently and have one or more unpaired electrons (Halliwell and Gutteridge 2007). On the other hand the term "oxidant" is used in reference to any substance that can abstract an electron or hydrogen atom from other molecules, regardless of having an unpaired electron. These chemical species readily react with macromolecules in the biological systems by oxidizing them. In addition, they can react with metals, other oxidants, and reducing substances found in the intracellular milieu and generate many other reactive species. Within cells, "free radicals" and other oxidants can be formed by several sources, include enzymatic and non-enzymatic and also as a byproduct of biochemical reactions. Because of the complexity of the chemistry of these species, especially in biological systems, the terms reactive oxygen species (ROS) and reactive nitrogen species (RNS) will be used in this chapter to refer to the species that are derived from oxygen or nitrogen respectively. ROS include oxygen radicals such as diatomic oxygen (O_2), superoxide anion ($O_2^{-\bullet}$), hydroxyl radical ($^{\bullet}OH$), and peroxide ion (O_2^{2-}). In addition to non-radicals, species such as hyperchlorous acid (HOCl), hydrogen peroxide (H_2O_2), and ozone (O_3) are commonly present in biological systems and are also considered ROS. RNS include nitrogen-derived molecules, represented by the nitric oxide (NO) and its more oxidized counterparts. In biological systems, NO is catalyzed by a family of NADPH-dependent enzymes known as nitric oxide synthases (NOS). In mammals, there are three NOS isoforms named as neuronal (nNOS or NOS1), inducible (iNOS or NOS2) and endothelial (eNOS or NOS3). Depending on the circumstances or amount that is generated, NO can act as signaling molecule ("low input NO") or as defense substance against pathogens ("high input NO"). As a signaling molecule NO is generated in small amounts and exerts its function through generally reversible mild chemical reactions with protein amino acids or prosthetic groups, including reactions with heme centers in metalloproteins and thiol groups of cysteine amino acid. However, when NO is generated in high amounts and/or accompanied by other ROS, such as $O_2^{-\bullet}$, it undergoes multiple and complex oxidative reactions forming more oxidative and detrimental molecules, such as peroxynitrite ($ONOO^-$), which is highly reactive to biomolecules (reaction 1).

$$^{\bullet}NO + O_2^{\bullet -} \longrightarrow ONOO^- \qquad (1)$$

The concentration of NO is regulated both by its consumption in chemical reactions as well as its production in the cellular microenvironment. Consequently, as important as the enzymes that generate NO directly are the enzymes that control NOS activity indirectly. One of the indirect control mechanisms for NOS activity, in particular for iNOS, is the availability of its required substrate, L-arginine. L-arginine is not only a substrate for NOS, but also for arginases, enzymes that hydrolyze L-arginine to L-ornithine and urea (Diagram 1) (Lerzynski et al. 2006).

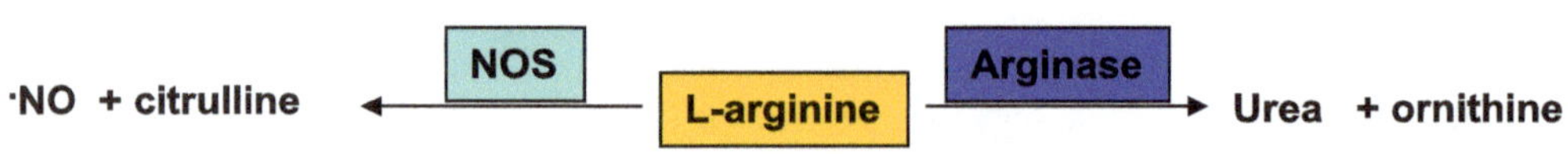

Diagram 1. Simplified reaction demonstrating substrate competition between the enzymes NOS and arginase.

Arginase, classically known as an enzyme within the urea cycle in the liver, is also found in many other cells and tissues including inflammatory cells (Munder 2009). There are two distinct isoforms of mammalian arginase, arginase I and arginase II (Morris 2009). The expression and activity of arginases are induced in murine models of allergic airways disease, as well as in patients with asthma (Zimmermann and Rothenberg 2006). It has been indicated that limitation of L-arginine availability, caused by activation of arginase, could contribute to the loss of NO bioactivity (Ricciardolo et al. 2005; Maarsingh et al. 2006). In fact, the inhibition of arginase by the pharmacological arginase inhibitor, *S*-(2-boronoethyl)-L-cysteine (BEC), decreased arginase activity and caused alterations in NO homeostasis, which were reflected by increases in NO-modified proteins in the lungs from inflamed mice. In addition, the same inhibitor enhanced perivascular and peribronchiolar lung inflammation, mucus metaplasia, genes of inflammatory chemokines, such as chemokine (C-C motif) ligand 20 (CCL20, which attracts neutrophils and dendritic cells) and keratinocyte chemoattractant (KC, responsible for attracting neutrophils). These results suggest that inhibition of arginase activity enhanced a variety of inflammatory parameters, possibly by altering NO homeostasis (Diagram 2) (Ckless et al. 2008). At the molecular level, arginase manipulation in lung epithelial cells can also impact NO homeostasis and affect inflammatory responses. In this scenario, the reduction of arginase activity enhances the general cellular content of NO and NO-modified proteins, including augmentation of NO-modified nuclear factor kappa B (NF-κB), which has a major role in regulating immune and inflammatory responses. Interestingly, the effects of arginase inhibition on NF-κB is reversed by the generic NOS inhibitor, N-ω-nitro-L-arginine methyl ester (L-NAME), suggesting a causal role for NO in the attenuation of NF-κB induced by arginase suppression. Conversely, overexpression of arginase I decreases cellular NO-derivative content which causes decrease of NO-modified NF-κB. The aforementioned NO-modification on NF-κB and other proteins includes S-nitrosylation, which will be discussed in more detail later in this chapter. Collectively, this study points out to a regulatory mechanism wherein NF-κB is controlled through arginase dependent regulation of NO levels, which may impact on chronic inflammatory diseases (Ckless et al. 2007).

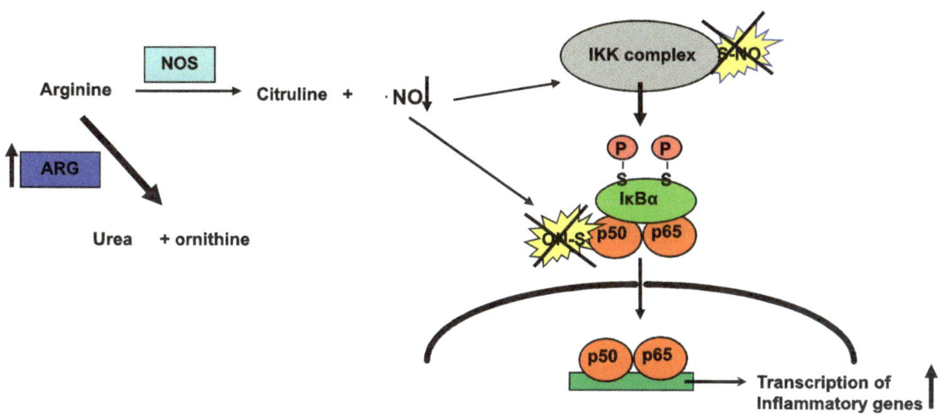

Diagram 2. Mechanism by which arginase might control NF-κB activity by decreasing NO availability.

ROS can also be generated endogenously by several enzymatic and non-enzymatic reactions. In pathological, and perhaps physiological states, the major non-mitochondrial ROS sources are the enzymes called oxidases, which includes NADPH oxidases, and cyclooxygenases among others. In general the production of ROS by these non-mitochondrial enzymes is dependent on a stimulus. Therefore in non-stimulated or in physiological conditions little is known about participation of these enzymes in ROS generation. The generation of ROS by these non-mitocondrial enzymes in inflamed states will be discussed further in this chapter.

The mitochondria can be a significant source of superoxide and nitric oxide in eukaryotic cells. The mitochondrial contribution to the pool of free radicals varies depending on cell function, and actively respiring mitochondria contribute more to the pool than do inactive mitochondria. Given that the standard reduction potential of O_2 to $O_2^{-\bullet}$ is -0.160 V and the standard reduction potentials of the redox centers in the respiratory chain range from -0.32 V to +0.39 V, and the presence of substantial transition metals in the redox centers, it comes as no surprise that there is significant reactive species generation in this environment (Halliwell and Gutteridge 2007). Superoxide is generated on the outer mitochondrial membrane, on both surfaces of the mitochondrial intermembrane space, and within the matrix. Although superoxide generated within the matrix is dismutated by the many antioxidant defenses within the matrix, superoxide generated in the intermembrane space and on the surface of the outermembrane of the mitochondria may be carried into the cytoplasm by voltage-dependent anion channels (Halliwell and Gutteridge 2007). Under normal physiological conditions, electrons flow through the respiratory chain generating a proton gradient, pumping protons into the intermembranous space between the inner and outer mitochondrial membrane. The gradient then creates ATP as the protons flow through the ATP synthase. During times of low ADP concentration, proton flow through the ATP synthase is disrupted causing electron flow through the respiratory chain to slow, and the chain to become more reduced. It seems that the reduced state of the chain increases the rate of autoxidation of the redox centers by O_2, forming $O_2^{\bullet-}$. It has been suggested that within the mitochondrial matrix, a unique form of NOS exists (Bustamante et al. 2007). The putative formation of NO in this environment has significant consequences due to its binding affinity to heme groups in the cytochromes of the respiratory chain. Additionally, the simultaneous production of O_2^- and NO can result in the production of peroxynitrite, which might inhibit important enzymes and disrupt mitochondrial integrity. Since the generation of NO requires oxygen, the rate of its generation is O_2 dependent (Halliwell and Gutteridge 2007).

Due to the increased ROS and RNS generation present in the mitochondria, antioxidant defenses have evolved to protect the integrity of the organelle. A family of metalloenzymes known as superoxide disumutases (SODs) catalyzes the formation of H_2O_2 and O_2 from O_2^- and water. Although the dismutation of O_2^- to H_2O_2 and water will occur spontaneously, SODs increase the rate of this diffusion in a controlled-manner. Within the mitochondrial matrix, a specific manganese containing SOD eliminates O_2^- from the matrix and the inner side of the inner mitochondrial membrane. Superoxide concentration in the intermembrane space is regulated by three mechanisms; a CuZnSOD, cytochrome c, and spontaneous dismutation induced by the lower pH of this area. In physiological conditions, H_2O_2 is rapidly decomposed by glutathione peroxidase and in some cell types by catalase. However if H_2O_2 accumulates it can be detrimental because it is the main precursor of the highly reactive hydroxyl radical, formed by interaction with reduced transition metals. In general the integrity of the mitochondrial membrane is maintained by a second glutathione peroxidase, known as phopholipid-hydroperoxide glutathione. This specialized peroxidase reduces lipid peroxides associated with the membrane. In addition to the "classical" antioxidant enzymes mitochondria integrity is also preserved by mitochondrial proteins that participate in the respiratory electron chain transport. It appears that the cytochrome c electron carriers have a detoxifying role against ROS, ubiquinol (QH_2) can act as a reducing agent in the elimination of peroxides in the presence of succinate, an intermediate of citric acid cycle. Non-enzymatic antioxidant systems also play a role in protecting mitochondrial integrity. The inner mitochondrial membrane contains high levels of vitamin E, a powerful antioxidant and inhibitor of free radical propagation reactions.

3. Redox chemistry in inflammation states

It is well known that chronic inflammatory diseases are associated with enhanced ROS and RNS production exemplified by elevated levels of NO and H_2O_2 in the site of inflammation (Antczak et al. 1997; Emelyanov et al. 2001). These oxidants can be generated by enzymes abundant not only in inflammatory cells but also in non-inflammatory cells (Janssen-Heininger et al. 2008). ROS and RNS generation in the inflammation site is typically induced as part of a defensive reaction intended to clear infectious and environmental threats, including microbial agents and particulate material. The resident and inflammatory hematopoietic-derived cells in the tissues possess oxidant-generating enzyme systems, including NADPH oxidase, which activity is mediated through the catalytic subunit gp91^{phox} (NOX2) (Bedard and Krause 2007; van der Vliet 2008). This enzyme is capable of generating $O_2^{\bullet-}$, which spontaneously or enzymatically dismutates to H_2O_2 to further induce oxidation. ROS generation by non-hematopoietic NOXs is also very important. The non-hematopoietic ROS are generated by a family of enzymes, including, NOX1, NOX3, and NOX4, which function distinct from gp91^{phox} (van de Veerdonk et al. 2010). In addition, some cell types such as epithelial cells have been described to produce active DUOX enzymes capable of generating H_2O_2 (van der Vliet 2008). Stimulated cells such as respiratory epithelium, neutrophils, and macrophages are also capable to produce NO in high amounts via iNOS (Janssen-Heininger et al. 2002). Induction of both iNOS and NADPH oxidases at the inflammation site leads to simultaneous increases in $O_2^{\cdot-}$ and NO that combine to form $ONOO^-$, which ultimately can react with tyrosine residues in protein, forming the more stable product, nitrotyrosine (Diagram 3) (Brennan et al. 2002). Indeed, increased levels of NO in exhaled breath and protein nitration have been observed in patients with asthma, correlating NO with inflammation (Reszka et al. 2011).

NO is highly diffusible, allowing it to potentially form $ONOO^-$ in areas spatially separated from the site of NO synthesis, limited only by its potent capacity to react with macromolecules (Lancaster and Gaston 2004). In addition, the reaction of NO with molecular oxygen (O_2) yields nitrite (NO), which can be oxidized by hemeperoxidases to form NO_2, thereby perpetuating the capacity for NO_2 reactivity. NO_2 is also formed when eosinophil peroxidase and myeloperoxidase, from eosinophils and neutrophils, respectively, consume NO and H_2O_2 (van der Vliet et al. 1999; Brennan et al. 2002). The environment can also be a source of NO_2. In fact high levels of this gas can be found in the atmosphere, and it is associated with poor air quality caused by pollution in highly industrialized areas. NO_2 primarily interacts with airway surface macromolecules, forming stable footprints of reactivity including the protein tyrosine modifications nitrotyrosine and dityrosine (Brennan et al. 2002), perhaps altering protein function. In addition, $ONOO^-$ or NO_2 can decompose to form $^{\bullet}OH$ and H_2O_2, which can facilitate further oxidation and participate in intracellular signaling events. Therefore, exogenous or endogenous-generated ROS and RNS may directly and indirectly affect cells that participate in the inflammatory and immune processes.

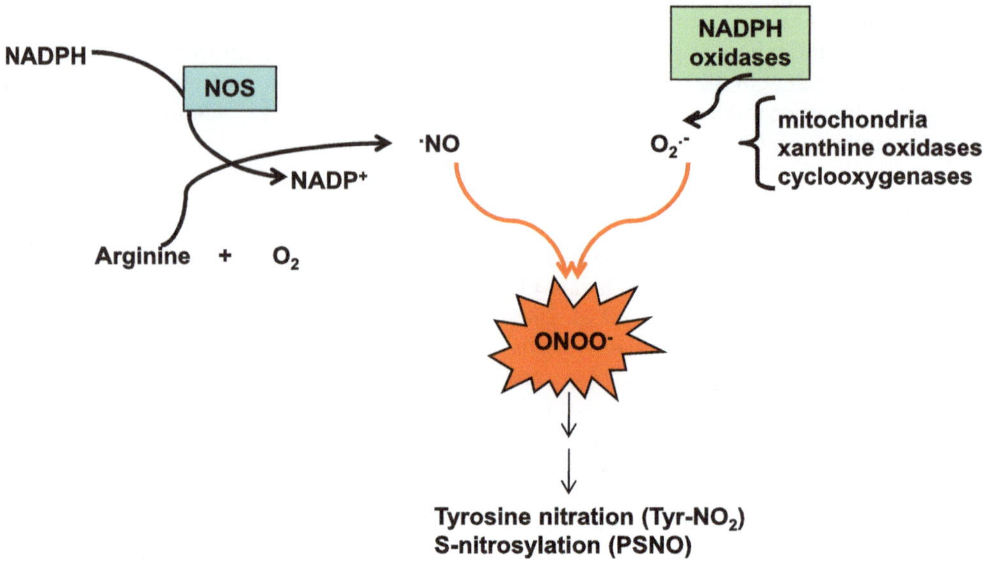

Diagram 3. Generation of peroxynitrite ($ONOO^-$) in the inflammation site and potential reactions with proteins.

The direct detection of ROS and RNS *in situ* of inflammation is an extremely challenging task. To overcome this difficulty, the detection of stable oxidation endproducts in proteins, such as nitrotyrosine, cysteine sulfenic (Cys-SOH), sulfinic (Cys-SO_2H) and sulfonic (Cys-SO_3H) acids is a feasible approach to indicate the presence of ROS and RNS. The chemistry of these oxidations is especially complex. NO generated endogenously by NOS can react indirectly with the tripeptide glutathione (GSH) and convert it to the S-nitrosothiol, called S-nitrosoglutathione (GSNO). Consequently, NO can exert its effects directly or through its derivatives (GSNO), by mediating protein S-nitrosylation (Diagram 4). By definition,

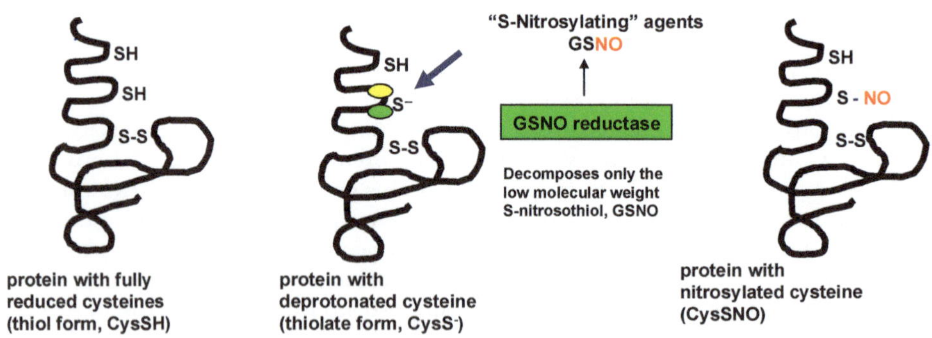

Diagram 4. Mechanism by which GSNO mediates S-nitrosylation of proteins and the role of enzyme GSNO reductase on the equilibrium of S-nitrosylated proteins.

protein S-nitrosylation is a covalent binding of NO to a cysteine residues in the proteins and it has been considered a mechanism of protein regulation (Numajiri et al. 2011). Up to date there is no identified enzyme that specifically and directly decomposes PSNO, however the enzyme GSNO reductase decomposes the S-nitrosothiol, GSNO and indirectly controls the protein S-nitrosylation. In more oxidized states, NO is further oxidized to ONOO- which is very well known as a nitrating agent of tyrosine residues in proteins (See above). The presence of these oxidized proteins has been considered "a biomarker" of inflammation.

The redox changes on cysteine residues are very dynamic and complex. In fact, S-nitrosothiols, such as GSNO can also mediate another Cys oxidation, called S-glutathionylation. Similar to S-nitrosylation, protein S-glutathionylation (PSSG) is the covalent modification of cysteines with the tri-peptide, glutathione (GSH). The formation of PSSG follows a more transient form of Cys-protein oxidation, which can by initiated by H_2O_2 which oxidizes protein cysteine to its thiolate state (Cys^-) and further to the unstable sulfenic acid (Cys-SOH). In the presence of high amounts of ROS, cysteine residues can also be further overoxidized to Cys-SO_2H and Cys-SO_3H. The susceptibility of cysteine to oxidation is proportionally dependent on the low *pKa* of this amino acid, indicating substantial specificity to these oxidation events. Different from protein S-nitrosylation, protein S-glutathionylation can be decomposed by specific enzymes. In physiologic settings, glutaredoxins act to specifically reverse S-glutathionylated proteins (Diagram 5). Similarly, the thioredoxin (Trx) system of enzymes catalyzes the reversible reduction of disulfides, thereby resulting in a reduced thiol on target protein, and a disulfide on Trx, which is subsequently reduced by thioredoxin reductase. The presence of these and other enzymes to

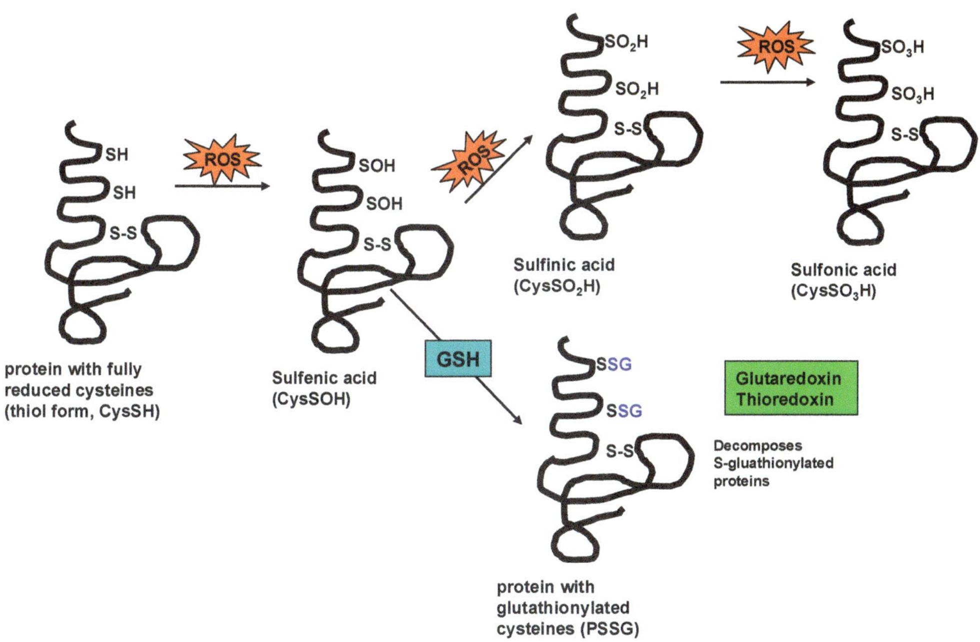

Diagram 5. Simplified mechanism by which protein S-glutathionylation is mediated in biological systems.

directly or indirectly regulate the oxidation state of protein cysteines gives additional acceptance to the relevance of protein oxidation events in cell biology and disease (Janssen-Heininger et al. 2008).

Since protein S-glutathionylation is reversible and perhaps regulated by specific enzymes, this post-translational modification has emerged as a regulatory mechanism of proteins. While certain redox changes that occur in the inflamed and adjacent cells may well contribute to the inflammatory disease process, the exact mechanisms by which ROS and RNS participate in the inflammatory and immune responses has remained unknown. One emerging scenario is centered on the role of oxidants as signaling molecules critical to tissue homeostasis and innate host defense. This concept of "redox biology" is based on the recently gained appreciation that NO and H_2O_2 cause specific oxidations in target cysteines within proteins, which exert regulatory functions, depending on the protein that is being targeted. Proteins with several functions, ranging from membrane proteins and proteases to transcription factors, are regulated via S-nitrosylation, S-glutathionylation, or other forms of cysteine oxidation. In this context, the NF-κB is the most represented transcription factor that is redox regulated.

4. Redox regulation of transcription factors controlling immune and inflammatory responses

The transcription factor NF-κB has been considered the master regulator of both innate and adaptive immune responses and has been demonstrated to play a critical role in allergic airways disease. In addition, this transcription factor has been known for a long time as a "redox sensitive transcription factor". Therefore, understanding the various facets of redox regulation of NF-κB and its targets offers the potential to advance our understanding of immune and inflammatory processes. The family of NF-κB comprises five related proteins: p50, p52, RelA (also known as p65), c-Rel, and RelB. These factors can homo- and heterodimerize through the rel homology domain. Only RelA, c-Rel, and RelB contain a transcriptional activation domain, while p50 and p52 lack this, and can only activate transcription through heterodimerization with RelA, c-Rel, or RelB (Hayden and Ghosh 2004; Pantano et al. 2006). NF-κB is sequestered in the cytoplasm of unstimulated cells bound to IκB proteins. In response to a wide array of stimuli, IκB proteins are phosphorylated by the serine kinase; inhibitor of kappa B kinase (IKK). Phosphorylated IκBs are ubiquitinated and degraded by the 26S proteosome, unmasking the NF-κB nuclear localization signal, allowing NF-κB to accumulate in the nucleus. At least two parallel pathways of IKK-induced NF-κB have been described. In the canonical pathway, activation of IKKβ by many stimuli, including cytokine TNF-α, TLR agonists, and IL-1β leads to the phosphorylation of IkBα at Serines 32 and 36 (DiDonato et al. 1997). In the noncanonical pathway, NF-κB–inducing kinase (NIK) phosphorylates IKKα. IKKα subsequently phosphorylates p100, which causes its proteolytic processing to p52 (Karin 1999), allowing p52/RelB dimeric complexes to translocate to the nucleus (Hayden and Ghosh 2008). Activators of the noncanonical pathway include subsets of stimuli that include B cell-activating factor (BAFF), lymphotoxin b (LTb), and CD40 ligand (CD40L), as well as lipopolysaccharide (LPS). It is generally held that the noncanonical pathway is necessary for the adaptive immune response, while the canonical pathway is required for the onset of the innate immune response (Bonizzi et al. 1999), although crosstalk between these pathways exists to control the strength and duration of the transcriptional response (Ghosh and Hayden 2008).

NF-κB activation, by diverse proinflammatory stimuli including IL-1β, has been demonstrated to require ROS in part after activation of NADPH oxidases (Bonizzi et al. 1999; Li and Engelhardt 2006), and mitochondrial ROS in certain contexts also can lead to activation of NF-κB (Chandel et al. 2001; Hughes et al. 2005). However, it is not clear whether the oxidative events triggered by those stimuli are temporal and therefore specific to components of the NF-κB pathway. In fact, the physiologic role for oxidants in the activation of NF-κB has been questioned by studies demonstrating that redox activation is cell type specific (Anderson et al. 1994; Brennan and O'Neill 1995), and that various antioxidants were nonspecific in their actions (Hayakawa et al. 2003). Evidence also exists that NADPH oxidase-induced ROS do not mediate NF-κB signaling, but lower the magnitude of its activation (Hayakawa et al. 2003). A number of reports demonstrate that oxidants can specifically inhibit the NF-κB pathway in lung epithelial cells via S-nitrosylation or S-glutathionylation of cysteine 179 of IKKβ (Reynaert et al. 2004; Reynaert et al. 2006), the same cysteine also targeted by anti-inflammatory cyclopentenone prostaglandins (Rossi et al. 2000). It is likely that additional cysteine oxidative events that include modification of p50 (Matthews et al. 1992) and RelA (Kelleher et al. 2007) also contribute to oxidative inhibition of NF-κB. These observations suggest that certain regulatory oxidative events could play important anti-inflammatory roles in tissues by limiting the activation of NF-κB. The redox regulation of NF-κB and perhaps other transcription factors and proteins involved in inflammatory and immune responses is extremely complex, and there are strong evidences that this process is cell type, ROS/RNS space-temporal dependent. A good illustration of this complexity is represented by several publications on post-translational modifications of the NF-κB pathway. In two separate studies, the same cell line but different sources of RNS were utilized to demonstrate that the NF-κB pathway is a target for redox regulation. In one study it has been demonstrated that exogenous S-nitrosothiols (an NO-derivative) cause S-nitrosylation of IKKβ inhibiting it and consequently inhibiting NF-κB (Reynaert et al 2004). In contrast, the second study demonstrated that increases in endogenous S-nitrosothiols caused by arginase inhibition do not affect the extent of IKKβ activity, but still attenuate the NF-κB pathway downstream of IKKβ (Ckless et al 2007). This apparent inconsistency may stem from potentially different chemical forms of NO, concentration, or subcellular localization that arose after arginase suppression (endogenous generation of S-nitrosothiols) compared with extracellularly delivered S-nitrosothiols and this different scenario may impact different targets of NF-κB pathways. In fact, in the study where the S-nitrosolthiols were generated endogenously, the target for S-nitrosylation was the p50 subunit of NF-κB complex. The NF-κB pathway is also a target for other type of posttranslational modification induced by ROS. Indeed in airway epithelial cells, cysteine-179 of the IKKβ regulatory kinase is a central target for oxidative inactivation by S-glutathionylation, caused by exogenous H_2O_2. The various conflicting mechanisms that are described for ROS and their role in NF-κB regulation and consequent antioxidants response to ROS generation may reflect on the complexity of the inflammatory processes. Recently it was suggested that acute inflammation possesses well balanced opposing arms, apoptosis and wound healing (Khatami 2008). Since NF-κB controls at least in part apoptotic/antiapoptotic events of this process, misregulation of this transcription factor caused by oxidative stress could lead to an unbalance between apoptosis and wound healing and in addition to the co-existence of death and growth factors in tissues, could create an dysfunctional immune response potentially leading to chronic inflammation, autoimmune diseases and cancer. (Khatami 2008; Khatami 2009; Khatami 2011).

5. RNS and ROS beyond transcription factors

The Interleukin 1 (IL-1) family of cytokines is critical to the host response to infection, playing a variety of roles not only in the acute phase response from the liver, but also in alterations of metabolism, induction of fever, and lymphocyte activation (Dinarello 2009). Overproduction of IL-1β, in particular, is thought to be responsible for a variety of autoinflammatory syndromes such as familial Mediterranean fever and Muckle-Wells syndrome, and is also a contributing factor in rheumatoid arthritis, gout, multiple sclerosis (in the animal model experimental autoimmune encephalomyelitis), Alzheimer's Disease, and diabetes (Gris et al.2010 ; Masters et al. 2010 ; Zhou et al. 2010 ; Griffin et al. 2006; Daheshia and Yao 2008; Clutterbuck et al. 2009). IL-1β is also a pathogenic mediator in several pulmonary disorders, including infection, asthma, ALI/ARDS, transplant rejection, COPD, PAH, sarcoidosis, asbestosis, and silicosis (Dorfmuller et al. 2003; Wanderer 2008; Soon et al. 2010). Setting IL-1β apart from other acute phase cytokines such as IL-6 and TNF-α is the requirement for processing from an inactive pro-form to an active secreted form by caspase-1 cleavage, which itself is activated by the assembly of cytoplasmic inflammasome complexes, which are multiprotein complexes that can activate caspase-1 and ultimately lead to the processing and secretion of interleukin (IL)-1β and IL-18 . A number of the NOD-like receptor (NLR) family members can form inflammasomes. One of the best-studied members of the NLR family is NLRP3 (NOD-like receptors pyrin domain-containing 3). The activation of NLRP3 inflammasome facilitates the formation of a molecular platform for caspase1-dependent secretion of IL-1β. It has been demonstrated that the mechanism of processing and secretion of mature IL-1β in myeloid cells is a multistep event. The initial event necessary is the synthesis and accumulation of the precursor proteins including pro-IL-1β and NLRP3 ("signal 1"), accomplished by a variety of stimuli, including danger- and pathogen- associated molecular pattern molecules (DAMPs and PAMPs, respectively). After priming, NLRP3 activation leads to recruitment of the adaptor protein ASC (apoptotic speck-like protein containing a CARD) and the enzyme caspase-1 to form the NLRP3 inflammasome complex ("signal 2"), which ultimately is responsible for the cleavage and secretion of IL-1β (Diagram 6) (Martinon et al. 2009). The cleavage and secretion of IL-1β can be enhanced by release of endogenous ATP that stimulates the purinergic receptor P2X7 (Piccini et al. 2008). Interestingly, several identified NLRP3 activators also trigger reactive oxygen species (ROS) production. It is well documented that activation of P2X7 is accompanied by production of ROS, produced at least in part by NADPH oxidases (Cruz et al. 2007; Dostert et al. 2008).

In the context of redox regulation of target proteins, what appears to be highly significant is the cellular location and quantity of ROS generated. Overall, several studies using antioxidants support a model in which ROS production by NLRP3 agonists drive inflammasome assembly (Tschopp and Schroder, 2010). The initial idea that NADPH oxidases are the primary source of ROS production during inflammasome activation is becoming less accepted. Two independent studies utilizing mononlucear phagocytes from patients with granulomatous disease, who because of mutation in $p47^{phox}$ have defective NADPH activity, demonstrated that there is IL-1β secretion from these inflammatory cells upon stimulation, despite the fact that these cells cannot generate NADPH oxidase-dependent ROS. (Meissner et al. 2010; van de Veerdonk et al.,2010). Since NADPH oxidase may not be the only source of ROS in the cells, the importance of mitochondrial-derived ROS has been recently explored. The mitochondria is the main source of ROS under physiological conditions, however under conditions of cellular stress, including increases in metabolic rates, hypoxia or cellular disruption, the mitochondria can generate increased amount of ROS (Brookes et al. 2004). In fact, blockage of key enzymes of the respiratory chain leads to ROS generation and consequent NLRP3 inflammasome activation (Zhou et al. 2010). Since NLRP3 de novo synthesis is an essential step in the activity of NLRP3, the temporal generation of ROS is also another important aspect to be considered to understand the role of these species in controlling NLRP3 inflammasome activation. In fact it has been recently published that ROS are important for de novo synthesis of NLRP3, but not activation. However, this evidence does not exclude a general role for ROS in the process of NLRP3-triggered inflammation (Bauernfeind et al. 2011). Despite several high profile publications in the field, the mechanisms of production and the nature of ROS involvement in inflammasome activation remain the subject of intense scrutiny.

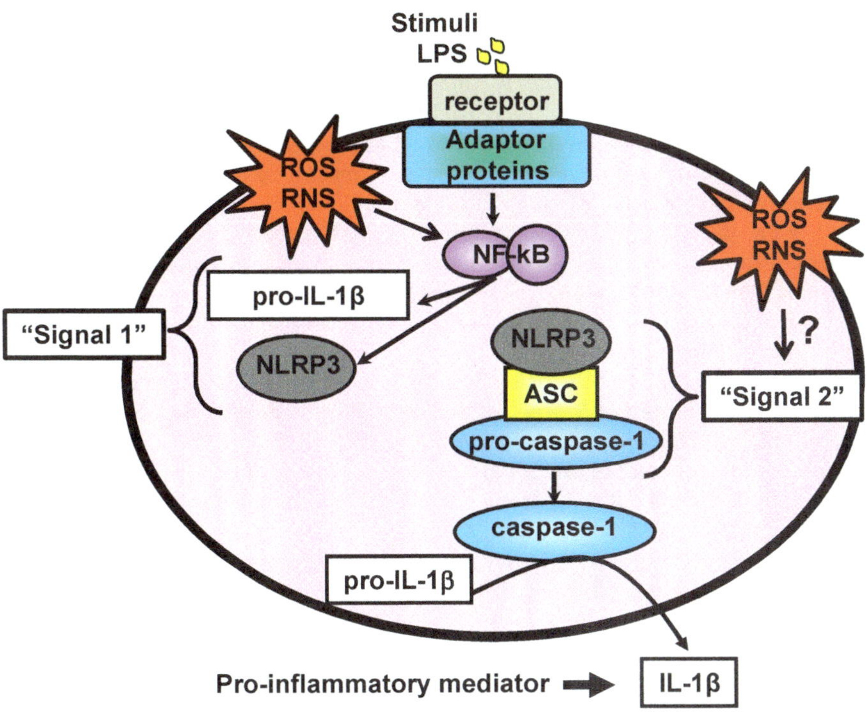

Diagram 6. Suggested mechanism of NLRP3 inflammasome activation and IL-1β secretion.

6. Conclusions

ROS and RNS are active participants in complex biological processes, including innate and immune responses. Whether the sources of ROS and RNS are environmental (exogenous sources) or are generated endogenously, they can affect several steps involved in these processes. It is critical to take in consideration that individual cells and multicellular organisms have developed intricate mechanisms to utilize ROS and RNS to modulate homeostasis and respond to threats. Therefore, generalized therapeutic and prophylactic approaches to modulate ROS and RNS generation and reactivity may not represent realistic tools to prevent or treat inflammatory diseases. Therefore, a better understanding of the sequence of events leading to specific immune and inflammatory responses, the temporal and spatial generation of ROS and RNS, and the potential molecular targets of oxidative modification, may provide crucial knowledge for the future development of more effective alternative therapeutic interventions in combination with the current ones to improve quality of life of patients with chronic inflammatory and auto-immune diseases

7. Acknowledgements

We thank Jennifer Ather and Edward Manna for editing the manuscript.

8. References

Anderson, M. T., F. J. Staal, et al. (1994). "Separation of oxidant-initiated and redox-regulated steps in the NF-kappa B signal transduction pathway." *Proceedings of the National Academy of Sciences of the United States of America* 91(24): 11527-11531.

Antczak, A., D. Nowak, et al. (1997). "Increased hydrogen peroxide and thiobarbituric acid-reactive products in expired breath condensate of asthmatic patients." *The European respiratory journal : official journal of the European Society for Clinical Respiratory Physiology* 10(6): 1235-1241.

Bauernfeind, F., E. Bartok, et al. (2011). "Cutting Edge: Reactive Oxygen Species Inhibitors Block Priming, but Not Activation, of the NLRP3 Inflammasome." *Journal of immunology* 187(2): 613-617.

Bedard, K. and K. H. Krause (2007). "The NOX family of ROS-generating NADPH oxidases: physiology and pathophysiology." *Physiological reviews* 87(1): 245-313.

Bonizzi, G., J. Piette, et al. (1999). "Reactive oxygen intermediate-dependent NF-kappaB activation by interleukin-1beta requires 5-lipoxygenase or NADPH oxidase activity." *Molecular and cellular biology* 19(3): 1950-1960.

Brennan, L. A., S. Wedgwood, et al. (2002). "The overexpression of copper-zinc superoxide dismutase protects NOS III from nitric oxide-mediated inhibition." *DNA and cell biology* 21(11): 827-838.

Brennan, P. and L. A. O'Neill (1995). "Effects of oxidants and antioxidants on nuclear factor kappa B activation in three different cell lines: evidence against a universal hypothesis involving oxygen radicals." *Biochimica et biophysica acta* 1260(2): 167-175.

Brookes, P. S., Y. Yoon, et al. (2004). "Calcium, ATP, and ROS: a mitochondrial love-hate triangle." *Am J Physiol Cell Physiol* 287(4): C817-833.

Bustamante, J., A. Czerniczyniec, et al. (2007). "Brain nitric oxide synthases and mitochondrial function." *Frontiers in bioscience : a journal and virtual library* 12: 1034-1040.

Chandel, N. S., P. T. Schumacker, et al. (2001). "Reactive oxygen species are downstream products of TRAF-mediated signal transduction." *The Journal of biological chemistry* 276(46): 42728-42736.

Ckless, K., A. Lampert, et al. (2008). "Inhibition of arginase activity enhances inflammation in mice with allergic airway disease, in association with increases in protein S-nitrosylation and tyrosine nitration." *Journal of immunology* 181(6): 4255-4264.

Ckless, K., A. van der Vliet, et al. (2007). "Oxidative-nitrosative stress and post-translational protein modifications: implications to lung structure-function relations. Arginase modulates NF-kappaB activity via a nitric oxide-dependent mechanism." *American journal of respiratory cell and molecular biology* 36(6): 645-653.

Clutterbuck, A. L., A. Mobasheri, et al. (2009). "Interleukin-1beta-induced extracellular matrix degradation and glycosaminoglycan release is inhibited by curcumin in an explant model of cartilage inflammation." *Ann N Y Acad Sci* 1171: 428-435.

Cruz, C. M., A. Rinna, et al. (2007). "ATP activates a reactive oxygen species-dependent oxidative stress response and secretion of proinflammatory cytokines in macrophages." *J Biol Chem* 282(5): 2871-2879.

Daheshia, M. and J. Q. Yao (2008). "The interleukin 1beta pathway in the pathogenesis of osteoarthritis." *J Rheumatol* 35(12): 2306-2312.

DiDonato, J. A., M. Hayakawa, et al. (1997). "A cytokine-responsive IkappaB kinase that activates the transcription factor NF-kappaB." *Nature* 388(6642): 548-554.

Dinarello, C. A. (2009). "Immunological and inflammatory functions of the interleukin-1 family." *Annu Rev Immunol* 27: 519-550.

Dorfmuller, P., F. Perros, et al. (2003). "Inflammation in pulmonary arterial hypertension." *Eur Respir J* 22(2): 358-363.

Dostert, C., V. Petrilli, et al. (2008). "Innate immune activation through Nalp3 inflammasome sensing of asbestos and silica." *Science* 320(5876): 674-677.

Emelyanov, A., G. Fedoseev, et al. (2001). "Elevated concentrations of exhaled hydrogen peroxide in asthmatic patients." *Chest* 120(4): 1136-1139.

Ghosh, S. and M. S. Hayden (2008). "New regulators of NF-kappaB in inflammation." *Nature reviews. Immunology* 8(11): 837-848.

Griffin, W. S., L. Liu, et al. (2006). "Interleukin-1 mediates Alzheimer and Lewy body pathologies." *J Neuroinflammation* 3: 5.

Gris, D., Z. Ye, et al. (2010)"NLRP3 plays a critical role in the development of experimental autoimmune encephalomyelitis by mediating Th1 and Th17 responses." *J Immunol* 185(2): 974-981.

Halliwell, B. and J. M. C. Gutteridge (2007). *Free radicals in biology and medicine*. Oxford ; New York, Oxford University Press.

Hayakawa, M., H. Miyashita, et al. (2003). "Evidence that reactive oxygen species do not mediate NF-kappaB activation." *The EMBO journal* 22(13): 3356-3366.

Hayden, M. S. and S. Ghosh (2004). "Signaling to NF-kappaB." *Genes Dev* 18(18): 2195-2224.

Hayden, M. S. and S. Ghosh (2008). "Shared principles in NF-kappaB signaling." *Cell* 132(3): 344-362.

Hughes, G., M. P. Murphy, et al. (2005). "Mitochondrial reactive oxygen species regulate the temporal activation of nuclear factor kappaB to modulate tumour necrosis factor-induced apoptosis: evidence from mitochondria-targeted antioxidants." *The Biochemical journal* 389(Pt 1): 83-89.

Janssen-Heininger, Y. M., R. L. Persinger, et al. (2002). "Reactive nitrogen species and cell signaling: implications for death or survival of lung epithelium." *American journal of respiratory and critical care medicine* 166(12 Pt 2): S9-S16.

Karin, M. (1999). "How NF-kappaB is activated: the role of the IkappaB kinase (IKK) complex." *Oncogene* 18(49): 6867-6874.

Kelleher, Z. T., A. Matsumoto, et al. (2007). "NOS2 regulation of NF-kappaB by S-nitrosylation of p65." *The Journal of biological chemistry* 282(42): 30667-30672.

Khatami, M. (2008). "'Yin and Yang' in inflammation: duality in innate immune cell function and tumorigenesis." *Expert Opin Biol Ther* 8(10): 1461-1472.

Khatami, M. (2009). "Inflammation, aging, and cancer: tumoricidal versus tumorigenesis of immunity: a common denominator mapping chronic diseases." *Cell Biochem Biophys* 55(2): 55-79.

Khatami, M. (2011). "Unresolved inflammation: 'immune tsunami' or erosion of integrity in immune-privileged and immune-responsive tissues and acute and chronic inflammatory diseases or cancer." *Expert Opin Biol Ther.*

Lancaster, J. R., Jr. and B. Gaston (2004). "NO and nitrosothiols: spatial confinement and free diffusion." *Am J Physiol Lung Cell Mol Physiol* 287(3): L465-466.

Lerzynski, G., C. V. Suschek, et al. (2006). "In hepatocytes the regulation of NOS-2 activity at physiological L-arginine levels suggests a close link to the urea cycle." *Nitric oxide : biology and chemistry / official journal of the Nitric Oxide Society* 14(4): 300-308.

Li, Q. and J. F. Engelhardt (2006). "Interleukin-1beta induction of NFkappaB is partially regulated by H2O2-mediated activation of NFkappaB-inducing kinase." *The Journal of biological chemistry* 281(3): 1495-1505.

Maarsingh, H., J. Leusink, et al. (2006). "Arginase strongly impairs neuronal nitric oxide-mediated airway smooth muscle relaxation in allergic asthma." *Respiratory research* 7: 6.

Martinon, F., A. Mayor, et al. (2009). "The inflammasomes: guardians of the body." *Annu Rev Immunol* 27: 229-265.

Masters, S. L., A. Dunne, et al. (2010). "Activation of the NLRP3 inflammasome by islet amyloid polypeptide provides a mechanism for enhanced IL-1beta in type 2 diabetes." *Nat Immunol* 11(10): 897-904.

Matthews, J. R., N. Wakasugi, et al. (1992). "Thioredoxin regulates the DNA binding activity of NF-kappa B by reduction of a disulphide bond involving cysteine 62." *Nucleic acids research* 20(15): 3821-3830.

Meissner, F., R. A. Seger, et al. (2010). "Inflammasome activation in NADPH oxidase defective mononuclear phagocytes from patients with chronic granulomatous disease." *Blood* 116(9): 1570-1573.

Morris, S. M., Jr. (2009). "Recent advances in arginine metabolism: roles and regulation of the arginases." *British journal of pharmacology* 157(6): 922-930.

Munder, M. (2009). "Arginase: an emerging key player in the mammalian immune system." *British journal of pharmacology* 158(3): 638-651.

Numajiri, N., K. Takasawa, et al. (2011). "On-off system for PI3-kinase-Akt signaling through S-nitrosylation of phosphatase with sequence homology to tensin (PTEN)." *Proceedings of the National Academy of Sciences of the United States of America* 108(25): 10349-10354.

Pantano, C., N. L. Reynaert, et al. (2006). "Redox-sensitive kinases of the nuclear factor-kappaB signaling pathway." *Antioxidants & redox signaling* 8(9-10): 1791-1806.

Piccini, A., S. Carta, et al. (2008). "ATP is released by monocytes stimulated with pathogen-sensing receptor ligands and induces IL-1beta and IL-18 secretion in an autocrine way." *Proc Natl Acad Sci U S A* 105(23): 8067-8072.

Reszka, K. J., L. Sallans, et al. (2011). "Airway peroxidases catalyze nitration of the {beta}2-agonist salbutamol and decrease its pharmacological activity." *The Journal of pharmacology and experimental therapeutics* 336(2): 440-449.

Reynaert, N. L., K. Ckless, et al. (2004). "Nitric oxide represses inhibitory kappaB kinase through S-nitrosylation." *Proceedings of the National Academy of Sciences of the United States of America* 101(24): 8945-8950.

Reynaert, N. L., A. van der Vliet, et al. (2006). "Dynamic redox control of NF-kappaB through glutaredoxin-regulated S-glutathionylation of inhibitory kappaB kinase beta." *Proceedings of the National Academy of Sciences of the United States of America* 103(35): 13086-13091.

Ricciardolo, F. L., J. Zaagsma, et al. (2005). "The therapeutic potential of drugs targeting the arginase pathway in asthma." *Expert opinion on investigational drugs* 14(10): 1221-1231.

Rossi, A., P. Kapahi, et al. (2000). "Anti-inflammatory cyclopentenone prostaglandins are direct inhibitors of IkappaB kinase." *Nature* 403(6765): 103-108.

Soon, E., A. M. Holmes, et al. (2010). "Elevated levels of inflammatory cytokines predict survival in idiopathic and familial pulmonary arterial hypertension." *Circulation* 122(9): 920-927.

Tschopp, J. and K. Schroder (2010). "NLRP3 inflammasome activation: The convergence of multiple signalling pathways on ROS production?" *Nat Rev Immunol* 10(3): 210-215.

van de Veerdonk, F. L., S. P. Smeekens, et al. (2010) "Reactive oxygen species-independent activation of the IL-1beta inflammasome in cells from patients with chronic granulomatous disease." *Proc Natl Acad Sci U S A* 107(7): 3030-3033.

van der Vliet, A. (2008). "NADPH oxidases in lung biology and pathology: host defense enzymes, and more." *Free radical biology & medicine* 44(6): 938-955.

van der Vliet, A., J. P. Eiserich, et al. (1999). "Reactive nitrogen species and tyrosine nitration in the respiratory tract: epiphenomena or a pathobiologic mechanism of disease?" *American journal of respiratory and critical care medicine* 160(1): 1-9.

Wanderer, A. A. (2008). "Interleukin-1beta targeted therapy in severe persistent asthma (SPA) and chronic obstructive pulmonary disease (COPD): proposed similarities between biphasic pathobiology of SPA/COPD and ischemia-reperfusion injury." *Isr Med Assoc J* 10(12): 837-842.

Zhou, R., A. Tardivel, et al. (2010) "Thioredoxin-interacting protein links oxidative stress to inflammasome activation." *Nat Immunol* 11(2): 136-140.

Zhou, R., A. S. Yazdi, et al. (2010) "A role for mitochondria in NLRP3 inflammasome activation." *Nature.*

Zimmermann, N. and M. E. Rothenberg (2006). "The arginine-arginase balance in asthma and lung inflammation." *European journal of pharmacology* 533(1-3): 253-262.

7

Regulatory T Cells and Viral Disease

Tanya LeRoith and S. Ansar Ahmed
Virginia Tech
USA

1. Introduction

The mammalian immune system has the ability to distinguish self from non-self-antigens, a phenomenon which begins in the thymus during T cell development. T cells that express a fully rearranged T cell receptor (TCR) with a high affinity for self-antigens presented in the thymus are deleted or undergo anergy in a process known as negative selection. Because of this mechanism, T cells in the periphery are primarily specific for non-self-antigens. However, this process is somewhat inefficient, because some self-reactive cells escape deletion therefore additional mechanisms are required to maintain peripheral immune tolerance. Regulatory T cells (T_{regs}) are a distinct subset of T cells that are critical for maintaining both immune homeostasis and peripheral immune tolerance. T_{regs} are typically identified by expression of the forkhead box 3 (FoxP3) transcription factor. The majority of FoxP3+ cells also express CD4 and express high levels of the IL-2 receptor (CD25). Additional subsets of T_{regs} that have been described in humans and mice include Tr1 cells, T helper 3 cells (Th3), NK cells, and CD8+ T_{regs} (Beissert S, 2006). CD4+ T cells that express high levels the IL-2α receptor ($CD25^{high}$) do not respond to T cell receptor (TCR) activation or mitogen stimulation, and inhibit IL-2 transcription in CD25- cells. Suppression of CD25- cells is contact dependent, and requires activation of the T_{regs} through the TCR; however, once activated, the suppressor effector function is nonspecific (Thornton AM, 2000). In mice and humans, FoxP3+ cells also express high levels of cytotoxic T lymphocyte-associated antigen 4 (CTLA-4) and glucocorticoid-induced tumor necrosis factor receptor (GITR) on the surface (Bacchetta R, 2005). CD4+CD25+ T cells suppress the immune response to some viruses, protozoa, and bacteria, and aid in the survival of intracellular pathogens (Sakaguchi, 2003) most likely by potent suppression of proliferation and IFN-γ production of both CD4+ and CD8+ T lymphocytes (Bacchetta R, 2005). Tr1 cells secrete high amounts of IL-10 and moderate amounts of TGF-β. Inhibiting IL-10 with neutralizing antibody blocks the suppressor effects of Tr1 cells (Beissert S, 2006). Th3 cells produce high concentrations of TGF-β and moderate amounts of IL-10, and the suppressor effects are not antigen specific (Beissert S, 2006). Interestingly, Th3 cells suppress the activation of both Th1 and Th2 cell clones while other subsets primarily inhibit Th1 cells and have no effect on Th2 cells (Beissert S, 2006). A number of studies have shown that T_{regs} affect the magnitude of immunity and outcome of viral infections, especially with persistent viruses that give rise to chronic lesions (Rouse BT, 2006). Depletion of T_{regs} prior to infection using a monoclonal antibody against the IL-2α receptor results in enhanced in vivo CD8+ and CD4+ T lymphocyte proliferation, and increased mucosal antibody levels in response to herpes simplex viral infection in mice (Rouse BT, 2006). Humans with chronic hepatitis C virus have IL-10-producing Tr1 cells, while those who control infection do not. The IL-10 - producing cells were shown to modulate the activity of protective IFN-γ producing T lymphocytes, and both the Th1 and regulatory T cells were induced against the same epitopes (MacDonald AJ, 2002). Additionally, immunosuppression induced by chronic retroviral infection in the absence of T cell depletion was shown to be mediated by CD4+ regulatory T lymphocytes in mice (Iwashiro M, 2001). Importantly, these regulatory T lymphocytes suppressed IFN-γ production by CD8+ T lymphocytes, contributing to virus persistence (Dittmer U, 2004). The ability of viruses to induce proliferation and activation of regulatory T cells likely contributes to delayed clearance and persistence in the host.

2. Regulatory T cell biology and development

Following infection, naïve CD4+ T cells recognize antigen presented on antigen presenting cells, bound to class II major histocompatibility complexes (MHC class II). These CD4+ T cells expand and differentiate into effector T cells that can become polarized into distinct subsets depending on the cytokine environment (McKinstry KK, 2010). The best characterized are Th1 and Th2 subsets that have been associated with cell-mediated (Th1) and humoral (Th2) immunity (reviewed in (Sakaguchi S, 2010). In addition to T cells, B cells, and plasma cells are vital in development of humoral immunity. The role of plasma cells in antibody development is beyond the scope of this discussion. Recently, additional subsets have been described, including Th9, Th17, Th22, T-follicular helper cells (Tfh), and regulatory T cells. Recent studies have shown that multiple CD4+ T cells are actually generated *in vivo*, rather than distinct subsets as previously thought. The effector cells secrete large amounts of cytokines, chemokines, and other proteins that can produce cytotoxicity to host tissues, or induce autoimmunity. Until recently, control of T_{reg} function was believed to have primarily been through cytokine signaling. However, there is evidence that T_{regs} can also sense pathogens through toll-like receptors (TLRs) which modifies their behavior (Sutmuller RPM, 2006). The role of cytokines and TLRs in controlling T_{reg} function will be discussed separately.

Th subset	Selected Key Transcription factors	Cytokines produced
Th1	T-bet	IFN-γ, TNF, IL-2
Th2	GATA-3	IL-4, IL-5, IL-13
Th17	ROR-γt	IL-17, IL-22
Tfh	Bcl-6	IL-4, IL-21
Treg	Foxp3	IL-10

Table 1. CD4+ T cell subsets (modified from (McKinstry KK, 2010))

Regulatory T cells function to provide a balance between combating pathogens and the risk of developing autoimmunity or overwhelming inflammation. Regulatory T cells can be divided into two groups - natural T_{regs} develop in the thymus, while inducible T_{regs} are generated in the periphery from conventional T cells in response to different stimuli. The natural T_{regs} are the best characterized of the two groups and make up approximately 5-10% of circulating T lymphocytes in mice and humans (Gückel E, 2011). Regulatory T cells are primarily characterized by the expression of the transcription factor FoxP3. FoxP3 maintains

T_{reg} gene expression induced by other transcription factors rather than actually driving T_{reg} development. However, FoxP3 is essential for T_{reg} function since loss of FoxP3 function results in severe lymphoproliferative disease and autoimmunity in humans and mice (Bennett CL, 2001). The role of FoxP3 in maintaining self-tolerance was first identified in scurfy mice, and then in humans with immunodysregulation, polyendocrinopathy, enteropathy, X-linked (IPEX) syndrome, both of which have a FoxP3 mutation as the underlying genetic defect. Humans express two isoforms of FoxP3 (A and B), either of which has regulatory function. FoxP3B contains a deletion of the proline-rich exon 2 which is required to bind to the retinoic acid receptor-related orphan receptor-α (RORα). In addition, FoxP3B lacks the amino-terminal residues that interact with nuclear factor of activated T cells (NFAT) (Sakaguchi S, 2010). In humans, FoxP3 expression on T_{regs} is transient, and downregulation of FoxP3 expression decreases the ability of these cells to suppress. In contrast, this transient expression has not been found in mice; however, mouse conventional T cells can be converted to FoxP3+ T regs following stimulation with TFGβ or retinoic acid. These adaptive T_{reg} cells also express FoxP3, CD25, and CTLA4 (Sakaguchi S, 2010). In humans, FoxP3+ T cells stimulated with TGFβ do not have suppressive activity and may require other factors to develop T_{reg} function. Both natural and induced T_{reg} cells have unique surface markers that differentiate them from conventional T cells. The surface marker expression is summarized in Figure 1.

2.1 Natural regulatory T cells

Natural regulatory T cells were first discovered in two animal models of autoimmunity. In the first, neonatal mice were thymectomized at 2-4 days of life. These mice developed autoimmune disease that could be abrogated by adoptive transfer of CD4+ T cells from normal mice. In the second, adult rats were thymectomized and subjected to X-ray irradiation. Adoptive transfer of CD4+ T cells from normal rats similarly abrogated the autoimmune disease, suggesting that CD4+ T cells within the thymus suppressed the development of autoimmunity. Later experiments showed that adoptive transfer of thymocytes depleted of CD4+CD25+ cells resulted in the development of autoimmune disease in syngeneic T cell deficient mice (reviewed in (Sakaguchi S, 2010)). Thymic stromal cells and dendritic cells are critical for nT_{reg} development. Natural regulatory T cells develop in the thymus through interactions between the high-affinity T cell receptor and cognate antigens on thymic epithelial cells. Co-stimulation through CD28 and common gamma (cγ) chain cytokines, especially IL-2 and IL-7 have also been shown to be necessary for nT_{reg} development. Signal transducer and activation of transcription 5 (STAT5) signaling through the cγ chain is also required. Thymic development of nT_{reg} cells follows a two-step process: 1), thymocytes upregulate CD25 and other IL-2 signaling molecules in response to TCR/CD28 co-stimulation and 2), CD4+CD25^{high}FoxP3- T_{regs} respond to IL-2 independent of the TCR, and induce FoxP3 expression in response to STAT5 activation (Gückel E, 2011). T_{reg} cell-intrinsic NF-κB activation is essential for thymic T_{reg} development (Gückel E, 2011). Naturally occurring T_{regs} cannot produce IL-2 and therefore rely on paracrine IL-2 production from conventional T cells. Mice deficient in IL-2 or CD25 have reduced numbers of FoxP3+ T cells and a dramatic reduction in peripheral and thymic T_{regs}. In humans, Hassall's corpuscles in the thymic medulla secrete thymic stroma lymphopoietin (TSLP) which activates immature dendritic cells and upregulates the expression of co-stimulatory molecules. The activated DCs induce FoxP3 expression in CD4+CD8-CD25- thymocytes (Sakaguchi S, 2010).

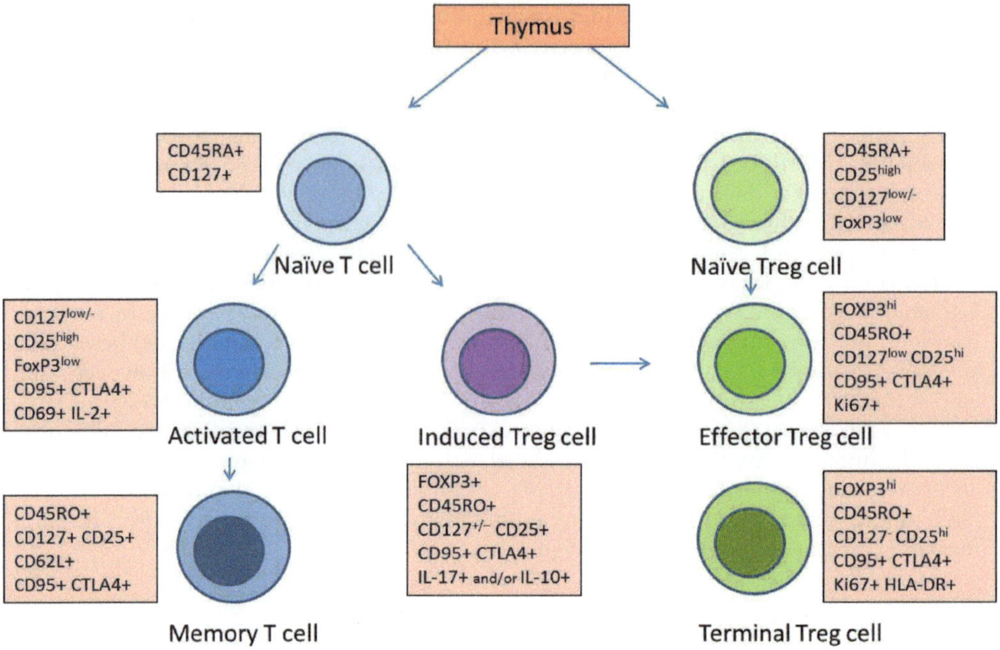

Fig. 1. Regulatory T cell development. The phenotype of different stages of CD4+ T cell differentiation into the conventional T cell and regulatory T cells are shown. The T cells originate in the thymus and emigrate as naïve CD45RA+ T cells to the periphery where they are activation. Activation induces differentiation into either conventional or regulatory T cells. Conventional T cells can then differentiate into memory T cells. Treg cells have not yet been shown to produce memory cells, but they do differentiate into terminal effector Tregs. Treg-like cells are induced from conventional T cells depending on cytokine stimulation. These converted Treg-like cells have cell surface markers similar to those expressed by natural Tregs. CTLA4, cytotoxic T lymphocyte antigen 4; FOXP3, forkhead box P3 (Modified from (Sakaguchi S, 2010)).

2.2 Inducible regulatory T cells

A less well-characterized subset of regulatory T cells is the inducible T_{regs} that develop from conventional T cells under certain conditions. iT_{regs} are induced by prolonged exposure to circulating antigen or weak co-stimulation in the periphery. Additionally, soluble factors such as the cytokines IL-4, IL-10 and TGF-β, retinoic acid or neuropeptides can enhance Foxp3 upregulation and iT_{reg} generation in the periphery. FoxP3 expression induces upregulation of other T_{reg} molecules including CTLA-4, GITR, and CD127. Tr1 cells secrete IL-10, while Th3 cells secrete TGF-β. Other cells with adaptive regulatory function include some CD4-CD8- and CD8+CD28- T cells (Sakaguchi S, 2010). Early after iT_{regs} are stimulated, they express high levels of cell-cycle progression and T cell activation-associated genes (Prots I, 2011), mimicking genes that are upregulated in activated effector T cells. As iTregs mature, expression of these genes diminishes while they remain high in mature effector T cells. By 10 days after differentiation into iT_{regs}, most cell cycle progression and T cell activation genes are expressed at levels approximately 3 times lower than in effector T cells. In addition, genes in the FoxO family of transcription factors are over-expressed in iT_{regs} compared to overexpression of the FoxM1 family in effector cells (Prots I, 2011).

2.3 Toll-like receptors

At the center of the balance between protective immunity and autoimmunity are the pattern recognition receptors on antigen presenting cells that activate innate immunity and provide the bridge between innate and adaptive immunity. Pattern recognition receptors include Toll-like receptor molecules (TLRs), Nod and Nod-like receptors, RIG-I-like receptors (RLRs), and C-type lectin receptors (Dai J., 2009). TLRs are critical for sensing pattern associated molecular patterns (PAMPs) such as those from bacteria, viruses, protozoa, and fungi, and act to bridge innate and acquired immunity. Stimulation of TLRs by PAMPs alerts the immune system to the presence of microbial infections, triggers maturation in dendritic cells, and allows them to initiate adaptive immunity. TLRs have recently been found to be expressed on T_{regs} as well, and may act to curtail excessive inflammation, autoimmunity, and sepsis (Sutmuller RPM, 2006). However, TLR signaling has also been shown to block T_{reg} activity, leading to an enhanced immune response. Therefore, the function of T_{regs} can be attenuated or enhanced depending on TLR activity in response to certain pathogens (Dai J., 2009). Of the thirteen TLRs that have been identified in mice and humans, T_{regs} express TLRs 7, 8, and 9 intracellularly, and 1, 2, 4, 5, 6, and 10 on the surface. Additionally, T_{reg} subsets express significantly more TLR4, TLR5, TLR7, and TLR8 than conventional T cells. TLR4 recognizes lipopolysaccharide (LPS), which is produced by gram negative bacteria, while TLR2 is activated by lipoteichoic acid (LTA) and bacterial lipoproteins. TLR7 and TLR8 recognize single stranded RNA, and TLR9 recognizes unmethylated CpG DNA motifs found primarily in DNA viruses and some prokaryotic genomes (Sutmuller RPM, 2006). Interestingly, bacterial product signaling through TLR 2, 4, and 5 results in increased T_{reg} function in a MyD88 and phosphatidylinositol 3-kinase (PI-3 kinase)-dependent fashion; while signaling through intracellular TLRs 7, 8, and 9 decreases T_{reg} function (Dai J., 2009). The reason for the dual function of T_{regs} in infection is unclear; however Dai et. al suggest that the dual response is a necessary pathogen-specific response. On the one hand, bacterial and fungal products are responsible for acute sepsis, and these products are recognized by cell surface TLRs 2, 4, and 5. A robust anti-inflammatory response is necessary to prevent overwhelming inflammation in septic individuals. On the other hand, viruses do not cause sepsis, and an adaptive immune response is necessary for protective immunity. Recognition of viruses through intracellular TLRs 7, 8, and 9 ensures a robust effector T cell response by inhibiting the function of T_{regs} (Dai J., 2009). Alternatively, changes in T_{reg} function may be a result of the expression levels, the density, or the subcellular localization of TLRs, or of differential expression of co-stimulatory or accessory molecules, or the cytokine milieu. Importantly, TLR2 seems to be crucial in expanding and regulating T_{reg} function. TLR-2 deficient mice have significantly fewer T_{reg} cells than control mice, and administering TLR2 ligands to wild-type mice increases T_{reg} numbers. TLR2 triggering, IL-2 treatment, and TCR ligation can overcome T_{reg} anergy *in vitro* and *in vivo*. Additionally, Foxp3 expression was decreased following TLR2 stimulation of T_{reg} cells. How TLR-signaling affects Foxp3 expression is still unknown. TLR2 ligand also increases IL-2 receptor expression on T_{regs} and induces IL-2 production by conventional T cells resulting in IL-2 mediated abrogation of suppression (Sutmuller RPM, 2006).

2.4 Cytokines

Recently, the Th1/Th2 paradigm has shifted to focus on other subsets of T cells. The focus has been on the relationship between regulatory T cells and CD4+ T cells that secrete IL-17 (Th17 cells). These cells are derived from a common progenitor cell, and develop in response to the cytokine milieu. T_{regs} and Th17 cells even share common chemokine receptors and homing properties (Kanwar B, 2010). The balance between these subsets is important in many immune disorders related to host-pathogen interaction, inflammatory syndromes, autoimmune disease, and immunodeficiency. T_{reg} cell development is dependent on cytokine production: the presence of TGF-β favors T_{reg} differentiation (Fig 2), while the addition of IL-6 favors Th17 development, and IL-4 and TGF-β favors Th9 development (Jutel M, 2011). TGF-β upregulates the retinoic acid receptor-related orphan receptor-γt (ROR-γt), which is a master transcription factor of Th17 differentiation. TGF-β also induces FoxP3 upregulation when IL-6 is not present. The presence of IL-6 inhibits T_{reg} development and induces development of Th17 cells. One of the first ways found to modify T_{reg} function was using high concentrations of IL-2. Adding extra IL-2 to *in vitro* suppression assays resulted in abrogation of suppression. It was then found that IL-2 can both overcome T_{reg}-mediated suppression, as well as enhance T_{reg} function by upregulating IL-10, FoxP3, and CTLA-4. IL-2 - deficient mice fail to generate functional regulatory T cells in the periphery, lose CD4+ T cell homeostasis, and suffer from lethal lymphoid hyperplasia,

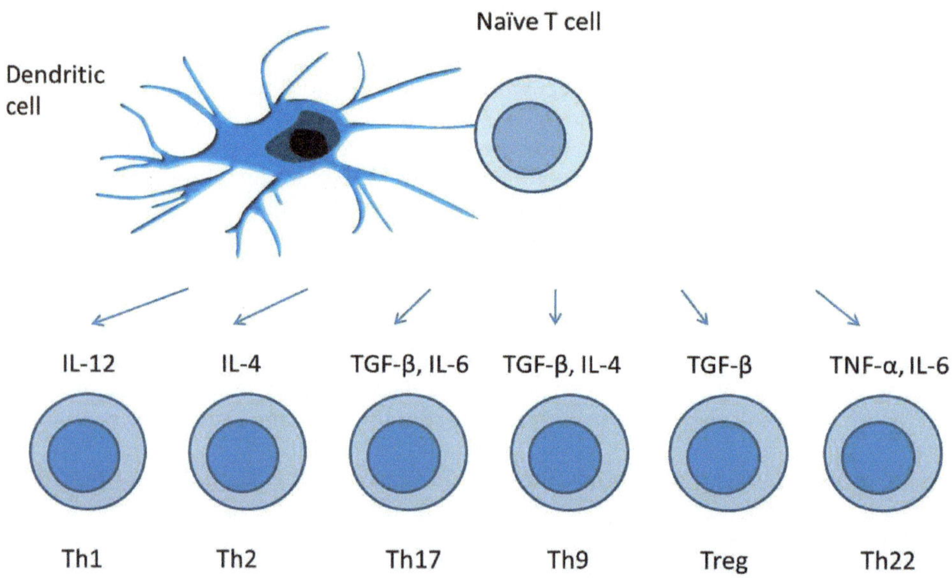

Fig. 2. The differentiation of naïve T cells into effector T cells is mediated by cytokines in the microenviroment. The resulting cytokine profiles, responses to chemokines, and interactions with other cells promote different types of inflammatory responses. In the presence of TGFβ alone, naïve T cells differentiate into regulatory T cells. However, if IL-4 or IL-6 is present, the naïve T cells differentiation into proinflammatory Th9 or Th17 cells. IFN, interferon; IL, interleukin; TGF, transforming growth factor; TNF, tumor necrosis factor (modified from (Jutel M, 2011))

underscoring the significance of IL-2 in T_{reg} development (Sutmuller RPM, 2006). Studies have shown that IL-2 production by effector T cells is not affected; however, T_{regs} act as an IL-2 sink, and sequester IL-2 from the supernatant. Therefore IL-2 likely plays a dual role in boosting T_{reg} function while allowing effector T cells to escape T_{reg}-mediated suppression (Walker, 2009). Interestingly, IL-15 can take over many of IL-2's functions as a growth factor *in vitro*, a phenomenon that may be related to the fact that IL-15 signals through the common IL-2 receptor β and γ chains. However, IL-15 deficient mice do not develop lymphoid hyperplasia, suggesting that IL-2 is more important in T_{reg} development (reviewed in (Sutmuller RPM, 2006)).

2.5 The suppressive activity of regulatory T cells

Currently, human T_{reg}-mediated suppression has only been studied *in vitro* and it is not yet clear if *in vitro* suppression translates to what occurs *in vivo*. Additionally, the exact molecular mechanism of suppression is not yet known. However; the mechanism of suppression has been studied both *in vivo* and *in vitro* in mice and may provide clues as to what occurs in humans. Even though conventional T cells in mice can be induced to express high levels of FoxP3 and have suppressive activity (unlike humans), mice nevertheless provide a valuable animal model to study the overall mechanism of T_{reg}-mediated immune suppression. From mouse studies, we know that several mechanisms may be involved, including cytokine expression, metabolic disruption of the target cell, the alteration of the ability of dendritic cell to activate conventional T cells, and cytolysis (Sakaguchi S, 2010). For example, CTLA4 expressed by T_{regs} can alter expression of CD80 and CD86 on dendritic cells and prevent activation of effector T cells (Wing K, 2008). T_{reg}-mediated suppression requires initial activation through the T cell receptor (Thornton AM, 2000). However, once activated, they do not require antigen-specific TCR activation. In fact, following TCR activation, T_{regs} typically undergo apoptosis yet remain suppressive. Surprisingly, even paraformaldehyde-fixed T_{regs} retain their suppressive function. Suppression also depends on the level of effector T cell activation. Those effector T cells that receive strong co-stimulatory signals remain refractory to T_{reg}-mediated suppression. Additionally, growth-promoting cytokines can overcome T_{reg} function. This suggests that inflammatory responses cannot be modulated in conditions where strong pro-inflammatory signals predominate (Sakaguchi S, 2010). The direct interaction between DCs and T_{reg} can also influence T_{reg} function. T_{reg} cells can downregulate co-stimulatory molecules on immature DCs; however, mature DCs are resistant to T_{reg} effects. Mature DCs express high levels of CD80, CD86, and CD40 which can increase T_{reg} numbers. DCs can also overcome T_{reg}-mediated suppression through the tumor necrosis factor receptor superfamily. Glucocorticoid-induced TNF receptor family-related gene (GITR), OX40, 4-1BB, and RANK can all block T_{reg} -mediated suppression. GITR is expressed at high levels on T_{regs}, and the ligand is expressed primarily on DCs and macrophages. Triggering through GITR induces T_{reg} proliferation but can also block suppression (Sutmuller RPM, 2006).

3. Regulatory T cells in cancer

T_{regs} play a dual role in preventing and enhancing disease in cancer. On one hand, T_{regs} have been shown to inhibit the activation of both CD4+ and CD8+ tumor-suppressor T lymphocytes, and suppress anti-tumor immunity (Zamarron BF, 2011). A correlation between greater numbers of FoxP3+ T cells and larger invasive breast ductal carcinomas was found in sentinel lymph nodes of patients (Gupta R, 2011). Similarly, depletion of FoxP3+ T cells enhances tumor rejection in mice (Zamarron BF, 2011). In these examples, strategies to prevent T_{reg} activation would be needed to enhance anti-tumor immunity. On the other hand, chronic inflammation can promote the development of cancers such as feline vaccine associated sarcomas, feline post-traumatic ocular sarcomas, and colon and hepatocellular carcinomas in humans. In these cases, activating T_{regs} may be necessary to prevent the progression to cancer. Anti-tumor immunity or immunosurveillance is necessary to prevent the development and progression of cancers, through the recognition and elimination of tumor cells. Elimination of tumor cells is primarily dependent on Th1 and CD8+ T cells, and pro-inflammatory cytokines like IFN-γ. It is well established that immunosuppression results in an increase in viral-associated neoplasia. CD4+ T_{regs} initially respond to limit chronic inflammation; however, once tumors are established, their immunosuppressive effect limits anti-tumor immunity and promotes tumor cell growth. Higher numbers of T_{regs} are associated with a shorter time to treatment in patients with chronic lymphocytic leukemia (Weiss L, 2011). Increased expression of FoxP3 and higher numbers of FoxP3+ T cells is associated with a poorer prognosis and shorter time to recurrence in ovarian cancer (Wolf D, 2005), metastatic melanoma (Knol AC, 2011), and gastric cancer (Shen Z, 2010). Paradoxically, in humans, hepatocellular carcinoma is often associated with chronic hepatitis B or C infection. The proposed mechanism is that chronic, unresolved inflammation triggers tumor growth, angiogenesis, and tumor survival (Grivennikov SI, 2010). Additionally, autoimmune diseases are associated with the development of lymphoma, and colon cancer is associated with chronic intestinal inflammation and ulcerative colitis (Grivennikov SI, 2010). Interestingly, T_{regs} within the tumor microenvironment of most cancers are associated with a poor prognosis; however, high T_{reg} infiltration in colon cancer is associated with a favorable prognosis (Ladoire S, 2011). Importantly, this favorable prognosis is not associated with inactivation or loss of function of mismatch repair genes (reviewed in Ladoire, et al, 2011 (Ladoire S, 2011)). While TGFβ is required for activation of FoxP3, the addition of IL-6 results in activation of Th17 cells through the transcription factor RORC. Th17 cells produce IL-17 in the tumor microenvironment. IL-17 has an angiogenic effect, promoting cancer growth and survival, which is necessary for tumor progression. In conditions of excessive inflammation, IL-6 and TGF-β may inhibit T_{reg} function and promote the development of Th17 cells. A recent study by Tosolini et. al demonstrated that colorectal cancers with high numbers of Th17 have a significantly worse prognosis than those with high numbers of T_{reg} cells (Tosolini M, 2011). Although strategies to block T_{reg} function in the treatment of cancer to enhance tumor immunity may be effective for some cancers, they cannot be used as widespread treatments because of the dual role of T_{regs} in the development and progression of cancer.

4. Viral-mediated regulatory T cell induction

Regulatory T cells typically increase late in chronic viral disease to prevent a persistent inflammatory response and viral-mediated immunopathology. In fact, tissue-protective effects of T_{reg} were shown in models of respiratory syncytial virus, Friend virus, and West Nile Virus infection. Additionally, T_{reg} responses to viruses (and bacteria) form the basis of the "hygiene hypothesis." Infection with influenza A in suckling mice protected these mice as adults against allergy induced airway hyperactivity due to the expansion of allergen-specific regulatory T cells (Chang YJ, 2011). Additionally, regulatory T cells responses to

Mycobacterium spp. may provide the explanation for the decreased incidence of asthma and autoimmune diseases in developing countries. However, some viruses have exploited the regulatory immune response, and trigger T_{reg} activation early in the course of disease, leading to immune suppression and viral persistence. Viruses activate endosomal TLRs 3, 7, 8, and 9 (Rouse BT, 2010). Of those, only TLR 7, 8, and 9 are expressed in T_{regs} (Dai J., 2009). Rather than triggering pro-inflammatory cytokines like IFN-α or IFN-γ, persistent viruses often trigger production of IL-10 and TGF-β. For example, dendritic cells infected with Japanese encephalitis virus have increased production of IL-10 and decreased production of IFN-α and TNF-α. In addition, when these infected DCs are cultured with allogenic T cells, they also expanded the population of regulatory T cells (Cao S, 2011). Dendritic cells from lymphocytic choriomeningitis virus-infected mice and monocytes from people infected with hepatitis B, hepatitis C, and human immunodeficiency virus similarly produce increased levels of IL-10 (reviewed in (Rouse BT, 2010)). IL-10 blocks production of pro-inflammatory cytokines and chemokines, and down-regulates MHC class II expression. IL-10 can also inhibit pro-inflammatory cytokine signaling pathways such as NF-κB. In addition, IL-10 suppresses phosphorylation of STAT1 and induces suppressor of cytokine signaling 3 (SOCS3) expression by neutrophils and macrophages (Rouse BT, 2010). Protective immunity against hepatitis C virus is associated with a robust Th1 response and production of IFN-γ. However, approximately 85% of patients respond with IL-10-producing CD8+ and CD4+ T cells, and occasionally FoxP3+ T_{regs} (Wang J-P, 2010). These patients develop chronic HCV infection, while those that respond with a Th1 response clear the virus (Rouse BT, 2010). Hall et al showed that HCV-infected hepatocytes are capable of inducing T_{regs}. HCV-infected hepatoma cell lines were co-cultured with activated CD4+ T cells resulting in decreased production of IFN-γ and increased expression of CD25, CTLA-4, FoxP3, and LAP. These T_{regs} were able to suppress effector T cells and upregulate production of TGF-β. T_{reg} function and phenotype was inhibited by blocking TGF-β, suggesting that this phenomenon is also TGF-β dependent (Hall CHT, 2010). Early in disease, T_{regs}, TGF-β, and IL-10 production in HCV infection are associated with development of chronic infection. On the other hand, in patients already chronically infected with HCV, IL-10 production does appear to have a protective effect since patients with the highest level of IL-10 tend to have a better prognosis. Disease progression in human and simian immunodeficiency virus infection is associated with the loss of Th17 cells, and an increase in CD4+FoxP3+ T_{regs}. Surprisingly, the loss of Th17 cells was associated with increased immune activation. Investigators found that because Th17 cells were responsible for maintaining the integrity of the mucosal barrier in the intestine, loss of Th17 cells resulted in increased microbial translocation across the gut (reviewed in (Kanwar B, 2010). Both HIV and SIV infection trigger an increase in regulatory T cells that produce TGF-β1. This in turn triggers TGF-β1 signaling in fibroblasts resulting in production of chitinase 3-like1 (CHI3L1) and pro-collagen. CHI3L1 enhances maturation of the procollagen into collagen in lymphoid tissue fibroblasts resulting in lymphoid tissue fibrosis. Lymphoid tissue fibrosis limits access of lymphocytes to reticular cells and IL-7 which depletes naïve CD4+ T cells. This may be one mechanism of CD4 depletion in HIV (Zeng M, 2011).

Further evidence of the role of T_{regs} in chronic viral infections is seen in the mouse model of infection with lymphocytic choriomeningitis virus (LCMV). Infections with different strains of LCMV can either cause acute infection that is cleared within a week (Armstrong strain), or chronic infection in which the mice are infected for life (variant clone 13). In variant clone 13-infected mice, mice with a specific TCR (Vβ5) have more prominent activation and expansion of T_{regs}. These T_{regs} expand from an existing T_{reg} -population and expansion is dependent on retrovirus-encoded superantigens in the mouse genome (Punkosdy GA, 2011). However, it is not known if the T_{reg} expansion is involved in establishing chronic infection in this model. These viruses and others have exploited the phenomenon of activation of T_{regs} in response to infection by triggering T_{reg} proliferation early in disease progression. T_{reg} activation allows them to evade the host immune response and persist in the host. Using animal models to understand the mechanism of T_{reg} activation and expansion is vital to developing strategies to combat some of the persistent viral diseases that are not controlled well by vaccination.

5. The pig as an immunological model

Pigs provide a powerful tool in viral immunology studies, including the study of both innate and adaptive immunity. Germ free and gnotobiotic pigs can be relatively easily derived by cesarean section, and since pigs have epitheliochorial placentation, there is no interference by maternal antibody if the pigs are removed from the dam before suckling (Butler JE, 2009),(Butler JE, 2007). Although outbred, the pig is large enough that all *in vitro* tests can be done using cells from the same animal. Additionally, litter sizes are very large, decreasing genetic diversity of individual animals. Like humans, each individual can be treated as a biological unit (Butler JE, 2009), and using isolator piglets can decrease environmental variables. Pigs have digestive and respiratory systems, as well as T cell receptor and light chain repertoires that are similar to humans (reviewed in Butler, et al., 2009(Butler JE, 2009)). Importantly, porcine dendritic cells (DC) resemble human DCs, making them ideal to study pathogen responses relevant to humans (Paillot R, 2001; Raymond CR, 2005; Summerfield A, 2009). Additionally, porcine regulatory T cells function similarly to humans.

6. Porcine regulatory T cells

While regulatory T cells had been described and characterized in humans and mice since 1995 (Sakaguchi S, 1995), they were not demonstrated in pigs until 2008 (Käser T, 2008a, b). Although FoxP3 expression has been found in cells without suppressive activity in mice (Chen X, 2011), FoxP3 remains the most relevant phenotypic marker for T_{regs} in pigs. Identification and characterization of these cells was made possible by the fact that the anti-mouse monoclonal antibody FJK-16s (eBiosciences, San Diego, CA) cross-reacts with porcine regulatory T cells (Käser T, 2008b). The majority of FoxP3+ cells are also CD25+; however, in contrast to the findings of Käser et. al, we identified a small percentage of porcine FoxP3+ cells that do not express CD25. Besides CD4+ T_{regs}, FoxP3 expression was also found on CD4-CD8α+ T cells, as well as CD4+ T_{regs} that also expressed CD45RC (Käser T, 2008a), CD8α, and MHC-II (Käser T, 2008b). Our understanding the mechanism of porcine T_{reg} suppression is still in its infancy. A recent publication by Käser et al demonstrated that T_{reg} suppression can occur in any one of three ways: 1) cell-contact dependent, 2) production of IL-10 or TGF-β, or 3) by competing for IL-2 (Käser T, 2011). Interestingly, the authors showed that IL-10 was produced by $CD4+CD25^{dim}$ cells, which have lower suppressive activity in swine (Käser T, 2008a). This suggests that IL-10 is likely produced by activated Th2 cells rather than regulatory T cells.

7. Regulatory T cells and pig viral diseases

7.1 The immune response to porcine reproductive and respiratory syndrome virus

Since the initial description of porcine reproductive and respiratory syndrome (PRRS) in the USA in 1987 (Collins JE, 1992; Keffaber, 1989), the disease has been shown to be endemic in many swine producing countries, and is now considered to be the most important disease of swine worldwide (www.prrs.org,(Xiao Z, 2004)). In the USA alone, economic losses caused by PRRS virus (PRRSV) infection are estimated to total $560 million (www.prrs.org). PRRSV is a single-stranded, positive sense RNA virus in the *Arteriviridae* family, order *Nidovirales* (Cavanaugh, 1997). Other *Arteriviridae* include lactate dehydrogenase-elevating virus, equine arteritis virus, and simian hemorrhagic fever virus (Cavanaugh, 1997). Within a susceptible herd, reproductive failure due to PRRSV infection can range from sporadic abortions to abortion storms that may persist within the herd for up to 6 months (Rossow, 1998). Third-trimester exposure may manifest as late-term abortion, or stillborn, partially autolyzed, or mummified fetuses (Rossow, 1998). Neonatal infection results in severe dyspnea and tachypnea, and mortality of up to 100%, while disease in weaned pigs is primarily due to pneumonia and secondary bacterial or viral infections (Rossow, 1998). In addition to clinical disease, PRRSV infection is associated with decreased local cellular immunity, resulting in increased susceptibility to secondary bacterial and viral infections, including *Streptococcus suis, Haemophilus parasuis, Mycoplasma hyopneumoniae, Salmonella choleraesuis,* and swine influenza virus (Riber U, 2004; Rossow KD, 1995; Zeman D, 1993). Piglets infected with PRRS in utero have a decreased innate immune response to bacterial pathogens (Riber U, 2004). Riber and colleagues showed that in utero infection with PRRSV inhibits the phagocytic ability of blood macrophages against *Salmonella* spp., and inhibits the oxidative burst capacity of alveolar macrophages (Riber U, 2004). Additionally, both PRRSV infection and vaccination decreases the efficiency of vaccines against *Mycoplasma hyopneumoniae* (Thacker EL, 2000) and porcine pestivirus (Suradhat S, 2006). Infection and vaccination with PRRSV induces a rapid, non-neutralizing antibody response, and an early, weak gamma interferon (IFN-γ) response (Meier WA, 2003; Wesley RD, 2006). The initial IFN-γ response is not PRRSV-specific and may be a result of activation of natural killer cells (Wesley RD, 2006). A PRRSV-specific T lymphocyte IFN-γ response does not appear until at least 2 weeks after infection (Xiao Z, 2004). The IFN-γ response gradually increases and plateaus at 6 months postinfection, and is associated with a slow increase in neutralizing antibody (Lopez OJ, 2004; Meier WA, 2003). Protective immunity is associated with both an IFN-γ and neutralizing antibody response; however, peak viremia and shedding occur before development of neutralizing antibody and IFN-γ (Lopez OJ, 2004). Acute infection is characterized by high viral load in alveolar and tissue macrophages, and may last up to one month. The acute infection is followed by persistence of lower levels of virus in lymphoid tissue and then clearance after several months (Lopez OJ, 2004). The cause of the delayed IFN-γ and neutralizing antibody response resulting in persistent infection is unknown. Meier et al. were unable to enhance the induction of PRRSV-specific IFN-γ secreting cells and generation of neutralizing antibody using an adjuvant that enhances the immune response to pseudorabies modified live vaccine (Meier WA, 2003). These data suggest that the virus somehow modulates the immune response to not only delay the response to the virus itself, but to also decrease the ability to mount a protective response against secondary infection. The ability to induce a rapid IFN-γ response is not only important for viral clearance, but also heterologous protection by vaccination (Díaz I, 2006; Martelli P, 2009).

Current vaccine strains do not provide adequate heterologous protection because of their inability to stimulate an adequate IFN-γ response. One reason for the inadequate IFN-γ may be due to the ability of PRRSV to stimulate regulatory T cells *in vitro* (Silva-Campa E, 2009). The mechanism of immune modulation by PRRSV is unknown. PRRSV infection results in a significant upregulation of IL-10 expression in peripheral blood mononuclear cells and pulmonary alveolar macrophages in vivo and in vitro, and the upregulation of IL-10 is increased significantly with concurrent *M. hyopneumoniae* infection (Suradhat S, 2003; Thanawongnuwech R, 2004). The increase in IL-10 expression correlates with an increased percentage of lymphocytes in bronchoalveolar lavage cells, suggesting that the lymphocytes are involved in cytokine production in the lungs (Suradhat S, 2003).

7.1.1 Immune modulation mediated by interleukin-10

Low levels of interleukin-10 (IL-10) stimulate the proliferation of B cells, and activate natural killer (NK) cells and CD8+ cytotoxic T cells (Vicari AP, 2004). However, the primary action of IL-10 is to inhibit inflammatory cytokines and antagonize the function of antigen presenting cells, including immature dendritic cells (DC) (Enk, 2005). In humans and mice, exposure of immature DCs to IL-10 in vitro results in decreased surface expression of MHC class I and II molecules, reduction of costimulatory molecules, and inhibition of pro-inflammatory cytokines including IL-1β, IL-6, TNFα, and IL-12 (Enk, 2005). Additionally, IL-10 inhibits the synthesis of pro-inflammatory cytokines, the production of nitric oxide, and MHC class II expression by macrophages (Fiorentino DF, 1991; Gazzinelli RT, 1992). Since IL-12-mediated production of IFN-γ by pulmonary alveolar macrophages reduces PRRS viral titers in the lungs and serum (Carter QL, 2005), inhibition of IL-12 synthesis by IL-10 likely enhances the occurrence of natural disease. IL-10 affects innate immunity by inhibiting the response to Toll-like receptors (TLR), including TLR7 and TLR8 that recognize single-stranded viral RNA (Vicari AP, 2004). IL-10 - treated DCs also induce the proliferation of regulatory T cells (T_{regs}) as well as antigen-specific anergy in CD4+ and CD8+ T lymphocytes (Enk, 2005). Importantly, IL-10 not only plays a role in the development of type 1 T_{regs} (Tr1), but is also one of the primary mechanisms by which T_{regs} inhibit effector T lymphocyte function (Vicari AP, 2004). In previous experiments, we have shown that PRRSV infection increases the number of CD4+CD25+FoxP3+ regulatory T cells in the lungs and PBMC of pigs (LeRoith, unpublished). Others have shown that the induced T_{regs} produce TGF-β, consistent with a Th3 phenotype,(Silva-Campa E, 2009) indicating that the cells are not only increased, but are also functional. Since intracellular viral ssRNA is recognized by TLR7 and 8, and TLR7- and 8-signalling downregulates T_{regs} (Dai J, 2009), it is unlikely that this increase in T_{reg} numbers is merely a result of infection.

Which components of the virus are responsible for T_{reg} proliferation are unknown, but are currently under investigation by our group. Importantly, we were able to demonstrate that T_{reg} induction by PRRSV results in increased susceptibility to natural *Mycoplasma hyopneumoniae* infection (LeRoith T, 2011). In this study, pigs were inoculated with a virulent strain of PRRSV and a modified live vaccine that was derived from the same strain. In attenuation of this virus to produce the vaccine strain, approximately 30% of the mutations were in the replicase region (ORF 1)(Yuan S, 2001) and the majority of the mutations in this region were silent. Another 35% of the mutations were in the structural proteins, and the majority of mutations resulted in conservative or non-conservative amino acid changes(Yuan S, 2001). We hypothesized that even with changes in the non-structural and structural proteins that decrease the pathogenicity, the mutations did not alter the virus's ability to stimulate T_{regs}. Consistent with our hypothesis, we found that, although attenuated, the vaccine strain did not differ from the parent strain in its ability to activate T_{regs}. Although the animals were protected against PRRS challenge, animals in the attenuated vaccine group did not differ from animals in the virulent group in the severity of *M. hyopneumonia*-mediated disease (Table 2) (LeRoith T, 2011). Similar to previous findings that infection with wild type PRRSV or vaccination with PRRS MLV vaccines has been shown to decrease the efficacy of *M. hyopneumoniae* vaccines (Thacker EL, 2000), inoculation with all three PRRSV in this study resulted in activation regulatory T cells and likely decreased the ability of the pigs to mount an effective anti-bacterial immune.

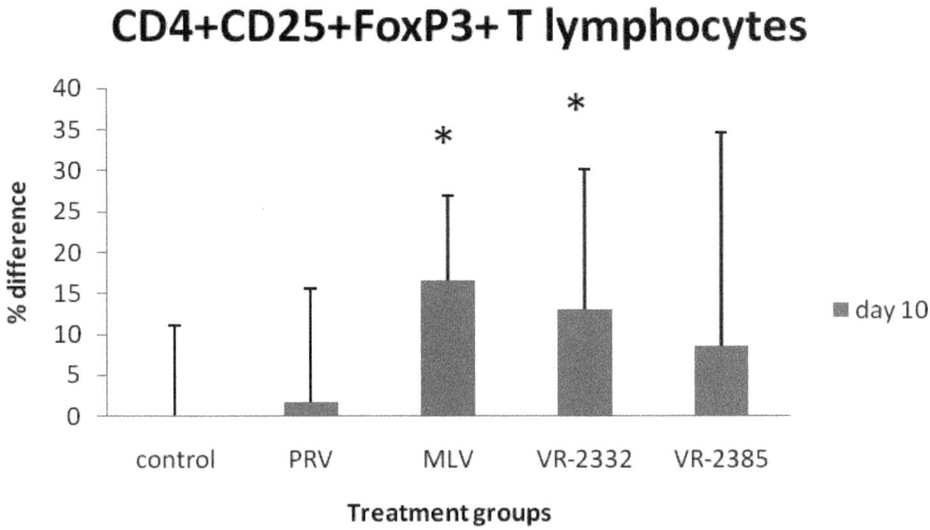

Fig. 3. Modified live virus vaccine and PRRSV infection significantly increases regulatory T cells 10 days post infection. The graph represents mean differences in regulatory T cells as determined by flow cytometry. Error bars represent standard errors. *= significantly different from the control ($p < 0.05$). PRV, pseudorabies virus; MLV, modified live virus vaccine; VR-2332, reference strain of porcine reproductive and respiratory syndrome virus; VR-2385, pathogenic strain of porcine reproductive and respiratory syndrome virus. (modified from (LeRoith T, 2011))

Importantly, vaccine efficacy appears to be related to the ability to stimulate IFN-γ production. Also, efficacy against heterologous virus challenge seems to correlate more with the ability to stimulate IFN-γ than homology of the vaccine strain to the infective strain. Current vaccines fail to protect against other strains (Mateu E, 2007), which may be due to their inability to stimulate IFN-γ production. Our study was the first to show the correlation between vaccine induction of T_{regs} and increased susceptibility to bacterial infection. Although T_{regs} that are induced by PRRS *in vitro* produce TGF-β (Silva-Campa E, 2009), the induction of T_{regs} may indirectly result in IL-10 production, a phenomenon that is well established in the PRRS literature (Feng WH, 2003; Suradhat S, 2003). Production of IL-10 instead of IFN-γ by the MLV vaccine strain would lead to a lack of heterologous protection, and decreased efficacy of other vaccines, as seen by other authors (Thacker EL, 2000). Our results suggest that mutations in the vaccine strain that result in attenuation of the virus do not alter the virus's ability to stimulate T_{regs} (LeRoith T, 2011). This information can help us design vaccines in which the T_{reg}-stimulating epitopes can be mutated or deleted in order to stimulate a robust virus-specific IFN-γ response, and provide protection against heterologous strains (LeRoith T, 2011).

Treatment Group	Number of pigs with lung lesions	Lung lesion scores
Control	3/5	2.2 ± 0.96
PRV vaccine	5/7	2.67 ± 0.78
PRRSV MLV vaccine	7/8	3.14 ± 0.78**
PRRSV VR-2332	8/8	3.75 ± 1.06*
PRRSV VR-2385	5/8	3 ± 1.2

* Significantly different from the control (p = 0.024)
**Trend towards a significant difference from the control (p = 0.086)

Table 2. Incidence and severity of *Mycoplasma hyopneumoniae* microscopic lung lesions ((LeRoith T, 2011))

7.2 Small single-stranded circular DNA viruses

Porcine circovirus 2 (PCV2) is a small, single stranded, non-enveloped, circular DNA virus in the family *Circoviridae*. PCV2-associated diseases are of the most economically important diseases in swine, and include post-weaning multisystemic wasting syndrome (PMWS) and porcine dermatitis and nephropathy syndrome (PDNS) (Allan GM, 2000). Porcine circoviruses are widespread in the United States pork industry, and can often be isolated from both pork products and human feces (Li L, 2009). The contamination of human rotavirus vaccines by porcine circovirus type 1 and type 2 led to the temporarily suspension of the licensed rotavirus vaccines [http://www.virology.ws/2010/03/22/porcine-circovirus-dna-in-rotavirus-vaccine/]. Although PCV2 has been recognized as necessary to produce PCVAD, it is difficult to experimentally reproduce the disease with PCV2 alone (Magar R, 2000),(Allan GM, 2003). Typically infection by other viruses, immune stimulation, or vaccination is required to reproduce clinical disease (Krakowka S, 2001). Other small, single stranded, circular DNA viruses infecting both humans and other animals are of the genus Anellovirus, including Torque teno virus (TTV) and TTV-like mini virus (TLMV) (Biagini, 2004). TTV is ubiquitous in the human population; however no specific disease has been linked to TTV infection. Interestingly, TTVs are more frequently reported in malignant biopsies from human compared to controls (zur Hausen H, 2009) and are associated, at least epidemiologically with liver disease, respiratory disease, cancer, and blood disorders (Okamoto, 2009). Additionally, higher TTV viral loads are found in patients with systemic lupus erythematosis (SLE) and idiopathic inflammatory myopathies (Gergely P Jr, 2006). Swine TTV in conjunction with a respiratory virus has also been shown to produce PDNS without PCV2 in gnotobiotic pigs (Krakowka S, 2008), producing lesions not seen with the respiratory virus alone. How TTV and other circoviruses contribute to disease is unknown, but there is evidence that anelloviruses affect both innate and adaptive immunity and can impact how the infected host can respond to other pathogens (Maggi F, 2009). Some authors suggest that the role of TTV in carcinogenesis may be due to its effect on antitumoral immunity (zur Hausen H, 2009). Other small, single-stranded DNA viruses include human bocavirus, human parvovirus 4, and parvovirus B19 (B19). B19, the causative agent of Fifth disease in children, typically causes self-limiting disease in immunocompetent individuals; however, virus has been shown to persist in the bone marrow several years after primary infection (Servant-Delmas A, 2010). The mechanism of persistence is unknown. PCV2 is ubiquitous in the swine industry, and genetically similar strains have been isolated from both diseased and healthy pigs. There is overwhelming evidence that PCV2 has an immunomodulatory effect by infecting macrophages and dendritic cells (DC's) and inducing DC maturation (Vincent IE, 2005). Pigs with PMWS have higher viral loads of PCV2 (Rosell C, 1999),(Rovira A, 2002),(Liu Q, 2000), suggesting that disease is associated with enhanced PCV2 replication. One of the major contributors to the development of PMWS is co-infection with porcine reproductive and respiratory syndrome virus (PRRSV). Pigs with PMWS have an increase in monocytes, the presence of low-density immature granulocytes in peripheral blood; and a decrease in CD4+ and CD4+CD8+ T lymphocytes and B lymphocytes (Darwich L, 2002), (Segalés J AF, 2001). Pigs co-infected with PCV2 and PRRSV have more severe lymphoid depletion and enhanced PCV2 replication and tissue distribution (Allan GM, 2000; Harms PA SS, 2001; Rovira A, 2002), suggesting that the interaction between the two viruses is important in the pathogenesis of clinical disease. The effect of the interaction between the two viruses on the immune system is not well understood. It has been suggested that immune stimulation by PRRSV enhances PCV2-mediated disease (Krakowka S, 2001). However; PRRSV, both infection and vaccination, has been shown to non-specifically dampen the immune response to other infectious agents (Suradhat S, 2003; Thacker EL, 2000). Additionally, a protective effect of porcine parvovirus and erysipelas vaccination against PMWS was shown in piglets born to PCV2 infected sows, further supporting the idea that factors other than immune stimulation may be involved in clinical disease. Importantly, when PMWS is produced by a combination of PCV2 and PRRSV, although current vaccines against PCV2 are able to decrease the severity of PMWS-associated lesions, the vaccines alone are ineffective at completely diminishing the lesions to those of PRRSV infection alone (Opriessnig T MD, 2008). The contribution of the immune effects of each virus in producing clinical PMWS is unknown. PRRSV infects and replicates in alveolar macrophages and dendritic cells, resulting in IL-10 production and proliferation of regulatory T cells. PCV2 is taken up by DCs and alveolar macrophages but does not replicate in these cells and has no effect on them other than to increase differentiation of DCs. Importantly, generally co-infection by both viruses is needed to produce PMWS. Presumably, PCV2 may enhance differentiation of DCs, thereby increasing the number of cells available for PRRSV infection, resulting in increased IL-10 production, and regulatory T cell activation. Since T_{reg} activation is associated with a decreased IFN-γ response, and IFN-γ is necessary for protective immunity against PCV2, PRRSV-mediated activation of regulatory T cells may then dampen the immune response to PCV2, resulting in increased virus replication and clinical disease. We are interested in determining if the effects of PCV2 on DC maturation and PRRSV-mediated activation of T_{regs} is enhanced in pigs with endemic PCV2 infection, or if PCV2 infection at the time of PRRSV infection is necessary for developing PMWS. Our data shows that PCV2 is able to induce regulatory T cells (T_{regs}) *in vitro* (Fig 4), and this effect is enhanced by the addition of a second virus, PRRSV (Cecere T, manuscript under review).

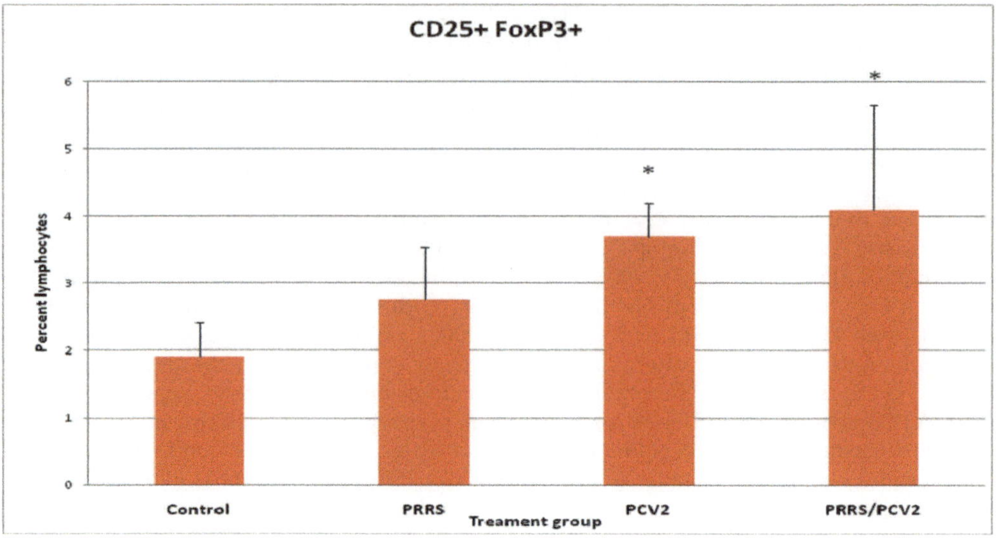

Fig. 4. PCV2 and PCV2/PRRSV co-infection of porcine dendritic cells results inactivation of CD25+FoxP3+ T lymphocytes *in vitro* compared to the control ($p < 0.05$).

What is unknown is whether or not chronic or persistent PCV2 or acute infection is associated with more severe pulmonary immunosuppression (as defined by T_{reg} activation and suppression of effector T cell function, IL-10 production, and suppression of IFN-γ production), leading to more severe manifestation of PMWS. It is also not yet clear if pigs persistently infected with PCV2 are at a higher risk of developing PMWS when infected with PRRSV than pigs acutely infected with PCV2 and PRRSV. Additionally, it is not known if acute PCV2 infection in pigs already persistenly infected with a different PCV2 genotype is associated with a higher incidence of PMWS when infected with PRRSV.

8. Conclusion

Regulatory T cells are critical for maintaining immune tolerance and immune homeostasis by protecting against devastating autoimmune disease and overwhelming inflammation. Without these subsets of T cells, animals quickly succumb to inflammatory or autoimmune diseases. The dual role of Tregs fits well into the perspectives proposed by Khatami that unresolved inflammation is the loss of balance between the "Yin" or tumoricidal and "Yang" or tumorigenic arms of acute inflammation (Khatami, 2008, 2009, 2011). Tregs play a vital role in preventing what Khatami terms "pathogen-induced immunological chaos," the "immune tsunami," or cytokine storm can then lead to inflammatory disease and cancer (Khatami, 2011). Immunologists are currently trying to identify strategies to enhance regulatory T cell activation to protect against inflammatory disease such as systemic lupus erythematosis and rheumatoid arthritis. However, some viruses, including PRRSV in pigs, have exploited these cells to enhance their survival and replication in the host. Activation of regulatory T cells by viruses dampens the immune response to the virus and allows them to replicate and persist in host tissues. Understanding the mechanism of T_{reg} activation by viruses is critical for identifying new strategies to prevent the effects on the host. In many cases, activation of T_{regs} not only dampens the immune response to the virus, but non-specifically dampens the immune response to other pathogens. While the initial immune suppression likely plays a role in virus persistence, the non-specific immune suppression is one of the mechanisms by which secondary infection can occur. The complete effects of these viruses on the immune response of the host are still under investigation. The ability of certain viruses to stimulate regulatory provides valuable insight as to how viruses modulate the immune system. Understanding the mechanisms of T_{reg} induction is important in determining the contribution of RNA and small single-stranded circular DNA virus like PCV2, TTV, and parvovirus to the development of disease. Understanding the contribution of the immune response to viruses is also essential for vaccine development. PRRSV and PCV2 infection in swine provide a valuable animal model to study the immune effects of viruses because pigs are outbred and are immunologically similar to humans. Additionally, germ-free and colostrum deprived pigs are relatively easy to derive and function well in the experimental environment. With these models, we may be able to uncover some of the mysteries of the contribution of T_{regs} in chronic infectious and inflammatory disease.

9. References

Allan GM, E.J., 2000, Porcine circoviruses: a review. Journal of Veterinary Diagnostic Investigation 12, 3-14.

Allan GM, M.F., Meehan BM, McNair I, Ellis JA, Krakowka SJ, Fossum C, Wattrang E, Wallgren P, Adair BM, 2003, Reproduction of postweaning multisystemic wasting syndrome in pigs experimentally inoculated with a Swedish porcine circovirus 2 isolate. Journal of Veterinary Diagnostic Investigation 15, 553-560.

Bacchetta R, G.S., Rocarolo M, 2005, CD4+ regulatory T cells: Mechanisms of induction and effector function. Autoimmunity Reviews 4, 491-496.

Beissert S, S.A., Schwarz T, 2006, Regulatory T Cells. The Society for Investigative Dermatology 126, 15-24.

Bennett CL, C.J., Ramsdell F, Brunkow ME, Ferguson PJ, Whitesell L, Kelly TE, Saulsbury FT, Chance PF, Ochs HD., 2001, The immune dysregulation, polyendocrinopathy, enteropathy, X-linked syndrome (IPEX) is caused by mutations of FOXP3. Nature Genetics 27, 20-21.

Biagini, 2004, Human circoviruses. Veterinary Microbiology 98, 95-101.

Butler JE, L.K., Splichal I, Francis D, Kacskovics I, Sinkora M, Wertz N, Sun J, Zhao Y, Brown WR, DeWald R, Dierks S, Muyldermans S, Lunney JK, McCray PB, Rogers CS, Welsh MJ, Navarro P, Klobasa F, Habe F, Ramsoondar J, 2009, The piglet as a model for B cell and immune system development. Veterinary Immunology and Immunopathology 128, 147-170.

Butler JE, S.M., 2007, The isolator piglet: a model for studying the development of adaptive immunity. Immunology Research 39, 33-51.

Cao S, L.Y., Ye J, Yang X, Chen L, Liu X, Chen H., 2011, Japanese encephalitis Virus wild strain infection suppresses dendritic cells maturation and function, and causes the expansion of regulatory T cells. Virology Journal, 39.

Carter QL, C.R., 2005, Interleukin-12 (IL-12) ameliorates the effects of porcine respiratory and reproductive syndrome virus (PRRSV) infection. Veterinary Immunology and Immunopathology 107, 105-118.

Cavanaugh, D., 1997, Nidovirales: a new order comprising coronaviridae and arteriviridae. Archives of Virology 142, 629-633.

Chang YJ, K.H., Albacker LA, Lee HH, Baumgarth N, Akira S, Savage PB, Endo S, Yamamura T, Maaskant J, Kitano N, Singh A, Bhatt A, Besra GS, van den Elzen P, Appelmelk B, Franck RW, Chen G, DeKruyff RH, Shimamura M, Illarionov P, Umetsu DT., 2011, Influenza infection in suckling mice expands an NKT cell subset that protects against airway hyperreactivity. Journal of Clinical Investigation 121, 57-69.

Chen X, O.J., 2011, Resolving the identity myth: Key markers of functional CD4(+)FoxP3(+) regulatory T cells. International Immunopharmacology Epub ahead of print.

Collins JE, B.D., Christianson WT, Harris L, Hennings JC, Shaw DP, Goyal SM, McCullough S, Morrison RB, Joo HS, Gorcyca DE, Chladek DW, 1992, Isolation of swine infertility and respiratory syndrome virus (isolate ATCC VR-2332) in North America and experimental reproduction of the disease in gnotobiotic pigs. Journal of Veterinary Diagnostic Investigation 4, 117-126.

Dai J, L.B., Li Z, 2009, Regulatory T cells and Toll-like receptors: what is the missing link? International Immunopharmacology 9, 528-533.

Dai J., L.B., Li Z, 2009, Regulatory T cells and Toll-like receptors: What is the missing link? International Immunopharmacology 9, 528-533.

Darwich L, S.J., Domingo M, Mateu E., 2002, Changes in CD4(+), CD8(+), CD4(+) CD8(+), and immunoglobulin M-positive peripheral blood mononuclear cells of postweaning multisystemic wasting syndrome-affected pigs and age-matched uninfected wasted and healthy pigs correlate with lesions and porcine circovirus type 2 load in lymphoid tissues. Clinical Diagnostic Laboratory Immunology 9, 236-242.

Díaz I, D.L., Pappaterra G, Pujols J, Mateu E., 2006, Different European-type vaccines against porcine reproductive and respiratory syndrome virus have different immunological properties and confer different protection to pigs. Virology 351, 249-259.

Dittmer U, H.H., Messer RJ, Schimmer S, Olbrich ARM, Ohlen C, Greenberg PD, Stromnes IM, Iwashiro M, Sakaguchi S, Evans LH, Peterson KE, Yang G, Hasenkrug KJ, 2004, Functional impairment of CD8+ T cells by regulatory T cells during persistent retroviral infection. Immunity 20, 293-303.

Enk, A., 2005, Dendritic cells in tolerance induction. Immunology Letters 99, 8-11.

Feng WH, T.M., Xu JS, Zhang HX, McCaw MB. , 2003, Analysis of constitutive cytokine expression by pigs infected in-utero with porcine reproductive and respiratory syndrome virus. Veterinary Immunology and Immunopathology 94, 35-45.

Fiorentino DF, Z.A., Mosmann TR, Howard M, O'Garra A, 1991, IL-10 inhibits cytokine production by activated macrophages. The Journal of Immunology 147, 3815-3822.

Gazzinelli RT, O.I., James SL, Sher A, 1992, IL-10 inhibits parasite killing and nitrogen oxide production by IFN-g-activated macrophages. The Journal of Immunology 148, 1792-1796.

Gergely P Jr, P.A., Poór G, 2006, Possible pathogenic nature of the recently discovered TT virus: does it play a role in autoimmune rheumatic diseases? Autoimmunity Reviews 6, 5-9.

Grivennikov SI, G.F., Karin M., 2010, Immunity, inflammation, and cancer. Cell 140, 883-899.

Gückel E, F.S., Zaiss MM, Schett G, Ghosh S, Voll RE., 2011, Cell-Intrinsic NF-κB Activation Is Critical for the Development of Natural Regulatory T Cells in Mice. PLoS One 5, e20003.

Gupta R, B.J., Singh B, Chiriboga L, Liebes L, Adams S, Demaria S., 2011, The Numbers of FoxP3+ Lymphocytes in Sentinel Lymph Nodes of Breast Cancer Patients Correlate With Primary Tumor Size but Not Nodal Status. Cancer Investigation 29, 419-425

Hall CHT, K.R., Tacke RS, Hahn YS, 2010, HCV+ Hepatocytes Induce Human Regulatory CD4+ T Cells through the Production of TGF-b. PLoS One 5, e12154.

Harms PA SS, H.P., Bolin SR, Lager KM, Morozov I, Paul PS, 2001, Experimental reproduction of severe disease in CD/CD pigs concurrently infected with type 2 porcine circovirus and porcine reproductive and respiratory syndrome virus. Veterinary Pathology 38, 525-539.

Iwashiro M, M.R., Peterson KE, Stromnes IM, Sugie T, Hasenkrug KJ, 2001, Immunosuppression by CD4+ regulatory T cells induced by chronic retroviral infection. PNAS 98, 9226-9230.

Jutel M, A.C., 2011, T-cell subset regulation in atopy. Current Allergy and Asthma Reports 11, 139-145.

Kanwar B, F.D., McCune JM., 2010, Th17 and regulatory T cells: implications for AIDS pathogenesis. Current Opinions in HIV and AIDs 5, 151-157.

Käser T, G.W., Hammer SE, Patzl M, Saalmüller A, 2008a, Detection of Foxp3 protein expression in porcine T lymphocytes. Veterinary Immunology and Immunopathology 125, 92-101.

Käser T, G.W., Hammer SE, Patzl M, Saalmüller A, 2008b, Phenotypic and functional characterisation of porcine CD4(+)CD25(high) regulatory T cells. Veterinary Immunology and Immunopathology 122, 153-158.

Käser T, G.W., Saalmüller A., 2011, Porcine regulatory T cells: Mechanisms and T-cell targets of suppression. Developmental and Comparative Immunology Epub ahead of print.

Keffaber, K., 1989, Reproductive failure of unknown etiology. American Association of Swine Practitioners Newsletter 1, 1-9.

Khatami, M., 2008, 'Yin and Yang' in inflammation: duality in innate immune cell function and tumorigenesis. Expert Opinion on Biological Therapy 8, 1461-1472.

Khatami, M., 2009, Inflammation, aging, and cancer: tumoricidal versus tumorigenesis of immunity: a common denominator mapping chronic diseases. Cell Biochemistry and Biophysics 55, 55-79.

Khatami, M., 2011, Unresolved inflammation: 'immune tsunami' or erosion of integrity in immune-privileged and immune-responsive tissues and acute and chronic inflammatory diseases or cancer. Expert Opinion on Biological Therapy Jun 11. [Epub ahead of print].

Knol AC, N.J., Quéreux G, Brocard A, Khammari A, Dréno B., 2011, Prognostic value of tumor-infiltrating Foxp3+ T-cell subpopulations in metastatic melanoma. Experimental Dermatology 20, 430-434.

Krakowka S, E.J., McNeilly F, Ringler S, Rings DM, Allan G., 2001, Activation of the immune system is the pivotal event in the production of wasting disease in pigs infected with porcine circovirus-2 (PCV-2). Veterinary Pathology 38, 31-42.

Krakowka S, H.C., Hamberg A, Shoup D, Rings M, Zhang Y, Allan G, Ellis JA., 2008, Evaluation of induction of porcine dermatitis and nephropathy syndrome in gnotobiotic pigs with negative results for porcine circovirus type 2. American Journal of Veterinary Research 69, 1615-1622.

Ladoire S, M.F., Ghiringhelli F., 2011, Prognostic role of FOXP3+ regulatory T cells infiltrating human carcinomas: the paradox of colorectal cancer. Cancer Immunology, Immunotheraphy Jun 5. [Epub ahead of print].

LeRoith T, H.S., Todd SM, Ni Y, Cecere T, Pelzer KD., 2011, A modified live PRRSV vaccine and the pathogenic parent strain induce regulatory T cells in pigs naturally infected with Mycoplasma hyopneumoniae. Veterinary Immunology and Immunopathology 140, 312-316.

Li L, K.A., Slikas B, Bamidele OS, Wang C, Shaukat S, Masroor MA, Wilson ML, Ndjango JB, Peeters M, Gross-Camp ND, Muller MN, Hahn BH, Wolfe ND, Triki H, Bartkus J, Zaidi SZ, Delwart E., 2009, Multiple diverse circoviruses infect farm animals and are commonly found in human and chimpanzee feces. Journal of Virology 84, 1674-1682.

Liu Q, W.L., Willson P, Babiuk LA., 2000, Quantitative, competitive PCR analysis of porcine circovirus DNA in serum from pigs with postweaning multisystemic wasting syndrome. Journal of Clinical Microbiology 38, 3474-3477.

Lopez OJ, O.F., 2004, Role of neutralizing antibodies in PRRSV protective immunity. Veterinary Immunology and Immunopathology 102, 155-163.

MacDonald AJ, D.M., Brady MT, McKiernan S, Hall W, Hegarty J, Curry M, Mills KHG, 2002, CD4 helper type 1 and regulatory T cells induced against the same epitopes on the core protein in hepatitis C virus-infected persons. The Journal of Infectious Diseases 185, 720-727.

Magar R, L.R., Thibault S, Lamontagne L, 2000, Experimental transmission of porcine circovirus type 2 (PCV2) in weaned pigs: a sequential study. Journal of Comparatiive Pathology 123, 258-269.

Maggi F, B.M., 2009, Immunobiology of the Torque teno viruses and other anelloviruses. Current Topics in Microbiology and Immunology 331, 65-90.

Martelli P, G.S., Ferrari L, Rosina S, De Angelis E, Quintavalla C, Bottarelli E, Borghetti P, 2009, Efficacy of a modified live porcine reproductive and respiratory syndrome virus (PRRSV) vaccine in pigs naturally exposed to a heterologous European

(Italian cluster) field strain: Clinical protection and cell-mediated immunity. Vaccine 27, 3788-3799.

Mateu E, D.I., 2007, The challenge of PRRS immunology. The Veterinary Journal 177, 345-351.

McKinstry KK, S.T., Swain SL, 2010, Regulation of CD4+ T-cell contraction during pathogen challenge. Immunological Reviews 236, 110-124.

Meier WA, G.J., Osorio FA, Husmann RJ, Schnitzlein WM, Zuckermann FA, 2003, Gradual development of the interferon-g response of swine to porcine reproductive and respiratory syndrome virus infection or vaccination. Virology 309, 18-31.

Okamoto, H., 2009, History of discoveries and pathogenicity of TT viruses. Current Topics in Microbiology and Immunology 331, 1-20.

Opriessnig T MD, P.J., Kuhar D, Lunney JK, Elsener J, Halbur PG, 2008, Effect of porcine circovirus type 2 (PCV2) vaccination on porcine reproductive and respiratory syndrome virus (PRRSV) and PCV2 coinfection. Veterinary Microbiology 131, 103-114.

Paillot R, L.F., Audonnet JC, Andreoni C, Juillard V., 2001, Functional and phenotypic characterization of distinct porcine dendritic cells derived from peripheral blood monocytes. Immunology 102, 396-404.

Prots I, S.A., Lipsky PE, Schulze-Koops H., 2011, Analysis of the transcriptional program of developing induced regulatory T cells. PLoS One 6, e16913.

Punkosdy GA, B.M., Glass DD, Lozano MM, O'Mara L, Dudley JP, Ahmed R, Shevach EM, 2011, Regulatory T-cell expansion during chronic viral infection is dependent on endogenous retroviral superantigens. PNAS 108, 3677-3682.

Raymond CR, W.B., 2005, Toll-like receptor, MHC II, B7 and cytokine expression by porcine monocytes and monocytederived dendritic cells in response to microbial pathogen-associated molecular patterns. Veterinary Immunology and Immunopathology 107, 235-247.

Riber U, N.J., Lind P, 2004, In utero infection with PRRS virus modulates cellular functions of blood monocytes and alveolar lung macrophages in piglets. Veterinary Immunology and Immunopathology 99, 169-177.

Rosell C, S.J., Plana-Durán J, Balasch M, Rodríguez-Arrioja GM, Kennedy S, Allan GM, McNeilly F, Latimer KS, Domingo M., 1999, Pathological, immunohistochemical, and in-situ hybridization studies of natural cases of postweaning multisystemic wasting syndrome (PMWS) in pigs. Journal of Comparative Pathology 120, 59-78.

Rossow, K., 1998, Porcine Reproductive and Respiratory Syndrome. Veterinary Pathology 35, 1-20.

Rossow KD, C.J., Goyal SM, Nelson EA, Christopher-Hennings J, Benfield DA 1995, Pathogenesis of procine reproductive and respiratory syndrome virus infection in gnotobiotic pigs. Veterinary Pathology 32, 361-373.

Rouse BT, S.P., Suvas S, 2006, Regulatory T cells in virus infections. Immunological Reviews 212, 272-286.

Rouse BT, S.S., 2010, Immunity and immunopathology to viruses: what decides the outcome? Nature Reviews 10.

Rovira A, B.M., Segalés J, García L, Plana-Durán J, Rosell C, Ellerbrok H, Mankertz A, Domingo M., 2002, Experimental inoculation of conventional pigs with porcine reproductive and respiratory syndrome virus and porcine circovirus 2. 76, 3232-3239.

Sakaguchi, S., 2003, Regulatory T cells: mediating compromises between host and parasite. Nature Immunology 4, 10-11.

Sakaguchi S, M.M., Costantino CM, Hafler DA, 2010, FOXP3+ regulatory T cells in the human immune system. Nature Reviews 10, 490-500.

Sakaguchi S, S.N., Asano M, Itoh M, Toda M., 1995, Immunologic self-tolerance maintained by activated T cells expressing IL-2 receptor alpha-chains (CD25). Breakdown of a single mechanism of self-tolerance causes various autoimmune diseases. Journal of Immunology 155, 1151-1164.

Segalés J AF, R.C., Pastor J, Chianini F, Campos E, López-Fuertes L, Quintana J, Rodríguez-Arrioja G, Calsamiglia M, Pujols J, Domínguez J, Domingo M., 2001, Changes in peripheral blood leukocyte populations in pigs with natural postweaning multisystemic wasting syndrome (PMWS). . Veterinary Immunology and Immunopathology 81, 37-44.

Servant-Delmas A, L.J., Morinet F, Pillet S, 2010, Advances in Human B19 Erythrovirus Biology. Journal of Virology 84, 9658-9665.

Shen Z, Z.S., Wang Y, Li RL, Zhong C, Liang C, Sun Y., 2010, Higher intratumoral infiltrated Foxp3+ Treg numbers and Foxp3+/CD8+ ratio are associated with adverse prognosis in resectable gastric cancer. Journal of Cancer Research and Clinical Oncology 136, 1585-1595.

Silva-Campa E, F.-M.L., Reséndiz M, Pinelli-Saavedra A, Mata-Haro V, Mwangi W, Hernández J, 2009, Induction of T helper 3 regulatory cells by dendritic cells infected with porcine reproductive and respiratory syndrome virus. Virology 387, 373-379.

Summerfield A, M.K., 2009, The porcine dendritic cell family. Developmental and Comparative Immunology 33, 299-309.

Suradhat S, K.S., Sada W, Buranapraditkun S, Wongsawang S, Thanawongnuwech R, 2006, Negative impact of porcine reproductive and respiratory syndrome virus infection of the efficacy of classical swine fever vaccine. Vaccine 24, 2634-2642.

Suradhat S, T.R., 2003, Upregulation of interleukin-10 gene expression in the leukocytes of pigs infected with porcine reproductive and respiratory syndrome virus. Journal of General Virology 84, 2755-2760.

Sutmuller RPM, M.M., Netea MG, Grauer O, Adema GJ2006, Toll-like receptors on regulatory T cells: expanding immune regulation. TRENDS in Immunology 27, 387-393.

Thacker EL, T.B., Young TF, Halbur PG, 2000, Effect of vaccination on the potentiation of porcine reproductive and respiratory syndrome virus (PRRSV)-induced pneumonia by *Mycoplasma hyopneumoniae*. Vaccine 18, 1244-1252.

Thanawongnuwech R, T.B., Halbur P, Thacker EL, 2004, Increased production of proinflammatory cytokines following infection with porcine reproductive and respiratory syndrome virus and *Mycoplasma hyopneumoniae*. Clinical and Diagnostic Laboratory Immunology 11, 901-908.

Thornton AM, S.E., 2000, Suppressor effector function of CD4+CD25+ immunoregulatory T cells is antigen nonspecific. The Journal of Immunology 164, 183-190.

Tosolini M, K.A., Mlecnik B, Fredriksen T, Mauger S, Bindea G, Berger A, Bruneval P, Fridman WH, Pages F, Galon J, 2011, Clinical impact of different classes of infiltrating T cytotoxic and helper cells (Th1, th2, treg, th17) in patients with colorectal cancer. Cancer Research 71, 1263-1271.

Vicari AP, T.G., 2004, Interleukin-10 in viral diseases and cancer: exiting the labyrinth? Immunological Reviews 202, 223-236.

Vincent IE, C.C., Guzylack-Piriou L, Herrmann B, McNeilly F, Allan GM, Summerfield A, McCullough KC., 2005, Subset-dependent modulation of dendritic cell activity by circovirus type 2. Immunology 115, 388-398.

Walker, L.S.K., 2009, Regulatory T cells overturned: the effectors fight back. Immunololgy 126, 466-474.

Wang J-P, Z.X., Wei X, Li J, Nan X-P, Yu H-T, Li Y, Wang P-Z, Bai X-F, 2010, Circulating Toll-like receptor (TLR) 2, TLR4, and regulatory T cells in patients with chronic hepatitis C. APMIS 118, 261-270.

Weiss L, M.T., Egle A, Grabmer C, Greil R, Tinhofer I, 2011, Regulatory T cells predict the time to initial treatment in early stage chronic lymphocytic leukemia. Cancer 117, 2163-2169.

Wesley RD, L.K., Kehrli ME, 2006, Infection with Porcine reproductive and respiratory syndrome virus stimulates an early gamma interferon response in the serum of pigs. The Canadian Journal of Veterinary Research 20, 176-182.

Wing K, O.Y., Prieto-Martin P, Yamaguchi T, Miyara M, Fehervari Z, Nomura T, Sakaguchi S., 2008, CTLA-4 control over Foxp3+ regulatory T cell function. Science 322, 271-275.

Wolf D, W.A., Rumpold H, Fiegl H, Zeimet AG, Muller-Holzner E, Deibl M, Gastl G, Gunsilius E, Marth C., 2005, The expression of the regulatory T cell-specific forkhead box transcription factor FoxP3 is associated with poor prognosis in ovarian cancer. Clinical Cancer Research 11, 8326-8331.

Xiao Z, B.L., Dee S, Halbur P, Murtaugh MP, 2004, The level of virus-specific T-cell and macrophage recruitment in porcine reproductive and respiratory syndrome virus infection in pigs is independent of virus load. Journal of Virology 78, 5923-5933.

Yuan S, M.D., Murtaugh MP, Faaberg KS., 2001, Complete genome comparison of porcine reproductive and respiratory syndrome virus parental and attenuated strains. Virus Research 79, 189-200.

Zamarron BF, C.W., 2011, Dual roles of immune cells and their factors in cancer development and progression. International Journal of Biological Sciences 7, 651-658.

Zeman D, N.R., Yaeger M, Nelson E, Benfield D, Leslie-Steen P, Thomson J, Miskimins D, Daly R, Minehart M, 1993, Laboratory investigation of PRRS virus in three swine herds. Journal of Veterinary Diagnostic Investigation 5, 522-528.

Zeng M, S.A., Wietgrefe SW, Southern PJ, Schacker TW, Reilly CS, Estes JD, Burton GF, Silvestri G, Lifson JD, Carlis JV, Haase AT., 2011, Cumulative mechanisms of lymphoid tissue fibrosis and T cell depletion in HIV-1 and SIV infections. Journal of Clinical Investigation 121, 998-1008.

zur Hausen H, d.V.E., 2009, TT viruses: oncogenic or tumor-suppressive properties? Current Topics in Microbiology and Immunology 331, 109-116.

8

The Role of Chemokines and Cytokines in the Pathogenesis of Periodontal and Periapical Lesions: Current Concepts

Gustavo P. Garlet et al.*
Department of Biological Sciences, School of Dentistry of Bauru,
Universidade de São Paulo
Brazil

1. Introduction

The oral cavity is a complex environment that may harbor more than 750 bacterial species. Proper oral hygiene is essential to maintain the equilibrium of microbial community and oral health. The ecological balance can be compromised in inadequate microbial control situations and an oral infection can be evoked. The bacteria can aid in the formation of dental plaque and caries, leading to periodontal disease (PD) and periapical lesion (PL). PD is the most common chronic inflammatory disorder of microbial origin that affects tooth-supporting tissues including the periodontal ligament and the alveolar bone. Dental caries is characterized by demineralization of enamel and dentine produced by microorganisms' acids. This process can cause pulp necrosis and root canal infection and the progression through the root apex can induce PL. PD and PLs constitute inflammatory and immune response against oral pathogens. Both processes encompass pathogenic mechanisms of inflammation-mediated soft tissue destruction and bone resorption. The etiopathogenesis of these diseases have been extensively investigated over the last decades and the role of several cell types, cytokines and pathways has been described (Graves, 2008, Graves et al., 2011a, Nair, 1997).

Last decades research have documented the importance and commitment of immune system to protect the host from pathogen and also the paradoxical effect accounting for the bone resorption observed in these diseases. More recently, the pattern of immune cell response involved in the lesions progression (i.e. Th1, Th2, Th17, Th9 or T regulatory) has received particular attention (Cardoso et al., 2009, Colic et al., 2009a, Gaffen & Hajishengallis, 2008, Ohlrich et al., 2009, Queiroz-Junior et al, 2011). Although chemokines and cytokines are pivotal to determine these Th patterns, not much is known regarding the expression of these markers in the regulation of bone resorption in sites of PD and PL. This

* Andreza M.F. Aranha[1], Elcia M. Silveira[1], Andreia Espindola Vieira[1], Celso M. Queiroz-Junior[2], Mila F.M. Madeira[2], Sandra Y. Fukada[3] and Tarcilia A. Silva[2]
[1]*Department of Biological Sciences, School of Dentistry of Bauru, Universidade de São Paulo, Brazil*
[2]*Department of Oral Pathology and Surgery, Faculty of Dentistry, Universidade Federal de Minas Gerais, Brazil*
[3]*Department of Physics and Chemistry, School of Pharmaceutical Sciences of Ribeirão Preto, Universidade de São Paulo, Brazil*

chapter will cover the findings regarding the pathways involved in soft and mineralized tissue destruction and present hypotheses that integrate this information into a context of inflammatory/immune host response.

2. Periodontal and periapical lesions etiology: Similarities and peculiarities

The oral cavity is replete with surface-associated communities of microorganisms - the biofilms - colonizing mucous membranes, dental materials and teeth, and these oral biofilms are strongly associated with the etiology of oral inflammatory diseases, such as PD and PL (Beikler & Flemming, 2011). Despite this association, bacteria alone are not sufficient to cause disease. Both lesions of periodontal and endodontic origin involve the host response to bacteria and the formation of osteolytic lesions. Also, additional factors that benefit the microbial community or make the host more susceptible are determinant for PD and PL to develop and progress (Graves, 2008, Nair, 1997).

PDs are the pathological manifestation of the host response against the bacterial challenge from the dental biofilm (Sanz & van Winkelhoff, 2011). PD is a chronic inflammatory condition of the attachment structures of the teeth - alveolar bone, periodontal ligament, connective tissues of gingiva - initiated and perpetuated by predominantly Gram-negative, anaerobe or microaerophilic bacteria that colonize subgingival area - such as *Porphyromonas gingivalis, Tannerella forsythia* and *Aggregatibacter actinomycetemcomitans*. These bacteria trigger the destruction of tooth supporting tissues leading to the formation of periodontal pockets, conversion of junctional epithelium to pocket epithelium which culminate with tooth loss (Page et al., 1997). But bacteria mostly cause such tissue destruction indirectly, through the perturbation of the homeostasis between the subgingival microbiota and the host defenses in susceptible individuals. Although bacteria are essential, they are insufficient for the disease to occur (Graves, 2008). For PD, both endogenous risk factors - genetics (Michalowicz et al., 2000), diabetes mellitus (Emrich et al., 1991), rheumatic disorders (Pablo et al., 2009) - and exogenous risk factors - cigarette smoking (Bergström, 2004) and psychological stress (Monteiro da Silva et al., 1996) - may even outweigh the bacteria as determinants of whether the disease occurs and of the severity of clinical outcome.

In the presence of the microbial challenge, the susceptible host responds with an immediate inflammatory and immune response in order to control the challenge. The initial host response comprises an innate recognition of microbial components - lipopolysaccharides (LPS), bacterial DNA - by host cells of the gingiva and the subsequent production of inflammatory mediators, such as eicosanoids (Offenbacher et al., 1986), reactive oxygen species (Chapple, 1997), matrix metalloproteinases (MMPs) (Garlet et al., 2006), chemokines (Silva et al., 2007) and cytokines (Garlet, 2010), which are directly responsible for PD pathogenesis. In addition, periodontal bacteria also lead to the polarization and activation of antigen-specific lymphocytes and migration of other inflammatory cells to periodontal tissues, characterizing an adaptive response (Cutler & Jotwani, 2004). In fact, the development of the PDs seems to be related to the progression of the inflammatory cell infiltrate into the deeper periodontal tissues since the blockade of such inflammation reduces disease process (Graves et al., 1998). These responses, although directed against bacteria, perpetuate and mediate the destruction of connective and mineralized periodontal tissues, being the main responsible for periodontal breakdown (Garlet, 2010).

As for PD, mounting evidence indicate that PLs are also biofilm-induced diseases influenced by the host immune response (Nair, 1997). The distinction for PD is that PLs are initiated as a response to microorganisms present inside the tooth, specifically in the dental pulp

(Ricucci & Siqueira, 2010). Thus, lesions of endodontic origin pose a particular challenge since that bacteria persist in a protected reservoir that is not readily accessible to the immune defenses. In healthy conditions, dental pulp is protected from microorganisms of the oral cavity by enamel and dentin. The exposure of dental pulp to microorganisms as a consequence of dental caries, fractures or operative procedures triggers a local inflammatory response. The progression of such infection and inflammation results in necrosis of the pulp and involvement of periapical tissues, generating a PL (Nair, 1997). An initial acute inflammatory response induces tissue changes in the apical region, such as hyperemia and neutrophil recruitment, which can shift to the formation of a granulation tissue with chronic inflammatory cells and fibroblasts, the apical granuloma. A granuloma can remain latent or be converted to an epithelium lined cavity, the inflammatory cysts. These pathological changes in periapical tissues are the clinical consequence of the host defensive reaction against bacterial products that egress through apical foramen from infected dental pulp (Nair, 1997), but inhibition of this inflammation tends to aggravate the formation of osteolytic lesions through impairment of the antibacterial activity of the host response, that is critical in endodontic lesions (Graves et al., 2000). Similarly to PD, this response is characterized by the persistent release of inflammatory mediators, such as chemokines and cytokines (Kawashima et al., 2007, Nair, 1997, Silva et al., 2007, Queiroz-Junior et al., 2011, Vernal et al., 2006), and migration of inflammatory cells (Liapatas et al., 2003, Stashenko et al., 1992) to infected sites (as stated in Table 1). It largely prevents microbial invasion into periapical tissues (Liapatas et al. 2003, Nair, 1997), but it also induces the resorption of the periapical alveolar bone (Stashenko et al., 1992). Although the commitment of immune cells and production of inflammatory mediators protect the host from pathogen invasion, it also accounts for periapical bone resorption (Nair, 1997, Takahashi, 1998).

Cytokine / Chemokine	Cellular Source	Receptor	Function	Levels in		Reference
				Homeostasis	Inflammation	
IL-1β	Phagocytes (Neutrophils, Macrophages) Epithelial cells Fibroblasts	IL-1R1 IL-1R2	Induces inflammatory cell migration Induces bone resorption	Absent or low	Increased in chronic inflammation	Bloemen et al., 2010
IL-4	Th2 cells	IL-4R	Prototypical Th2 cytokine Anti-inflammatory properties Induces IL-10 production B cell stimulatory factor Humoral immune response Suppressing the polarization of Th1 cells Inhibit the transcription of pro-inflammatory cytokines Inhibits production of MMPs and RANKL Induces the upregulation of its respective inhibitors TIMPs and OPG	Absent or low	Low to high, depending on the nature of inflammatory immune response	Cronstein, 2007 Kawashima et al., 1999 Fukada et al., 2009 Ihn et al., 2002 Pestka et al., 2004 Agnello et al., 2003, Appay et al., 2008, Bluestone et al., 2009
IL-6	Phagocytes (Neutrophils, Macrophages) T and B cells Epithelial cells	IL-6R	Osteoclastogenesis processes Promotes bone resorption Pro-inflammatory properties	Absent or low	Increased in chronic inflammation	Pestka et al., 2004 Cronstein, 2007

Cytokine / Chemokine	Cellular Source	Receptor	Function	Levels in Homeostasis	Levels in Inflammation	Reference
	Fibroblasts Osteoblasts		Inflammatory cell migration Humoral immune response			
IL-9	Th2 cells	IL-9R	Promotes allergic inflammation associated with various Th2 responses Promotes Th17 cells development Increasing the activity of Treg cells	Absent or low	Low to high, depending on the nature of inflammatory immune response	Hauber et al., 2009 Elyaman et al., 2009, Novak et al., 2009
IL-10	Th2 cells Treg cells	IL-10R1 IL-10R2	Anti-inflammatory properties Protective role in tissue destruction Stimulates OPG production	Absent or low	Increased	Pestka et al., 2004 Chou et al., 2006 Zhang & Teng, 2006
IL-12	Monocytes/ Macrophages Dendritic cells	IL-12Rβ1 IL-12Rβ2	Mediates alveolar bone resorption via IFN-γ Inhibits osteoclast activation *in vitro*	Absent or low	Low to high, depending on the nature of inflammatory immune response	Sasaki et al., 2008 Queiroz-Junior et al., 2010
IL-17	T cells Th17 cells Mast cells	IL-17RA/ IL-17R IL-17RB/ IL-15R IL-17RC IL-17RD/ SEF IL-17RE	Osteoclastogenic properties Upregulates IL-1β and TNF-α Inducer of RANKL production Neutrophil mobilization	Absent or low	Low to high, depending on the nature of inflammatory immune response	Yago et al., 2009 Kotake et al., 1999 Sato et al.,2006 Yu et al., 2007
IL-22	T cells Dendritic cells	IL-22Rα1	Anti-inflammatory properties Positively correlated to OPG, IL-10 and TGF-β Participates in adaptive response	Absent or low	Low to high, depending on the nature of inflammatory immune response	Brand et al., 2006 Valencial et al., 2006
TNF-α	Phagocytes (Neutrophils, Macrophages) Epithelial cells Fibroblasts	TNFR1 TNFR2	Upregulates adhesion molecules Upregulates chemokine production Regulates production of IL-1β and IL-6 Induces cell migration Increases of MMPs and RANKL expression	Absent or low	Increased in chronic inflammation	Dinarello, 2000 Kindle et al., 2006 Garlet et al., 2007a Wajant et al., 2003 Graves, 2008 Peschon et al., 1998
TGF-β	Treg cells Monocytes/ Macrophages	TGF-βRI TGF-βRII	Pleiotropic cytokine Regulates cell growth Regulates differentiation and matrix production Potent immunosuppressive factor Downregulates IL-1β, TNF-α, MMPs production	Increased	Low to high, depending on the nature of inflammatory immune response	Cardoso et al., 2008 Okada & Murakami, 1998 Steinsvoll et al., 1999 Dutzan,

Cytokine / Chemokine	Cellular Source	Receptor	Function	Levels in Homeostasis	Levels in Inflammation	Reference
			Protective role against tissue destruction			2009a, Dutzan, 2009b
IFN-γ	Th1 cells NK cells		Induces inflammatory cytokines Induces chemokines Stimulates osteoclast formation Main phagocyte-activating cytokine bone loss described by in vivo inhibit osteoclastogenesis in vitro	Absent or low	Low to high, depending on the nature of inflammatory immune response	Appay et al., 2008 Murphy & Reiner, 2002 Garlet et al., 2008 Sallusto and Lanzavecchia, 2011, Schroder et al., 2004 Repeke et al., 2010 Ji et al., 2009, Takayanagi et al., 2005
CXCL8 (IL-8)	Phagocytes (Neutrophils/ Polymorphonuclear leukocytes Monocytes/ Macrophages) Lymphocytes, Mast cells Epithelial cells Fibroblasts Endothelial cells, Osteoclasts.	CXCR1	Inflammatory chemokine Neutrophil chemotaxis activating factor (Enhances production of Leucotrien B4) Induces osteoclast differentiation and activity	Absent or low	Increased	Yoshimura et al., 1987 Tonetti et al., 1998 Darveau, 2010 Rossi, 2003 Traves & Donnelly, 2005 Bendre et al., 2003
CCL2 (MCP-1)	Phagocytes (Neutrophils/ Polymorphonuclear leukocytes Monocytes/ Macrophages) Lymphocytes, Mast cells Epithelial cells Fibroblasts Endothelial cells, Osteoblasts Osteoclasts.	CCR2 CCR11	Chemoattracts monocytes Inflammatory bone remodeling Limits infiltration of PMNs Chemoattracts for osteoclast precursors	Absent or low	Increased	Koch et al., 1992 Bonecchi et al., 2009 Garlet et al., 2010
CCL3 (MIP-1α)	Phagocytes (Neutrophils/ Polymorphonuclear leukocytes Monocytes/	CCR1 CCR5	Chemotatic for lymphocytes, monocytes / macrophages, basophils, eosinophils, dendritic cells. Stimulates bone resorption Homologus chemokines	Absent or low	Increased	Koch et al., 2005 Gemmel et al., 2001 Alnaeeli et al., 2007

Cytokine / Chemokine	Cellular Source	Receptor	Function	Levels in Homeostasis	Levels in Inflammation	Reference
	Macrophages) Lymphocytes, Mast cells Epithelial cells Fibroblasts Endothelial cells, Osteoclasts.		CCL4 and CCl5			Taub, 1996 Repeke et al., 2010 Graves et al., 2011
CCL5 (RANTES)	Phagocytes (Neutrophils/ Polymorphonuclear leukocytes Monocytes/ Macrophages) Lymphocytes, Mast cells Epithelial cells Fibroblasts Endothelial cells, Osteoclasts.	CCR1 CCR5	Chemoattracts for lymphocytes, monocytes Induces CXCL8 and IL-6 production	Absent or low	Increased	Koch et al., 2005 Yu et al., 2004 Garlet et al., 2003 Gemmel et al., 2001 Gamonal et al., 2001 Nanki et al., 2001
MMPs	Phagocytes (Neutrophils/ Polymorphonuclear leukocytes Monocytes/ Macrophages) Lymphocytes Epithelial cells Fibroblasts Endothelial cells	TIMPs[1]	Remodeling of extracelleular matrix	Absent or low	Increased	Garlet, 2010 Garlet et al., 2006 Hannas et al., 2007 Verstappen and Von, 2006 Birkedal-Hansen, 1993
TIMPs		MMPs[1]	Regulates matrix remodeling	Low	Decreased or Increased	Garlet, 2010 Garlet et al., 2006 Hannas et al., 2007
RANKL	Osteoblasts[2] Osteocytes[2] Leukocytes[3]	RANK	Differentiation and activation of osteoclasts	Low	Increased	Teitelbaum, 200 Katagiri and Takahashi, 2002
OPG	T cells Osteoblasts	RANKL[1]	Inhibits bone resorption by preventing RANK-RANKL engagement	Low	Decreased or Increased	Teitelbaum, 2000 Katagiri and Takahashi, 2002

Notes:

1 – in the absence of a "receptor", the coupling molecules were listed

2 – under homeostatic conditions

3 – under inflammatory conditions

Table 1. Cytokines and chemokines involved in the pathophysiology of periodontal and periapical diseases

Therefore, the etiology of PD and PL shares the paradoxical condition in which the same host systems that provide protection against distinct pathogens are responsible for tissue destruction. Activation of these systems to achieve defense virtually always results in some degree of destruction which, if not controlled, will lead to tooth loss as the end result (Garlet, 2010, Nair, 1997, Page et al., 1997, Silva et al., 2007).

3. Periodontal and periapical tissues under homeostatic and inflammatory conditions

A normal periodontium is a complex and dynamic structure composed of soft and hard tissues, encompassed cementum and self-renewing tissues including the gingival mucosa (epithelium and connective), periodontal ligament, alveolar bone which, together, provide attachment apparatus for teeth into the jaw (Potempa et al., 2000, Bosshardt & Lang, 2005). The periodontal tissues are constantly exposed to multiple assaults by microbes that live harmoniously in the oral niche. The homeostasis of these tissues depends on a dynamic equilibrium of bacteria-host interactions. Besides the overall periodontal tissues, the pulp tissue, usually free of microbial challenge in healthy conditions, play an important role in the initial host responses that can lead to the development of PLs, and therefore will be also considered in the sequence.

3.1 Periodontal and pulpar tissues under homeostatic conditions

Gingival epithelium is the first line of host defense, represented not only by its barrier function that physically hamper microbial invasion in gingival sulcus and periodontal soft and mineralized connective tissues, but also by its antimicrobial properties that biologically suppress the propagation of putative pathogens (Darveau et al., 1997, Lu et al., 2004, Page et al., 1997). This epithelium adjacent to a tooth can be classified into three anatomical types: the oral gingival epithelium, the sulcular epithelium, and the junctional epithelium (Hatakeyama et al., 2006).

The oral gingival epithelium is composed of a keratinizing stratified epithelium and covers the external surface of the gingiva, while the sulcular epithelium is a nonkeratinizing epithelium that lines the inner aspect of the gingival sulcus. In contrast, the junctional epithelium is structurally and functionally unique. Namely, the junctional epithelium is located at a strategically important interface between the gingival sulcus and the underlying soft and mineralized connective tissues of the periodontium (Hatakeyama et al., 2006, Hormia et al., 2001), contains a nonkeratinizing epithelial layer at the free surface. The gingival epithelium, in particular, the junctional epithelium is highly porous and the epithelial cells are interconnected by a few desmosomes and the occasional gap junction, resulting in wider intercellular spaces that may provide a pathway for fluid and transmigrating leukocytes from the gingival connective tissue to the gingival sulcus (Hashimoto et al., 1986, Bosshardt & Lang 2005, Hatakeyama et al., 2006), and even for microorganisms moving in the opposite direction (Bosshardt & Lang 2005, Darveau, 2010, Darveau et al., 1997, Marra & Isberg, 1996, Page & Schroeder, 1976, Tonetti et al., 1998). In the absence of clinical signs of inflammation, approximately 30,000 polymorphonuclear leukocytes (PMNs) migrate *per* minute through the junctional epithelia of all human teeth into the oral cavity (Darveau, 2010, Schiött & Löe, 1970). The tissue fluid transports a variety of molecules through the junctional epithelium to the bottom of the gingival sulcus. These molecules, together with the leukocytes, represent a host defense system against the bacterial challenge. Its interposition between the underlying soft and mineralized connective tissues of the periodontium points to its important roles in tissue homeostasis and defense against micro-organisms and their products (Schroeder & Listgarten, 1997). Moreover, the highly dynamic nature of the junctional epithelium indicates an important role for the cells themselves in the maintenance of tissue integrity, being essential for its protective and regenerative functions (Schiött & Löe, 1970).

In health condition, the connective tissue components are subject to a tightly controlled cycle of synthesis and breakdown (Potempa et al., 2000). At clinically healthy sites, a balanced and dynamic equilibrium challenge of bacteria–host may be beneficial, resulting in resistance to colonization by periodontopathogens and triggering other less-well-defined responses of the host. By contrast, this delicate balance in connective tissue turnover continuously challenged by the accumulation of bacteria on the tooth surface, if excessive, can ignite an inflammatory reaction aimed to eradicate the microbial intruders. Although indispensable for host defense against pathogens, this response may upset homeostasis within the periodontium, leading first to gingivitis and then to periodontitis (Bosshardt & Lang, 2005, Potempa et al., 2000), as will be described in the sequence. In addition, the extracellular matrix (ECM) and collagen type I of the connective tissue help stabilize periodontal tissues, and fibronectins affect cell morphology, migration and differentiation (Darveau, 2010, Mussig et al., 2005). The coordinated regulation of cell proliferation and differentiation events is controlled by host signaling mechanisms and is referred to as tissue homeostasis. These signaling mechanisms maintain homeostasis of the periodontal tissue by regulating epithelial cell functions as well as connective-tissue resident cells and hematopoietic cells (Darveau, 2010).

Among the host proteases that target the ECM, the matrix metalloproteinases (MMPs) have been especially associated with the remodeling of periodontal tissues (Garlet, 2010, Garlet et al., 2006, Hannas et al., 2007, Verstappen & Von den Hoff, 2006) during different physiological and pathological processes (Birkedal-Hansen, 1993, Garlet, 2010, Garlet et al., 2006). MMPs, a family of zinc- and calcium-dependent proteases, are usually found in balance with a group of endogenous proteins named tissue inhibitors of metalloproteinases (TIMPs), to keep matrix remodeling highly regulated (Garlet, 2010, Garlet et al., 2006, Hannas et al., 2007). In fact, MMPs and TIMPs are regularly expressed in healthy periodontal tissues, where they are supposed to control the ECM physiological turnover (Garlet et al., 2006, Gonçalves et al., 2008). It is thought that MMPs and TIMPs are involved in the physiological turnover of periodontal tissues, and MMPs appear to be involved in tissue destruction in PDs (Birkedal-Hansen, 1993, Garlet et al., 2006, Golub et al., 2001, Reynolds et al., 1994, Van der Zee et al., 1997). However, there are contradictory results regarding the balance of MMPs/TIMPs in pathological versus healthy gingival samples (Aiba et al., 1996, Dahan et al., 2001, Garlet et al., 2006, Garlet et al., 2004, Ingman et al., 1996, Kubota et al., 1996, Nomura et al., 1998). Some studies show a decrease in the levels of TIMPs in diseased periodontal tissues, supporting the idea that an imbalance in the levels of TIMPs/MMPs occurs in PDs and results in tissue destruction (Garlet et al., 2006, Soell et al., 2002, Tuter et al., 2002). Conversely, other studies detected an increased expression of TIMPs in diseased periodontal tissues (Alpagot et al., 2001, Garlet et al., 2006, Garlet et al., 2004, Haerian et al., 1995, Nomura et al., 1998) which could reflect an attempt to maintain the tissue homeostasis, in view of the increased expression of MMPs. However, such up-regulation of TIMPs may not be enough to compensate for the even higher upregulation of MMPs, and such an imbalance may result in periodontal destruction. Nevertheless, imbalances in the MMP/TIMP system (i.e. lower levels of TIMPs and/or higher levels of MMPs) are involved in the pathogenesis of several diseases including rheumatoid arthritis (Garlet et al., 2006, Katrib et al., 2003, Lanchou et al., 2003, Romas et al., 2002, Schulze et al., 2003, Yoshihara et al., 2000), which share several features with PDs, including the chronic nature of the inflammatory reaction and tissue destruction (Garlet et al., 2006, Mercado et al., 2003).

In the soft tissues context, it is also important to consider the features that characterize the dental pulp. The dental pulp consists of a connective tissue with a complex and rich neuronal and vascular networks surrounded by dentin walls, which lacks epithelium, differing from others connective tissues (Goldberg et al., 2004, Shroder, 1985). The pulp tissue is composed by heterogeneous cell populations responsible for its maintenance, defense, and repair. The cell types identified within the pulp include fibroblasts, which are the predominant cell type, as well as inflammatory and immune system cells, including dendritic cells, neutrophils, histiocytes/macrophages, T-/B- lymphocytes and odontoblasts (Izumi et al., 1995). Several niche environments for latent or dormant pulpal stem cells (progenitors), necessary for repair and regenerative processes, have been identified within the components of dental pulp (Huang et al., 2009, Shi et al., 2003, Sloan et al., 2007). Interestingly, while periodontal tissues are directly exposed to a microbial challenge even both health and disease conditions, dental pulp features comprise a special situation where the tissue is enclosed by a rigid, mineralized tissue shell, and thus the microbial challenge only will reach the host tissue after significant enamel and dentin matrix degradation, or in other words, in already established pathological process. While the mineralized structure may present an initial protective role, in the course of pathological process the tubular structure of dentin confers significant permeability properties on the tissue (Pashley et al., 2002) and bacterial products may diffuse down the dentinal tubules and invoke cellular responses (Bergenholtz, 1990, Smith et al., 2001). After dental tissue damage by caries lesions, odontoblasts are the first pulp cells to encounter both products of the infectious process, including the invading pathogens and their components, as well as detecting dentine matrix constituents released during demineralization. Although odontoblasts provide barrier function by protecting the underlying tissue from the invading bacteria, they are also immunocompetent and capable of coordinating an inflammatory response (Veerayutthwilai et al., 2007). Progression of the carious infection deeper into the underlying dental tissue results in changes in the composition of the bacterial biofilm (Takahashi et al., 2008) and also deleterious effects on the host cells, including death of pulp cells. Certainly, further molecular interactions between bacteria and stem cells at the core of the pulp arise, resulting in exacerbation of inflammatory events.

Finally, it is important to consider the structure and properties of the periodontal ligament (PDL), which is responsible for supporting the teeth and can be affected by inflammatory conditions of periodontal and pulpar origin. The PDL is critical for teeth positioning within the alveolar bone and for absorbing forces generated by chewing. The main components of the PDL are blood vessels, fibroblasts, and collagen fibers, composed primarily of collagen type I. Several previous studies have demonstrated that mesenchymal stem cells associated with the vasculature within the PDL have the potential to differentiate into cell types that populate bone and cementum (McCulloch & Bordin, 1991, Trombetta & Bradshaw, 2010). Thereby, resident cells of the PDL are postulated to play an important role in periodontal health and disease by providing cellular source for regeneration of the primary tissues injured in PD. It is because of their ability to proliferate, migrate and synthesize several components of the periodontium, and also participate in both protective and destructive mechanism that prevents periodontitis or impede its progression, and initiates lesions and promotes progressive disease by various biological mechanisms, respectively (Benatti et al., 2009, Gemmell & Seymour, 2004).

PDLC (periodontal ligament cells) proliferation is considered one of the major events for periodontal homeostasis, because of their capacity to proliferate and differentiate into all the other periodontal tissues (Benatti et al., 2009). Another key event critical for periodontal tissue homeostasis in which PDLC play a significant role is the bone remodeling process. PDLC play a major role in alveolar bone metabolism in periodontal health and disease, because of their ability to secrete factors that regulate the homeostasis of connective and osseous tissue, including inflammatory cytokines such as interleukins (ILs), and the major osteoclast regulators receptor activator of nuclear factor-kB ligand (RANKL) and osteoprotegerin (OPG) (Ogasawara et al., 2004, Benatti et al., 2009).

In addition to the soft connective tissue elements, alveolar bone loss is a key structure of periodontal and periapical environments. Bone homeostasis depends on the maintenance of a delicate equilibrium between bone resorption by osteoclasts and bone formation by osteoblasts. The major mechanism that regulates bone remodeling is driven by the receptor RANK (receptor activator of nuclear factor-κB, also known as TNFRSF11A), its ligand RANKL (also known as TNFSF11), and its soluble counterpart OPG (also known as TNFRSF11B) (Boyle et al., 2003, Cochran, 2008, Darveau, 2010, Garlet, 2010, Leibbrandt & Penninger, 2008, Nagasawa et al., 2007). RANKL binding to the receptor RANK, present on the surfaces of pre-osteoclasts, drives their maturation and activation, while OPG acts as a decoy receptor and inhibits RANK-RANKL engagement (Leibbrandt & Penninger, 2008). Therefore, the balance between RANKL and OPG expression is essential for bone remodeling, but the expression of such system is usually investigated in the viewpoint of pathological changes (Baud'huin et al., 2007, Garlet, 2010, Garlet et al., 2006, Menezes et al., 2008, Rodan & Martin, 2000, Romas et al., 2002), and the exact participation of such mediators in homeostatic bone remodeling of alveolar bone remain unclear.

It is important to make clear that tissue homeostasis represents a delicate balance between anabolic and catabolic activities, and that a wide range of stimuli can disrupt this balance and compromise the tissue integrity. Along such stimuli, inflammation-related molecules can result in pathological changes in periodontal, periapical and pulpar tissues, as discussed in the next section. However, it is important to consider that even in clinical health conditions, the periodontium continuously expresses cytokines, chemokines and cell adhesion molecules, associated with a basal level of inflammation, thought to be responsible for providing protection against bacterial challenge without resulting in tissue damage. Indeed, as previously cited, periodontal tissues are directly exposed to a microbial challenge even in healthy subjects. To cope with such microbial stimulation, the periodontium has a highly orchestrated expression of select innate host defence mediators (Darveau, 2010). Periodontal tissue, unlike the intestine, does not have a large mucous layer to prevent contact between the microbial community and the epithelial cell surface (Bosshardt & Lang, 2005, Darveau, 2010). In fact, although both periodontal and intestinal tissues are in close proximity to polymicrobial communities, it seems that they use two completely different strategies to contend with the constant presence of microbial stimulation. The intestinal epithelium is a single layer of cells connected by tight junctions that channels bacteria and their components to the highly specialized Peyers patches, where a localized, fully developed lamina propria can recognize microorganisms and respond accordingly

(Darveau, 2010, Duerkop et al., 2009). Like the intestinal epithelium, clinically healthy human gingival tissue expresses a wide range of toll-like receptors (TLRs), including TLR1–TLR9 (Darveau, 2010, Mahanonda & Pichyangkul, 2007, Ren et al., 2005, Sugawara et al., 2006,). Innate host protective mechanisms are coupled with regenerative and biomechanical signalling systems, resulting in tissue homeostasis. The status of healthy periodontal tissue results in the coordinated expression of E-selectin, intercellular adhesion molecules (ICAMs) and interleukin-8 (IL-8) which facilitates neutrophil transit through the tissue, where they form a wall between the host tissue and the dental-plaque biofilm (Tonetti et al., 1998, Darveau, 2010). Interestingly, some cytokines usually associated with chronic inflammation and tissue damage, such as IL-1, IL-6, TNF-α, are found in gingival crevicular fluid from clinically healthy sites, but in lower levels than in diseased sites. In this context, the transition from a healthy-related to a disease-related inflammatory condition seems to be associated with quantitative and qualitative changes in the host inflammatory immune response, whose characteristics have been investigated usually in a pathological context, which will be discussed in the sequence.

3.2 Periodontal and periapical tissues under inflammatory conditions – Pathways involved in tissue destruction

Cytokines play a major role in inflammatory and immune responses within the bone microenvironment. The balance between pro- and anti-inflammatory mediators determines the outcome of resorption in bone destructive diseases, as in periodontitis (Garlet et al., 2006, Menezes et al., 2008) and periapical granulomas (Silva et al., 2005, Silva et al., 2007) (Table 1). However, before specific discussion on host response to periodontal and periapical diseases outcome modulation, it is important to review the molecular pathways associated with periodontal and periapical tissues destruction. As previously considered, MMPs have been associated with remodeling of the periodontal tissues with special interest (Hannas et al., 2007, Shin et al., 2002, Verstappen & von den Hoff, 2006), and are usually found in balance with TIMPs in order to keep matrix remodeling in a highly regulated fashion (Hannas et al., 2007). However, unbalanced MMPs/TIMPs ratio was described in diseased periodontal and periapical tissues, and is thought to account for the soft and mineralized tissue destruction associated to periodontal and periapical diseases (Garlet et al., 2004, Gonçalves et al., 2008, Shin et al., 2002, Verstappen & von den Hoff, 2006). In accordance, the disarray of the MMPs/TIMPs model is involved in the pathogenesis of osteolytic diseases (Malemud, 2006), and the MMPs inhibition is proposed as an adjuvant therapy to control PD (Giannobile, 2008).

Besides the connective tissue destruction, alveolar bone loss is a key event in bone inflammatory diseases, as in periodontitis and chronic PLs. The integrity of bone tissues depends on the maintenance of a delicate equilibrium between osteoclasts and osteoblasts. It has been proposed that proinflammatory cytokines play a fundamental role in periapical bone destruction through the induction of RANKL, while OPG synthesis is supposed to attenuate lesion progression (Garlet et al., 2006, Menezes et al., 2008). As previously cited, the major regulatory mechanism of osteoclasts activity is driven by the receptor RANK, its ligand RANKL and its soluble counterpart OPG (Leibbrandt & Penninger, 2008). Being the balance between RANKL and OPG expression essential to determine the overall bone loss outcome. Regarding periodontal and periapical diseases, an increased RANKL expression in diseased periodontal and periapical tissues are described (Cochran, 2008, Garlet et al., 2004).

Interestingly, the patterns of RANKL/OPG expression present a high variation between inactive PD (i.e. chronic gingivitis) and active PLs (i.e. periapical granulomas) (Menezes et al., 2008) and also significantly differ between clinical forms of periodontitis (i.e. aggressive versus chronic periodontitis) (Garlet et al., 2004). For that reason, it is possible that RANKL/OPG balance may be associated with the stable or progressive nature of periodontal lesions. Previous human studies showed that RANKL/OPG balance was associated with osteolytic activity and the experimental disease progression (Garlet et al., 2006). Accordingly, the blockade of RANKL by OPG leads to a reduction of alveolar bone loss throughout experimental PD in mice (Jin et al., 2007). Appropriately, the coupled bone formation, which takes place under homeostatic conditions (Parfitt, 1982), seems to contribute to the conventional increased bone resorption in overall bone loss in PD (Behl et al., 2008). It has long been assumed that the host defense against microbial invasion and subsequent tissue destruction involves both innate and adaptive immunity cytokines. We are going to discuss both immune response mechanisms, separately, in this chapter.

4. Classic inflammatory cytokines role in periodontal and periapical inflammatory lesions

As previously discussed in this chapter, the presence of pathogens is required, but not sufficient for bone inflammatory diseases initiation, being the host response a critical determinant of periodontal and periapical tissues breakdown (Graves, 2008, Nair, 2004). The innate host response initially involves the recognition of microbial components as "danger signals" by host cells and the subsequent production of inflammatory mediators. The TLRs are expressed by resident cells and leukocytes in periodontal habitat, and activate the innate immune response, binding to various bacterial components (i.e., LPS, bacterial DNA, diacyl lipopeptides, peptidoglycan, etc) (Mahanonda & Pichyangkul, 2007). TLR-2 and TLR-4 seem to participate in the recognition of periodontopathogens such as *A. actinomycetemcomitans, P. gingivalis and T. forsythia* (Nussbaum et al., 2009). After TLRs activation, an intracellular signaling cascade is initiated. This signalling cascade involves activation of transcription factors and the subsequent inflammatory cytokines expression, leukocyte migration and osteoclastogenesis (Lima et al., 2010, Nakamura et al., 2008, Ukai et al., 2008). In accordance, the absence of TLR2 or TLR4 results in reduction of alveolar bone loss in mice after *P. gingivalis* infection (Costalonga et al., 2009, Lima et al., 2010, Nakamura et al., 2008). Besides TLRs, the nucleotide-binding oligomerization domain (NOD) receptors and the inflammasome system have been described as potential accessory molecules in triggering innate host response against periodontal pathogens (Okugawa & Bostanci, 2009, Uehara & Takada, 2007). The first mediators to have their role related to PD pathogenesis were innate immunity cytokines produced after microbial recognition, such as TNF-α, IL-1 and IL-6. These cytokines are produced by both resident cells (i.e. epithelial cells and fibroblasts) and phagocytes (i.e. neutrophils and macrophages) in periodontal environment. While the exact contribution of each cell type remains to be elucidated, previous studies described that a hyper-reactive phenotype of phagocytes is related to increased pro-inflammatory cytokines production in both aggressive and chronic PD (Gustafsson et al., 2006, Shaddox et al., 2010). Recent evidence also points to important roles of resident cells in periodontal bone loss, since the periodontal ligament fibroblasts and osteoclast precursors contact synergistically increases the expression of genes related to osteoclastogenesis, such as RANKL, TNF-α and IL-1 (Bloemen et al., 2010).

TNF-α is responsible for cell migration process at multiple levels, inducing the upregulation of adhesion molecules and the production of chemokines, which are chemotactic cytokines involved in cell migration to infected and inflamed sites (Dinarello, 2000, Kindle et al., 2006, Peschon et al., 1998, Wajant et al., 2003). TNF-α is present at high levels in gingival crevicular fluid (GCF), diseased periodontal tissues (Garlet et al., 2004, Graves, 2008, Graves & Cochran, 2003), and radicular cysts (Teixeira-Salum et al., 2010), it is positively correlated with MMPs and RANKL expression. Supporting the data from human studies, experimental PD in rats and primates clearly demonstrated that TNF-α plays a central role in the inflammatory reaction, alveolar bone resorption and in the loss of connective tissue attachment (Graves, 2008, Graves & Cochran, 2003). Accordingly, experimental periodontitis in TNF-α p55 receptor deficient mice (TNFp55KO) was characterized by a significant decrease in MMPs and RANKL expression, which was associated with a significant decrease in the alveolar bone loss (Garlet et al., 2007a).

However, recent studies from mouse models point to important roles of cytokines in the control of periodontal infection. While the destructive roles of TNF-α in periodontal environment led to the proposal of anti-TNF therapies to control PD (Mayer et al, 2009), it was also demonstrated a dual role for TNF-α in the pathogenesis of experimental PD, since this cytokine present an important role in the control of experimental *A. actinomycetemcomitans* infection, as demonstrated by the increased bacterial load and acute phase response presented by TNFp55-KO infected mice (Garlet et al., 2007a). Accordingly, TNFp55-KO mice characteristically present severe pathogen clearance impairment (Pfeffer et al., 1993). Besides its role in inflammatory cell migration previously cited, TNF-α plays a critical role in both innate and adaptive immune responses, upregulating antigen presentation and the bactericidal activity of phagocytes (Dinarello, 2000).

Besides the direct effect on the pathogenesis of periodontal and periapical diseases, TNF-α upregulates the production of other classic pro-inflammatory innate immune cytokines, such as IL-1β and IL-6 (Dinarello, 2000, Garlet et al., 2007a, Graves, 2008, Okada & Murakami, 1998, Wajant et al., 2003,). IL-1β and IL-6 have also been characteristically associated with inflammatory cell migration and osteoclastogenesis processes (Graves, 2008, Fonseca et al., 2009). Curiously, the individual absence of innate immunity cytokines attenuates inflammatory bone loss; however their simultaneous inhibition results in more effective protection leading to almost complete remission of bone loss rate (Sartori et al., 2009, Graves & Cochran, 2003).

In addition to a direct action toward bone resorption, innate immune cytokines also interfere with the coupled bone formation process (Behl et al., 2008). In fact, recent studies confirmed the early hypothesis that proinflammatory cytokines inhibit osteogenic differentiation (Ding et al., 2009, Lacey et al., 2009), and also demonstrate that activation of TLRs in osteoblasts induces the production of osteoclastogenic cytokines (Bar-Shavit, 2008).

5. T helper cytokines role in periodontal and periapical inflammatory lesions

Complementarily to the innate immune response, periodontal and endodontic bacteria result in mobilization of adaptive immunity mechanisms. The host adaptive response starts with the recognition of the putative pathogens (using a similar set of TLRs and NODs as described to innate immunity cells) by antigen presenting cells, such as dendritic cells (Cutler & Jotwani, 2004). After activation, mature dendritic cells express co-stimulatory molecules and produce distinct patterns of cytokines that will determine the subsequent polarization and activation of antigen specific lymphocytes (Cutler & Jotwani, 2004). The immune response polarization is determined by prototypical cytokines of each pattern, and also involves the selective migration of CD4 T helper subsets and the subsequent production of characteristic cytokines at the response foci (Bluestone et al., 2009, Kalinski & Moser, 2005, Murphy & Reiner, 2002).

It has long been assumed that the pathogenesis of inflammatory diseases is mainly mediated by CD4 T cells subsets, Th1 and Th2 cells, contrasting in their pattern of cytokine production (Brand et al., 2006, Colic et al., 2007, Gaffen & Hajishengallis, 2008, Murphy & Reiner, 2002, Stashenko et al., 2008). As a general rule, immune responses mediated by T cells polarized into a Th1-type phenotype are characteristically cellular and pro-inflammatory, while Th2 cells are associated with humoral immunity and present anti-inflammatory properties (Jankovic et al., 2001, Murphy & Reiner, 2002). This has been supported by increased levels of Th1 cytokines (IFN-γ, IL-12) in bone destruction involved in the progression of chronic periapical and periodontitis diseases (Kawashima et al., 1999, Trombone et al., 2010). Under normal condition, proinflammatory mechanisms must be controlled in order to prevent excessive tissue destruction and promote autoimmune processes. Th2 cytokines (IL-4, IL-10) are classic antagonist of Th1 responses and associated to the humoral immune response and antibody production, leading to the restriction of inflammatory/immune mechanisms (Kawashima et al., 1999, Fukada et al., 2009).

IFN-γ is the signature cytokine of Th1-type responses, being considered the main phagocyte-activating cytokine and characteristically associated with the production of inflammatory cytokines and chemokines (Appay et al., 2008, Murphy & Reiner, 2002, Sallusto & Lanzavecchia, 2011, Schroder et al., 2004). Concerning periapical diseases of endodontic origin and periodontitis, IFN-γ is present at high levels in chronic PLs, and is associated with progressive lesions or higher severity (Colic et al., 2006, Colic et al., 2009, Dutzan et al., 2009, Garlet et al., 2003, Honda et al., 2006). In agreement, studies in rodents demonstrated that IFN-γ is involved in the development of inflammatory reaction and bone resorption in response to *A. actinomycetemcomitans and P. gingivalis* (Baker et al., 1999, Garlet et al., 2008, Teng et al., 2005). Interestingly, a controversial role for IFN-γ in bone lytic lesions have been described, since the association with increased bone loss described *in vivo* (human and experimental) is not confirmed by *in vitro* experiments, in which IFN-γ is described to systematically inhibit osteoclastogenesis (Ji et al., 2009, Takayanagi et al., 2005). In fact, *in vitro* data clearly demonstrated that IFN-γ induces rapid degradation of the RANK adapter protein TRAF6 by the ubiquitin-proteasome system, resulting in the inhibition of the RANKL-signaling and its subsequent osteoclastogenic events (Takayanagi et al., 2000). The *in vitro* data support a previous hypothesis that Th1 cells are associated with the stable lesions while Th2 cells are associated with disease progression (Gemmell et al., 2007). However, the pro-inflammatory effect of IFN-γ demonstrated *in vivo*, leading to the upregulation of TNF-α and IL-1β levels (and consequently RANKL) seems to overcome the direct anti-osteoclastogenic effect described *in vitro* (Gao et al., 2007, Garlet et al., 2008). In addition, IFN-γ also stimulates osteoclast formation and bone loss *in vivo* via antigen-driven T cell activation or through the chemoattraction of RANKL+ cells (Gao et al., 2007, Garlet et al., 2008, Repeke et al., 2010). This finding is supported by a recent study, which demonstrates that Th1 cells (characterized as CD3+CCR5+CXCR3+ cells) are an important source of RANKL throughout experimental periodontitis (Repeke et al., 2010). An additional evidence of the adverse effect of Th1 response concerning periodontal tissue destruction indicates the role of IL-12 (the major Th1-inducing cytokine) mediating alveolar bone loss in mice after *P. gingivalis* challenge (Sasaki et al., 2008). However, as observed with IFN-γ, data from human periodontitis concerning the role of IL-12 in PD pathogenesis is controversial. Although studies demonstrate that IL-12 concentrations are lower within diseased than healthy gingival tissues (Johnson et al., 2005), a recent report showed that IL-12 levels decrease in gingival crevicular fluid following initial periodontal therapy (Thunell et al., 2009).

Meantime, similarly as described earlier to TNFp55-KO strain, IFN-γKO mice presented a severe impairment of protective immunity to *A. actinomycetemcomitans* infection, as demonstrated by the higher bacterial load in periodontium, increased acute phase response, and bacterial dissemination followed by mice death (Garlet, et al., 2008). The immune protection mediated by IFN-γ characteristically involves leukocyte recruitment and its subsequent activation at inflammatory foci (Schroder et al., 2004). Indeed, IFN-γ is considered the main phagocyte-activating cytokine by enhancing phagocytosis, antigen uptake and stimulating the production of inflammatory cytokines, chemokines and microbicidal molecules (Schroder et al., 2004). In fact, IFN-γ plays an essential role in clearing a wide range of infections (Schroder et al., 2004). As a result, further studies are required to determine the exact effect of Th1 cytokines, IFN-γ and IL-12, in the immunopathogenesis of periapical inflammatory diseases.

An extra possibility for a destructive role for T cells all over periodontitis and periapical diseases brings up the Th2 subset, also present in PDs and PLs (Gemmell & Seymour, 2004). Th2 cells commitment and action is primarily dependent of IL-4, the prototypical Th2 cytokine, which also acts as a B cell stimulatory factor (Appay et al., 2008, Murphy, 2002, Sallusto & Lanzavecchia, 2011). In addition to IL-4, IL-6 is further believed to contribute to B cell differentiation and antibody production (Cronstein, 2007). Previous studies demonstrated that B cells produce RANKL as a result of periodontal pathogens stimulation (Han et al., 2009), and also that the majority of B cells in periodontal lesions are RANKL+ (Kawai et al., 2006). Considering the hypothesis that B cells outnumber T cells in periodontal lesions, the predominance of a Th2-type response in periodontal lesions potentially leads to the accumulation RANKL producing cells and consequently to tissue destruction (Gemmell, 2002, Kawai et al., 2006). In fact, B cell deletion was recently demonstrated to prevent bone loss in mice after oral *P. gingivalis* infection (Baker et al., 2009). However, while B cells seem to contribute to alveolar bone loss, they are not essential since T cells are able to promote LPS-induced bone resorption in the absence of B cells (Yamaguchi et al., 2008). An additional possibility for a destructive role for Th2/B cell pole is the expression of autoantibodies against periodontal tissue components (such as collagen, heat shock proteins, vimentin, spectrin, filamin, actin, lamin, keratin, and tubulin), described in both aggressive and chronic PD patients (Koutouzis et al., 2009).

On the other hand, some studies propose that the Th2-type cytokine IL-4 may attenuate periodontitis progression, in contrast to its putative destructive role previously discussed. Although there is no evidence of the role of IL-4 in periapical diseases, this cytokine has been asssociated to control other inflammatory diseases, such as periodontitis and rheumatoid arthritis (Bozkurt et al., 2006). IL-4 presents marked suppressive and anti-inflammatory properties mediated by its capacity to inhibit the transcription of pro-inflammatory cytokines and IFN-γ, then suppressing the polarization of Th1 cells (Agnello et al., 2003, Appay et al., 2008, Bluestone et al., 2009). Moreover, IL-4 induces the production of cytokines with similar or complementary suppressive properties, such as IL-10 (Pestka et al., 2004). In addition, IL-4 is also able to inhibit the production of MMPs and RANKL, and concomitantly induce the upregulation of its respective inhibitors TIMPs and OPG (Ihn et al., 2002), reinforcing its potential protective role in PD pathogenesis (Giannopoulou, 2003). Indeed, the concentration of IL-4 in GCF was demonstrated to decrease from periodontal health to disease, suggesting that this cytokine could mediate the remission or improvement of periodontal lesions (Bozkurt et al., 2006, Pradeep et al., 2009). The protective role for Th2-biased humoral immunity also refers to the prevention of alveolar bone loss after immunization protocols, which are usually associated with increase in serum immunoglobulin levels (Zhang, et al., 2009). Accordingly, a longitudinal human study demonstrated that serum levels of IgG antibodies against *A. actinomycetemcomitans* or *P. gingivalis* in periodontitis-stable patients were higher than those in patients with active periodontitis, suggesting a protective role for IgG (Rams et al., 2006).

Also in the tissue protection context, the prototypical anti-inflammatory cytokine IL-10 (Pestka et al., 2004) described to be widely expressed in inflamed periodontal and periapical tissues, is thought to be associated with lower disease severity (Colic et al., 2010, Garlet et al., 2006, Garlet et al., 2004, Rossi et al., 2008). Genuinely, IL-10 knockout mouse is highly susceptible to *P. gingivalis*-induced alveolar bone loss (Sasaki et al., 2004), and great PLs may be developed, reinforcing the important role of IL-10 in the pathogenesis of experimentally induced pulp infection as endogenous suppressor of PL development (Rossi et al., 2008). Studies suggest that IL-10 can act on multiple ways to restrain periodontitis severity. The control of inflammatory signaling mediated by IL-10 may involve the inhibition of inflammatory mediators mRNA transcription after TLR or cytokine signaling (Yoshimura et al., 2003). This control can be exerted by the suppressors of cytokine signaling (SOCS), which act to attenuate signal transduction as part of a negative feedback loop to inhibit the response to subsequent stimuli (Yoshimura et al., 2007). Accordingly, a recent study demonstrates that the upregulation of SOCS expression after the challenge with DNA from PD-associated bacteria significantly suppressed the response to a subsequent bacterial challenge (Taubman et al., 2007). Aside from the suppression of innate immunity cytokines, IL-10 interferes directly with IFN-γ and IL-17 production by T cells, demonstrating a broad role for this immunoregulatory cytokine (Jovanovic et al., 1998, Naundorf et al., 2009). Hence, in PLs, a previous study demonstrated that macrophages are able to control periapical tissue and alveolar bone destruction by inhibiting the DC-mediated production of IFN-γ by CD4+ T cells and by augmenting the secretion of IL-10 (Colic et al., 2010). Therefore, it is possible that IL-10 may reduce the inflammatory signaling that leads to inflammatory and Th1 cytokine mRNA transcription, which in turn could downregulate downstream pathways under its influence (Hosokawa et al., 2009). In accordance, the expression of SOCS-1 and SOCS-3 is significantly higher in inactive versus active periodontal lesions (Garlet et al., 2006).

In addition to the control of inflammatory reaction, IL-10 also presents a direct protective role in tissue destruction, modulating both MMPs and RANK systems. IL-10 characteristically induces the upregulation of TIMPs, which are capable of inhibiting almost every member of the MMP family in a non-specific way (Chou et al., 2006, Claudino et al., 2008, Garlet et al., 2004). In fact, increased TIMPs levels in periodontal and periapical tissues are thought to effectively counteract MMPs, and have been associated with the attenuation of disease severity (Garlet et al., 2004, Lin et al., 2002, Ramamurthy et al., 2005, Sato et al., 2009). Moreover, IL-10 stimulates the production of OPG, which consequently inhibits bone resorption by preventing RANK-RANKL engagement (Zhang & Teng, 2006). Concurring, IL-10 modulates the levels of both TIMPs and OPG *in vitro* and *in vivo* (Kumada et al., 2004, Liu et al., 2006, Zhang & Teng, 2006). IL-10 was also described to suppress osteoclastogenesis by selectively inhibiting calcium signaling downstream of RANK and by inhibiting transcription of the osteoclast co-stimulatory molecule triggering receptor expressed on myeloid cells 2 (TREM-2) (Park-Min et al., 2009). Indeed, IL-10 are thought to present a direct effect over bone formation, since the alveolar bone loss in the absence of IL-10 is associated with a reduced expression of osteoblast and osteocyte markers, independently of microbial, inflammatory or bone-resorptive pathways (Claudino et al., 2008).

Interestingly, IL-10 was initially considered to be produced by Th2 cells in periodontal and PLs, but the discovery of Tregs as an important IL-10-producing T helper subset resulted in an evaluation of such concept. Indeed, while the association of Th2 cells with inflammatory diseases outcome remains controversial, Tregs have been described as a protective T cell subset concerning the tissue damage in periodontal and periapical environment. Natural Tregs are CD4+CD25+ T cells that specifically regulate the activation, proliferation, and effector function of activated conventional T cells determining the outcome of several immunological settings, ranging from infectious diseases to immunopathology and autoimmunity (Appay et al., 2008, Belkaid et al., 2009, Sallusto & Lanzavecchia, 2009, Shevach et al., 2009). Tregs seem to be essential for the maintenance of peripheral tolerance and to control the immune response (Kotake et al., 2001), presenting a suppressive effect on osteoclasts differentiation (Zaiss et al., 2007) and controlling bone resorption (Zaiss et al., 2010). Tregs characteristically express as phenotypic markers the transcription factor forkhead box P3 (FOXp3), CD103, the glucocorticoid-inducible TNF receptor (GITR), the inhibitory molecule cytotoxic T-lymphocyte-associated molecule 4 (CTLA-4) and cell surface TGF-β1, among other surface molecules (Li & Flavell, 2008, Shevach et al., 2009). Regarding PD, immunohistological, flow-cytometry and molecular analysis characterized Tregs in periodontal tissues by the expression of its phenotypic markers (FOXp3, CTLA-4, IL-10, GITR, CD103 and CD45RO), demonstrating therefore its presence in periodontal environment (Nakajima et al., 2005, Cardoso et al., 2008). Similarly, the presence of CD4+ CD25hi Foxp3+ Tregs was also observed in PLs, which inhibited the proliferation of responder T-cells *in vitro*, at least in part, by stimulating the production of IL-10 (Colic et al., 2010). A recent study demonstrates that CD4+Foxp3+ cells migrate to periodontal tissues after experimental infection, while its inhibition resulted in increased alveolar bone loss and inflammatory cell migration (Garlet, 2010). Interestingly, recent data demonstrated that Tregs inhibition throughout *A. actinomycetemcomitans*-induced experimental periodontitis in mice does not compromise the control of infection (Garlet, 2010). This apparent inconsistency may rely on the uniqueness of PDs, as previously discussed regarding the characteristics of host response against the subgingival biofilm and to individual invasive periodontal pathogens, and the still unknown degree and nature of host response required to restrain the periodontal infection.

Besides IL-10, Tregs-associated cytokine TGF-β and the inhibitory molecule CTLA-4 are also supposed to attenuate PD progression (Cardoso et al., 2008). Regarding CTLA-4, this classic Tregs marker is expressed by leukocytes in diseased periodontium, and was found to be increased in CD4+ cells of periodontitis patients when compared to healthy subjects (Aoyagi et al., 2000, Orima et al., 1999). Additionally, CTLA-4 suppresses the proliferation of T cells in response to periodontopathogens (Aoyagi et al., 2000). TGF-β can also play important roles in the attenuation of inflammatory damage in periodontal tissues. TGF-β is a pleiotropic cytokine that regulates cell growth, differentiation and matrix production, and is a potent immunosuppressive factor that downregulates the transcription of pro-inflammatory factors (such as IL-1β and TNF-α) and MMPs (Okada & Murakami, 1998, Steinsvoll, et al., 1999). Moreover, in active periodontal lesions and stable granulomas, TGF-β levels are negatively correlated with RANKL levels, reinforcing its protective role against tissue destruction (Dutzan, 2009a, Dutzan, 2009b, Steinsvoll et al., 1999).

Subsequently to the discovery of Tregs subsets, the identification of a Th17 subset that present effector antagonic roles for Treg-suppressive cells (Appay et al., 2008, Cardoso et al., 2008, Garlet, 2010, Sallusto & Lanzavecchia, 2009, Weaver, & Hatton, 2009), had an immediate impact not only on the understanding of T-cell function and regulation, but also has encouraged many researchers to re-examine the dichotomic Th1/Th2 model in bone inflammatory disorders, such as periodontal and periapical diseases.

Th17 lymphocytes is an osteoclastogenic cell subset (Yago et al., 2009), characterized as an IL-17-producing CD4 T cell subset, which have been implicated in numerous autoimmune and inflammatory conditions (Annunziato et al., 2008, Colic et al., 2008, Colic et al., 2007, Gaffen and Hajishengallis, 2008, Sallusto & Lanzavecchia, 2009). Th17 cells develop through cytokine signals distinct from, and antagonized by, products of the Th1 and Th2 lineages (Appay et al., 2008, Dong et al., 2008, Sallusto & Lanzavecchia, 2009). Although IL-23 is important for the final differentiation of Th17 cells (Kastelein et al. 2007), it is not the only cytokine responsible for their development and activation, IL-1, IL-6 and TGF-β seem to be also involved (McGeachy and Cua, 2008). It has been reported that T cells are involved in the bone destruction via IL-17 production, which in their turn is described as an inducer of RANKL production (Kotake et al., 1999, Sato et al., 2006). While some studies suggest that IL-17 seems to be less potent as a direct MMP inducer than classic innate immunity cytokines, the ability of Th17 cells to produce IL-6 and to upregulate IL-1β and tumor necrosis factor-α (TNF-α) production may generate an inflammation amplification loop, with a consequent increase of MMPs and RANKL expression. Recent reports demonstrated the presence of IL-17, in periodontitis and chronic PLs (Cardoso et al., 2008, Colic et al., 2007, Takahashi et al, 2005, Vernal et al., 2005). In consequence, Th17 cells are thought to exacerbate inflammatory diseases by activating adjacent cells to produce inflammatory mediators, generating therefore a positive loop for inflammatory reaction amplification that leads to lesion exacerbation. In accordance, recent evidences demonstrate that the Th17/IL-17 axis, by itself or along with pro-inflammatory and Th1 cytokines, mobilize macrophages and neutrophils against extracellular and intracellular pathogens. IL-17 was described to play a role in neutrophil mobilization after *P. gingivalis* infection (Yu et al., 2007). Interestingly, experimental studies in rodents demonstrate the IL-17 deficient mice may present increased or decreased bone lesions in response to periodontal pathogens challenge (Oseko et al., 2009, Yu et al., 2007). However, we must consider that experimental periodontitis or PLs models may not reflect perfectly the chronic nature of human disease,

and that alveolar bone loss in aged mice is associated to an increased expression of IL-17A. Curiously, IL-17 was also recently described to increase TLR responsiveness in human gingival epithelial cells, suggesting that this cytokine can play a supporting role in the innate immunity sensing of pathogens and in the subsequent host response.
Recently, it has been shown the involvement of others cytokines and Th subsets than Th1, Th2, Tregs and Th17 in the complex process of inflammatory diseases development and progression (Brand et al., 2006, Cardoso et al., 2009, Colic et al., 2007, Colic et al., 2008, Gaffen et al., 2008, Seiderer et al., 2008). IL-9 has long been thought to be a Th2 cytokine, as it promotes allergic inflammation and is associated with various Th2 responses (Hauber et al., 2009). However, reports have described an IL-9-secreting population T cell, Th9 cells, which are differentiated in culture with a combination of TGF-β1 and IL-4 (Dardalhon et al., 2008). IL-9 has also been shown to promote Th17 cells development, while increasing the activity of Treg cells (Elyaman et al., 2009, Novak et al., 2009). In addition, Th22, a novel Th cell population characterized by IL-22 expression, was identified in epidermis of patients with skin inflammatory disorders (Brand et al., 2006). Although, unpublished data from our group suggests a anti-inflammatory function for IL-22, since IL-22 was positively correlated to OPG, IL-10 and TGF-β in chronic periapical granulomas, exhibiting anti-inflammatory properties, in accordance to other studies in intestinal inflammatory diseases (Valencial et al., 2006). The opposite result could reinforce the theory proposed that IL-22 presents bi-directional function (Seiderer & Brand, 2009). In Chron's disease, an intestinal inflammatory disease, IL-22 was capable at the same time to stimulate proinflammatory mediators expression and to mediate the intestinal barrier function. Based on opposite effects of IL-22, it can be suggested the Th22 participation in adaptative immune response in PLs.
At this point, it is possible to propose that the differential expression of T helper cytokines in periodontal and periapical tissues determine the PD and PLs outcome. However, the discovery of new T cell subsets lead to a more complex scenario regarding the role of cytokines in periapical inflammatory diseases pathogenesis. In fact, the Th1/Th2 and Th17/Tregs paradigms provided interesting frameworks, but further studies are still required to integrate them in a string theory to unravel the destructive and protective role of cytokines from the tissue destruction viewpoint. Although the lipid mediators do not fit in the classic definition of cytokines (usually comprising proteins, peptides or glycoproteins), they may modulate or be modulated by them. However, recent reports suggest that the concept of "protective and destructive" mediators in the control of periodontal and periapical infection is an obviously simplified model, and that cytokines may present dual and apparently conflicting protective or destructive roles. Hence, a different perspective is that the spatial orientation of the inflammatory infiltrate to the bone and the periodontal ligament is an important component of determining whether the destructive influence is reversible as in the case of gingivitis or irreversible as in the case of periodontitits and pulp necrosis (Graves et al., 2011).

6. Chemokines as determinants of host response nature

Leukocytes are an essential part of the host's inflammatory response and are fundamental to antibacterial defense (Bellingan, 2000, Kantarci et al., 2003, Nathan, 2006). Their chemotaxis can be induced by several inflammatory mediators, including IL-1 and TNF-α, which in turn induce the production of specific chemoattractants, the chemokines. Chemokines are a family of potent chemotatic cytokines that regulate the trafficking and recruitment of leukocytes to distant sites of inflammation (Zlotnik & Yoshie, 2000). The fine tuning of the regulation of the chemokine system is essential for host homeostasis and defense, and its abnormal expression is often associated with pathological processes (Garin & Proudfoot, 2011). The first cytokine identified to have chemotactic activity was IL-8, which proved to be a selective neutrophil chemoattractant (Yoshimura et al., 1987). The discovery of IL-8 triggered the search for other chemokines, stimulating a search for new family members with considerable interest in mediators responsible for the selective recruitment and activation of all leukocyte subsets (Murphy et al., 2000, Silva et al., 2007, Ward et al., 1998). Today, several chemokines have been described and they can be subclassified into four groups, according to their structure and spacing of conserved cysteine residues present in their molecules, namely CXC, CC, C and CX_3C (Murphy et al., 2000, Rossi et al., 2000, Zlotnik & Yoshie, 2000). This relatively new classification system was introduced in 2000, in which chemokines were considered as chemokine ligands, and each chemokine has been assigned a designation of CXCL or CCL (Rossi et al., 2000, Bacon et al., 2002). These ligands mediated their effects via 7-transmembrane domain receptors comprising a subset of G protein-coupled receptors (GPCRs) (Zlotnik & Yoshie, 2000). There is a great deal of redundancy and binding promiscuity between chemokine ligands and their receptors because some chemokines can bind multiple receptor subtypes, and some receptors can bind multiple chemokines (Murphy et al., 2000). Although most chemokine receptors recognize more than one chemokine, they are almost always restricted to a single subclass. Thus, the nomenclature system is rooted by the chemokine subclass specificity of the receptor been referred to as CC chemokines receptor (CCR) and CXC chemokine receptor (CXCR) followed by a number (Bacon et al., 2002, Murphy et al., 2000). Engagement of chemokine receptors with their respective ligands affects leukocyte migration by regulation of cytoskeletal re-arrangement, integrin-dependent adhesion, as well as by the binding and detachment of cells from their substrate (Silva et al, 2007).

Among the mediators potentially involved in leukocyte migration to periodontal and periapical environment, chemokines have been investigated with special interest (Silva et al., 2007). Chemokines are found in gingival tissue and crevicular fluid and are produced by a number of cell types in the periodontium, such as fibroblasts, endothelial cells, macrophages, osteoclasts, epithelial cells, polymorphonuclear leukocytes, monocytes, lymphocytes, and mast cells and exert their effects locally in paracrine or autocrine fashion (Baggiolini, 2001, Traves & Donnelly, 2005). Some chemokines have important proinflammatory effects and are related to periodontal tissue destruction that involves the stimulation of bone resorption and induction of tissue damage. Chemokines can also affect the recruitment, differentiation, or fusion of precursor cells to form osteoclasts or enhance osteoclast survival (Pradeep et al., 2009, Silva et al., 2007). They could also interfere with PD by recruiting cells, such as neutrophils, which protect host against bacterial invasion (Graves et al., 2011, Kantarci et al., 2003).

CXCL8 (IL-8) is an inflammatory chemokine which functions mainly as a neutrophil chemoattractant and activating factor. CXCL8 is able to upregulate the expression of adhesion molecules on the surface of neutrophils, enhancing leukotriene B4 (LTB4) production, inducing neutrophil chemotaxis and increasing neutrophils adherence to endothelial and epithelial cells (Rossi, 2003, Traves & Donnelly, 2005). CXCL8 is found at higher levels in gingival crevicular fluid prior to clinical signs of inflammation (Graves et al., 2011). As PD seems to be related to the progression of the inflammatory process to deeper periodontal tissues, chemokines found in both gingival tissue and crevicular fluid may play an important role on its pathogenesis. In this regard, subjects with a history of periodontitis have high levels of CXCL8 in gingival tissue and crevicular fluid and these levels are correlated with disease severity (Graves et al., 2011, Tsai et al., 1995). Moreover, CXCL8 has a direct effect on osteoclast differentiation and activity by signaling through the specific receptor, CXCR1 (Bendre et al., 2003). Analysis of the chemokines KC/CXCL1 (the analogue of the human CXCL8), in an experimental model of PD in mice, revealed their expression in diseased tissues, preferentially in the junctional epithelium, and their correlation with the migration of PMNs (Garlet et al., 2005). Furthermore, there was a significant increase in the expression of CXCL8 by epithelial cells from periapical granulomas, suggesting that those cells also could increase vascular permeability and leukocyte chemotaxis (Takeichi et al., 2008).

Other abundant chemokine expressed in the connective tissue subjacent to gingival epithelium is Macrophage Inflammatory Protein-1α (MIP-1α)/CCL3 (Gemmell et al., 2001). CCL3 chemoattracts a variety of cells, including lymphocytes, monocytes, basophils and eosinophils (Koch et al., 2005, Taub, 1996). It is a ligand for the receptors CCR1 and CCR5 and is associated with the recruitment of monocytes/macrophages and dendritic cells via CCR1, and lymphocytes polarized into the Th1 phenotype by CCR5 (Alnaeeli et al., 2007). Thus, CCL3 has a potential role in stimulating bone resorption through effects on macrophages and Th1 cells (Graves et al., 2011). The number of CCL3-positive cells increases in periodontal tissues with increasing severity of PD. On the other hand, the absence of CCL3 does not affect the development of experimental PD in mice, probably due to the presence of homologous chemokines CCL4 and CCL5 which share the receptors CCR1 and CCR5 with CCL3 and present a similar kinetics of expression than CCL3 (Repeke et al., 2010).

Regulated upon Activation Normal T-cell Expressed and Secreted (RANTES/CCL5) is found in greater levels in active periodontal lesions compared to inactive sites (Gamonal et al., 2001, Gemmell et al., 2001) and it chemoattracts lymphocytes and monocytes as well as other cell types (Koch et al., 2005, Schall et al., 1990). The involvement of CCL5 in periodontal bone resorption is supported by findings that it binds to CCR1 and/or CCR5 (Garlet et al., 2003), inducing chemotaxis and the formation of osteoclasts *in vitro* (Yu et al., 2004). Fibroblasts from patients with rheumatoid arthritis, which shares some inflammatory features with PD, produce CCL5 mRNA upon stimulation with TNF-α, IL-1, or IFN-γ (Koch et al., 2005, Volin et al., 1998) and this production of CCL5 can participate in cytokine networks by inducing the production of CXCL8 and IL-6 (Nanki et al., 2001). Nevertheless, findings in a model of PL implicated CCR5 as a negative regulator of bone resorption, as mice lacking CCR5 presented larger PL than wild-type mice (Rossi et al., 2008). Accordingly, an increased amount of orthodontic tooth movement, correlated with increased alveolar bone resorption, was observed in the absence of CCR5 in mice (Andrade Jr. et al., 2009). Interestingly, an intermediate phenotype of PD development was observed after individual blockage of CCR1 and CCR5 (using genetically deficient mice strains) (Repeke et al., 2010). Thus, supported by findings that showed CCR1 expression in pre-osteoclasts and its increase expression in RANKL differentiated osteoclasts (Yu et al., 2004), it seems that the bone resorptive activity of CCL5 in PD and PL might be mediated by its engagement with CCR1, while it seems to be controlled by CCR5, although lack direct evidence to support this hypothesis.

Monocyte chemoattractant protein-1 (MCP-1/CCL2) is a potent chemoattractant for monocytes (Koch et al., 1992), detectable in the sera of patients with rheumatoid arthritis

(Koch et al., 2005). CCL2 is produced by a variety of cell types, either constitutively or after induction by oxidative stress, cytokines, or growth factors (Yada et al., 2010). CCL2 binds to CCR2 and CCR11 receptors, however, binding to CCR11 does not result in increased intracellular calcium mobilization, which is essential for chemotaxis (Schweickart et al., 2000). Some evidence indicates that CCL2 may contribute to periodontitis once its levels are directly correlated with gingival inflammation. It has been demonstrated that IL-1β and TNF-α induce and synergistically stimulate CCL2 expression by fibroblasts from human periodontal ligament contributing to the infiltration of monocytes into inflammatory sites (Hanazawa et al., 1993, Ozaki et al., 1996, Yu et al., 1995). The monocytes/macrophages accumulation at sites of bone injury and bone remodeling may play a significant role in the regulation of bone metabolism (Rahimi et al., 1995, Williams et al., 1992, Yada et al., 2010). CCL2 also has been implicated as chemoattractant for osteoclast precursors (Bonecchi et al., 2009, Garlet et al., 2003) while limiting the infiltration of PMNs (Garlet et al., 2010). Accordingly, it was demonstrated that the mean concentration of CCL2 in GCF in chronic periodontitis patients reduced after treatment (Pradeep et al., 2009). Thus, a variety of evidence that support the role of CCL2 in inflammatory bone remodeling conditions, such as PD and PL, include: 1) CCL2 is the principal monocyte chemoattractant produced by osteoblastic cells *in vitro*, 2) CCL2 is not expressed in normal bone, but is induced during bone inflammation, 3) The induction of CCL2 in inflamed bone is temporally and spatially correlated with the recruitment of monocytes, 4) CCL2 production is associated with the recruitment of monocytes to areas of both bone formation and resorption during developmentally regulated bone remodeling (reviewed by Yada et al., 2010).

Altogether, these findings indicate that chemokines orchestrate a large proportion of the cellular and molecular events observed in inflammatory oral diseases. In PD and PL, chemokines are directly involved in the recruitment of cells to control infection, but also contribute to the pathways involved in bone resorption. Thus, the control of this highly tuned system is essential in the determination of tissue homeostasis or disease when an infectious challenge disturbs the natural host balance.

7. Clinical implications and future directions

Periodontal disease and periapical lesion progression remain significant aspects of dentistry today. Extensive efforts to understand the etiology and pathogenesis of the oral inflammatory diseases concluded that they share common pathogenic mechanisms. Both diseases are mainly mediated by the perpetuation of infection and destruction of connective and mineralized tissues. This information gives us a clue that certain therapeutic strategies may be beneficial to both diseases and a number of mediators may have therapeutical potential. Ironically, the same host systems that defend against diverse pathogens are also responsible for tissue destruction. Hence, the spatial orientation of the inflammatory infiltrate to the bone and the periodontal tissue is an important component that can determine whether the destructive influence is predominant over the infection control. Despite recent technological advances in curative treatment, the disease prevention are still elusive. Deeper knowledge of the etiology and pathogenesis to uncover predictive biomarkers may well be important to provide safe host-modulating approaches, which can reveal real possibility of early intervention and prevention of alveolar bone loss.

8. Concluding remarks (Summary)

The past 20 years have seen major advances in our understanding of the role of cytokine networks and chemokines orchestrating cellular and molecular events in the complex process of inflammatory disease development and progression. In fact, the development of oral inflammatory diseases is characterized by the persistent release of inflammatory mediators, such as cytokines and chemokines and migration of inflammatory cells to infected sites. These responses, although directed against bacteria, perpetuate and mediate the destruction of connective and mineralized periodontal tissues, being the main responsible for periodontal breakdown. Moreover, ongoing research results let us to conclude that the discovery of new T cell subsets lead to a more complex scenario regarding the role of cytokines in inflammatory oral diseases pathogenesis. Recent reports suggest that the control of periodontal and periapical infection by "protective and destructive" mediators is an obviously simplified concept and several cytokines may present dual and apparently conflicting protective and destructive roles. Thus, string theories to unravel the destructive and protective role of cytokines and chemokines from the tissue destruction viewpoint make the development of effective therapies a very interesting challenge.

9. References

Agnello, D., Lankford, C.S., Bream, J., Morinobu, A., Gadina, M., O'Shea, J.J. & Frucht DM (2003). Cytokines and transcription factors that regulate T helper cell differentiation: new players and new insights. *J Clin Immunol,* Vol 23, No.3 (May 2003), pp.147-61, ISSN 12797537.

Aiba, T., Akeno, N., Kawane, T., Okamoto, H. & Horiuchi, N. (1996). Matrix metalloproteinases-1 and -8 and TIMP-1 mRNA levels in normal and diseased human gingivae. *European Journal of Oral Sciences*, Vol. 104, No. 5-6, (October-December 1996), pp. 562-569, ISSN 1600-0722.

Akira, S., Hirano, T., Taga, T. & Kishimoto, T. (1990) Biology of multifunctional cytokines: IL 6 and related molecules (IL 1 and TNF). *The FASEB Journal*, Vol. 4, No 11 (August 1990). ,pp. 2860–2867, ISSN 2199284.

Alnaeeli, M., Park, J., Mahamed, D., Penninger, J. M. & Teng, Y. T. (2007). Dendritic cells at the osteo-immune interface: implications for inflammation-induced bone loss. *Journal of Bone and Mineral Research,* Vol. 22, No. 6, (June 2007), pp. 775-780, ISSN 0884-0431.

Alpagot, T., Bell, C., Lundergan, W., Chambers, D. W. & Rudin, R. (2001). Longitudinal evaluation of GCF MMP-3 and TIMP-1 levels as prognostic factors for progression of periodontitis. *Journal of Clinical Periodontology,* Vol. 28, No. 4, (April 2001), pp. 353-359, ISSN 1600-051X.

Andrade, Jr., I., Taddei, S. R. A., Garlet, G. P., Garlet, T. P., Teixeira, A. L., Silva, T. A. & Teixeira, M. M. (2009). CCR5 down-regulates osteoclast function in orthodontic tooth movement. *Journal of Dental Research,* Vol. 88, No. 11, (November 2009), pp. 1037-1041, ISSN 1544-0591.

Annunziato, F., Cosmi, L., Liotta, F. & (2008). The phenotype of human Th17 cells and their precursors, the cytokines that mediate their differentiation and the role of Th17 cells in inflammation. *International Immunol,* Vol. 20, No. 11 (November 2008), pp.1361-1368, ISSN 18820263.

Appay, V., van Lier, R.A., Sallusto, F., Roederer, M. (2008). Phenotype and function of human T lymphocyte subsets: consensus and issues. *Cytometry A,* Vol. 73, No.11 (November 2008), pp.975-83, ISSN 18785267.

Aranami, T. & Yamamura, T. Th17 cells and autoimmune encephalomyelitis (2008). *Allergol Int.,* Vol. 57, No. 2 (June 2008), pp.115-20, ISSN 18427164.

Bacon, K., Baggiolini, M., Broxmeyer, H., Horuk, R., Lindley, I., Mantovani, A., Maysushima, K., Murphy, P., Nomiyama, H., Oppenheim, J., Rot, A., Schall, T., Tsang, M., Thorpe, R., Van Damme, J., Wadhwa, M., Yoshie, O., Zlotnik, A., Zoon, K. & IUIS/WHO Subcommittee on Chemokine Nomenclature. (2002). Chemokine/chemokine receptor nomenclature. *Journal of Interferon and Cytokine Research,* Vol. 22, No. 10, (October 2002), pp. 1067–1068, ISSN 1079-9907.

Baggiolini, M. (2001). Chemokines in pathology and medicine. *Journal of Internal Medicine,* Vol. 250, No. 2, (August 2001), pp. 91-104, ISSN 1365-2796.

Baker, P.J., Boutaugh, N.R., Tiffany, M., Roopenian, D.C. (2009). B Cell IgD Deletion Prevents Alveolar Bone Loss Following Murine Oral Infection. *Interdiscip Perspect Infect Dis,* 2009:864359. ISSN19859584 (in process).

Baker, P.J., Dixon, M., Evans, R.T., Dufour, L., Johnson, E. & Roopenian, D.C, (1999). CD4(+) T cells and the proinflammatory cytokines gamma interferon and interleukin-6 contribute to alveolar bone loss in mice. *Infect Immunol.,* Vol. 67, No. 6 (June 1999), p.2804-2809, ISSN 10338484.

Bar-Shavit, Z. (2008). Taking a toll on the bones: regulation of bone metabolism by innate immune regulators. *Autoimmunity,* Vol. 41, No.3 (April 2008), pp.195-203, ISSN 18365832.

Bartold, P. M. & Marshall, R. I..(2005). Periodontitis and rheumatoid arthritis: a review. *Journal of Periodontology,* Vol. 76, No. suppl11 (November 2005), pp.2066-2074, ISSN 16277578.

Baud'huin, M., Lamoureux, F., Duplomb, L., Rédini, F. & Heymann, D. (2007). RANKL, RANK, osteoprotegerin: key partners of osteoimmunology and vascular diseases. *Cellular and Molecular Life Sciences,* Vol. 64, No. 18, (September 2007), pp. 2334-2350, ISSN 1420-9071.

Beertsen, W., McCulloch, C. A. & Sodek, J. (1997). The periodontal ligament: a unique, multifunctional connective tissue. *Periodontology 2000,* Vol. 13, No. 1, (February 1997), pp. 20-40, ISSN 0906-6713.

Behl, Y., Siqueira, M., Ortiz, J., Li, J., Desta, T., Faibish, D., & Graves, D. T. (2008). Activation of the acquired immune response reduces coupled bone formation in response to a periodontal pathogen. *J Immunol,* Vol. 181, No. 12(December 2008), pp. 8711-8718, ISSN 19050291.

Beikler, T. & Flemming, T. F. (2011). Oral biofilm-associated diseases: trends and implications for quality of life, systemic health and expenditures. *Periodontology 2000,* Vol. 55, No. 1, (February 2011), pp. 87-103, ISSN 1600-0757.

Bellingan, G. (2000). Leukocytes: friend or foe. *Intensive Care Medicine,* Vol. 26, pp. S111-S118, ISSN: 1432-1238, ISSN 0342-4642.

Benatti, B. B., Silverio, K. G., Casati, M. Z., Sallum, E. A. & Nociti, F. H. Jr. (2009). Inflammatory and bone-related genes are modulated by aging in human periodontal ligament cells. *Cytokine*, Vol. 46, No. 2, (May 2009), pp. 176-181, ISSN 1043-4666.

Bendre, M. S., Montague, D. C., Peery, T., Akel, N. S., Gaddy, D. & Suva, L. J. (2003). Interleukin-8 stimulation of osteoclastogenesis and bone resorption is a mechanism for the increased osteolysis of metastatic bone disease. *Bone*, Vol. 33, No. 1, (July 2003), pp. 28-37, ISSN 8756-3282.

Bergenholtz, G (1990). Pathogenic mechanisms in pulpal disease. *J Endod.*, Vol. 16, No. 2 (February 1990), pp. 98-101, ISSN 2388024.

Bergström, J. (2004). Tobacco smoking and chronic destructive periodontal disease. *Odontology*, Vol. 92, No. 1, (September 2004), pp. 1-8. ISSN 1618-1255.

Birkedal-Hansen, H. (1993). Role of matrix metalloproteinases in human periodontal diseases. *Journal of Periodontology*, Vol. 64, No. Suppl 5, (May 1993), pp. 474-484, ISSN 0022-3492.

Bloemen, V., Schoenmaker, T., de Vries, T.J., Everts, V. (2010). Direct cell-cell contact between periodontal ligament fibroblasts and osteoclast precursors synergistically increases the expression of genes related to osteoclastogenesis. *J Cell Physiol*, Vol. 222, No. 3(March 2010), pp. 565-573, ISSN 19927302.

Bluestone, J.A., Mackay, C.R., O'Shea, J.J. & Stockinger, B. (2009). The functional plasticity of T cell subsets. *Nat Rev Immunol*, Vol. 9, No. 11 (November 2009), pp. 811-816, ISSN 19809471.

Bosshardt, D. D. & Lang, N. P. (2005). The junctional epithelium: from health to disease. *Journal of Dental Research*, Vol. 84, No. 1, (January 2005), pp. 9-20, ISSN 1544-0591.

Bostanci, N., Emingil, G., Saygan, B., Turkoglu, O., Atilla, G., Curtis, M.A. & Belibasakis G.N. (2009). Expression and regulation of the NALP3 inflammasome complex in periodontal diseases. *Clin Exp Immunol*, Vol. 157, No. 3 (September 2009), pp. 415-422, ISSN 19664151.

Botero, T.M., Son, S.J., Vodopyanov, D., Hasegawa, M., Shelburne, C.E. & Nor, J.E. (2010). MAPK signaling is required for LPS-induced VEGF in pulp stem cells. *Journal of Dental Research*, Vo. 89, No. 3 (March 2010), pp. 264–269, ISSN 20110511.

Boyle, W. J., Simonet, W. S. & Lacey, D. L. (2003). Osteoclast differentiation and activation. *Nature*, Vol. 423, No. 6937, (May 2003), pp. 337-342, ISSN 0028-0836.

Bozkurt, F.Y., Yetkin, A. Z., Berker, E., Tepe, E., Akku, S. (2006). Anti-inflammatory cytokines in gingival crevicular fluid in patients with periodontitis and rheumatoid arthritis: a preliminary report. *Cytokine*, Vol. 35, No. 3-4 (August 2006), pp. 180-185, ISSN 16982199.

Brand, S., Beigel, F., Olszak, T. & (2006). IL-22 is increased in active Crohn's disease and promotes proinflammatory gene expression and intestinal epithelial cell migration. *Am J Physiol Gastrointest Liver Physiol*, Vol. 290; No. 4 (April 2006), pp.G827-838, ISSN 16537974.

Cardoso, C.R., Garlet, G.P., Crippa, G.E., Rosa, A.L., Júnior, W.M., Rossi, M.A. & Silva, J.S. (2009). Evidence of the presence of T helper type 17 cells in chronic lesions of human periodontal disease. *Oral Microbiol Immunol.*, Vol 24, No.1 (February 2009), pp.1-6, ISSN 19121062.

Cardoso, C.R., Garlet, G.P., Moreira, A.P., Júnior, W.M., Rossi, M.A. & Silva, J.S. (2008). Characterization of CD4+CD25+ natural regulatory T cells in the inflammatory infiltrate of human chronic periodontitis. *J Leukoc Biol,*Vol. 84, No.1 (July 2008), pp.311-318, ISSN 18451325.

Caviedes-Bucheli, J., Muñoz, H.R., Azuero-Holguın, M.M. & Ulate, E. (2208). Neuropeptides in dental pulp: the silent protagonists. *Journal of Endodontics* , Vol. 34, No. 34 (July 2008), pp.773–788, ISSN 18570980.

Chapple, I. L. (1997). Reactive oxygen species and antioxidants in inflammatory diseases. *Journal of Clinical Periodontology,* Vol. 24, No. 5, (May 1997), pp. 287-296, ISSN 1600-051X.

Claudino, M., Trombone, A.P., Cardoso, C.R., Ferreira Jr., S.B., , Martins Jr., W., Assis, G.F., Santos, C.F., Trevilatto, P.C., Campanelli, A.P., Silva, J.S. & Garlet, G.P. (2008). The broad effects of the functional IL-10 promoter-592 polymorphism: modulation of IL-10, TIMP-3, and OPG expression and their association with periodontal disease outcome. *Journal of Leukoc Biology,* Vol. 84, No.6 (December 2008), pp.1565-73, ISSN 18725394.

Cochran, D. L. (2008). Inflammation and bone loss in periodontal disease. *Journal of Periodontology,* Vol. 79, Vol. Suppl 8, (August 2008), pp. 1569-1576, ISSN 0022-3492.

Colic, M., Gazivoda. D., Vasilijic. S., Vucevic. D. & Lukic, A. (2010). Production of IL-10 and IL-12 by antigen-presenting cells in periapical lesions. *J Oral Pathol Med,* Vol. 39, No. 9 (October 2010), pp. 690-696, ISSN 20819132.

Colic, M., Gazivoda. D., Vucevic. D., Majstorovic, I., Vasilijic, S., Rudolf, R., Brkić, Z., & Milosavljević, P. (2009a). Regulatory T-cells in periapical lesions. Journal of Dental *Research,* Vol. 88, No. 11 (November 2009), pp. 997–1002, ISSN 19828886.

Colic, M., Gazivoda, D., Vucevic, D., Vasilijić, S., Rudolf, R. & Lukić, A. (2009b). Proinflammatory and immunoregulatory mechanisms in periapical lesions. *Molec Immunol,* Vol. 47, No. 1 (November 2009), pp. 101-113, ISSN 19232436. Colic, M., Lukic, A., Vucevic, D., Milosavljevic, P., Majstorovic, I., Marjanovic, M. & Dimitrijevic, J. (2006). Correlation between phenotypic characteristics of mononuclear cells isolated from human periapical lesions and their in vitro production of Th1 and Th2 cytokines. *Archives of Oral Biology,* Vol. 51, No. 12 (December 2006), pp. 1120-1130, ISSN 16797478.

Colic, M., & Vasilijic, S. (2007). Interleukin-17 plays a role in exacerbation of inflammation within chronic periapical lesions. *European Journal of Oral Sciense,* Vol 115, No. 4, (August 2007), pp. 315-320, ISSN 17697172.

Cornelis, P. (2009). Shielding, a new pathogen defense mechanism against PMNs. *Microbiology,* Vol. 155, No. 11(November 2009), pp. 3474-3475, ISSN 19729405.

Costalonga, M., Batas, L. & Reich, B.J. (2009). Effects of Toll-like receptor 4 on Porphyromonas gingivalis-induced bone loss in mice. *Journal of Periodontal Research,* Vol. 44, No. 4 (August 2009), pp. 537-542, ISSN 18752565.

Cronstein, B.N. (2007). Interleukin-6--a key mediator of systemic and local symptoms in rheumatoid arthritis. *Bull NYU Hosp Jt Dis,* Vol. 65, No. Suppl 1 (2007), pp. S11-S15, ISSN 17708739.

Cutler, C. W. & Jotwani, R. (2004). Antigen-presentation and the role of dendritic cells in periodontitis. *Periodontology 2000*, Vol. 35, No. 1, (June 2004), pp. 135-157, ISSN 0906-6713.

Dahan, M., Nawrocki, B., Elkaïm, R. Soell, M., Bolcato-Bellemin, A. L., Birembaut, P. & Tenenbaum, H. (2001). Expression of matrix metalloproteinases in healthy and diseased human gingiva. *Journal of Clinical Periodontology*, Vol. 28, No. 2, (February 2001), pp. 128-136, ISSN 1600-051X.

Dardalhon, V., Awasthi, A., Kwon, H., Galileos, G., Gao, W., Sobel, R.A., Mitsdoerffer, M., Strom, T.B., Elyaman, W., Ho, I.C., Khoury, S., Oukka, M. & Kuchroo, V.K. (2008). IL-4 inhibits TGF-β-induced FoxP3+ T cells and, together with TGF-β, generates IL-9+IL10+Foxp3- effector T cells. *Nat Immunol*, Vol 9, No. 12 (December 2008), pp.1347-1355, ISSN 18997793.

Darveau, R. P. (2010). Periodontitis: a polymicrobial disruption of host homeostasis. *Nature Reviews. Microbiology*, Vol. 8, No. 7, (July 2010), pp. 481-490, ISSN 1700-1526.

Darveau, R. P., Tanner, A. & Page, R. C. (1997). The microbial challenge in periodontitis. *Periodontology 2000*, Vol. 14, No. 1, (June 1997), pp. 12-32, ISSN 0906-6713.

De Rossi, A., Rocha, L.B., Rossi, M.A. (2008). Interferon-gamma, interleukin-10, Intercellular adhesion molecule-1, and chemokine receptor 5, but not interleukin-4, attenuate the development of periapical lesions. *J Endod*, Vol. 34, No. 1 (January 2008), pp. 31-38, ISSN 18155488.

Delany, A. M. & Hankenson, K. D. (2009). Thrombospondin-2 and SPARC/osteonectin are critical regulators of bone remodeling. *Journal of Cell Communication and Signaling*, Vol. 3, No. 3-4, (December 2009), pp. 227-238, ISSN 1873-961X.

Dinarello, C.A. (2000). Proinflammatory cytokines. *Chest*, Vol. 118, No.2 (August 2000), pp.503-508, ISSN 10936147.

Ding, J., Ghali, O., Lencel, P., Broux,O., Chauveau, C., Devedjian, J.C., Hardouin, P. & Magne, D. (2009). TNF-alpha and IL-1beta inhibit RUNX2 and collagen expression but increase alkaline phosphatase activity and mineralization in human mesenchymal stem cells. *Life Sci*, Vol. 84, No.15-16 (April2009), pp. 499-504, ISSN 19302812.

Duerkop, B. A., Vaishnava, S. & Hooper, L. V. (2009). Immune responses to the microbiota at the intestinal mucosal surface. *Immunity*, Vol. 31, No. 3, (September 2009), pp. 368-376, ISSN 1074-7613.

Dutzan, N., Gamonal, J., Silva, A., Sanz, M. & Vernal, R. (2009a). Over-expression of forkhead box P3 and its association with receptor activator of nuclear factor-kappa B ligand, interleukin (IL) -17, IL-10 and transforming growth factor-beta during the progression of chronic periodontitis. *Journal of Clinical of Periodontology*, Vol. 36, No. 5 (May 2009), pp. 396-403, ISSN 19419438.

Dutzan, N., Vernal, R., Hernandez, M., Dezerega, A., Rivera, O., Silva, N. & . (2009b). Levels of interferon-gamma and transcription factor T-bet in progressive periodontal lesions in patients with chronic periodontitis. *Journal of Periodontology*, Vol. 80, No. 2(February 2009), pp. 290-296, ISSN 19186970.

Elyaman, W., Bradshaw, E.M., Uyttenhove, C., Dardalhon, V. & (2009). IL-9 induces differentiation of Th17 cells and enhances function of FoxP3+ natural regulatory T cells. *Proc Natl Acad Sci USA,* Vol. 106, No. 31 (August 2009), pp. 12885-12890, ISSN 19433802.

Emrich, L. J., Shlossman, M. & Genco, R. J. (1991). Periodontal disease in non-insulin-dependent diabetes mellitus. *Journal of Periodontology,* Vol. 62, No. 2, (February 1991), pp. 123-131, ISSN 0022-3492.

Fine, D.H., Kaplan, J.B., Kachlany, S.C. & Schreiner, H.C. (2006). How we got attached to Actinobacillus actinomycetemcomitans: A model for infectious diseases. *Periodontol 2000,* Vol. 42, pp.114-157, ISSN 16930309.

Fonseca, J.E., Santos, M.J., Canhao, H. & Choy, E. (2009). Interleukin-6 as a key player in systemic inflammation and joint destruction. *Autoimmun Rev,* Vol. 8, No. 7 (June 2009), pp. 538-542, ISSN 19189867.

Fristad, I., Bletsa, A. & Byers, M. (2010). Inflammatory nerve responses in the dental pulp. *Endodontic Topics*, Vol. 17, No. 11 (November 2010), pp. 12–41, ISSN 19732182.

Fukada, S.Y., Silva, T.A., Garlet, G.P., Rosa, A.L., da Silva, J.S. & Cunha, F.Q. (2009). Factors involved in the T helper type 1 and type 2 cell commitment and osteoclast regulation in inflammatory apical diseases. *Oral Microbiol Immunol*, Vol. 24, No. 1 (February 2009), pp. 25–31, ISSN 19121066.

Fukui, M., Hinode, D., Yokoyama, M., Tanabe, S. & Yoshioka, M. (2006). Salivary immunoglobulin A directed to oral microbial GroEL in patients with periodontitis and their potential protective role. *Oral Microbiol Immunol,* Vol. 21, No. 5 (October 2006), pp. 289-295, ISSN 16922927.

Gaffen, S.L. & Hajishengallis, G. (2008). A new inflammatory cytokine on the block: re-thinking periodontal disease and the Th1/Th2 paradigm in the context of Th17 cells and IL-17. *Journal of Dental Research,* Vol. 87, No. 9 (September 2008), pp. 817-828, ISSN 18719207.

Gamonal, J., Acevedo, A., Bascones, A., Jorge, O. & Silva, A. (2001). Characterization of cellular infiltrate, detection of chemokine receptor CCR5 and interleukin-8 and RANTES chemokines in adult periodontitis. *Journal of Periodontal Research,* Vol. 36, No. 3, (June 2001), pp. 194-203, ISSN 0022-3484.

Gao, Y., Grassi, F., Ryan, M.R., Terauchi, M., Page, K., Yang, X. & . (2007). IFN-gamma stimulates osteoclast formation and bone loss in vivo via antigen-driven T cell activation. *Journal of Clinical Investigation,* Vol. 117, No. 1 (January 2007), pp. 122-132, ISSN 17173138.

Garin, A. & Proudfoot, A. E. I. (2011). Chemokines as targets for therapy. *Experimental Cell Research,* Vol. 317, No. 5, (March 2011), pp. 602-612, ISSN 0014-4827.

Garlet, G.P., Cardoso, C.R., Campanelli, A.P., Ferreira, B.R., Avila-Campos, M.J., Cunha, F.Q. &,. (2007). The dual role of p55 tumour necrosis factor-alpha receptor in Actinobacillus actinomycetemcomitans-induced experimental periodontitis: host protection and tissue destruction. *Clin Exp Immunol,* Vol. 147, No.1 (January 2007), pp. 128-138, ISSN 17177972.

Garlet, G.P., Cardoso, C.R., Campanelli, A.P., Martins, W., Jr. & Silva, J.S. (2006a). Expression of suppressors of cytokine signaling in diseased periodontal tissues: a stop signal for disease progression? *Journal of Periodontal Research,* Vol. 41, No. 6, (December 2006), pp. 580-584, ISSN 17076785.

Garlet, G.P., Cardoso, C.R., Campanelli, A.P., Garlet, T. P., Avila-Campos, M. J., Cunha, F. Q. & Silva, J. S. (2008).The essential role of IFN-γ in the control of lethal Aggregatibacter actinomycetemcomitans infection in mice. *Microbes and Infection,* Vol. 10, No. 5 (April 2008), pp., ISSN 18403243.

Garlet, G. P. (2010). Destructive and protective roles of cytokines in periodontitis: a re-appraisal from host defense and tissue destruction viewpoints. *Journal of Dental Research,* Vol. 89, No. 12, (December 2010), pp. 1349-1363, ISSN 1544-0591.

Garlet, G. P., Avila-Campos, M. J., Milanezi, C. M., Ferreira, B. R., Silva, J. S. (2005). *Actinobacillus actinomycetemcomitans*-induced periodontal disease in mice: patterns of cytokine, chemokine, and chemokine receptor expression and leukocyte migration. *Microbes and Infection,* Vol. 7, No. 4, (April 2005), pp. 738-747, ISSN 1286-4579.

Garlet, G. P., Cardoso, C. R., Silva, T. A., Ferreira, B. R., Ávila-Campos, M. J., Cunha, F. Q. & Silva, J. S. (2006b). Cytokine pattern determines the progression of experimental periodontal disease induced by *Actinobacillus actinomycetemcomitans* through the modulation of MMPs, RANKL, and their physiological inhibitors. *Oral Microbiology Immunology,* Vol. 21, No. 1, (February 2006), pp. 12-20, ISSN 1399-302X.

Garlet, G. P., Martins, W. Jr., Ferreira, B. R., Milanezi, C. M. & Silva, J. S. (2003). Patterns of chemokines and chemokine receptors expression in different forms of human periodontal disease. *Journal of Periodontal Research,* Vol. 38, No. 2, (April 2003), pp. 210-217, ISSN 0022-3484.

Garlet, G. P., Martins, W. Jr., Fonseca, B. A., Ferreira, B. R. & Silva, J. S. (2004). Matrix metalloproteinases, their physiological inhibitors and osteoclast factors are differentially regulated by the cytokine profile in human periodontal disease. *Journal of Clinical Periodontology,* Vol. 31, No. 8, (August 2004), pp. 671-679, ISSN 1600-051X.

Garlet, T. P., Coelho, U., Silva, J. S. & Garlet, G. P. (2007). Cytokine expression pattern in compression and tension sides of the periodontal ligament during orthodontic tooth movement in humans. *European Journal of Oral Sciences,* Vol. 115, No. 5, (October 2007), pp. 355-362, ISSN 1600-0722.

Gemmell, E., Carter, C.L., Grieco, D.A., Sugerman, P.B. & Seymour, G.J. (2002a). *P. gingivalis*-specific T-cell lines produce Th1 and Th2 cytokines. *Journal of Dental Research,* Vol. 81, No.5 (May 2002), pp. 303-307, ISSN 12097441.

Gemmell, E., Yamazaki, K. & Seymour, G.J. (2002b). Destructive periodontitis lesions are determined by the nature of the lymphocytic response. *Crit Rev Oral Biol Med,* Vol. 13, No.1 (2002), pp. 17-34, ISSN 12097235.

Gemmell, E. & Seymour, G. J. (2004). Immunoregulatory control of Th1/Th2 cytokine profiles in periodontal disease. *Periodontology 2000,* Vol. 35, No. 1, (June 2004), pp. 21-41, ISSN 0906-6713.

Gemmell, E., Carter, C. L. & Seymour G. J. (2001). Chemokines in human periodontal disease tissues. *Clinical and Experimental Immunology,* Vol. 125, No. 1, (July 2001), pp.134-141, ISSN 0009-9104

Giannobile, W.V. (2008). Host-response therapeutics for periodontal diseases. *Journal of Periodontology,* Vol. 79, No. 8 Suppl (August 2008), pp. 1592-1600, ISSN 18673015.

Giannopoulou, C., Kamma, J.J. & Mombelli, A. (2003). Effect of inflammation, smoking and stress on gingival crevicular fluid cytokine level. *Journal of Clinical of Periodontology,* Vol. 30, No.2 (February 2003), pp.145-153, ISSN 12622857.

Gibson 3rd, F.C., Savelli, J., Van Dyke, T.E. & Genco, C.A. (2005). Gingipain-specific IgG in the sera of patients with periodontal disease is necessary for opsonophagocytosis of Porphyromonas gingivalis. *Journal of Periodontology,* Vol. 76, No.10 (October 2008), pp.1629-1636, ISSN 16253083.

Giudici, C., Raynal, N., Wiedemann, H., Cabral, W. A., Marini, J. C., Timpl, R., Bächinger, H. P., Farndale, R. W., Sasaki, T. & Tenni, R. (2008). Mapping of SPARC/BM-40/osteonectin-binding sites on fibrillar collagens. *The Journal of Biological Chemistry*, Vol. 283, No. 28, (July 2008), pp. 19551-19560, ISSN 1083-351X.

Goldberg, M. & Smith, A.J. (2004). Cells and extracellular matrices of dentin and pulp: a biological basis for repair and tissue engineering. *Critical Reviews in Oral Biology and Medicine,* Vol. 15, No. 1 (January 2004), pp. 13–27, ISSN 14761897.

Golub, L. M., McNamara, T. F., Ryan, M. E., Kohut, B., Blieden, T., Payonk, G., Sipos, T. & Baron, H. J. (2001). Adjunctive treatment with subantimicrobial doses of doxycycline: effects on gingival fluid collagenase activity and attachment loss in adult periodontitis. *Journal of Clinical Periodontology*, Vol. 28, No. 2, (February 2001), pp. 146-156, ISSN 1600-051X.

Gonçalves, L. D., Oliveira, G., Hurtado, P. A., Feitosa, A., Takiya, C. M., Granjeiro, J. M., Trackman, P. C., Otazú, I. & Feres-Filho, E. J. (2008). Expression of metalloproteinases and their tissue inhibitors in inflamed gingival biopsies. *Journal of Periodontal Research*, Vol. 43, No. 5, (October 2008), pp. 570-577, ISSN 1600-0765.

Graves, D.T. & Cochran, D. (2003). The contribution of interleukin-1 and tumor necrosis factor to periodontal tissue destruction. *Journal of Periodontology,* Vol. 74, No. 3 (March 2003), pp. 391-401, ISSN 12710761.

Graves, DT, Li J, Cochran DL. (2011a). Inflammation and uncoupling as mechanisms of periodontal bone loss. *Journal of Dental Research,* Vol. 90, No. 2 (February 2011), pp. 143-53, ISSN 21135192.

Graves, DT (2008). Cytokines that promote periodontal tissue destruction. *Journal of Periodontology*, Vol. 79, No. Suppl 8, (August 2008), pp. 1585-1591, ISSN 0022-3492.

Graves, D.T., Delima, A.J., Assuma, R., Amar, S., Oates, T. & Cochran, D. (1998). Interleukin-1 and tumor necrosis factor antagonists inhibit the progression of inflammatory cell infiltration toward alveolar bone in experimental periodontitis. *Journal of Periodontology*, Vol. 69, No. 12, (December 1998), pp. 1419-1425, ISSN 0022-3492.

Graves, D.T., Chen, C., Douville, C. & Jiang, Y. (2000). Interleukin-1 receptor signaling rather than that of the tumor necrosis factor is critical in protecting the host from the severe consences of a polymicroe anaerobic infection. *Infection and Immunity*, Vol. 68, No. 8, (August 2000), pp. 4746-4751, ISSN 1098-5522.

Graves, D.T., Oates, T. & Garlet, G.P. (2011b). Review of osteoimmunology and the host response in endodontic and periodontal lesions. *Journal of Oral Microbiology,* Vol. 3, (January 2011), DOI: 10.3402/jom.v3i0.5304, ISSN 2000-2297.

Guentsch, A., Puklo, M., Preshaw, P.M., Glockmann, E., Pfister, W., Potempa, J. & Eick, S. (2009). Neutrophils in chronic and aggressive periodontitis in interaction with

Porphyromonas gingivalis and Aggregatibacter actinomycetemcomitans. *Journal of Periodontal Research,* Vol. 44, No. 3(June 2009), pp. 368-377, ISSN 19210340.

Guha, M. & Mackman, N. (2001) LPS induction of gene expression in human monocytes. *Cellular Signalling,* Vol. 13, No. 2 (February 2001), pp. 85–94, ISSN 11257452.

Gustafsson, A., Ito, H., Asman, B. & Bergstrom, K. (2006). Hyper-reactive mononuclear cells and neutrophils in chronic periodontitis. *Journal of Clinical of Periodontology,* Vol. 33, No. 2 (February 2006), pp. 126-129, ISSN 16441737.

Haerian, A., Adonogianaki, E., Mooney, J., Docherty, J. P. & Kinane, D. F. (1995). Gingival crevicular stromelysin, collagenase and tissue inhibitor of metalloproteinases levels in healthy and diseased sites. *Journal of Clinical Periodontology,* Vol. 22, No. 7, (July 1999), pp. 505-509, ISSN 1600-051X.

Haffajee, A.D. & Socransky, S.S. (2005). Microbiology of periodontal diseases: introduction. *Periodontol 2000,* Vol. 38, (2005), pp. 9-12, ISSN 15853934.

Haffajee, A.D., Teles, R.P. & Socransky, S.S. (2206) The effect of period- ontal therapy on the composition of the subgingival micro- biota. *Periodontology 2000,* Vol. 42, (2006), pp. 219-258, ISSN 16930312.

Hagemann, C. & Blank, J.L. (2008). The ups and downs of MEK kinase interactions. *Cellular Signalling,* Vol. 13, No. 12 (December 2008), pp. 863–875, ISSN 11728826.

Hajishengallis, G., Wang, M., Liang, S., Triantafilou, M. & Triantafilou, K. (2008). Pathogen induction of CXCR4/TLR2 cross-talk impairs host defense function. *Proc Natl Acad Sci U S A,* Vol 105, No. 36 (September 2008), pp. 13532-13537, ISSN18765807.

Han, X., Lin, X., Seliger, A.R., Eastcott, J., Kawai, T. & Taubman, M.A. (2009). Expression of receptor activator of nuclear factor-kappaB ligand by B cells in response to oral bacteria. *Oral Microbiol Immunology,* Vol. 24, No.3 (June 2009), pp. 190-196, ISSN 19416447.

Hanazawa, S., Kawata, Y., Takeshita, A., Kumada, H., Okithu, M., Tanaka, S., Yamamoto, Y., Masuda, T., Umemoto, T. & Kitano, S. (1993). Expression of monocyte chemoattractant protein 1 (MCP-1) in adult periodontal disease: increased monocyte chemotactic activity in crevicular fluids and induction of MCP-1 expression in gingival tissues. *Infection and Immunity,* Vol. 61, No. 12, (December 1993), pp. 5219-5224, ISSN 0019-9567.

Hannas, A. R., Pereira, J. C., Granjeiro, J. M. & Tjäderhane, L. (2007). The role of matrix metalloproteinases in the oral environment. *Acta Odontologica Scandinavica,* Vol. 65, No. 1, (February 2007), pp. 1-13, ISSN 0001-6357.

Hashimoto, S., Yamamura, T. & Shimono, M. (1986). Morphometric analysis of the intercellular space and desmosomes of rat junctional epithelium. *Journal of Periodontal Research,* Vol. 21, No. 5, (September 1986), pp. 510-520, ISSN 1600-0765.

Hatakeyama, S., Yaegashi, T., Oikawa, Y., Fujiwara, H., Mikami, T., Takeda, Y. & Sato, M. (2006). Expression pattern of adhesion molecules in junctional epithelium differs from that in other gingival epithelia. *Journal of Periodontal Research,* Vol. 41, No. 4, (August 2006), pp. 322-328, ISSN 1600-0765.

Hauber, H.P., Bergeron, C. & Hamid, Q. (2004) IL-9 in alergic inflammation. *International Archives Allergy Immunol,* Vol. 134, No. 1 (May 2004), pp. 79-87, ISSN 15133304.

Hirao, K., Yumoto, H., Takahashi, K., Mukai, K., Nakanishi, T. & Matsuo, T. (2009). Roles of TLR2, TLR4, NOD2, and NOD1 in pulp fibroblasts. *Journal of Dental Research,* Vol. 88, No. 8 (August 2009), pp. 762–767, ISSN 19734466.

Honda, T., Domon, H., Okui, T., Kajita, K., Amanuma, R. & Yamazaki, K. (2006). Balance of inflammatory response in stable gingivitis and progressive periodontitis lesions. *Clinical Exp Immunol,* Vol. 144, No.1 (April 2006), pp. 35-40, ISSN 16542362.

Hormia, M., Owaribe, K. & Virtanen, I. (2001). The dento-epithelial junction: cell adhesion by type I hemidesmosomes in the absence of a true basal lamina. *Journal of Periodontology,* Vol. 72, No. 6, (June 2001), pp. 788-797, ISSN 0022-3492.

Hosokawa, Y., Hosokawa, I., Ozaki, K., Nakae, H. & Matsuo, T. (2009). Cytokines differentially regulate CXCL10 production by interferon-gamma-stimulated or tumor necrosis factor-alpha-stimulated human gingival fibroblasts. *Journal of Periodontal Research,* Vol. 44, No. 2 (April 2009), pp. 225-231, ISSN 18973545.

Huang, G.T., Gronthos, S. & Shi, S. (2009). Mesenchymal stem cells derived from dental tissues vs. those from other sources: their biology and role in regenerative medicine. *Journal of Dental Research,* Vol. 88, No. 9 (September 2009), pp. 792–806, ISSN 19767575.

Ihn, H., Yamane, K., Asano, Y., Kubo, M. & Tamaki, K. (2002). IL-4 up-regulates the expression of tissue inhibitor of metalloproteinase-2 in dermal fibroblasts via the p38 mitogen-activated protein kinase dependent pathway. *J Immunol,* Vol. 168, No. 4 (February 2002), pp. 1895-1902, ISSN 11823524.

Ingman, T., Tervahartiala, T., Ding, Y., Tschesche, H., Haerian, A., Kinane, D. F., Konttinen, Y. T. & Sorsa, T. (1996). Matrix metalloproteinases and their inhibitors in gingival crevicular fluid and saliva of periodontitis patients. *Journal of Clinical Periodontology,* Vol. 23, No. 12, (December 1996), pp. 1127-1132, ISSN 1600-051X.

Izumi, T., Kobayashi, I., Okamura, K. & Sakai, H. (1995). Immunohistochemical study on the immunocompetent cells of the pulp in human non-carious and carious teeth. *Arch Oral Biol* , Vol. 40, No. 7 (july1995), pp. 609–614, ISSN 7575232.

Jankovic, D., Liu, Z., Gause, W.C. (2001). Th1- and Th2-cell commitment during infectious disease: asymmetry in divergent pathways. *Trends Immunol,* Vol. 22, No. 8 (August 2001), pp. 450-457, ISSN 11473835.

Jenkinson, H.F., Lamont, R.J. (2005). Oral microbial communities in sickness and in health. *Trends Microbiol,* Vol. 13, No. 12 (December 2005), pp. 589-595, ISSN 16214341.

Ji, J.D., Park-Min, K.H., Shen, Z., Fajardo, R.J., Goldring, S.R., McHugh, K.P. & (2009a). Inhibition of RANK expression and osteoclastogenesis by TLRs and IFN-gamma in human osteoclast precursors. *J Immunol,* Vol. 183, No. 11 (December 2009), pp. 7223-7233, ISSN 19890054.

Ji, S., Hyun, J., Park, E., Lee, B.L., Kim, K.K. & Choi, Y. (2007). Susceptibility of various oral bacteria to antimicrobial peptides and to phagocytosis by neutrophils. *Journal of Periodontal Research,* Vol. 42, No. 5 (October 2007), pp. 410-419, ISSN 17760818.

Ji, S., Shin, J.E., Kim, Y.S., Oh, J.E., Min, BM. & Choi, Y. (2009b). Toll-like receptor 2 and NALP2 mediate induction of human beta-defensins by fusobacterium nucleatum in gingival epithelial cells. *Infect Immun,* Vol. 77, No. 3 (March 2009), pp. 1044-1052, ISSN 19103770.

Jin, Q., Cirelli, J.A., Park, C.H., Sugai, J.V., Taba, M., Jr., Kostenuik, P.J. . (2007). RANKL inhibition through osteoprotegerin blocks bone loss in experimental periodontitis. *Journal of Periodontology*, Vol. 78, No.7 (July 2007), pp.1300-1308, ISSN 17608585.

Jorgensen, G.H., Arnlaugsson, S., Theodors, A., Ludviksson, B.R. (2010). Immunoglobulin A deficiency and oral health status: a case-control study. *Journal of Clinical of Periodontology*, Vol. 37, No. 1 (January 2010), pp. 1-8, ISSN 19968742.

Kalinski, P. & Moser, M. (2005). Consensual immunity: success-driven development of T-helper-1 and T-helper-2 responses. *Nat Rev Immunol*, Vol. 5, No. 3 (March 2005), pp. 251-260, ISSN 15738955.

Kantarci, A., Oyaizu, K. & Van Dyke, T. E. (2003). Neutrophil-mediated tissue injury in periodontal disease pathogenesis: findings from localized aggressive periodontitis. *Journal of Periodontology*, Vol. 74, No. 1, (January 2003), pp. 66-75, ISSN 0022-3492.

Kastelein, R.A., Hunter, C.A. & Cua, D.J. (2007). Discovery and biology of IL-23 and IL-27:related but functionally distinct regulators of inflammation. *Annu. Rev. Immunol*, Vol. 25, (2007), pp. 221-242, ISSN 17291186.

Katagiri, T. & Takahashi N. (2002). Regulatory mechanisms of osteoblast and osteoclast differentiation. *Oral Dis*, Vol. 8, No. 3, pp. 147-159.

Katoh, M., Saito, S., Takiguchi, H.& Abiko, Y. (2000). Bactericidal activity of a monoclonal antibody against a recombinant 40-kDa outer membrane protein of Porphyromonas gingivalis. *Journal of Periodontology*, Vol. 71, No. 3 (March 2000), pp. 368-375, ISSN 10776923.

Katrib, A., Smith, M. D., Ahern, M. J., Slavotinek, J., Stafford, L., Cuello, C., Bertouch, J. V., McNeil, H. P. & Yussef, P. P. (2003). Reduced chemokine and matrix metalloproteinase expression in patients with rheumatoid arthritis achieving remission. *Journal of Rheumatology*, Vol. 30, No. 1, (January 2003), pp. 10-21, ISSN 1499-2752.

Kawai, T., Matsuyama, T., Hosokawa, Y., Makihira, S., Seki, M., Karimbux, N.Y. & . (2006). B and T lymphocytes are the primary sources of RANKL in the bone resorptive lesion of periodontal disease. *Am J Pathol*, Vol. 169, No. 3 (September 2006), pp. 987-998, ISSN 16936272.

Kawashima, N. & Stachenko, P. (1999). Expression of bone-resorptive and regulatory cytokines in murine periapical inflammation. *Arch Oral Biol* , Vol. 44, No. 1 (January 1999), pp. 55-66, ISSN 10075151.

Kawashima, N., Suzuki, N., Yang, G., Ohi, C., Okuhara, S., Nakano-Kawanishi, H. & Suda, H. (2007). Kinetics of RANKL, RANK and OPG expressions in experimentally induced rat periapical lesions. *Oral Surgery, Oral Medicine, Oral Pathology, Oral Radiology and Endodontics*, Vol. 103, No. 5, (May 2007), pp. 707-711, ISSN 1528-395X.

Kelchtermans, H., Schurgers, E., Geboes, L., Mitera, T., Van Damme, J., Van Snick, J. & (2009). Effector mechanisms of interleukin-17 in collagen-induced arthritis in the absence of interferon-gamma and counteraction by interferon-gamma. *Arthritis Res Ther*, Vol. 11, No. 4 (2009), pp. R122, ISSN 19686583.

Kindle, L., Rothe, L., Kriss, M., Osdoby, P.& Collin-Osdoby, P. (2006). Human microvascular endothelial cell activation by IL-1 and TNF-alpha stimulates the adhesion and transendothelial migration of circulating human CD14+ monocytes that develop with RANKL into functional osteoclasts. *Journal of Bone Miner Research,* Vol. 21, No. 2 (February 2006), pp. 193-206, ISSN 16418775.

Koch, A. E. (2005). Chemokines and their receptors in rheumatoid arthritis. *Arthritis and Rheumatism,* Vol. 52, No. 3, pp. 710-721, ISSN 0004-3591.

Koch, A. E., Kunkel, S. L., Harlow, L. A., Johnson, B., Evanoff, H. L., Haines, G. K., Burdick, M. D., Pope, R. M. & Strieter, R. M. (1992). Enhanced production of monocyte chemoattractant protein-1 in rheumatoid arthritis. *Journal of Clinical Investigation,* Vol. 90, No. 3, (1992), pp.772-779, ISSN 0021-9738.

Kotake, S., Udagawa, N., Hakoda, M., Mogi, M., Yano, K., Tsuda, E., Takahashi, K., Furuya, T., Ishiyama, S., Kim, K.J., Saito, S., Nishikawa, T., Takahashi, N., Togari, A., Tomatsu, T., Suda, T. & Kamatani, N. (2001). Activated human T cells directly induce osteoclastogenesis from human monocytes: possible role of T cells in bone destruction in rheumatoid arthritis patients. *Arthritis Rheumathoide,* Vol. 44, No. 5 (May 2001), pp. 1003–1012, ISSN 11352231.

Kotake, S., Udagawa, N., Takahashi, N., Matsuzaki, K., Itoh, K., Ishiyama, S., Saito, S., Inoue, K., Kamatani, N., Gillespie, M.T., Martin, T.J. & Suda, T. (1999). IL-17 in synovial fluids from patients with rheumatoid arthritis is a potent stimulator of osteoclastogenesis. *J Clin Invest,* Vol. 103, No. 9 (May 1999), pp. 1345-52, ISSN 10225978.

Koutouzis, T., Haber, D., Shaddox, L., Aukhil, I. & Wallet, S.M. (2009). Autoreactivity of serum immunoglobulin to periodontal tissue components: a pilot study. *Journal of Periodontology,* Vol. 80, No. 4 (April 2009), pp. 625-633, ISSN 19335083.

Krauss, J.L., Potempa, J., Lambris, J.D. & Hajishengallis, G. (2010). Complementary Tolls in the periodontium: how periodontal bacteria modify complement and Toll-like receptor responses to prevail in the host. *Periodontol 2000,* Vol. 52, No. 1 (February 2010), pp. 141-162, ISSN 20017800.

Kubota, T., Nomura, T., Takahashi, T. & Hara, K. (1996). Expression of mRNA for matrix metalloproteinases and tissue inhibitors of metalloproteinases in periodontitis-affected human gingival tissue. *Archives of Oral Biology,* Vol. 41, No. 3, (March 1996), pp. 253-262, ISSN 0003-9969.

Kumada, M., Kihara, S., Ouchi, N., Kobayashi, H., Okamoto, Y., Ohashi, K., Maeda, K., Nagaretani, H., Kishida, K., Maeda, N., Nagasawa, A., Funahashi, T. & Matsuzawa, Y. (2004). Adiponectin specifically increased tissue inhibitor of metalloproteinase-1 through interleukin-10 expression in human macrophages. *Circulation,* Vol. 109, No. 17 (May 2004), pp. 2046-2049, ISSN 15096450.

Kupper, T.S., Horowitz, M., Birchall, N., Mizutani, H., Coleman, D., McGuire, J., Flood, P., Dower, S. & Lee, F. (1998). Hematopoietic, lymphopoietic, and pro- inflammatory cytokines produced by human and murine keratinocytes. *Annals of the New York Academy of Sciences,* Vol. 548, (1998), pp. 262–270, ISSN 2470299.

Lacey, D.C., Simmons, P.J., Graves, S.E. & Hamilton, J.A. (2009). Proinflammatory cytokines inhibit osteogenic differentiation from stem cells: implications for bone repair during inflammation. *Osteoarthritis Cartilage,* Vol. 17, No. 6 (June 2009), pp. 735-742, ISSN 19136283.

Lanchou, J., Corbel, M., Tanguy, M., Germain, N., Boichot, E., Theret, N., Clement, B., Lagente, V. & Malledant, Y. (2003). Imbalance between matrix metalloproteinases

(MMP-9 and MMP-2) and tissue inhibitors of metalloproteinases (TIMP-1 and TIMP-2) in acute respiratory distress syndrome patients. *Critical Care Medicine*, Vol. 31, No. 2, (February 2003), pp. 536-542, ISSN 1530-0293.

Lane, T. F. & Sage, E. H. (1994). The biology of SPARC, a protein that modulates cell-matrix interactions. *The FASEB Journal*, Vol. 8, No. 2, (February 1994), pp. 163-173, ISSN 1530-6860.

Leibbrandt, A. & Penninger, J. M. (2008). RANK/RANKL: regulators of immune responses and bone physiology. *Annals of the New York Academy of Sciences*, Vol. 1143, (November 2008), pp. 123-150, ISSN 1749-6632.

Li, M.O. & Flavell, R.A. (2008). TGF-beta: a master of all T cell trades. *Cell*, Vol.134, No. 3 (August 2008), pp. 392-404, ISSN 18692464.

Liapatas, S., Nakou, M. & Rontogianni, D. (2003). Inflammatory infiltrate of chronic periradicular lesions: an immunohistochemical study. *International Endodontic Journal*, Vol. 35, No. 7 (July 2003), pp. 464-471, ISSN 12823701.

Liapatas, S., Nakou, M. & Rontogianni, D. (2003). Inflammatory infiltrate of chronic periradicular lesions: an immunohistochemical study. *International Endodontic Journal*, Vol. 36, No. 7, (July 2003), pp. 464-471, ISSN 1365-2591.

Lima, H.R., Gelani, V., Fernandes, A.P., Gasparoto, T.H., Torres, S.A., Santos, C.F. & (2010). The essential role of toll like receptor-4 in the control of Aggregatibacter actinomycetemcomitans infection in mice. *Journal of Clinical of Periodontology*, Vol. 37, No. 3 (March 2010), pp. 248-254, ISSN 20149215.

Lin, S.K., Kok, S.H, Kuo, M.Y., Wang, T.J., Wang, J.T., Yeh, F.T., Hsiao, M., Lan, W.H. & Hong, C.Y. (2002) Sequential expressions of MMP-1, TIMP-1, IL-6, and COX-2 genes in induced periapical lesions in rats. *European Journal of Oral Sciense*, Vol. 110, No. 3 (June 2002), pp. 246-53, ISSN 12120711.

Liu, D., Yao, S. & Wise, G.E. (2006). Effect of interleukin-10 on gene expression of osteoclastogenic regulatory molecules in the rat dental follicle. *European Journal of Oral Sciense*, Vol. 114, No. 1 (February 2006), pp. 42-49, ISSN 16460340.

Liu, Y.C., Lerner, U.H. & Teng, Y.T. (2010). Cytokine responses against periodontal infection: protective and destructive roles. *Periodontol 2000*, Vol. 52, No. 1 (February 2010), pp. 163-206, ISSN 20017801.

Lu, Q., Jin, L., Darveau, R. P. & Samaranayake, L. P. (2004). Expression of human beta-defensins-1 and -2 peptides in unresolved chronic periodontitis. *Journal of Periodontal Research*, Vol. 39, No. 4, (August 2004), pp. 221-227, ISSN 1600-0765.

Mahanonda, R. & Pichyangkul, S. (2007). Toll-like receptors and their role in periodontal health and disease. *Periodontology 2000*, Vol. 43, No. 1, (February 2007), pp. 41-55, ISSN 0906-6713.

Malemud, C.J. (2006). Matrix metalloproteinases (MMPs) in health and disease: an overview. *Front Biosci*, Vol. 11, (May 2006), pp. 1696-1701, ISSN 16368548.

Marra, A. & Isberg, R. R. (1996). Common entry mechanisms. Bacterial pathogenesis. *Current Biology*, Vol. 6, No. 9, (September 1996), pp. 1084-1086, ISSN 0960-9822.

Mayer, Y., Balbir-Gurman, A. & Machtei, E.E. (2009). Anti-tumor necrosis factor-alpha therapy and periodontal parameters in patients with rheumatoid arthritis. *Journal of Periodontology*, Vol. 80, No. 9 (September 2009), pp. 1414-1420, ISSN 19722791.

McCulloch, C. A. & Bordin, S. (1991). Role of fibroblast subpopulations in periodontal physiology and pathology. *Journal of Periodontal Research*, Vol. 26, No. 3 Pt 1, (May 1991), pp. 144-154, ISSN 1600-0765.

McCurdy, S., Baicu, C. F., Heymans, S. & Bradshaw, A. D. (2010). Cardiac extracellular matrix remodeling: fibrillar collagens and Secreted Protein Acidic and Rich in Cysteine (SPARC). *Journal of Molecular and Cellular Cardiology*, Vol. 48, No. 3, (March 2010), pp. 544-549, ISSN 0022-2828.

McGeachy, M.J. & Cua, D.J. (2008). Th17 cell differentiation: the long and winding road. *Immunity*, Vol. 28, No. 4 (April 2008), pp. 445-453, ISSN 18400187.

Medzhitov, R. (2001). Toll-like receptors and innate immunity. *Nature Reviews Immunology*, Vol. 1, No. 2 (November 2001), pp. 135–145, ISSN 11905821.

Menezes, R., Garlet, T. P., Letra, A., Bramante, C. M., Campanelly, A. P., Figueira, R. C., Sogayar, M. C., Granjeiro, J. M. & Garlet, G. P. (2008). Differential patterns of receptor activator of nuclear factor kappa B ligand/osteoprotegerin expression in human periapical granulomas: possible association with progressive or stable nature of the lesions. *Journal of Endodontics*, Vol. 34, No. 8, (August 2008), pp. 932-938, ISSN 0099-2399.

Mercado, F. B., Marshall, R. I. & Bartold, P. M. (2003). Inter-relationships between rheumatoid arthritis and periodontal disease. A review. *Journal of Clinical Periodontology*, Vol. 30, No. 9, (September 2003), pp. 761-772, ISSN 1600-051X.

Michalowicz, B. S., Diehl, S. R., Gunsolley, J. C., Sparks, B. S., Brooks, C. N., Koertge, T. E., Califano, J. V., Burmeister, J. A. & Schenkein, H. A. (2000). Evidence of a substantial genetic basis for risk of adult periodontitis. *Journal of Periodontology*, Vol. 71, No. 11, (November 2000), pp. 1699-1707, ISSN 0022-3492

Momoi, F., Hashizume, T., Kurita-Ochiai, T., Yuki, Y., Kiyono, H. & Yamamoto, M. (2008). Nasal vaccination with the 40-kilodalton outer membrane protein of Porphyromonas gingivalis and a nontoxic chimeric enterotoxin adjuvant induces long-term protective immunity with reduced levels of immunoglobulin E antibodies. *Infect Immun*, Vol. 76, No. 6 (June 2008), pp. 2777-2784, ISSN 18411288.

Monteiro da Silva, A. M., Oakly, D. A., Newman, H. N., Nohl, R. S. and Lloyd, H. M. (1996). Psychosocial factors and adult onset rapidly progressive periodontitis. *Journal of Clinical Periodontology*, Vol. 23, No. 8, (August 1996), pp. 789-794, ISSN 1600-051X.

Murphy, K.M.& Reiner, S.L. (2002). The lineage decisions of helper T cells. *Nat Rev Immunol*, Vol. 2, No. 12 (December 2002), pp. 933-944, ISSN 12461566.

Murphy, P. M, Baggiolini, M., Charo, I. F., Hebert, C. A., Horuk, R., Matsushima, K., Miller, L. H., Oppenheim, J. J. & Power, C. A. (2000). International union of pharmacology. XXII. Nomenclature for chemokine receptors. *Pharmacological Reviews*, Vol. 52, No. 1, (March 2000), pp. 145-176, ISSN 0031-6997.

Mussig, E., Tomakidi, P. & Steinberg, T. (2005). Molecules contributing to the maintenance of periodontal tissues. Their possible association with orthodontic tooth movement. *Journal of Orofacial Orthopedics*, Vol. 66, No. 6, (November 2005), pp. 422-433, ISSN 1615-6714.

Nagasawa, T., Kiji, M., Yashiro R., Hormdee, D., Lu, H., Kunze, M., Suda, T., Koshy, G., Kobayashi, H., Oda, S., Nitta, H. & Ishikawa, I. (2007). Roles of receptor activator of nuclear factor-kappaB ligand (RANKL) and osteoprotegerin in periodontal health and disease. *Periodontology 2000*, Vol. 43, No. 1, (February 2007), pp. 65-84, ISSN 0906-6713.

Nair, P.N. R. (2004). Pathogenesis of apical periodontitis and the causes of endodontic failures. *Crit Rev Oral Biol Med*, Vol.15, No. 6 (November 2004), pp.348-381, ISSN 15574679.

Nair, P. N. R. (1997). Apical periodontitis: a dynamic encounter between root canal infection and host response. *Periodontology 2000*, Vol. 13, No. 1, (February 1997), pp. 121-148, ISSN 0906-6713.

Nakajima, T., Ueki-Maruyama, K., Oda, T., Ohsawa, Y., Ito, H., Seymour, G.J. & Yamazaki, K. (2005). Regulatory T-cells infiltrate periodontal disease tissues. *Journal of Dental Research*, Vol. 84, No. 7 (July 2005), pp. 639-643, ISSN 15972593.

Nakamura, H., Fukusaki, Y., Yoshimura, A., Shiraishi, C., Kishimoto, M., Kaneko, T. & Hara, T. (2008). Lack of Toll-like receptor 4 decreases lipopolysaccharide-induced bone resorption in C3H/HeJ mice in vivo. *Oral Microbiology Immunology*, Vol. 23, No. 3 (June 2008), pp. 190-195, ISSN 18402604.

Nanki, T., Nagasaka, K., Hayashida, K., Saita, Y. & Miyasaka, N. (2001). Chemokines regulate IL-6 and IL-8 production by fibroblast-like synoviocytes from patients with rheumatoid arthritis. *Journal of Immunology*, Vol. 167, No. 9, (November 2001), pp. 5381-5385, ISSN 0022-1767.

Nathan, C. (2006). Neutrophils and immunity: challenges and opportunities. *Nature Reviews Immunology*, Vol. 6, No. 3, (March 2006), pp. 173-182, ISSN 1474-1733.

Naundorf, S., Schroder, M., Hoflich, C., Suman, N., Volk, H.D. & Grutz, G. (2009). IL-10 interferes directly with TCR-induced IFN-gamma but not IL-17 production in memory T cells. *European Journal of Immunology*, Vol. 39, No. 4 (April 2009), pp. 1066-1077, ISSN 19266486.

Nomura, T., Ishii, A., Oishi, Y., Kohma, H. & Hara, K. (1998). Tissue inhibitors of metalloproteinases level and collagenase activity in gingival crevicular fluid: the relevance to periodontal diseases. *Oral Diseases*, Vol. 4, No. 4, (December 1998), pp. 231-240, ISSN 1354-523X.

Novak, E.C., Weaver, C.T., Turner, H., Begum-Haque, S., Becher, B., Schreiner, B., Coyle, A.J., Kasper, L.H. & Noelle, R.J. (2009). IL-9 as a mediator of Th17-driven inflammatory disease. *Journal of Exp Med*, Vol. 206, No. (2009), pp. 1653-1660, ISSN 19596803.

Nussbaum, G., Ben-Adi, S., Genzler, T., Sela, M. & Rosen, G. (2009). Involvement of Toll-like receptors 2 and 4 in the innate immune response to Treponema denticola and its outer sheath components. *Infect Immun*, Vol. 77, No.9 (September 2009), pp. 3939-3947, ISSN 19596768.

Offenbacher, S., Odle, B. M. & Van Dyke, T. E. (1986). The use of crevicular fluid prostaglandin E2 levels as a predictor of periodontal attachment loss. *Journal of Periodontal Reserach*, Vol. 21, No. 2, (March 1986), pp. 101-112, ISSN 1600-0765.

Ogasawara, T., Yoshimine, Y., Kiyoshima, T., Kobayashi, I., Matsuo, K., Akamine, A. & Sakai, H. (2004). In situ expression of RANKL, RANK, osteoprotegerin and cytokines in osteoclasts of rat periodontal tissue. *Journal of Periodontal Research*, Vol. 39, No. 1, (February 2004), pp. 42-49, ISSN 1600-0765.Ohlrich, E.J., Cullinan, M.P. & Seymour, G.J. (2009). The immunopathogenesis of periodontal disease. *Australian*

Dental Journal, Vol. 54, No. suppl 1 (September 2009), pp. S2-S10, ISSN 19737265.Okada, H. & Murakami, S. (1998). Cytokine expression in periodontal health and disease. *Critical Reviews in Oral Biology and Medicine*, Vol. 9, No. 3,pp 248-266, ISSN 1045-4411.

Okugawa, T., Kaneko, T., Yoshimura, A., Silverman, N. & Hara, Y. (2010) NOD1 and NOD2 mediate sensing of periodontal pathogens. *Journal of Dental Research*, Vol. 89, No. 2 (February 2010), pp. 186-191, ISSN 20040739.

Orima, K., Yamazaki, K., Aoyagi, T. & Hara, K. (1999). Differential expression of costimulatory molecules in chronic inflammatory periodontal disease tissue. *Clin Exp Immunology*, Vol. 115, No. 1 (January 1999), pp.153-160, ISSN 9933436.

Oseko, F., Yamamoto, T., Akamatsu, Y., Kanamura, N., Iwakura, Y., Imanishi, J. & Kita, M. (2009). IL-17 is involved in bone resorption in mouse periapical lesions. *Microbiology Immunology*, Vol. 53, No. 5 (May 2009), pp. 287-294, ISSN 19457170.

Otte, J. M., Cario, E. & Podolsky, D. K. (2004). Mechanisms of cross hyporesponsiveness to Toll-like receptor bacterial ligands in intestinal epithelial cells. *Gastroenterology*, Vol. 126, No. 4, (April 2004), pp. 1054-1070, ISSN 0016-5085.

Ouhara, K., Komatsuzawa, H., Yamada, S., Shiba, H., Fujiwara, T., Ohara, M., Sayama, K., Hashimoto, K., Kurihara, H. & Sugai, M. (2005). Susceptibilities of periodontopathogenic and cariogenic bacteria to antibacterial peptides,{beta}-defensins and LL37, produced by human epithelial cells. *Journal of Antimicrob Chemother*, Vol. 55, No. 6 (June 2005), pp. 888-896, ISSN 15886266.

Ozaki, K., Hanazawa, S., Takeshita, A., Chen, Y., Watanabe, A., Nishida, K., Miyata, Y. & Kitano, S. (1996). Interleukin-1beta and tumor necrosis factor-alpha stimulate synergistically the expression of monocyte chemoattractant protein-1 in fibroblastic cells derived from human periodontal ligament. *Oral Microbiology and Immunology*, Vol. 11, No. 2, (April 1996), pp. 109-114, ISSN 0902-0055.

Pablo, P., Chapple, I. L. C., Buckley, C. D. & Dietrich, T. (2009). Periodontitis in systemic rheumatic diseases. *Nature Reviews Rheumatology*, Vol. 5, No. 4, (April 2009), pp. 218-224, ISSN 1759-4790.

Page, R.C., Lantz, M.S., Darveau, R., Jeffcoat, M., Mancl, L., Houston, L. &. (2007). Immunization of Macaca fascicularis against experimental periodontitis using a vaccine containing cysteine proteases purified from Porphyromonas gingivalis. *Oral Microbiol Immunol*, Vol. 22, No. 3 (2007), pp. 162-168, ISSN.

Page, R. C. & Schroeder, H. E. (1976). Pathogenesis of inflammatory periodontal disease. A summary of current work. *Laboratory Investigation*, Vol. 34, No. 3, (March 1976), pp. 235-249, ISSN 0023-6837

Page, R. C., Offenbacher, S., Schroeder, H. E., Seymour, G. J. & Kornman, K. S. (1997). Advances in the pathogenesis of periodontitis: summary of developments, clinical implications and future directions. *Periodontology 2000*, Vol. 14, No. 1, (June 1997), pp. 216-248, ISSN 0906-6713.

Parfitt, A.M. (1982). The coupling of bone formation to bone resorption: a critical analysis of the concept and of its relevance to the pathogenesis of osteoporosis. *Metab Bone Dis Relat Research*, Vol. 4, No. 1 (1982), pp. 1-6, ISSN 7121250.

Park-Min, K.H., Ji, J.D., Antoniv, T., Reid, A.C., Silver, R.B., Humphrey, M.B., Nakamura, M. & Ivashkiv, L.B. (2009). IL-10 suppresses calcium-mediated costimulation of receptor activator NF-kappa B signaling during human osteoclast differentiation by inhibiting TREM-2 expression. *Journal of Immunology,* Vol. 183, No. 4 (August 2009), pp. 2444-2455, ISSN 19625651.

Pashely, D.H., Pashley, E.L., Carvalho R.M. & Tay, F.R. (2002). The effects of dentin permeability on restorative dentistry. *Dent Clin North Am,* Vol. 46, No. 2 (April 2002), pp. 211-245, ISSN 12014033.

Peschon, J.J., Torrance, D.S., Stocking, K.L., Glaccum, M.B., Otten, C., Willis, C.R., Charrier, K., Morrissey, P.J., Ware, C.B., Mohlerm K.M. (1998). TNF receptor-deficient mice reveal divergent roles for p55 and p75 in several models of inflammation. *J Immunology,* Vol. 160, No. 2 (January 1998), pp. 943-952, ISSN 9551933.

Pestka, S., Krause, C.D., Sarkar, D., Walter, M.R., Shi, Y. & Fisher, P.B. (2004). Interleukin-10 and related cytokines and receptors. *Annu Rev Immunol,* Vol. 22, pp. 929-979, ISSN 15032600.

Pfeffer, K., Matsuyama. T., Kundig. T.M., Wakeham. A., Kishihara. K., Shahinian. A., Wiegmann, K., Ohashi, P.S., Krönke, M. & Mak, T.W. (1993). Mice deficient for the 55 kd tumor necrosis factor receptor are resistant to endotoxic shock, yet succumb to L. monocytogenes infection. *Cell,* Vol. 73, No. 3 (May 1993), pp. 457-467, ISSN 8387893.

Potempa, J., Banbula, A. & Travis, J. (2000). Role of bacterial proteinases in matrix destruction and modulation of host responses. *Periodontology 2000,* Vol. 24, No. 1, (October 2000), pp. 153-192, ISSN 0906-6713.

Pradeep, A.R., Roopa. Y. & Swati, P.P. (2008). Interleukin-4, a T-helper 2 cell cytokine, is associated with the remission of periodontal disease. *Journal of Periodontal Research,* Vol. 43, No. 6 (December 2008), pp. 712-716, ISSN 18624944.

Pradeep, A. R., Daisy, H. & Hadge, P. (2009). Gingival crevicular fluid levels of monocyte chemoattractant protein-1 in periodontal health and disease. *Archives of Oral Biology,* Vol. 54, No. 5, (May 2009), pp. 503-509, ISSN 0003-9969.

Puklo, M., Guentsch, A., Hiemstra, P.S., Eick, S. & Potempa, J. (2008). Analysis of neutrophil-derived antimicrobial peptides in gingival crevicular fluid suggests importance of cathelicidin LL-37 in the innate immune response against periodontogenic bacteria. *Oral Microbiol Immunol,* Vol. 23, No. 4 (August 2008), pp. 328-335, ISSN 18582333.

Queiroz-Junior, C. M., Silva, M. J., Corrêa, J. D., Madeira, M. F., Garlet, G. P., Cunha, F. Q., Teixeira, M. M. & da Silva, T. A. (2011). A controversial role for IL-12 in immune response and bone resorption at apical periodontal sites. *Clinical and Developmental Immunology,* Vol. 2010, 327417, ISSN 1740-2522

Rahimi, P., Wang, C. Y., Stashenko, P., Lee, S. K., Lorenzo, J. A. & Graves, D. T. (1995). Monocyte chemoattractant protein-1 expression and monocyte recruitment in osseous inflammation in the mouse. *Endocrinology,* Vol. 136, No. 6, (June 1995), pp. 2752-2759, ISSN 1945-7170.

Rams, T.E., Listgarten, M.A. & Slots, J. (2006). Actinobacillus actinomycetemcomitans and Porphyromonas gingivalis subgingival presence, species-specific serum immunoglobulin G antibody levels, and periodontitis disease recurrence. *Journal of Periodontal Research,* Vol. 41, No. 3 (June 2006), pp. 228-234, ISSN 16677293.

Ren, L., Leung, W. K., Darveau, R. P. & Jin, L. (2005). The expression profile of lipopolysaccharide-binding protein, membrane-bound CD14, and toll-like receptors 2 and 4 in chronic periodontitis. *Journal of Periodontology*, Vol. 76, No. 11, (November 2005), pp. 1950-1959, ISSN 0022-3492.

Rentz, T. J., Poobalarahi, F., Bornstein, P., Sage, E. H. & Bradshaw, A. D. (2007). SPARC regulates processing of procollagen I and collagen fibrillogenesis in dermal fibroblasts. *The Journal of Biological Chemistry*, Vol. 282, No. 30, (July 2007), pp. 22062-22071, ISSN 1083-351X.

Repeke, C. E., Ferreira, S. B. Jr., Claudino, M., Silveira, E. M., de Assis, G. F., Avila-Campos, M. J., Silva, J. S. & Garlet, G. P. (2010). Evidences of the cooperative role of the chemokines CCL3, CCL4 and CCL5 and its receptors CCR1+ and CCR5+ in RANKL+ cell migration throughout experimental periodontitis in mice. *Bone*, Vol. 46, No. 4, (April 2010), pp. 1122-1130, ISSN 8756-3282.

Reynolds, J. J., Hembry, R. M. & Meikle, M. C. (1994). Connective tissue degradation in health and periodontal disease and the roles of matrix metalloproteinases and their natural inhibitors. *Advances in Dental Research*, Vol. 8, No. 2, (July 1994), pp. 312-319, ISSN 1544-0737.

Ricucci, D. & Siqueira, J. F. Jr. (2010). Biofilms and apical periodontitis: study of prevalence and association with clinical and histopathologic findings. *Journal of Endodontics*, Vol. 36, No. 8, (August 2010), pp. 1277-1288, ISSN 0099-2399.

Rodan, G. A. & Martin, T. J. (2000). Therapeutic approaches to bone diseases. *Science*, Vol. 289, No. 5484, pp. 1508-1514, ISSN 1095-9203.

Romas, E., Sims, N. A., Hards, D. K., Lindsay, M., Quinn, J. W., Ryan, P. F., Dunstan, C. R., Martin, T. J. & Gillespie, M. T. (2002). Osteoprotegerin reduces osteoclast numbers and prevents bone erosion in collagen-induced arthritis. *The American Journal of Pathology*, Vol. 161, No. 4, (October 2002), pp. 1419-1427, ISSN 0002-9440.

Rossi, A., Rocha, L. B. & Rossi, M. A. (2008). Interferon-gamma, interleukin-10, intercellular adhesion molecule-1, and chemokine receptor 5, but not interleukin-4, attenuate the development of periapical lesions. *Journal of Endodontics*, Vol. 34, No. 1, (January 2008), pp. 31-38. ISSN 0099-2399.

Rossi, D. & Zlotnik, A. (2000). The biology of chemokines and their receptors. *Annual Review of Immunology*, Vol. 18, pp. 217–242, ISSN 0732-0582.

Rossi, G. A. (2003). COPD patients or "healthy smokers": is IL-8 synthesis and release the borderline? *Respiration*, Vol. 70, No. 5, (September-October 2003), pp. 457-459, ISSN: 0025-7931.

Sakamoto, M., Umeda, M. & Benno, Y. (2005). Molecular analysis of human oral microbiota. *Journal of Periodontal Research*, Vol. 40, No. 3 (June2005), pp. 277-285, ISSN 15853975.

Sallusto, F. & Lanzavecchia, A. (2009). Heterogeneity of CD4+ memory T cells: functional modules for tailored immunity. *European Journal of Immunology*, Vol. 39, No. 8 (August 2009), pp.2076-2082, ISSN 19672903.

Sanz, M. & van Winkelhoff, A. J. (2011) Periodontal infections: understanding the complexity – Consensus of the Seventh European Workshop on Periodontology. *Journal of Clinical Periodontology*, Vol. 38, No. Suppl 11, (March 2011), pp. 3-6, ISSN 1600-051X.

Sartori, R., Li, F. & Kirkwood, K.L. (2009). MAP kinase phosphatase-1 protects against inflammatory bone loss. *Journal of Dental Research,* Vol. 88, No. 12, (December 2009), pp. 1125-1130, ISSN 19864641.

Sasaki, H., Okamatsu, Y., Kawai, T., Kent, R., Taubman, M. & Stashenko, P. (2004). The interleukin-10 knockout mouse is highly susceptible to Porphyromonas gingivalis-induced alveolar bone loss. *Journal of Periodontal Research,* Vol. 39, No. 6 (December 2004), pp. 432-441, ISSN 15491348.

Sasaki, H., Suzuki, N., Kent, R., Jr., Kawashima, N., Takeda, J. & Stashenko, P. (2008). T cell response mediated by myeloid cell-derived IL-12 is responsible for Porphyromonas gingivalis-induced periodontitis in IL-10-deficient mice. *Journal of Immunology,* Vol. 180, No. 9 (May 2008), pp. 6193-6198, ISSN 18424741.

Sato, Y., Kishi, J., Suzuki, K., Nakamura, H. & Hayakawa, T. (2009). Sonic extracts from a bacterium related to periapical disease activate gelatinase A and inactivate tissue inhibitor of metalloproteinases TIMP-1 and TIMP-2. *International of Endodontic Journal,* Vol. 42, No. 12 (December 2009), pp. 1104-11, ISSN 19912382.

Sato, K., Suematsu, A &. Th17 functions as an osteoclastogenic helper T cell subset that links T cell activation and bone destruction. *Journal of Exp Med,* Vol203, No. 12 (November 2006), pp. 2673-2682, ISSN 17088434.

Schall, T. J., Bacon, K., Toy, K. J. & Goeddel, D. V. (1990). Selective attraction of monocytes and T lymphocytes of the memory phenotype by cytokine RANTES. *Nature,* Vol. 347, No. 6294, (October 1990), pp. 669-671, ISSN 0028-0836.

Schiott, C. R. & Loe H. (1970). The origin and variation in number of leukocytes in the human saliva. *Journal of Periodontal Research,* Vol. 5, No. 1, pp. 36-41, ISSN 1600-0765.

Schroder, K., Hertzog, P.J., Ravasi, T. & Hume, D.A. (2004). Interferon-gamma: an overview of signals, mechanisms and functions. *Journal of Leukoc Biology,* Vol. 75, No. 2 (February 2004), pp. 163-189, ISSN 14525967.

Schroder, U. (1985). Effects of calcium hydroxide-containing pulp-capping agents on pulp migration, proliferation and differentiation. *Journal of Dental Research,* Vol. 64, No. Special Issue (April 1985), pp. 541:548, ISSN 3857254.

Schroeder, H. E. & Listgarten, M. A. (1997). The gingival tissues: the architecture of periodontal protection. *Periodontology 2000,* Vol. 13, No. 1, (February 1997), pp. 91-120, ISSN 0906-6713.

Schulze, C. J., Wang, W., Suarez-Pinzon, W. L., Sawicka, J., Sawicki, G. & Schulz, R. (2003). Imbalance between tissue inhibitor of metalloproteinase-4 and matrix metalloproteinases during acute myocardial [correction of myoctardial] ischemia-reperfusion injury. *Circulation,* Vol. 107, No. 19, (May 2003), pp. 2487-2492, ISSN 0009-7322.

Schweickart, V. L., Epp, A., Raport, C. J. & Gray, P. W. (2000). CCR11 is a functional receptor for the monocyte chemoattractant protein family of chemokines. *The Journal of Biological Chemistry,* Vol. 275, No. 13, (March 2000), pp. 9550-9556, ISSN 0021-9258.

Seiderer, J.& Brand, S. (2009) IL-22: A two-headed cytokine in IBD? *Inflammatory Bowel Disease,* Vol. 15, No. 3 (March 2009), pp. 473-474, ISSN 18668680.

Shaddox, L., Wiedey, J., Bimstein, E., Magnuson, I., Clare-Salzler, M., Aukhil, I. & Wallet, S. M. (2010). Hyper-responsive phenotype in localized aggressive periodontitis.

Journal of Dental Research, Vol. 89, No. 2 (February 2010), pp. 143-148, ISSN 20042739.

Shao, H. & Demuth, D.R. (2010). Quorum sensing regulation of biofilm growth and gene expression by oral bacteria and periodontal pathogens. *Periodontology 2000,* Vol. 52, No. 1 (February 2010), pp. 53-67, ISSN 20017795.

Shevach, E.M. (2009). Mechanisms of foxp3+ T regulatory cell-mediated suppression. *Immunity,* Vol. 30, No. 5 (May 2009), pp. 636-645, ISSN 19464986.

Shi, S. & Gronthos, S. (2003). Perivascular niche of postnatal mesenchymal stem cells in human bone marrow and dental pulp. *Journal of Bone and Mineral Research,* Vol. 18, No. 4 (April 2003), pp. 696–704, ISSN 12674330.

Shin, J.E., Kim, Y.S., Oh, J.E., Min, B.M. & Choi, Y. (2010). Treponema denticola suppresses expression of human {beta}-defensin-3 in gingival epithelial cells through inhibition of the toll-like receptor 2 axis. *Infect Immun,* Vol. 78, No. 2 (February 2010), pp. 672-679, ISSN 19995893.

Shin, S.J., Lee, J.I., Baek, S.H. & Lim, S.S.Tissue levels of matrix metalloproteinases in pulps and periapical lesions. *Journal of Endodontic,* Vol. 28, No. 4 (April 2002), pp. 313-315, ISSN 12043871.

Silva, T.A., Garlet, G.P., Lara, V.S., Martins, W. Jr., Silva, J.S. & Cunha, F.Q. (2005). Differential expression of chemokines and chemokine receptors in inflammatory periapical diseases. *Oral Microbiology Immunology,* Vol. 20, No. 5 (October 2005), pp. 310-316, ISSN 16101967.

Silva, T. A., Garlet, G. P., Fukada, S. Y., Silva, J. S. & Cunha, F. Q. (2007). Chemokines in oral inflammatory diseases: apical periodontitis and periodontal disease. *Journal of Dental Research,* Vol. 86, No. 4, (April 2007), pp. 306-319, ISSN 1544-0591.

Sloan, A.J. & Smith, A.J. (2007). Stem cells and the dental pulp: potential roles in dentine regeneration and repair. *Oral Diseases,* Vol. 13, No. 2 (March 2007), pp. 151–157, ISSN 17305615 .

Smith, A.J., Tobias, R.S. & Murray, P.E. (2001). Transdentinal stimula- tion of reactionary dentinogenesis in ferrets by dentine matrix components. *Journal of Dentistry,* Vol. 29, No. 5 (July 2001), pp. 341-346, ISSN 11472806.

Soell, M., Elkaim, R. & Tenenbaum, H. (2002). Cathepsin C, matrix metalloproteinases, and their tissue inhibitors in gingiva and gingival crevicular fluid from periodontitis-affected patients. *Journal of Dental Research,* Vol. 81, No. 3, (March 2002), pp. 174-178, ISSN 1544-0591.

Stashenko, P., Teles, R. & D'Souza, R. (1998). Periapical inflammatory responses and their modulation. Crit *Rev Oral Biol Med,* Vol. 9, No. 4 (1998), pp. 498-521, ISSN 9825224.

Stashenko, P., Yu, S. M. & Wang, C. Y. (1992). Kinetics of immune cell and bone resorptive responses to endodontic infections. *Journal of Endodontics,* Vol. 18, No. 9, (September 1992), pp. 422-426, ISSN 0099-2399.

Steinsvoll, S., Halstensen, T.S. & Schenck, K. (1999). Extensive expression of TGF-beta1 in chronically-inflamed periodontal tissue. *Journal of Clinical Periodontology,* Vol. 26, No. 6 (June 1999), pp. 366-373, ISSN 10382576.

Sugawara, Y., Uehara, A., Fujimoto, Y., Kusumoto, S., Fukase, K., Shibata, K., Sugawara, S., Sasano, T. & Takada, H. (2006). Toll-like receptors, NOD1, and NOD2 in oral epithelial cells. *Journal of Dental Research*, Vol. 85, No. 6, (June 2006), pp. 524-529, ISSN 1544-0591.

Takahashi, K., Azuma, T., Motohira, H., Kinane, D.F. & Kitetsu, S. (2005). The potential role of interleukin-17 in the immunopathology of periodontal disease. *Journal of Clinical Periodontology*, Vol. 32, No. 4 (April 2005), pp. 369-374, ISSN 15811054.

Takahashi, N. & Nyvad, B. (2008). Caries ecology revisited: microbial dynamics and the caries process. *Caries Research*, Vol. 42, No. 6 (2008), pp. 409–418, ISSN 18832827.

Takahashi, K. (1998). Microbiological, pathological, inflammatory, immunological and molecular biological aspects of periradicular disease. *International Endodontic Journal*, Vol. 31, No. 5, (September 1998), pp. 311-325, ISSN

Takayanagi, H., Sato, K., Takaoka, A. & Taniguchi, T. (2005). Interplay between interferon and other cytokine systems in bone metabolism. *Immunology Rev*, Vol. 208, (December 2005), pp. 181-193, ISSN 16313349.

Takeichi, O., Hama, S., Iwata, K. & Ito, K. (2008). Confocal immunolocalization of VE-cadhering- and CXC chemokine-expressing endothelial cells in periapical granulomas. *International Endodontic Journal*, Vol. 41, No. 5, (May 2008), pp. 401-407, ISSN 1365-2591

Taub, D. D. (1996). C-C chemokines: an overview, In: *Chemokines in disease*, Koch A.E., Strieter R.M., (Ed.), pp. 27-54. R. G. Landes, Austin (TX).

Taubman, M.A., Han, X., Larosa, K.B., Socransky, S.S. & Smith, D.J. (2007). Periodontal bacterial DNA suppresses the immune response to mutans streptococcal glucosyltransferase. *Infect Immun*, Vol. 75, No. 8 (August 2007), pp. 4088-4096, ISSN 17517867.

Teitelbaum, S. L. (2000). Bone resorption by osteoclasts. *Science*, Vol. 289, No. 5484, pp. 1504-1508.

Teixeira-Salum, T.B., Rodrigues, D.B.R., Gervásio, A.M.G., Souza, C.J.A., Rodrigues, Jr. V. & Loyola, A.M. (2010). Distinct Th1, Th2 and Treg cytokines balance in chronic periapical granulomas and radicular cysts. *Journal of Oral Pathology Med*, Vol. 39, No. 3 (March 2010), pp. 250–256, ISSN 20102461.

Teng, Y.T., Mahamed, D. & Singh, B. (2005). Gamma interferon positively modulates Actinobacillus actinomycetemcomitans-specific RANKL+ CD4+ Th-cell-mediated alveolar bone destruction in vivo. *Infect Immun*, Vol. 73, No. 6 (June 2005), pp. 3453-3461, ISSN 15908374.

Tonetti, M. S., Imboden, M. A. & Lang, N. P. (1998). Neutrophil migration into the gingival sulcus is associated with transepithelial gradients of interleukin-8 and ICAM-1. *Journal of Periodontology*, Vol. 69, No. 10, (October 1998), pp. 1139-1147, ISSN 0022-3492.

Traves, S. L. & Donnelly, L. E. (2005). Chemokines and their receptors as targets for the treatment of COPD. *Current Respiratory Medicine Reviews*, Vol. 1, No. 1, pp. 15-32, ISSN 1573-398X.

Trombetta, J. M. & Bradshaw A. D. (2010). SPARC/osteonectin functions to maintain homeostasis of the collagenous extracellular matrix in the periodontal ligament. *The Journal of Histochemistry and Cytochemistry*, Vol. 58, No. 10, (October 2010), pp. 871-879, ISSN 0022-1554.

Trombone, A.P., Cardoso, C.R., Repeke, C.E., Ferreira, S.B. Jr, Martins, W. Jr., Campanelli, A.P., Avila-Campos, M.J., Trevilatto, P.C., Silva, J.S. & Garlet, G.P. Tumor necrosis factor-alpha -308G/A single nucleotide polymorphism and red-complex periodontopathogens are independently associated with increased levels of tumor necrosis factor-alpha in diseased periodontal tissues. *Journal of Periodontal Research*, Vol. 44, No. 5 (October 2009), pp. :598-608, ISSN 19076989.

Trombone, A.P., Claudino, M., Colavite, P., de Assis, G.F., Avila-Campos, M.J., Silva, J.S., Campanelli, A.P., Ibanez, O.M., de Franco, M. & Garlet, G.P. Periodontitis and arthritis interaction in mice involves a shared hyper-inflammatory genotype and functional immunological interferences. *Genes and Immunity* , Vol. 11, No. 6 (September 2010), pp. 479–489, ISSN 20428191.

Tsai, C. C., Ho, Y. P. & Chen, C. C. (1995). Levels of interleukin-1 beta and interleukin-8 in gingival crevicular fluids in adult periodontitis. *Journal of Periodontology,* Vol. 66, No. 10, (October 1995), pp. 852-859, ISSN 0022-3492.

Tuter, G., Kurtis, B., Serdar, M., Yücel, A., Ayhan, E., Karaduman, B. & Ozcan, G. (2002). Effects of phase I periodontal treatment on gingival crevicular fluid levels of matrix metalloproteinase-1 and tissue inhibitor of metalloproteinase-1. *Journal of Periodontology*, Vol. 73, No. 5, (September 2005), pp. 487-493, ISSN 0022-3492.

Uehara, A. & Takada, H. (2007). Functional TLRs and NODs in human gingival fibroblasts. *Journal of Dental Research,* Vol. 86, No. 3 (March 2007), pp.249-254, ISSN 17314257.

Uehara, A. & Takada, H. (2008). Synergism between TLRs and NOD1/2 in oral epithelial cells. *Journal of Dental Research,* Vol. 87, No. 7 (July 2008), pp. 682-686, ISSN 18573991.

Ukai, T., Yumoto, H., Gibson, F.C., 3rd & Genco, C.A. (2008). Macrophage-elicited osteoclastogenesis in response to bacterial stimulation requires Toll-like receptor 2-dependent tumor necrosis factor-alpha production. *Infect Immun,* Vol. 76, No. 2 (February 2008), pp. 812-819, ISSN 17998311.

Valencia, X., Stephens, G., Goldbach-Mansky, R. &. TNF downmodulates the function of human CD4+CD25hi T-regulatory cells. *Blood,* Vol. 108, No. 1 (July 2006), pp. 253-261, ISSN 16537805.

Van der Zee, E., Everts, V. & Beertsen, W. (1997). Cytokines modulate routes of collagen breakdown. Review with special emphasis on mechanisms of collagen degradation in the periodontium and the burst hypothesis of periodontal disease progression. *Journal of Clinical Periodontology,* Vol. 24, No. 5, (May 1997), pp. 297-305, ISSN 1600-051X.

Veerayutthwilai, O., Byers. M.R., Pham. T.T., Darveau. R.P. & Dale, B.A. (2007). Differential regulation of immune responses by odontoblasts. *Oral Microbiology and Immunology,* Vol. 22, No. 1 (February 2007), pp. 5–13, ISSN 17241164.

Vernal, R., Dutzan, N., Chaparro, A., Puente, J., Antonieta Valenzuela, M. & Gamonal, J. (2005). Levels of interleukin-17 in gingival crevicular fluid and in supernatants of cellular cultures of gingival tissue from patients with chronic periodontitis. *Journal of Clinical Periodontology,* Vol. 32, No. 4 (April 2005), pp. 383-389, ISSN 15811056.

Vernal, R., Dezerega, A., Dutzan, N., Chaparro, A., León, R., Chandía, S., Silva, A. & Gamonal, J. (2006). RANKL in human periapical granuloma: possible involvement in periapical bone destruction. *Oral Diseases*, Vol. 12, No. 3, (May 2006), pp. 283-289, ISSN 1601-0825.

Verstappen, J. & Von den Hoff J. W. (2006). Tissue inhibitors of metalloproteinases (TIMPs): their biological functions and involvement in oral disease. *Journal of Dental Research*, Vol. 85, No. 12, (December 2006), pp. 1074-1084, ISSN 1544-0591.

Volin, M. V., Shah, M. R., Tokuhira, M., Haines, G. K., Woods, J. M. & Koch, A. E. (1998). RANTES expression and contribution to monocyte chemotaxis in arthritis. *Clinical Immunology and Immunopathology*, Vol. 89, No. 1, (October 1998), pp. 44-53, ISSN 0090-1229.

Wajant, H., Pfizenmaier, K. & Scheurich, P. (2003). Tumor necrosis factor signaling. *Cell Death Differentiation*, Vol. 10, No. 1 (January 2003), pp. 45-65, ISSN 12655295.

Wakabayashi, H., Yamauchi, K., Kobayashi, T., Yaeshima, T., Iwatsuki, K. & Yoshie, H. (2009). Inhibitory effects of lactoferrin on growth and biofilm formation of Porphyromonas gingivalis and Prevotella intermedia. *Antimicrob Agents Chemotherapie*, Vol. 53, No. 8 (August 2009), pp. 3308-3316, ISSN 19451301.

Wang, M. & Hajishengallis, G. (2008). Lipid raft-dependent uptake, signalling and intracellular fate of Porphyromonas gingivalis in mouse macrophages. *Cell Microbiol*, Vol. 10, No. 10 (October 2008), pp. 2029-2042, ISSN 18547335.

Ward, S. G., Bacon, K. & Westwick, J. (1998). Chemokines and T lymphocytes: more than attraction. *Immunity*, Vol. 9, No. 1, (July 1998), pp. 1-11, ISSN 1074-7613.

Weaver, C.T. & Hatton, R.D. (2009). Interplay between the TH17 and TReg cell lineages: a (co-)evolutionary perspective. *Natural Rev Immunology*, Vol. 9, No. 12 (December 2009), pp. 883-889, ISSN 19935807.

Williams, S. R., Jiang, Y., Cochran, D., Dorsam, G. & Graves, D. T. (1992). Regulated expression of monocyte chemoattractant protein-1 in normal human osteoblastic cells. *American Journal of Physiology*, Vol. 263, No. 1, (July 1992), pp. 194-199, ISSN 0363-6143.

Yadav, A., Saini, V. & Arora, S. (2010). MCP-1: Chemoattractant with a role beyond immunity: a review. *Clinica Chimica Acta*, Vol. 411, No. 21-22, (November 2010), pp. 1570-1579, ISSN 0009-8981.

Yago, T., Nanke, Y., Ichikawa, N., Kobashigawa, T., Mogi, M., Kamatani, N. & Kotake, S. (2009). IL-17 induces osteoclastogenesis from human monocytes alone in the absence of osteoblasts, which is potently inhibited by anti-TNF-alpha antibody: a novel mechanism of osteoclastogenesis by IL-17. *Journal of Cell Biochemistry*, Vol. 108, No. 4 (November 2009), pp. 947-955, ISSN 19728295.

Yamaguchi, M., Ukai, T., Kaneko, T., Yoshinaga, M., Yokoyama, M., Ozaki, Y. & Hara Y. (2008). T cells are able to promote lipopolysaccharide-induced bone resorption in mice in the absence of B cells. *Journal of Periodontal Research*, Vol. 43, No. 5 (October 2008), pp. 549-55, ISSN 18624940.

Yoshihara, Y., Nakamura, H., Obata, K., Yamada, H., Hayakawa, T., Fujikawa, K. & Okada, Y. (2000). Matrix metalloproteinases and tissue inhibitors of metalloproteinases in synovial fluids from patients with rheumatoid arthritis or osteoarthritis. *Annals of the Rheumatic Diseases*, Vol. 59, No. 6, (June 2000), pp. 455-461, ISSN 0003-4967.

Yoshimura, A., Mori, H., Ohishi, M., Aki, D. & Hanada, T. (2003). Negative regulation of cytokine signaling influences inflammation. *Curr Opin Immunology,* Vol. 15, No. 6 (December 2003), pp. 704-708, ISSN 14630206.

Yoshimura, A., Naka, T. & Kubo, M. (2007). SOCS proteins, cytokine signalling and immune regulation. *Natural Rev Immunology,* Vol. 7, No. 6 (June 2007), pp. 454-465, ISSN 17525754.

Yoshimura, T., Matsushima, K., Tanaka, S., Robinson, E. A., Appella, E., Oppenheim, J. J. & Leonard, E. J. (1987). Purification of a human monocyte-derived neutrophil chemotactic factor that has peptide sequence similarity to other host defense cytokines. *Proceedings of the National Academy of Sciences of the United States of America,* Vol. 84, No. 24, (December 1987), pp. 9233-9237, ISSN-0027-8424.

Yu, J.J., Ruddy, M.J., Wong, G.C., Sfintescu, C., Baker, P.J., Smith, J.B., Evans, R.T. & Gaffen, S.L. (2007). An essential role for IL-17 in preventing pathogen-initiated bone destruction: recruitment of neutrophils to inflamed bone requires IL-17 receptor-dependent signals. *Blood,* Vol. 109, No. 9 (May 2007), pp. 3794-3802, ISSN 17202320.

Yu, X. & Graves, D. (1995). Fibroblasts, mononuclear phagocytes and endothelial cells express MCP-1 in inflamed human gingiva. *Journal of Periodontology,* Vol. 66, No. 1, (January 1995), pp. 80-88, ISSN 0022-3492.

Yu, X., Huang, Y., Collin-Osdoby, P. & Osdoby, P. (2004). CCR1 chemokines promote the chemotactic recruitment, RANKL development, and motility of osteoclasts and are induced by inflammatory cytokines in osteoblasts. *Journal of Bone and Mineral Research,* Vol. 19, No. 12, (December 2004), pp. 2065-2077, ISSN 0884-0431.

Zaiss, M.M.R., Axmann, J., Zwerina, K., Polzer, E. & (2007). Treg cells suppress osteoclast formation: a new link between the immune system and bone. *Arthritis Rheumathoide,* Vol. 56. No. 12 (December 2007), pp. 4104-4112, ISSN 18050211.

Zeichner-David, M. (2006). Regeneration of periodontal tissues: cementogenesis revisited. *Periodontology 2000,* Vol. 41, No. 1, (June 2006), pp. 196-217, ISSN 0906-6713.

Zhang, T., Hashizume, T., Kurita-Ochiai, T. & Yamamoto, M. (2009). Sublingual vaccination with outer membrane protein of Porphyromonas gingivalis and Flt3 ligand elicits protective immunity in the oral cavity. *Biochemistry Biophysics Res Community,* Vol. 390, No. 3 (December 2009), pp. 937-941, ISSN 19852927.

Zhang, X. & Teng, Y.T. (2006). Interleukin-10 inhibits gram-negative-microbe-specific human receptor activator of NF-kappaB ligand-positive CD4+-Th1-cell-associated alveolar bone loss in vivo. *Infectology Immunity,* Vol. 74, No. 8 (August 2006), pp. 4927-4931, ISSN 16861684.

Zlotnik, A. & Yoshie, O. (2000). Chemokines: a new classification system and their role in immunity. *Immunity,* Vol. 12, No. 2, (February 2000), pp. 121-127, ISSN 1074-7613.

9

Complement Receptors in Inflammation

Priyanka Pundir[1,2] and Marianna Kulka[1,3]
[1]*Institute for Nutrisciences and Health, National Research Council, Charlottetown, PE*
[2]*Department of Biomedical Sciences, Atlantic Veterinary College, University of Prince Edward Island, Charlottetown, PE*
[3]*Allergy-Immunology Division, Northwestern University, Feinberg School of Medicine, Chicago, IL*
[1,2]*Canada*
[3]*USA*

1. Introduction

Complement was first discovered in 1889 as a bactericidal protein, distinct from heat stable antibodies present in normal serum. Since that time, it has been shown that the complement system is a biochemical cascade, comprised of more than 30 fluid phase and membrane-associated proteins, normally present as inactive forms. The complement system can be activated by different sequential cascades of enzymatic reactions (described below) in which proteins are sequentially cleaved and activated. The resulting effector molecules, C3a and C5a (also known as anaphylatoxins) are the most potent complement activation products, showing diverse activities on many cell types ranging from chemoattraction to apoptosis. The main target cells carry specialized complement receptors through which anaphylatoxins participate in host defense, inflammatory processes, and immune responses.

The complement system plays an essential role in innate immunity by defending the host against bacterial, viral, and parasitic invasion. Complement proteins promote opsonisation and/or phagocytosis and intracellular killing of these pathogens by immune effector cells such as macrophage and neutrophils. Complement proteins, particularly those of the classical pathway, aid in the processing of immune complexes and in protection against the development of immune complex diseases such as systemic lupus erythematosus (SLE). Recently, it has become evident that the complement system also regulates adaptive immunity involving B and T cells that help in the elimination of pathogens. Furthermore, the engagement of complement receptors on antigen-presenting cells (APC) and other immune cells leads to production of immunoregulatory cytokines. Not only is complement involved in innate and adaptive immunity, it is also involved in pathological conditions. For example, in allergic disease complement proteins participate in the development of an inflammatory reaction. The complement pathways are also activated in patients with sepsis, allergic rhinitis, allergic asthma, and allergic skin conditions such as urticaria. This chapter will outline how complement proteins, C3a and C5a, and their complement receptors regulate inflammation.

2. Complement system

2.1 Complement activation pathways

Pattern recognition receptors (PRRs) in the complement system such as specific antibody, C1q, C3, mannose-binding lectin (MBL), and ficolins recognize exogenous as well as endogenous pattern-associated molecular patterns (PAMPs) leading to the activation of complement (Wills-Karp, 2007). The complement system can be activated by four different pathways: the classical, alternative, lectin and extrinsic protease pathway. Although each of these pathways is activated by distinct PRRs, they all culminate in activation of C3, the central step in complement activation.

2.1.1 Classical pathway

The classical pathway is activated when immune complexes are formed. These immune complexes are formed when antibodies (released during a humoral immune response (immunoglobulin (Ig)G or IgM)) bind to pathogens or other foreign and non-self antigens. The Fc portion of the antigen-antibody complex is engaged by the C1q molecule of the C1 complex (a multimeric complex consisting of C1q, C1r and C1s molecules) leading to activation of C1s and C1r. C1 then cleaves C4 and C2 to form C3 convertase (C4bC2a; Figure 1) (Wagner and Frank, 2010).

C3 convertase enzyme activates C3, the most abundant complement protein found freely in blood plasma, by proteolytic cleavage. This reaction results in the generation of: (1) complement proteins C3a, C4a and C5a; (2) membrane attack complex (MAC) consisting of C5b, C6, C7, C8 and C9; and (3) opsonisation molecule C3b (Wagner and Frank, 2010; Wills-Karp, 2007).

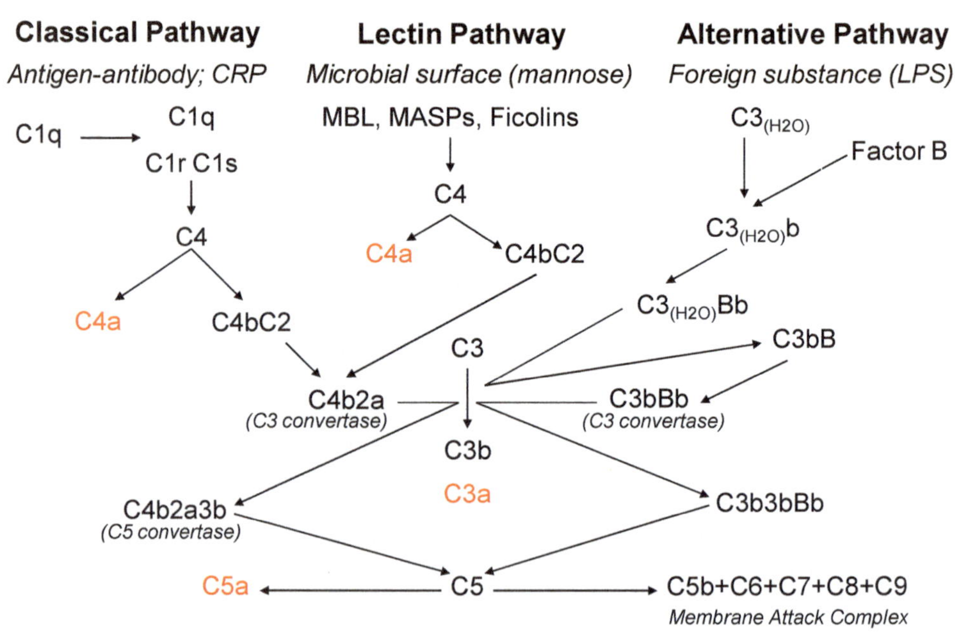

Fig. 1. Complement activation pathways

2.1.2 Lectin pathway

The lectin pathway is initiated when PRRs, MBL, H-, M- and L-ficolin, recognize and bind sugar moieties on yeast, bacteria, parasites and viruses. In the circulation, these PRRs associate with MBL-associated serine protease 1 (MASP1), MASP2 and MASP3, and a truncated MASP2 known as MAP19. Binding of the MBL-MASP complex to pathogen results in the cleavage of C4 and C2 and the generation of a C3 convertase (C4bC2a; Figure 1), similar to that of the classical pathway (Wagner and Frank, 2010).

2.1.3 Alternative pathway

The alternative pathway is triggered by carbohydrates, lipids and proteins found on pathogen. Slow and constant hydrolysis of circulating C3 (C3 tickover) and its interaction with complement factors B, and D leads to formation of a C3 convertase (C3bBb; Figure 1) (Wagner and Frank, 2010).

2.1.4 Extrinsic protease pathway

In addition to the above three pathways, a C3 independent pathway can also activate the complement system. An extrinsic protease pathway involves direct cleavage of C3 and C5 by a series of proteolytic enzymes released by neutrophils and macrophages; and factors such as Kallikrein, plasmin and factor XIIa. Thrombin, a coagulation factor, can directly cleave C5 to generate biologically active C5a in C3-deficient mice in which C5 convertase cannot be formed (Ricklin et al., 2010).

2.2 Complement proteins C3a, C4a and C5a

The complement proteins, C3a, C4a and C5a, are components of the complement system that are produced from C3, C4 and C5, respectively, as part of the complement activation cascade. C3a is a 9 kiloDalton (kDa) peptide fragment released during selective proteolytic cleavage of the C3 α chain by a C3 convertase of the classical or the alternative pathway. C4a is a 8.7 kDa peptide released from the α chain of C4 by C2a cleavage in an early step of the classical pathway. C5a is an 11 kDa peptide released from the α chain of C5 by action of either classical or alternative pathway C5 convertase (Ember and Hugli, 1997).

Although C3a, C4a and C5a are genetically related, they have marked structural differences in their sequences. Only 13 residues are conserved between C3a, C4a and C5a molecules from several species examined. Six of the conserved residues are cysteines whose side chains participate in forming three intrachain disulfide linkages that stabilize the folded alpha-helical peptide chain. The three disulfide bonds in C3a are Cys 22-Cys 49, Cys 23-Cys 56 and Cys 36-Cys 57. The four-helix bundle of C5a is stabilized by Cys 21-Cys 47, Cys 22-Cys 54 and Cys 34-Cys 55 disulfide bonds. Further structural similarities include a flexible carboxyl terminal tail -L-G-L-A-R in C3a, -A/V-G/H-L-A/Q-R in C4a, and -M/I/V-Q-L-G-R in C5a, which forms a helical turn connected by a short loop, which is important for effector functions of these proteins (Ember and Hugli, 1997).

C3a, C4a and C5a are potent inflammatory peptides with diverse activities on many cell types. They act as chemoattractants for immune cells such as neutrophils, eosinophils, mast cells, and monocytes recruiting to sites of injury or inflammation. They also regulate vasodilation, increase the permeability of blood vessels, and induce smooth muscle contraction. Anaphylatoxin stimulation can induce oxidative burst in neutrophils, histamine release from mast cells and basophils, production of eosinophil cationic protein (ECP) from

eosinophils, and production of pro-inflammatory cytokines from monocytes, B cells and T cells. Characterization of the inflammatory activities of complement proteins indicate relative activities in the order of C5a>C3a>C4a on most tissues examined (Hugli, 1981).
The complement proteins generated as a result of the complement activation damage host tissues. It is therefore obvious that control mechanisms are needed to tightly regulate these potent peptides and maintain homeostatic balance. Indeed, once C3a and C5a are cleaved from C3 and C5 respectively, they are rapidly degraded by plasma enzyme carboxypeptidases. The resulting C3a desArg lacks any pro-inflammatory activity; however, C5a desArg exhibits a reduced inflammatory activity of 1-10% compared with C5a. Interestingly, C3a desArg, also known as acylation stimulating protein (ASP), has been described as possessing metabolic hormone activity that drives triglyceride synthesis and glucose update. This suggests a regulatory role of C3a desArg in cell apoptosis and lipid metabolism (Cianflone et al., 1989).

3. Complement receptors for C3a and C5a: C3aR, C5aR and C5L2

The complement proteins C3a and C5a exert their pleiotropic effects by binding to a family of three receptors belonging to the G protein-coupled receptor (GPCR) superfamily. These receptors are the C3a receptor (C3aR), the C5a receptor (C5aR) and the C5a receptor-like 2 (C5L2).

3.1 C3a receptor (C3aR)

C3aR is a membrane glycoprotein of approximately 54 kDa (Ames et al., 1996). This receptor displays high affinity for C3a with a dissociation constant (K_d) of about 1 nM, but not for C3a desArg or C5a (Crass et al., 1996). Human platelets express a high molecular weight (95-105 kDa) variant of C3aR that binds C3a with K_d of 8×10^{-10} M.

3.1.1 Structure

As a GPCR, C3aR contains seven transmembrane domains within its 482 amino acids sequence. C3aR distinctively possesses a large second extracellular loop between the fourth and fifth transmembrane domain that is indispensable for ligand binding. This loop contains 175 amino acid residues; in most GPCR the corresponding extracellular loop is 30-40 amino acids long. Sulfation of tyrosine 174 in this loop is essential for binding C3a (Chao et al., 1999). The genes encoding C3aR have been mapped to p13.2-3 of chromosome 12 in humans and 6F1 in mouse (Hollmann et al., 1998). C3aR displays 50-60% homology between various species, with 65% sequence identity between human and murine counterparts (Hollmann et al., 1998).

3.1.2 Expression

C3aR is expressed on cells of myeloid origin, including monocytes/macrophages, neutrophils, eosinophils, basophils, mast cells, dendritic cells and microglia. Additionally, C3aR is also expressed on non-myeloid cells, such as astrocytes, endothelial cells, epithelial cells, smooth muscle cells, and activated T cells. One paper has described the receptor's expression on human tonsillar B cells; while others have confirmed the absence of C3aR on human B cells. The receptor is also expressed in tissues from lung, liver, kidney, brain, heart, muscle and, testis.

3.1.3 Biological role

C3aR mediates chemotaxis of eosinophils (Daffern et al., 1995), mast cells (Nilsson et al., 1996), dendritic cells (Gutzmer et al., 2004) and monocytes, but not neutrophils (Daffern et al., 1995). It can also trigger oxidative burst in macrophages, neutrophils and eosinophils (Burg et al., 1996). In addition, basophils (Bischoff et al., 1990) and mast cells (Johnson et al., 1975, Venkatesha et al., 2005) undergo degranulation and release histamine upon C3a-C3aR interaction. C3aR stimulates production of ECP from eosinophils (Takafuji et al., 1994), as well as upregulation of β_2-integrins and shedding of L-selectins, thereby promoting eosinophil adhesion to endothelial and epithelial cells (Jagels et al., 2000). Human monocytes and mast cells exhibit increased intracellular calcium (Ca^{2+}) levels when stimulated with C3a (Venkatesha et al., 2005). C3a also stimulates smooth muscle contraction (Stimler et al., 1983), lysozyme release from immune cells (Showell et al., 1982), platelet aggregation (Becker et al., 1978), and triglyceride synthesis in adipocytes (Baldo et al., 1993).

3.1.4 Signaling

Upon C3a binding to the C3aR, intracellular signal transduction is promoted via heterotrimeric guanosine triphosphate (GTP)-binding proteins (G proteins). C3aR mediates its effect on immune cells via coupling to the pertussis toxin (PTX)-sensitive and –insensitive G proteins $G\alpha_i$ and $G\alpha_{16}$, respectively. In endothelial cells, C3aR also couples to PTX-insensitive $G\alpha_{12}$ and $G\alpha_{13}$ (Schraufstatter et al., 2002). Downstream signaling events involve activation of phosphoinositol-3-kinase gamma (PI3K-γ), which in turn activates phospholipase C (PLC)β and PLCγ. This leads to generation of inositol triphosphate (IP3) and diacylglycerol (DAG), leading to Ca^{2+} mobilization and phosphokinase C (PKC) activation, respectively. PI3K can also activate Raf/mitogen-activated protein kinase (MAPK)/extracellular-signal regulated kinase (ERK) kinase (MEK)/ERK cascade inducing expression of various pro-inflammatory cytokines and chemokines.

3.2 C5a receptor (C5aR or CD88)

First cloned in 1991 (Boulay et al., 1991, Gerard and Gerard, 1991), C5aR is a membrane glycoprotein of approximately 42 kDa (Richardson et al., 1998), displaying high affinity for C5a and C5a desArg. Human C5aR binds C5a with a K_d of 1 nM, and with 10 to 100-fold lower affinity to C5a desArg (K_d of 412-660 nM) whereas C3a and C3a desArg are not recognized (Monk et al., 2007).

3.2.1 Structure

Similar to C3aR, C5aR is a seven transmembrane GPCR that belongs to the rhodopsin-like family. Based on the analysis of transmembrane domain sequences, C5aR is clustered with other chemoattractant receptors, such as C3aR, formyl peptide receptor family, ChemR23, platelet activating factor (PAF) receptor, IL-8 receptor, and bradykinin receptor (Methner et al., 1997, Samson et al., 1998). The C5aR gene is localized to q13.3-13.4 of human chromosome 19 (Gerard et al., 1998). Murine C5aR exhibits 65% sequence identity with its human counterpart (Gerard et al., 1992). The N terminus of C5aR is required for high affinity binding of C5a, but not for receptor activation (DeMartino et al., 1994, Mery and Boulay, 1993). A second distinct binding site is formed by charged residues in the second and third extracellular loops and the external faces of the transmembrane helical bundle and hydrophobic residues in the core of the C5aR. Unlike the N terminal binding site, the second site is responsible for receptor activation (Gerber et al., 2001). Current evidence suggests that at least three different discontinuous regions exist within the C5a molecule for interaction with C5aR (Huber-Lang et al., 2003).

3.2.2 Expression

C5aR is expressed on cells of myeloid origin such as neutrophils, eosinophils, basophils, mast cells, dendritic cells and monocytes, as well as on non-myeloid cells, including bronchial and alveolar epithelial cells, endothelial cells, Kupffer cells, stellate cells, astrocytes and microglial cells (Monk et al., 2007).

3.2.3 Biological role

C5aR is a powerful chemoattractant receptor for monocytes (Pieters et al., 1995), neutrophils (Webster et al., 1980), eosinophils (DiScipio et al., 1999), basophils (Lett-Brown and Leonard, 1977), mast cells (Hartmann et al., 1997), B cells (Kupp et al., 1991) and T cells (Nataf et al., 1999). It also stimulates mast cell degranulation (Subramanian et al., 2011), mast cell chemotaxis in specific mast cell subtypes (Hartmann et al., 1997, McCloskey et al., 1999), oxidative burst in granulocytes and the production of reactive oxygen species (ROS) in neutrophils (Guo et al., 2003), secretion of lysosomal enzymes from macrophages (McCarthy and Henson, 1979) and polymorphonuclear (PMN) cells as well as the secretion of pro-inflammatory mediators from monocytes, eosinophils (Takafuji et al., 1994) and mast cells (Hartmann et al., 1997). C5a is also responsible for upregulation of vascular adhesion molecules such as E-selectin, inter-cellular adhesion molecule 1 (ICAM-1) and vascular cell adhesion molecule 1 (VCAM-1) after systemic activation of complement (Albrecht et al., 2004, Jagels et al., 2000). Our preliminary findings suggest that C5a can promote human mast cell adhesion to extracellular matrix protein, as well as human mast cell migration *in vitro*, indicating a critical role of C5a/C5aR in inflammation.

3.2.4 Signaling

C5aR signaling depends on heterotrimeric G proteins. C5aR mainly couples to $G\alpha_{i2}$, a PTX-sensitive G protein (Skokowa et al., 2005). However, ectopically expressed C5aR, and C5aR on cells of the hematopoietic lineage, can also couple to PTX-insensitive $G\alpha_{16}$ (Amatruda et al., 1993, Monk and Partridge, 1993). C5a-C5aR interaction leads to activation of several components of signaling pathway, including PI3K-γ, PLCβ2, and phospholipase D (PLD) (Rabiet et al., 2007). C5aR can activate the transcription factor, cyclic AMP (cAMP) response element-binding protein (CREB), by phosphorylation at the convergence of two pathways, PI3K/Akt and ERK (Perianayagam et al., 2006). CREB activation has been proposed to be a part of the mechanism by which C5a can delay neutrophil apoptosis and prolong an inflammatory response (Perianayagam et al., 2004). In neutrophils, C5a causes downstream activation of p21-activated kinases (PAK), which are downstream effectors of cdc42 and rac (small guanosine triphosphate (GTP)-binding proteins (GTPases)), as well as Gγ subunits (Huang et al., 1998). PAK family members are involved in altering cell morphology/chemotaxis, activation or potentiation of several distinct MAPK cascades and the activation of nuclear factor (NF)-kB in macrophages. p38 MAPK is activated by PAK1/PAK2 and, in turn, activates MAPK-activated protein kinase 2 (MAPKAP-K2). In primary macrophages from MAPKAP-K2-deficient mice, chemotaxis to C5a is impaired.

Furthermore, the p38 MAPK inhibitor, SB203580, can inhibit C5a-induced migration in a mouse acute lung injury model (Rousseau et al., 2006).
C5aR also couples directly or indirectly to a small range of other intracellular proteins. The Wiskot–Aldrich syndrome protein (WASP) was detected as a binding partner of the C-terminus of C5aR using a yeast two-hybrid assay. WASP binding was strongly potentiated in the presence of active cdc42, suggesting that the association occurs after C5aR activation (Tardif et al., 2003). WASP is a multifunctional protein with a role in the regulation of actin dynamics, and so could be involved in the chemotactic response to C5a. In human erythroleukaemia cells, signal transducers and activators of transcription (STAT3) phosphorylation can be stimulated by C5a in a PTX-insensitive manner, most likely through $G\alpha_{16}$ and the Ras/Raf/MEK/ERK and janus kinase (JAK) pathways (Lo et al., 2006). In contrast, STAT3 phosphorylation occurs only through an ERK pathway in C5a-stimulated neutrophils (Kuroki and O'Flaherty, 1999).

3.3 C5a receptor-like 2 (C5L2)

First discovered in 2000 as a putative orphan receptor (GPR77), (Ohno et al., 2000) C5L2 has since been identified as a second C5a receptor. It is a 37 kDa protein and binds C5a with high affinity (K_d of 2.5 nM). Unlike C5aR, C5L2 binds C5a desArg with a 20-30 fold higher affinity (Cain and Monk, 2002).

3.3.1 Structure

C5L2 consists of 337 amino acids with asparagine 3 as a potential glycosylation site (Ohno et al., 2000). In the conserved transmembrane regions, C5L2 shares 58% sequence identity with C5aR and 55% with C3aR (Lee et al., 2001). Unlike C5aR, C5L2 uses critical residues in its N terminal domain for binding only to C5a desArg. In addition to C5a and C5a desArg binding, C5L2 has been considered a binding partner for C3a, C3a desArg (Kalant et al., 2005), C4a and C4a desArg; however the available data is not very convincing (Johswich et al., 2006, Okinaga et al., 2003).
Although C5L2 has the conventional structure of a GPCR, studies have found that C5L2 does not couple to G proteins. This may be due to a structural difference in the third transmembrane domain. In GPCR, a highly conserved DRY motif in the third transmembrane domain is important for its interaction with the corresponding G proteins. The DRY motif is DRC in C3aR and DRF in C5aR, but DLC in C5L2. Moreover, the third transmembrane domain of C5L2 is truncated. Mutation of DLC in human C5L2 to DRC has been shown to increase coupling to $G\alpha_{16}$ in co-transfected human embryonic kidney (HEK)293 cells and induce a functional response (Okinaga et al., 2003). Interestingly, no functional response occurs in rat basophilic leukemia cells (RBL-2H3) using a C5L2-mutant where the DRY-motif and two additional regions typically involved in G protein coupling are replaced by the corresponding C5aR sequences (Scola et al., 2009). Taken together, these findings strongly suggest that C5L2 completely lacks the potential to couple with G proteins.

3.3.2 Expression

C5L2 is expressed in various tissues of myeloid and non-myeloid origin and transcripts are detected in brain, placenta, ovary, testis, spleen and colon. Surface expression of C5L2 has been detected in lung, liver, heart, kidney, adipose tissue, skin fibroblasts, neutrophils, and immature, but not mature dendritic cells. In the presence of a C5aR antagonist, binding of C5a has been demonstrated on differentiated myeloblastic HL-60, U937, and epithelial HeLa-cells. C5L2 and C5aR seem to be frequently co-expressed in most cells or tissues (Monk et al., 2007).

3.3.3 Biological role and signaling

C5L2 is an enigmatic receptor as available data suggest opposing roles. On the one hand, C5L2 has been described as a non-signaling decoy receptor for C5a and C5a desArg. In contrast, some studies suggest that C5L2 serves as a signaling functional receptor. In support of a role as a decoy receptor, no mobilization of intracellular Ca^{2+} occurs in C5L2 transfected cells after C5a administration (Cain and Monk, 2002, Okinaga et al., 2003). Moreover, no Ca^{2+} mobilization occurs in neutrophils from C5aR-deficient mice after stimulation with C5a (Hopken et al., 1996) or in C5L2 expressing epithelial and myeloid cell lines (Johswich et al., 2006). In the presence of C5a and C5a desArg, C5L2 transfected RBL-2H3 cells do not degranulate (Cain and Monk, 2002). Further, C5a binding to C5L2 in bone marrow cells derived from C5aR-deficient mice fails to induce any changes in messenger RNA (mRNA) expression (Okinaga et al., 2003).

Nevertheless, there is accumulating evidence that C5L2 is a functional receptor capable of regulating C5aR function *in vitro* and *in vivo*. Neutrophils and macrophages from C5L2-deficient mice produce more tumor necrosis factor (TNF)α and interleukin (IL)6 in response to stimulation with C5a and lipopolysaccharide (LPS) than their wildtype (WT) counterparts. Further, C5a+LPS stimulation drive more IL-6 production from rat neutrophils when C5L2 is blocked (Gao et al., 2005). *In vivo*, C5L2-deficient mice suffer from augmented inflammatory responses and higher numbers of infiltrating neutrophils in a model of pulmonary immune complex injury (Gerard et al., 2005), indicating an anti-inflammatory function of C5L2. The anti-inflammatory role of C5L2 is further supported by a study in which LPS-injected C5L2-deficient mice show higher IL-1β levels and decreased survival rates (Chen et al., 2007). Similarly, C5L2-deficient mice display higher serum concentrations of IL-6 as compared to WT and C5aR-deficient mice in a model of septic peritonitis (Rittirsch et al., 2008).

In contrast, under the same conditions, a strong reduction of other inflammatory mediators, such as IL-1β, macrophage inflammatory protein (MIP)-1α and MIP-2 is observed in C5L2-deficient mice compared to WT mice. Indeed, the plasma concentrations of these mediators are comparable to those found in C5aR-deficient mice. Furthermore, C5L2-deficient mice, like C5aR-deficient mice, or mice in which either of the receptors are blocked by anti-receptor antibodies, show a higher survival rate in mid-grade sepsis (Rittirsch et al., 2008). Contrasting the *in vitro* findings that C5a+LPS-driven IL-6 production by mouse neutrophils is increased when C5L2 is blocked by antibodies (see above), Chen et al. found that IL-6 release is reduced from C5L2-deficient neutrophils (Chen et al., 2007). Moreover, C5a+LPS-induced Mac-1 surface expression on these neutrophils also diminishes, suggesting neutrophils chemotaxis may be impacted. Likewise, whereas C5a or C5a+LPS stimulation can lead to strong ERK1/2- and AKT-phosphorylation in neutrophils from WT mice, there is only a weak effect in the absence of C5L2. Additionally, C5L2-deficient macrophages have an impaired induction of co-stimulatory molecules (CD40, CD86). Even C3a mediated effects such as ERK1/2- and Akt-phosphorylation or F-actin formation on neutrophils are impaired in C5L2-deficient mice (Chen et al., 2007). In addition to these *in vitro* findings, inflammatory responses are reduced *in vivo* in models of thioglycollate induced peritonitis, thioglycollate induced migration into dorsal air pouches, and ovalbumin (OVA) induced airway hyperresponsiveness (AHR) (Chen et al., 2007). Thus, these studies point to a more complex role of C5L2 in inflammation with C5L2 acting not only as a decoy receptor but also as positive modulator of C5aR and even C3aR. Although C3a desArg does not bind directly to C5L2, overexpression of C5L2 or its downregulation by antisense oligonucleotides influences the effects of C3a desArg (Kalant et al., 2005), suggesting that C5L2 can modulate signaling pathways of other receptors.

Although C5L2 does not appear to signal using the traditional mechanisms employed by GPCRs, several studies suggest that C5L2 has the ability to induce cellular effects. A recent study has found that noradrenaline upregulates C5L2 message and protein in rat astrocytes, and this correlates with an anti-inflammatory response induced by noradrenaline. Transfection of astrocytes by C5L2 down regulates NF-kB activity, whereas antisense oligonucleotides against C5L2 induce the reverse effect (Gavrilyuk et al., 2005). These observations suggest that the presence of C5L2 may exert some inhibitory effects within the cell, although the mechanisms behind such responses are currently unknown.

4. Regulation of complement receptor signaling

GPCR represent the largest family of cell surface receptors in the human genome, allowing extracellular signals to regulate a vast number of physiological events. Following ligand binding, GPCR undergo a conformational change which activates heterotrimeric G proteins. G proteins exist as a complex of Gα and Gβγ subunits. Upon activation, GDP is displaced by GTP from the Gα subunit resulting in disassociation of Gα subunit from the Gβγ subunits. This facilitates the free subunits interactions with various effector molecules and initiates downstream signaling (Pundir and Kulka, 2010). In the immune system, GPCRs play a role in innate, adaptive and pathological responses. In allergic diseases, stimulation of the GPCRs, C3aR and C5aR, by C3a and C5a, respectively produces a diverse array of effector functions, ranging from inflammatory cell migration to pro-inflammatory mediator production, thus contributing towards the pathophysiology of the diseases.

Given that the activation of C3aR and C5aR can induce massive inflammation and tissue destruction, there are mechanisms in place to limit complement activation where and when it occurs. As mentioned before, after generation, C3a and C5a are quickly degraded by plasma carboxypeptidases. The enzyme cleave the C-terminal arginine, resulting in C3a desArg and C5a desArg formation, each having less than 10% of their original biological activity (Bokisch and Muller-Eberhard, 1970). Formation of C3a and C5a is also regulated by either preventing the assembly of C3 convertase or, once it is formed, by inhibiting its activity. This is accomplished through the actions of decay acceleration factor (DAF), C4 binding protein (C4BP) and Factor H (Sarma and Ward, 2011). In addition, desensitization to prolonged or repeated exposure to high agonist concentration is another important mechanism of GPCR regulation. Furthermore, G proteins may terminate their own activation by Gα hydrolysis of GTP, thereby allowing Gα-GDP to reunite with Gβγ and form an inactive heterotrimer (Tsang et al., 1998). As this reaction proceeds at a slow rate (Tsang et al., 1998), additional cofactors come into play that aid in GPCR desensitization. Indeed, there are around 30 isoforms of Regulator of G protein signaling (RGS) proteins, which bind to activated Gα subunit and accelerate their intrinsic GTPase activity (Willars,

2006). RGS13 can regulate human mast cell lines, HMC-1 and laboratory of allergic diseases (LAD)2, response to C5a. RGS13-deficient HMC-1 cells have more cytosolic Ca^{2+} in response to C5a, indicating that RGS13 regulates C5aR-stimulated events in immune cells (Bansal et al., 2008).

GPCR desensitization is also achieved by the G protein-coupled receptor kinase (GRK)-arrestin pathway. There are seven GRKs in humans, GRK1-7, and four arrestins, arrestin 1-4. Most GPCRs are regulated by only four GRKs: GRKs 2, 3, 5, or 6, and two arrestins: arrestin-2 (β-arrestin1) and arrestin-3 (β-arrestin2) (Premont and Gainetdinov, 2007). Agonist-induced desensitization of GPCRs occurs via a multistep process. Just as G proteins recognize activated GPCR, GRKs also recognize activated GPCR, which leads to receptor phosphorylation at various serine/threonine residues on the intracellular loops and the carboxyl-terminal tail (Langkabel et al., 1999). Upon phosphorylation by GRK, GPCR's affinity for arrestin proteins is increased, which prevents the receptor from activating additional G proteins. The β-arrestins interact with clathrin and the adaptor protein complex AP-2 and target the agonist occupied receptors to pre-existing clathrin-coated pits for internalization. Thus GRK phosphorylation and arrestin binding result in termination of GPCR signaling, despite the continued presence of agonist (Santini et al., 2002, Scott et al., 2002).

A study by Ahamed et al. has shown that C3a stimulates degranulation and chemokine monocyte chemotactic protein-1 (MCP-1) production in RBL-2H3 cells expressing C3aR. Stimulation with C3a causes phosphorylation of WT C3aR but not of phosphorylation-deficient C3aR (ΔST-C3aR). In addition, C3a stimulation increases degranulation only in RBL-2H3 cells expressing ΔST-C3aR, suggesting that receptor phosphorylation provides an "off" signal for degranulation. Overexpression of GRK2 in C3aR-transfected cells results in increased C3a-induced C3aR phosphorylation. This increase in receptor phosphorylation is associated with a significant inhibition of degranulation. Furthermore, C3a causes a rapid translocation of β-arrestin2 from the cytosol to the membrane in RBL-2H3 cells expressing C3aR but not in cells expressing ΔST-C3aR, indicating that GRK2-induced C3aR phosphorylation is required for β-arrestin recruitment following C3a stimulation (Ahamed et al., 2001). Similarly, in transfected COS cells, overexpression of GRK2, GRK3, GRK5 or GRK6 results in enhanced C3a-induced C3aR phosphorylation (Langkabel et al., 1999). Knockdown of GRK2 or GRK3 expression in HMC-1 and LAD2 cells, causes higher Ca^{2+} mobilization, attenuated C3aR desensitization, and enhanced degranulation, thus indicating GRK2 and GRK3 involvement in C3aR desensitization. On the other hand, GRK5 or GRK6 knockdown in HMC-1 and LAD2 cells has no effect on C3aR desensitization, but instead promotes C3a-mediated degranulation, suggesting a complex role for GRKs in regulating human mast cells (Guo et al., 2011).

A recent study has identified the roles of β-arrestin1 and β-arrestin2 on C3aR desensitization and internalization (Vibhuti et al., 2011). By stably knocking down their expression in HMC-1 cells, this study shows that β-arrestin2, but not β-arrestin1, is required for C3aR desensitization and internalization. Interestingly, β-arrestin1-deficient, but not β-arrestin2-deficient, HMC-1 cells show reduced NF-κB activation and chemokine MIP-1β generation in response to C3a. Similar knock-down study with LAD2 cells shows that the absence of β-arrestin1, but not β-arrestin2, significantly inhibits C3a-induced degranulation. This demonstrates that β-arrestin1 and β-arrestin2 play a distinct role on C3aR desensitization, internalization and mediator generation in human mast cells (Vibhuti et al., 2011).

Upon ligand binding, C5aR undergoes rapid phosphorylation of the six serine residues located in the carboxyl-terminal tail (Giannini et al., 1995). This phosphorylation is a critical step in the termination of the C5aR signaling since a phosphorylation-deficient C5aR mutant triggers sustained intracellular signaling leading to increased C5a-induced superoxide production by HL-60 cells (Christophe et al., 2000). A study by Braun et al. shows that a persistent complex between activated/phosphorylated C5aR and β-arrestins is necessary for receptor desensitization and internalization. WT C5aR and β-arrestin1-transfected RINm5F cells exhibit significant β-arrestin1 recruitment to the plasma membrane when stimulated with C5a. Moreover, in resting RINm5F cells, the C5aR is mainly located in the plasma membrane, and both β-arrestin1 and β-arrestin2 are evenly distributed throughout the cytoplasm. Upon addition of C5a, β-arrestin1 and β-arrestin2 rapidly move from the cytosol to the plasma membrane, co-localize with C5aR, promote endocytosis of C5aR and remain associated to C5aR-containing vesicles. Furthermore, this study also indicates that C5aR is mainly internalized via the classical clathrin-dependent pathway (Braun et al., 2003). Interestingly, an observation by Bamberg et al. reveals that in resting neutrophils C5L2 is distributed throughout the cytoplasm co-localized with β-arrestin, while C5aR is expressed on their surface. Following stimulation with C5a, association of both C5aR and C5L2 with β-arrestin is greatly increased. Cells treated with an anti-C5aR antibody when activated with C5a fail to translocate C5L2 to β-arrestin, indicating that the activation of C5L2 is a consequence of C5aR activation. Moreover, C5L2-β-arrestin complex is a negative regulator of C5aR signaling in neutrophils (Bamberg et al., 2010).

Thus, a number of mechanisms have evolved to efficiently regulate complement activation; however, these regulatory mechanisms seem to fail in various clinical and experimental situations underlining the important role of complement proteins and their complement receptors in the pathogenesis of inflammatory diseases. These include airway inflammation and asthma (Wagner et al., 1999), sepsis (Gao et al., 2005), multiple organ dysfunction (Mastellos et al., 2005), hyperactute graft rejection (Link et al., 1999), ischemic injuries of various organs (Arumugam et al., 2004), autoimmune disorders such SLE (Karp, 2005) or multiple sclerosis (Rus et al., 2005), neurological diseases such as stroke (Yanamadala and Friedlander), and cancer (Yan et al., 2008).

5. Diseases associated with complement function

5.1 Allergic inflammation: Allergic asthma

Asthma is a chronic inflammatory disorder of the airways characterized by variable airflow obstruction, and associated increase in airway responsiveness to a variety of stimuli. The clinical features of asthma include dyspnea, wheezing and coughing. It is thought to be mediated primarily by allergen-specific $CD4^{+}$ T cells, T helper (Th)2 cytokines, and allergen-specific IgE, leading to pulmonary inflammation and AHR. Complement is well recognized as an important factor in the pathophysiology of asthma.

In allergic asthma and allergic rhinitis conditions, the complement system is activated by several pathways leading to the cleavage of C3 and/or C5 into their active fragments. First, the presence of preexisting allergen-specific antibodies in asthmatic patients can activate the classical pathway through formation of immune complexes. Second, the alternative pathway can be initiated by nucleophilic attack of C3 directly on the surface of allergen or by Factor B (Taube et al., 2006). Third, the recognition of PAMPs and danger-associated molecular patterns (DAMPs), such as nucleic acids on apoptotic cells (Elward et al., 2005) or allergen polysaccharide, (Bito, 1977, Zimmermann et al., 1989) can activate the lectin pathway. Fourth, proteases released from inflammatory cells (Huber-Lang et al., 2002) or direct protease activity of allergens (Maruo et al., 1997) can drive the generation of C3a and C5a. Indeed, a variety of allergens have been shown to activate the complement and generate C3a and C5a in the airways. Ragweed extracts activate the complement cascade in both allergic individuals and healthy controls; however, generation of C3a is much stronger in allergic patients (Gonczi et al., 1997, Hidvegi et al., 1995). Ragweed allergen challenge also promotes C3a generation in the nasal mucosa of patients with allergic rhinitis. House dust mite (HDM), *Aspergillus fumigatus* and perennial ryegrass extracts induce serum C3a and C5a production in a dose and time-dependent manner (Nagata and Glovsky, 1987). Proteases from Dermatophagoides spp. (in particular, Der p 3 and Der f 3) can cleave C3 and C5 into their active fragments (Castro et al., 1991, Maruo et al., 1997). During an ongoing allergic reaction the Th2 cytokine IL-4 induces C3 mRNA production in human and murine epithelial cells (Khirwadkar et al., 1993).

Collectively, these studies provide strong evidence that major complement activation, and C3a and C5a generation occurs in asthmatic individuals. C3a and C5a are important contributing factors in the pathophysiology of asthma, because of their ability to recruit and activate inflammatory immune cells such as mast cells, eosinophils, macrophages, neutrophils, and basophils, increase vascular permeability, stimulate smooth muscle contraction, and trigger mast cell degranulation (Wust et al., 2006). Several studies have reported marked anaphylatoxins production under asthmatic condition. In the serum of asthmatic patients, an increase in C3a and C5a levels have been observed after allergen-induced bronchospasm (Arroyave et al., 1977, Smith et al., 1990). The levels of C3a, and to a lesser extent C5a increase in the bronchoalveolar lavage fluid (BALF) of asthmatic patients after segmental allergen provocation. Similarly, allergen-challenged lung lobes show significantly higher C3a levels in comparison to diluent (sham)-challenged lobes from asthmatic individuals (Humbles et al., 2000). In addition, sputum from patients with asthma exhibit increased C5a/C5a desArg concentrations (Marc et al., 2004). Infact, plasma C5a desArg levels reflect allergic disease severity (Bowser et al., 2010). Complement C3a and C4a concentrations increase in plasma of patients with aspirin-induced asthma (Lee et al., 2006). Studies with animal models of AHR have also indicated that C3a and C5a are crucial for asthma pathogenesis (Abe et al., 2001, Bautsch et al., 2000, Drouin et al., 2002, Lukacs et al., 2001).

In addition to allergen-mediated mechanisms, environmental stimuli can also trigger complement activation. Airborne pollutants such as diesel exhaust particles or airborne particulate matter can activate complement through the alternative pathway in human serum and airway epithelium, respectively (Walters et al., 2002). Moreover, acute ozone exposure can induce AHR and neutrophil infiltration, accompanied by elevated C3 levels in BALF in mice (Lambrecht and Hammad, 2009, Park et al., 2004). Cigarette smoke has been shown to directly activate the alternative pathway through cleavage of the internal thioester bond in C3 (Kew et al., 1987). Consistent with these studies, elevated levels of C3 have been found in children from smoking homes compared to those from non-smoking homes (Shima and Adachi, 1996).

Candidate gene and genome-wide screens for asthma susceptibility loci have identified C5 (9q34) (Ober et al., 1998, Wjst et al., 1999) and C5aR (19q.13.3) gene-containing chromosomal regions to be linked to asthma susceptibility (CSGA, 1997, Ober et al., 1998). One study reports an association between a single nucleotide polymorphism (SNP) in the *C3* gene and atopic asthma in children and adults in a Japanese population. On the other hand, SNPs in the human *C5* gene are associated with protection against both childhood and adult asthma. The authors also report a significant association between a SNP in the C3a receptor (*C3ar1*) gene and childhood asthma (Hasegawa et al., 2004). These observations may explain the opposing role of C3 and C5 in animal-based asthma studies. C3-deficient mice when challenged with an allergen to induce pulmonary allergy exhibit diminished AHR and lung eosinophilia. Furthermore, these mice show markedly reduced IL-4 secreting cells and attenuated allergen-specific IgE response (Drouin et al., 2002). Collectively, these results demonstrate that C3 promotes Th2 effector function in asthma. On the other hand, the A/J mouse strain in which allergic inflammation and AHR can be easily induced, are deficient in C5 (Karp et al., 2000), demonstrating that C5-deficient mice are more susceptible to experimental asthma. Furthermore, in vitro experiments have shown that peritoneal macrophages from C5-deifcient A/J mice produce significantly less IL-12, because IL-12 is critical for promotion of Th1 immune response (Karp et al., 2000), these studies suggest that dysfunction in C5 cleavage may influence susceptibility to asthma. In contrast, a study by Peng et al. has demonstrated the contribution of C5 in the development of airway inflammation, AHR and ongoing allergic response in OVA-sensitized mice (Peng et al., 2005). Pharmacological inhibition of C5 using a monoclonal antibody against C5, BB5.1, markedly attenuates airway obstruction, perivascular and peribronchial infiltration of inflammatory cells, and BALF levels of inflammatory mediators such as eotaxin, regulated upon activation, normal T-cell expressed and secreted (RANTES), TNFα, and matrix metalloproteinase (MMP)9 (Peng et al., 2005).

The paradoxical effects of C5 and C5a observed in allergic asthma may be due to C5 behaving differently during allergen sensitization as opposed to during established allergic inflammation. Evidence to this effect was provided by Kohl et. al in a study utilizing two models of pulmonary asthma: a) OVA sensitization and challenge of mice leading to inhalation tolerance; and b) HDM sensitization and challenge of mice which induce Th2 sensitization, airway inflammation, and AHR. Ablation of C5aR signaling by pharmacological targeting prior to initial pulmonary OVA challenge, using a neutralizing anti-C5aR monoclonal antibody, induces significant production of Th2 cytokines (IL-5, IL-13, and IL-10), high serum IgE levels, marked influx of inflammatory cells (eosinophils, neutrophils, and lymphocytes) into BALF, mucus production, and AHR. Similar results are observed when C5aR is blocked prior to initial pulmonary HDM challenge. Together, this data suggests that the presence of C5a in the airways at the time of initial allergen encounter serves to prevent the development of Th2-mediated immune response (Kohl et al., 2006).

Protection against allergic sensitization by C5aR activation is a complex process involving alterations in the function of APCs, in particular dendritic cells. Dendritic cells strategically located in the upper layers of the epithelium and lamina propria of the airways, are specialized for the recognition and internalization of PAMPs. Once loaded with allergen, dendritic cells migrate to draining lymph nodes and present antigen to naïve T cells, which under appropriate polarizing cytokine signals, differentiate into effector T cells (Banchereau and Steinman, 1998). Dendritic cells are composed of several subsets, some of which drive the development of an aberrant adaptive immune response. The two dendritic cell subsets which have been found in the bronchial airways are myeloid dendritic cells (mDCs) and plasmacytoid dendritic cells (pDCs) (GeurtsvanKessel and Lambrecht, 2008). Pulmonary mDCs function as the major APCs in mouse models of allergic asthma, preferentially inducing Th2 immune response towards inhaled allergen (Lambrecht et al., 2000). Pulmonary pDCs are immature dendritic cells, which induce respiratory tolerance by directly suppressing mDC-mediated activation of $CD4^+$ T effector cells or by inducing regulatory T cells (T_{regs}, a heterogeneous population of T cells that can suppress allergic immune responses) (GeurtsvanKessel and Lambrecht, 2008).

Several studies suggest that the ratio between mDCs and pDCs is critical for the development of the dysregulated Th cell response and that C5a regulates this ratio, thereby modulating the development of the allergic phenotype during allergen sensitization. $CD4^+$ T cells from mice challenged with HDM allergen in presence of an anti-C5aR monoclonal antibody produce higher levels of Th2 cytokines in co-culture with mDCs, but not with pDCs. Importantly, in the same setting, pDCs suppress the mDC-induced production of Th2 cytokines (Kohl et al., 2006). Furthermore, exposure to HDM leads to an increased number of mDCs, whereas the number of pDCs remains unaffected. These findings demonstrate that C5aR signaling controls the accumulation of pulmonary mDCs and pDCs in lungs, keeping the mDC:pDC ratio low, which facilitates the suppressive effects of pDCs on the mDC-mediated activation of T cells. In addition, C5aR blockade positively regulates the production of thymus and activation regulated chemokine (TARC) and macrophage-derived chemokine (MDC), thus promoting the recruitment of Th2 effector cells into the lungs (Kohl et al., 2006). Data obtained from C5-deficient mice indicate that C5aR signaling is required to keep mDC susceptible to suppression T_{regs}, thereby controlling the immunogenic effect of mDC (Lewkowich et al., 2005).

A study by Zhang et al. demonstrates that regulation of co-stimulatory molecules on mDCs and pDCs is an important mechanism underlying the protective impact of C5aR signaling on the development of the Th2 immune response. HDM exposure increases the frequency of pulmonary mDCs expressing B7-H1 and B7-DC. In vivo ablation of C5aR signaling dramatically reduces the frequency of pDCs expressing B7-H1 and B7-DC. In the presence of C5aR signaling, blockade of B7-H1 or B7-DC results in enhanced Th2 cytokine production by T cells, suggesting that B7-H1 and B7-DC are critical for pDC-driven regulation of mDCs, and protection against allergic sensitization (Zhang et al., 2009). Interestingly, C5aR expression on dendritic cells might be downregulated in the Th2 cytokine-dominated environment, thus dampening the negative regulatory effect of C5aR signaling, in particular on pDCs. Indeed, high levels of IL-4 downregulates C5aR expression in monocyte-derived dendritic cells (Soruri et al., 2003).

In the absence of C5aR, C5a binds C5L2, which has a similar distribution in lung tissue as C5aR. The pro-allergic role of C5L2 in experimental asthma has been demonstrated recently. OVA-sensitized C5L2-deficient mice exhibit reduced AHR, inflammatory cell infiltration, and airway inflammation (Chen et al., 2007). Similarly, HDM-sensitized C5L2-deficient mice show significantly attenuated AHR and airway inflammation that is associated with decreased mucus production, Th2 cytokine production, and serum IgE levels (Zhang et al., 2010), confirming the pro-inflammatory role of C5L2 in the development of asthma. The available data further indicates that C5L2 also has a regulatory impact on mDCs. Adoptive transfer of C5L2-deficient mDCs into WT mice results in decreased eosinophilic and lymphocytic inflammation and a decreased IgE response. Importantly, C5L2-deficient mDCs still promote production of large amounts of Th2 cytokines from lung cells; however, in contrast to their WT counterparts, the production of Th1 and Th17 cytokines is also enhanced, and is associated with an increased neutrophil influx. Moreover, HDM stimulation of C5L2-deficient mDCs results in production of the Th17-promoting cytokine IL-23. Collectively, this suggests a complex role of C5L2 in asthma; controlling the development of Th1 and Th17 cells in response to allergen challenge as well as driving the Th2 immune response (Zhang et al., 2010).

Th17 are IL-17A-producing subset of $CD4^+$ T cells which have received much interest recently in allergy research. Several reports suggest that in addition to Th2 cells, Th17 cells contribute to the development of allergic inflammation. Sputum IL-17A mRNA is significantly elevated in asthmatic patients, and correlates with increase in sputum neutrophil counts (Bullens et al., 2006). Bronchial biopsies taken from patients with severe asthma show massive infiltration of IL-17 producing Th17 cells (Pene et al., 2008). In experimental asthma, IL-17A (Hellings et al., 2003) and Th17 (McKinley et al., 2008) cells have been shown to promote bronchial influx of neutrophils and induce airway inflammation and AHR. Th17 cells not only mediate neutrophilic airway inflammation, they also upregulate airway eosinophilia, together with IL-23 (Wakashin et al., 2008). Recent studies have highlighted an important dual role for C5a in Th17 cell development. C5aR-deficient mDCs show elevated production of Th17 promoting cytokines (transforming growth factor (TGF)-β, IL-6, and IL-23) and Th17 cell differentiation (Weaver et al., 2010). Furthermore, A/J mice (lacking C5) develop severe AHR associated with elevated levels of IL-17A and Th2 cytokines in comparison to C3H/HeJ strain of mice (mice manifesting less severe AHR). HDM challenge induces increased frequency of Th17 cells, as well as IL-17A in lungs of A/J mice. *In vivo* blockade of IL-17A with an anti-IL-17A antibody reduces AHR and BALF neutrophilia in HDM challenged A/J mice. Furthermore, an inverse relationship is found between the serum C5a concentration and the frequency of Th17 cells and IL-17A staining in lungs of HDM challenged A/J mice. Pharmacological inhibition of C5aR in BALB/c mice leads to enhanced influx of Th17 cells into the lungs after HDM challenge, and increased production of IL-17A per cell. Also, dendritic cells from these mice produce more HDM-driven IL-23. Taken together this suggests that C5a/C5aR complex controls IL-17A by limiting IL-23 production (Lajoie et al., 2010). As described above, Th17 development in experimental asthma is not only regulated by C5aR but by C5L2 as well (Zhang et al. 2010).

In addition to its impact on Th17 cells, C5a may also regulate the development of T_{regs} (Palomares et al., 2010). Lack of C5aR signaling in mDCs results in T_{regs} differentiation (Lajoie et al.. 2010). Thus, C5aR signaling in APCs can modulate Th cell differentiation at several levels in allergic asthma.

The development of asthma is not only regulated by C5a-C5aR/C5L2 interactions, but also by C3a-C3aR; however the role is less clear. In contrast to C5a, several studies suggest that C3a mainly contributes to the pathogenesis of asthma. When challenged with allergen, C3-deficient mice exhibit diminished AHR and lung eosinophilia (Drouin et al., 2001). C3aR-deficient mice challenged with *Aspergillus fumigatus* and OVA show attenuated/decreased AHR, airway eosinophilia, lung IL-4 producing cells, BALF levels of Th2 cytokines, serum IgE, and mucus production (Drouin et al., 2002). Similarly, C3a is also involved in the development of the late asthmatic response and AHR; the mechanism being related to the production of IL-1β in the lung of OVA-challenged mice in response to C3a (Mizutani et al., 2009). However, in a model of particulate matter-induced pulmonary allergy, C3-deficient mice develop dramatically reduced AHR, but they are not protected from airway inflammation (Walters et al., 2002). Similarly, OVA-sensitized C3aR-deficient mice show markedly reduced bronchoconstriction and AHR, but IgE production and Th2 cytokine levels remains the same when compared to WT mice (Humbles et al., 2000).

Differences in mice strains, nature of the allergens used for sensitization and route of allergen administration may account for the conflicting results generated in different animal models. The study by Zhang at al. compared Th2 immune responses in C5aR- and C3aR-deficient mice side-by-side. As mentioned earlier, in the absence of C5aR signaling HDM-challenged mice suffer from an enhanced Th2 immune response. However, C3aR-deficient mice are protected against a Th2 immune response under same settings, delineating the opposing roles of C5aR and C3aR signaling in asthma. Interestingly, blocking C5aR-mediated signaling in C3aR-deficient mice significantly increases AHR, airway eosinophilia, and Th2 cytokines production, indicating that the decreased Th2 immune response in the absence of C3aR signaling results from a shift towards protective C5aR signaling (Zhang et al., 2009). Cross-talk between the two receptors is further supported by the fact that C5a negatively regulates C3aR internalization. Pulmonary C5aR-deficient dendritic cells exhibit dramatically higher expression of C3aR in comparison to WT dendritic cells. In contrast, C5aR expression significantly decreases in HDM-pulsed WT dendritic cells, but less so in C3aR-deficient dendritic cells, further confirming that there is a reciprocal regulation between C5aR and C3aR (Settmacher et al., 1999).

Recently, it has been shown that AHR, lung eosinophilia and mucus production are significantly increased in C5-deficient mouse model of Respiratory Syncytial Virus disease. C3aR expression in bronchial epithelial and smooth muscle cells of these mice are elevated as compared with WT mice. Ablation of C3aR signaling in C5-deficient mice significantly attenuates the disease phenotype, suggesting that C5 plays a crucial role in modulating AHR and eosinophilic inflammation by affecting expression of C3aR in the lungs (Melendi et al., 2007). C3a also has an impact on Th17 cell development. C3aR-deficient mice exhibit diminished AHR, fewer Th17 cells and decreased IL-17 compared to WT counterparts, which correlates with reduced IL-23 production. This suggests that unlike C5a, C3a mediates IL-23 production, IL-17 production and susceptibility to AHR (Lajoie et al., 2010).

It is clear that in experimental models of allergic asthma, C5a-C5aR signaling seems to protect against the development of Th2 immune response during allergen exposure, whereas C3a-C3aR signaling contributes to the development of maladaptive immune responses. However, the strong evidence that suggests C5a and C3a synergistically contribute to the development of allergic inflammation and asthma can not be overlooked. As mentioned earlier, the contradictory nature of this evidence may be due to the fact that once allergic inflammation is established (effector phase of allergic asthma), both C3a and C5a act on circulating and tissue resident inflammatory immune cells such as mast cells, eosinophils, basophils, and lymphocytes leading to the induction of a pro-allergic immune response. Indeed, pharmacological targeting of C3aR and C5aR during the effector phase suppresses AHR, airway inflammation and Th2 cytokines production (Baelder et al., 2005). Thus, complement C3a and C5a, and their receptors display diverse activities during the course of disease progression. Reagents that specifically targets C3a, C3aR, C5, C5a or C5aR could serve as potential therapy for asthma.

5.2 Sepsis

Sepsis is a life-threatening medical condition characterized by dysregulated systemic inflammatory responses followed by immunosuppression. Despite advances in medical health care, sepsis remains one of the leading causes of death, accounting for more than 1.5 million deaths annually in Europe and North America. Systemic inflammation in sepsis can be triggered by various infectious agents, including bacteria (leading cause of sepsis), fungi, parasites and viruses. Over recent years, efforts to better understand the pathophysiology of sepsis, has given rise to enough convincing evidence to suggest that the activation of the complement system and production of C3a and C5a occurs in sepsis.

Infectious agents activate the complement system through their interaction with C1q, MBL, or ficolins leading to local and/or systemic complement activation with subsequent production of C3a and C5a. Indeed, patients with sepsis syndrome show elevated plasma or serum levels of C3a/C3a desArg, C4a and C5a/C5a desArg (Bengtson and Heideman, 1988, Cole et al., 2002, Nakae et al., 1994, Nakae et al., 1996, Selberg et al., 2000, Solomkin et al., 1985, Weinberg et al., 1984), and circulating levels of C3a and C5a are inversely proportional to patient survival (Groeneveld et al., 2003, Hack et al., 1989, Hecke et al., 1997, Selberg et al., 2000). In humans, C5a levels can rise as high as 100 nM (Ward, 2004).

In vivo generation of C3a and C5a and their inflammatory effects in sepsis have been studied using three major animal models: a) intravenous injection of an exogenous toxin (e.g. anaphylatoxins); b) intravenous infusion of exogenous bacteria; and c) cecal ligation and puncture (CLP). Infusion of C5a into rabbits and rats produces the typical septic shock symptoms, including a rapid drop in mean arterial pressure and reduced circulation of granulocytes, monocytes and platelets in peripheral blood. Infusion of *Escherichia coli (E. coli)* in rabbits leads to severe septicemia with enhanced levels of C5a in the plasma, indicating that the degree of complement activation determines the severity of sepsis (Bergh et al., 1991). Administration of an anti-C5a desArg antibody to *E. coli*-infused primates confers protection against mortality and attenuates systemic manifestations of sepsis (Stevens et al., 1986), highlighting the importance of C5a in the septic shock pathology. Most of the studies dealing with the role of C5a in pathology of sepsis have been done using the rat and rodent models of CLP. This model of sepsis closely mimics the pathophysiology of sepsis in humans. Intravenous infusion of a neutralizing polyclonal antibody to rat C5a in CLP rats is highly protective, causing reduced evidence of multiorgan failure and resulting improved survival rates (from 0% survival in the unprotected to 50% survival in rats treated with an anti-C5a antibody). Moreover, CLP rats treated with an antibody against C5a show profound reduction (98% compared to unprotected rats) in bacterial colony forming units (CFUs), indicating that C5a is associated with the development of bacteremia in sepsis (Czermak et al., 1999).

Successive studies with anti-C5a antibody-treated CLP rats and mice have further revealed that the survival rate of these animals depends on amount of antibody infused at the time of CLP, as well as the time of administration of the antibody. For instance, the infusion of 600 g of antibody targeted against the mid region of C5a remarkably improves survival in CLP rats (83-90% survival rate compared to 23% survival rate in CLP rats receiving pre-immune IgG or 100-220 g of anti-C5a antibody). Moreover, when 600 g of antibody is given at time 0 of CLP, the survival rate is 90%; when infusion is delayed until 6 hr. post CLP, survival is around 60%; and when delayed until 12 hr. post CLP, the survival drops to 40% (Huber-Lang et al., 2001). These results suggest that neutralization of C5a during a specific time window after the onset of sepsis may be efficacious in the treatment of sepsis.

In sepsis, excessive production of C3a and C5a subsequently leads to dysfunction of neutrophils. Blood neutrophils display suppressed chemotactic responsiveness (Goya et al., 1994, Solomkin et al., 1981), depressed enzyme release (Goya et al., 1994, Solomkin et al., 1981, Utoh et al., 1989), alteration of intracellular pH (Sachse et al., 2000), and a defective respiratory burst (Czermak et al., 1999, Goya et al., 1994, Solomkin et al., 1981), resulting in impaired bactericidal activity. For instance, during experimental sepsis, blood neutrophils show a decreased ability to bind C5a, impaired chemotactic response to C5a and a loss of H_2O_2-generating capacity. Exposure of rat neutrophils to C5a induces a defect in phagocytic function (Huber-Lang et al., 2002). Treatment of CLP rats with an anti-C5a antibody reverses these functional defects in neutrophils (Huber-Lang et al., 2002). Early after CLP, blood neutrophils from septic mice exhibit enhanced expression of the CC chemokine receptors (CCR1, CCR2, and CCR5) (Speyer et al., 2004), which may contribute to a stronger neutrophilic inflammatory response in sepsis. Moreover, CLP causes blood neutrophils to show an increased expression of β1 integrins (CD29) and β2 integrins (CD18), indicating a hyperresponsiveness to the receptors for these integrins (Guo et al., 2002). Collectively, this demonstrates that neutrophils develop an exaggerated response to various inflammatory mediators in the early stages of sepsis.

Besides neutrophil dysfunction, C5a also affects other components of innate immunity leading to exacerbation of septicemia and immunosuppression. Systemic activation of complement in CLP model of sepsis induces C5a-dependent apoptosis of thymocytes (Guo et al., 2000), inducing a significant loss of thymus in first few days following CLP (Riedemann et al., 2002). C5aR expression on thymocytes rises rapidly after CLP and increased binding of C5a to CLP thymocytes can be found as early as 3 hr. post CLP. Administration of an anti-C5a neutralizing antibody at the time of CLP preserves the thymic mass and abolishes the apoptosis of thymocytes (Riedemann et al., 2002). Moreover, CLP in mice induces significant apoptosis of adrenomedullary cells 24 hr. post CLP, which is diminished after dual blockade of both C5aR and C5L2 (Flierl et al., 2008), indicating a role of C5a in multiorgan apoptosis during sepsis. C5a also promotes septic cardiomyopathy (Niederbichler et al., 2006) and consumptive coagulopathy (Laudes et al., 2002). The intensity of the coagulopathy of sepsis is greatly attenuated in CLP rats (for example, clotting times are minimally prolonged, thrombocytopenia is reduced and plasma levels of fibrin split products as well as thrombin-antithrombin complexes are greatly reduced) as a result of neutralization of C5a after CLP (Laudes et al., 2002).

It seems clear that excessive C5a produced during sepsis has harmful effects, as described above and it is obvious that the effects are mediated via the interaction of C5a with its receptors. Indeed, experimental studies in animals with CLP suggest a dynamic balance between C5aR and C5L2 on immune cells and in organs. C5aR expression is markedly increased in lung, liver, kidney, and heart early in septic mice (Riedemann et al., 2002). C5L2 mRNA is highly expressed in liver and thyroid of CLP rat, and weakly expressed in CLP rat brain, spleen, kidney, large intestine, eye as well as lung alveolar macrophages and peripheral blood neutrophils (Gao et al., 2005). Increased expression of C5aR and C5L2 in lung, liver, heart, and kidney after CLP-induced sepsis strongly implies the role of complement receptors in multiple organ failure.

In vitro exposure of neutrophils to C5a reduces surface C5aR expression suggesting that following interaction C5a/C5aR complex undergo internalization, suggesting a possible cause for compromised neutrophil function (Huber-Lang et al., 2002). During experimental sepsis C5aR content on blood neutrophils reduces 2.5-fold 24 hr. after CLP and increases steadily thereafter. On contrary, C5L2 content on blood neutrophils increases significantly 24 and 36 hr. after onset of CLP. Moreover, confocal microscopy on blood neutrophils from CLP rats show cytoplasmic distribution of C5aR, but not C5L2, indicating that C5a/C5L2 complex do not undergo internalization as C5a/C5aR after CLP (Gao et al., 2005), and that C5aR and C5L2 are independently regulated during sepsis. In presence of a cyclic peptide antagonist (C5aRa) to the C5aR, the binding of C5a to mice peritoneal neutrophils is diminished, and the *in vitro* chemotactic response of neutrophils to C5a is decreased, C5a-induced defect in the oxidative burst of neutrophils is reversed, and the lung vascular permeability index is markedly diminished. CLP mice treated with C5aRa show improved survival rates (from 10% survival in the sham to 60% survival in mice treated with C5aRa) (Huber-Lang et al., 2002). Using a combination of C5aR and C5L2 blocking antibodies, and mice lacking one of the two C5a receptors, considerable improvement in survival following CLP has been shown in a study by Rittirsch et al. In mid-grade CLP, WT, C5aR-deficient and C5L2-deficient mice show 31%, 80% and 100% survival by day 7, respectively, indicating harmful roles for both C5a receptors in the CLP model of sepsis. All WT mice show 100% and 80% survival after treatment with anti-C5aR and anti-C5L2 serum, respectively, compared to 40% survival in mice treated with preimmune serum. In high-grade CLP, none of the WT mice treated with preimmune serum, C5L2-deficient mice treated with anti-C5aR serum and C5aR-deficient mice survived. Interestingly, when C5L2-deficient mice are treated with anti-C5aR serum the survival rate improves significantly (80%). Similarly, treatment of C5aR-deficient mice with anti-C5L2 serum greatly improves survival (87% compared to 17% for C5aR-deficient mice treated with preimmune serum or 0% for WT mice treated with anti-C5L2 serum). Dual blockade of C5aR and C5L2 by a polyclonal antibody is also protective against the lethal outcome after high-grade CLP. Moreover, if the high-grade CLP mice are treated with anti-C5aR and anti-C5L2 serum after a delay of 12 hr. or 24 hr. post CLP there is no protective effect against mortality. The combined blockade of the C5a receptors during sepsis is most effective when given before the onset of sepsis. In summary, both C5aR and C5L2 contribute cooperatively to mortality in sepsis. Evaluation of plasma cytokine and chemokine concentrations after CLP shows a reduction in the levels of IL-1β, MIP-1α, and MIP-2 in C5aR-deficient and C5L2-deficient mice in comparison to WT mice. However, the plasma concentration of IL-6 is significantly increased in C5L2-deficient CLP mice in comparison to WT mice. In contrast, plasma IL-6 is markedly reduced in C5aR-deficient CLP mice when compared to WT mice, as observed by Gao et al. (Gao et al., 2005), suggesting that the sepsis-induced cytokine and chemokine production may occur in a sequential fashion which requires C5a engagement of both C5a receptors. Another important observation obtained from this study is that C5L2-deficient CLP mice have greatly reduced levels of high-mobility group protein 1 (HMGB1, a late mediator in sepsis) in plasma. Interestingly, CLP in C5aR-deficient CLP mice has no effect on plasma HMGB1 levels when compared to WT CLP mice. Furthermore, C5a-stimulated macrophages from WT and C5aR-deficient mice produce significant amounts of HMGB1, whereas C5a-stimulated macrophages from C5L2-deficient mice produce very little HMGB1 (Rittirsch et al., 2008), supporting the fact that C5a mediates the pathophysiology of sepsis by acting on C5a receptors and that C5L2 has a functional role in sepsis.

Recently, a study has shown that γδT cells are involved in the pathogenesis of sepsis by producing large amounts of IL-17 (Xu et al., 2010), express C5aR, and the expression of C5aR increases in mice following sepsis. Neutralization of C5a partially prevents the upregulation of C5aR on γδT cells in septic mice. Furthermore, C5a promotes the IL-17 expression by γδT cells which can be attenuated by blocking PI3K/Akt signaling pathway, demonstrating that C5a acts on C5aR expressed on γδT cells, resulting in the pathophysiology of sepsis (Han et al.).

In summary, C5a binding to C5aR and C5L2 receptors seem to contribute to cytokine storm, associated multiple organ dysfunction and subsequent lethal outcome in the setting of experimental sepsis. C5aR and C5L2 both contribute synergistically to the harmful events in sepsis. A maximal beneficial effect can be achieved by the blockade or absence of both receptors, which might have implication in complement-based therapy for inflammatory diseases.

5.3 Chronic urticaria

Chronic urticaria is a debilitating skin condition characterized by the near daily occurrence of pruritic wheals for at least six weeks (Kaplan, 2004). While the pathogenesis of chronic urticaria is not completely understood, mast cell and basophils degranulation and histamine release are believed to be of central importance. Recent studies suggest that this activation of mast cells and basophils could in part be initiated by the C3a and C5a or these complement proteins can augment allergen-antibody mediated cell activation. Indeed, heating serum from patients with chronic urticaria, which heat-inactivates complement proteins, reduces the ability of serum to induce histamine release from basophils. Similarly, decomplemented sera deficient in C5 is incapable of releasing histamine from dermal mast cells (Kikuchi and Kaplan, 2002).

C5a may play a key role in the pathogenesis of chronic urticaria as it can degranulate mast cells and basophils following its interaction with the C5aR present on these cells (Fureder et al., 1995). C5a can also chemoattract neutrophils, basophils, eosinophils and mast cells, which are present in chronic urticaria lesions. Korosec et al. showed that patients with chronic urticaria have enhanced basophil activation in response to C5a. However, C5aR antagonist-treated serum from these patients show decreased histamine release from basophil. Furthermore, the release of histamine from basophils by anti-FcεRI autoantibodies can be augmented by C5a activation (Korosec et al., 2009). Taken together these studies suggest that complement proteins and their receptors contribute towards the pathology of chronic urticaria.

5.4 Cancer

The complement system has also been well recognized as a promoter of tumor development. The deposition of complement component C3 is associated with the tumor vasculature in mice; C3-deficient mice show reduced tumor growth. The anaphylatoxin C5a promotes the growth of malignant tumors in a mouse model of cervical carcinoma. C5aR-deficient mice treated with a C5a antagonist exhibit reduced tumor growth, as well as enhanced infiltration of tumor tissue with $CD8^+$ cytotoxic T cells in comparison to WT mice, suggesting that C5a promotes tumor growth by inhibiting the response of $CD8^+$ cytotoxic T cells against tumors. Elimination of $CD8^+$ cytotoxic T cells from C5aR-deficient increases the rate of tumor growth, confirming that C5a modulates the $CD8^+$ T cells-mediated anti-tumor immune responses (Markiewski et al., 2008).

The interplay between $CD8^+$ cytotoxic T cells and myeloid-derived suppressor cells (MDSCs) play a significant role in determining the fate of tumors. MDSCs are a heterogeneous population of regular myeloid cells, also referred to as immature counterparts of monocytes and neutrophils, which express C5aR. C5aR is partially internalized in tumor-associated MDSCs, suggesting that MDSCs are constantly exposed to and activated by C5a generated in the tumor microenvironment. C5a chemoattracts MDSCs to the tumor, partly by upregulating adhesion molecules on MDSCs. C5a also enhances the production of ROS and reactive nitrogen species (RNS) from MDSC, which are known to suppress $CD8^+$ cytotoxic T cell anti-tumor responses. C5aR-deficient mice or mice treated with a C5aR antagonist show reduced numbers of MDSCs within the tumor tissue, increased numbers of $CD8^+$ cytotoxic T cells and decreased tumor growth. MDSCs from C5a-deficient mice are unable to inhibit T cell proliferation in vivo (Markiewski et al., 2008). These observations highlight the potential of anaphylatoxins and their receptors as novel targets for anti-cancer immunotherapy.

5.5 Ischemia-reperfusion injury

Ischemia-reperfusion (I/R) injury is defined as cellular injury occurring after the reperfusion of previously vascularised tissue following an extended period of ischemia. The augmentation of tissue injury after reperfusion results from an intense inflammatory response that develops simultaneously with tissue reperfusion (Eltzschig and Collard, 2004). Several pathological conditions can lead to I/R injury including myocardial infarction, stroke, hemorrhagic shock, severe trauma, and organ transplantation resulting in associated morbidity and mortality (Eltzschig and Collard, 2004).

Numerous studies have shown that ischemic tissue activates the complement system, which remarkably contributes to the development of tissue damage by enhancing inflammation (Hart et al., 2004). The first evidence for involvement of complement in I/R injury was proposed by Hill and Ward in 1971 (Hill and Ward, 1971). During I/R injury the complement system can be activated by the classical, alternative, and lectin pathways. For instance, skeletal muscle injury resulting from I/R likely occurs through the complement activation via the classical and lectin pathways (Weiser et al., 1996). Lectin pathway may be involved in myocardial (Jordan et al., 2001) and gastrointestinal I/R-induced complement activation (Hart et al., 2004). However, the amplification of complement activation in gastrointestinal I/R occurs through the alternative pathway (Hart et al., 2004). Alternative pathway of complement activation may contribute to renal I/R injury in mice (Thurman et al., 2003).

Studies suggest that complements C3a and C5a are major complement factors responsible for the induction of the reperfusion-associated inflammatory response. C3a and C5a activate endothelial cells and inflammatory leukocytes. C5a upregulates the expression of adhesion molecules on human umbilical vein endothelial cells (Foreman et al., 1996) and induces release of various cytokines, including IL-1, IL-6, MCP-1, and TNFα (Schindler et al., 1990). C5aR expression is upregulated following cold I/R injury in a mouse model of syngenic kidney transplantation, suggesting that C5aR may contribute to tissue damage, tubular apoptosis and dysfunction of donor organs. Furthermore, upregulation of C5aR expression in cadaveric kidneys correlates with cold ischemia time. Ablation of C5aR signaling during cold ischemia has a protective effect on kidney graft survival (Lewis et al., 2008). Animals treated with a C5aR antagonist show dramatically reduced accumulation of neutrophils in the post-ischemic livers and sustain less injury during reperfusion (Arumugam et al., 2003). In a mouse model of I/R muscle injury, mice treated with a C5aR antagonist exhibit decreased levels of circulating creatinine kinase, lactate dehydrogenase, alanine and aspartate aminotransferase, creatinine, blood urea nitrogen, muscle edema, lung and liver myeloperoxidase, and lung TNFα following hind limb injury (Woodruff et al., 2004).

Studies targeting C5a/C5aR complex have further confirmed the role played by C5a in the pathogenesis of I/R injury. Blocking C5aR signaling using an anti-C5aR antibody markedly decreases leukocyte adherence, microvascular permeability in the ischemic myocardial area (Zhang et al., 2007), myocardial neutrophil infiltration and arteriolar endothelial injury

(Park et al., 1999). Knocking down C5aR expression with small interference (si)RNA preserves renal function from I/R injury, reduces chemokine production and neutrophil infiltration (Zheng et al., 2008). Treatment with an anti-C5 neutralizing antibody reduces apoptosis and necrosis in heart allografts (Ferraresso et al., 2008).

In contrast to C5a, the role of C3a/C3aR in I/R injury is not properly established. Systemic inhibition of C3a with a C3aR antagonist minimally resolves myocardial I/R injury, and neutropenia rather than C3aR antagonism appears to be responsible for C3aR antagonist-associated improvement in myocardial I/R injury (Busche and Stahl, 2010). These results confirm similar observations from previous studies (Ames et al., 2001, Proctor et al., 2004), indicating that C3aR antagonist-mediated neutrophil tissue sequestration during I/R injury may account for the protective effects observed. Overall, the data indicate while C3a/C3aR inhibition in the clinical setting of I/R injury does not appear to be therapeutic, targeting C5a as well as C5aR may be a promising approach to prevent I/R injury.

5.6 Transplantation

The activation products of complement system play an important role in allograft rejection as evidenced by the fact that the lack of C3 in donor kidneys is associated with long-term graft survival in experimental transplantation (Pratt et al., 2002). A study in human kidney transplantation has shown that donor C3 polymorphisms are associated with late graft failure. Thus donor expression of C3 influences the alloimmune response and the fate of the transplantation (Brown et al., 2006). APCs are the source of C3 and macrophages from C3-deficient mice have an impaired potency to stimulate alloreactive T cell response and to drive Th1-biased adaptive immune responses supporting graft survival (Peng et al., 2006, Zhou et al., 2006). It is now clear that this effect of C3 is mediated via the interaction of C3a with the C3aR on APCs. C3a-deficient dendritic cells show reduced surface expression of major histocompatibility complex (MHC) class II and co-stimulatory molecules and elicit a defective T cell priming against alloantigen expressed on the dendritic cells (Peng et al., 2008). Mechanistically, C3a-C3aR interaction on surface of dendritic cells decreases the level of intracellular cAMP, which in turn promotes allergen uptake and T cell priming (Li et al., 2008).

As mentioned in previous section, complement activation is critically involved in I/R injury; C5a and C5aR blockade has been shown attenuate organ damage, improve graft function and transplantation outcome. In human kidney transplants with acute rejection, C5aR expression is increased in renal tissue and in cells infiltrating the tubulointerstitium. Treatment of recipient mice with a C5aR antagonist before transplantation markedly improves renal allograft survival and reduces alloreactive T cell priming. Similarly, inhibition of C5aR in murine model of renal allotransplantation substantially improved graft survival from 11 days to 12 weeks. In addition, C5aR inhibition reduces kidney inflammation, apoptosis, and priming of alloreactive T cells (Gueler et al., 2008). Pharmacological targeting of C5aR during organ preservation significantly improves kidney graft survival (Lewis et al., 2008). Baboons treated with an anti-C5a monoclonal antibody exhibit prolonged pulmonary xenografts survival, indicating that C5a exacerbates pulmonary xenografts injury (Gaca et al., 2006). A recent study by Vieyra et al. have shown that dendritic cell-derived C3a and C5a regulates $CD4^+$ T cell help to $CD8^+$ T cell responses required for murine allograft rejection (Vieyra et al., 2011). These results demonstrate that C3aR and C5aR signaling contribute towards the innate and adaptive inflammatory responses following solid organ transplantation, suggesting that pharmaceutical targeting of C3aR and C5aR may have an application in transplantation medicine.

5.7 Stroke

Stroke is the second leading cause of death worldwide, which is defined as a rapidly developing loss of brain function(s) due to inadequate blood flow in a localized area. When blood flow is interrupted to part of the brain, brain cells quickly begin to die leading to stroke development. There are many elements that contribute to the development of stroke, of which neuroinflammation is a major one. However, the precise roles of various pro-inflammatory mediators, including cytokines, chemokines and immune cells, are still largely unknown. Increasing evidence suggests that the activation of the complement cascade contributes to pathological inflammatory events in brain (upregulation of adhesion molecules, immune cell activation, chemotaxis, expression of IL-8 and MCP-1 by endothelial cells) (D'Ambrosio et al., 2001), resulting in ischemic insult, neurodegeneration and stroke development.

Following brain I/R injury ROS, RNS as well as oxygen free radicals are generated by activated brain cells and infiltrating immune cells, which stimulate stroke-associated brain injury (Elsner et al., 1994, McColl et al., 2009). Brain cells such as astrocytes, microglia, neurons, and endothelial cells and infiltrating immune cells produce various pro-inflammatory mediators following ischemia, further contributing towards cell death (Yilmaz et al., 2006). Ischemic stroke enhances interaction between endothelial cells, brain cells, and immune cells that may aggravate the injury process (Urra et al., 2009). All these stroke-associated brain pathologies are function of C3a-C3aR and C5a-C5aR interactions (D'Ambrosio et al., 2001). Strong C3a and C5a activation is observed in patients with acute ischemic stroke, which correlates with disease severity (Szeplaki et al., 2009). Regional brain I/R injury induces an inflammatory reaction that involves generation of C3a and C5a, upregulation and enhanced activation of their receptors C3aR and C5aR.

In the brain, C3aR and C5aR are expressed by astrocytes (Gasque et al., 1995, Gasque et al., 1997, Gasque et al., 1998, Lacy et al., 1995, Sayah et al., 1997), glial cells (Davoust et al., 1999, Gasque et al., 1997, Lacy et al., 1995) and neurons (Davoust et al., 1999). Experimental models of permanent and transient middle cerebral artery occlusion (MCAO) have demonstrated an increase in the expression of complement receptors. The expression of C3aR and C5aR is enhanced in mouse ischemic cortex following permanent MCAO. In addition, the expression is also induced on endothelial cells within ischemic core, suggesting that the complement receptors are important in leukocyte recruitment and neuroinflammation (Van Beek et al., 2000). Expression of C3aR and C5aR is significantly increased after transient MCAO in rats (Nishino et al., 1994) and mice (Barnum et al., 2002). In the later study, C5aR expression dramatically increases within 3 hr. after MCAO, whereas C3aR expression reduces to 25% of control animals. By 24 hr. post-occlusion, expression of both receptors is highest. This increased expression at the later time points after occlusion is most likely the result of a massive infiltration of immune cells expressing C3aR and C5aR (Barnum et al., 2002).

Early attempts at complement inhibition using cobra venom factor (CVF) have further revealed that abrogation of the complement system can provide protection for the brain during I/R injury and stroke. Pretreatment of rats with CVF (complement-depleted rats) prior to temporary cerebral ischemia significantly enhances the magnitude of reactive hyperemia and increases preservation of somatosensory evoked potentials (SSEPs), demonstrating that depleting the complement system can improve blood flow and clinical outcome following cerebral I/R (Vasthare et al., 1998). Similarly, complement depletion via CVF significantly reduces post-ischemic cerebral infarct volume in adult rats and post-hypoxic-ischemic cerebral atrophy in neonates (Figueroa et al., 2005). However, the lack of specificity of CVF did not give any information regarding complement components that are most relevant in the pathogenesis of brain injury and stroke.

Recent studies using genetic knockouts of C3 and C5 and inhibitors of C3a-C3aR, and C5a-C5aR signaling have better our understanding of the role of anaphylatoxins in stroke. C3-deficient mice are protected against cerebral I/R injury, as demonstrated by significant reductions in both infarct volume and neurological deficit score. C3-deficient mice also exhibit diminished granulocyte infiltration and oxidative stress. The administration of a C3aR antagonist reduces stroke volume leading to neurological improvement (Mocco et al., 2006), implicating the involvement of C3a and C3aR in acute stroke. Studies with genetic knockouts of C5 in stroke have yielded conflicting data. C5-deficient animals show increased vulnerability to intracerebral hemorrhage (ICH) (Nakamura et al., 2004) and ischemic stroke (Mocco et al., 2006). In contrast, C5-deficient mice subjected to brain I/R injury exhibits improved functional outcome and less brain damage (Arumugam et al., 2007). A recent study by Rynkowski et al. have shown that blocking C3a-mediated signaling using a C3aR antagonist is protective in a mouse model if ICH (Rynkowski et al., 2009). Similarly, mice treated with C5aR antagonist alone or C3aR and C5aR antagonists exhibit improvement in neurological functions following ICH, suggesting that blockade of C3aR and C5aR represents a promising therapeutic strategy in stroke.

6. Conclusion

The complement system is composed of a network of proteins that play an important role in innate and adaptive immunity. Originally discovered as antimicrobial agents, the main function of C3a and C5a was considered to be the opsonization of pathogens and chemoattraction to remove apoptotic and necrotic cells. However, today complement proteins, C3a and C5a, are considered as crucial immunoregulatory molecules with pleiotropic biological functions on immune cells which help to shape the immune response. Activation of complement system is exquisitely regulated, while improper activation or under certain conditions the effect can lead to adverse consequences. Similar to dysregulation of the adaptive immune system in hypersensitivity reactions, the pathological role of C3a, C5a and their receptors in inflammatory diseases as well as tumor growth is well defined. Due to their strong inflammatory properties, C3a/C3aR and C5a/C5aR are considered attractive pharmacological targets for the development of therapeutic agents. Given that many therapeutic agents targeting the interaction of C3a-C3aR and C5a-C5aR are already under investigation, the advances made in the field of complement and complement receptors discussed in this book chapter will better our understanding of the disease process and help develop new therapeutic approaches to modulate immune response

7. Acknowledgement

This work was supported by intramural funds from the National Research Council-Institute for Nutrisciences and Health, Canada and the Department of Biomedical Sciences, Atlantic

Veterinary College, Canada. Priyanka Pundir is a recipient of Innovation PEI Graduate Student Fellowship from the Department of Innovation and Advanced Learning, Prince Edward Island, Canada.

8. References

A genome-wide search for asthma susceptibility loci in ethnically diverse populations. The Collaborative Study on the Genetics of Asthma (CSGA). *Nature Genetics*, Vol.15, No.4, (April 1997), pp. 389-392, ISSN 1061-4036

Abe, M., Shibata, K., Akatsu, H., Shimizu, N., Sakata, N., Katsuragi, T. and Okada, H. (2001). Contribution of anaphylatoxin C5a to late airway responses after repeated exposure of antigen to allergic rats. *Journal of Immunology*, Vol.167, No.8, (October 2001), pp. 4651-4660, ISSN 0022-1767

Ahamed, J., Haribabu, B. and Ali, H. (2001). Cutting edge: Differential regulation of chemoattractant receptor-induced degranulation and chemokine production by receptor phosphorylation. *Journal of Immunology*, Vol.167, No.7, (October 2001), pp. 3559-3563, ISSN 0022-1767

Albrecht, E. A., Chinnaiyan, A. M., Varambally, S., Kumar-Sinha, C., Barrette, T. R., Sarma, J. V. and Ward, P. A. (2004). C5a-induced gene expression in human umbilical vein endothelial cells. *The American Journal of Pathology*, Vol.164, No.3, (March 2004), pp. 849-859, ISSN 0002-9440

Amatruda, T. T., 3rd, Gerard, N. P., Gerard, C. and Simon, M. I. (1993). Specific interactions of chemoattractant factor receptors with G-proteins. *Journal of Biological Chemistry*, Vol.268, No.14, (May 1993), pp. 10139-10144, ISSN 0021-9258

Ames, R. S., Li, Y., Sarau, H. M., Nuthulaganti, P., Foley, J. J., Ellis, C., Zeng, Z., Su, K., Jurewicz, A. J., Hertzberg, R. P., Bergsma, D. J. and Kumar, C. (1996). Molecular cloning and characterization of the human anaphylatoxin C3a receptor. *Journal of Biological Chemistry*, Vol.271, No.34, (August 1996), pp. 20231-20234, ISSN 0021-9258

Ames, R. S., Lee, D., Foley, J. J., Jurewicz, A. J., Tornetta, M. A., Bautsch, W., Settmacher, B., Klos, A., Erhard, K. F., Cousins, R. D., Sulpizio, A. C., Hieble, J. P., McCafferty, G., Ward, K. W., Adams, J. L., Bondinell, W. E., Underwood, D. C., Osborn, R. R., Badger, A. M. and Sarau, H. M. (2001). Identification of a selective nonpeptide antagonist of the anaphylatoxin C3a receptor that demonstrates antiinflammatory activity in animal models. *Journal of Immunology*, Vol.166, No.10, (May 2001), pp. 6341-6348, ISSN 0022-1767

Arroyave, C. M., Stevenson, D. D., Vaughan, J. H. and Tan, E. M. (1977). Plasma complement changes during bronchospasm provoked in asthmatic patients. *Clinical Allergy*, Vol.7, No.2, (March 1977), pp. 173-182, ISBN 978-1-58829-616-0

Arumugam, T. V., Shiels, I. A., Strachan, A. J., Abbenante, G., Fairlie, D. P. and Taylor, S. M. (2003). A small molecule C5a receptor antagonist protects kidneys from ischemia/reperfusion injury in rats. *Kidney International*, Vol.63, No.1, (January 2003), pp. 134-142, ISSN 0085-2538

Arumugam, T. V., Shiels, I. A., Woodruff, T. M., Granger, D. N. and Taylor, S. M. (2004). The role of the complement system in ischemia-reperfusion injury. *Shock*, Vol.21, No.5, (May 2004), pp. 401-409, ISSN 1073-2322

Arumugam, T. V., Tang, S. C., Lathia, J. D., Cheng, A., Mughal, M. R., Chigurupati, S., Magnus, T., Chan, S. L., Jo, D. G., Ouyang, X., Fairlie, D. P., Granger, D. N.,

Vortmeyer, A., Basta, M. and Mattson, M. P. (2007). Intravenous immunoglobulin (IVIG) protects the brain against experimental stroke by preventing complement-mediated neuronal cell death. *Proceedings of the National Academy of Science of the United States of America*, Vol.104, No.35, (August 2007), pp. 14104-14109, ISSN 0027-8424

Baelder, R., Fuchs, B., Bautsch, W., Zwirner, J., Kohl, J., Hoymann, H. G., Glaab, T., Erpenbeck, V., Krug, N. and Braun, A. (2005). Pharmacological targeting of anaphylatoxin receptors during the effector phase of allergic asthma suppresses airway hyperresponsiveness and airway inflammation. *Journal of Immunology*, Vol.174, No.2, (January 2005), pp. 783-789, ISSN 0022-1767

Baldo, A., Sniderman, A. D., St-Luce, S., Avramoglu, R. K., Maslowska, M., Hoang, B., Monge, J. C., Bell, A., Mulay, S. and Cianflone, K. (1993). The adipsin-acylation stimulating protein system and regulation of intracellular triglyceride synthesis. *The Journal of Clinical Investigation*, Vol.92, No.3, (September 1993), pp. 1543-1547, ISSN 0021-9738

Bamberg, C. E., Mackay, C. R., Lee, H., Zahra, D., Jackson, J., Lim, Y. S., Whitfeld, P. L., Craig, S., Corsini, E., Lu, B., Gerard, C. and Gerard, N. P. (2010). The C5a receptor (C5aR) C5L2 is a modulator of C5aR-mediated signal transduction. *Journal of Biological Chemistry*, Vol.285, No.10, (March 2010), pp. 7633-7644, ISSN 0021-9258

Banchereau, J. and Steinman, R. M. (1998). Dendritic cells and the control of immunity. *Nature*, Vol.392, No.6673, (March 1998), pp. 245-252, ISSN 0028-0836

Bansal, G., Xie, Z., Rao, S., Nocka, K. H. and Druey, K. M. (2008). Suppression of immunoglobulin E-mediated allergic responses by regulator of G protein signaling 13. *Nature Immunology*, Vol.9, No.1, (January 2008), pp. 73-80, ISSN 1529-2908

Barnum, S. R., Ames, R. S., Maycox, P. R., Hadingham, S. J., Meakin, J., Harrison, D. and Parsons, A. A. (2002). Expression of the complement C3a and C5a receptors after permanent focal ischemia: An alternative interpretation. *Glia*, Vol.38, No.2, (April 2002), pp. 169-173, ISSN 1098-1136

Bautsch, W., Hoymann, H. G., Zhang, Q., Meier-Wiedenbach, I., Raschke, U., Ames, R. S., Sohns, B., Flemme, N., Meyer zu Vilsendorf, A., Grove, M., Klos, A. and Kohl, J. (2000). Cutting edge: guinea pigs with a natural C3a-receptor defect exhibit decreased bronchoconstriction in allergic airway disease: evidence for an involvement of the C3a anaphylatoxin in the pathogenesis of asthma. *Journal of Immunology*, Vol.165, No.10, (November 2000), pp. 5401-5405, ISSN 0022-1767

Becker, S., Meuer, S., Hadding, U. and Bitter-Suermann, D. (1978). Platelet activation: a new biological activity of guinea-pig C3a anaphylatoxin. *Scandinavian Journal of Immunology*, Vol.7, No.2, pp. 173-180, ISSN 1365-3083

Bengtson, A. and Heideman, M. (1988). Anaphylatoxin formation in sepsis. *Archives of Surgery (Chicago, Ill.: 1960)*, Vol.123, No.5, (May 1988), pp. 645-649, ISSN 0004-0010

Bergh, K., Olsen, P. O., Halgunset, J. and Iversen, O. J. (1991). Complement activation and pulmonary dysfunction in experimental Escherichia coli septicaemia. *Acta Anaesthesiologica Scandinavica*, Vol.35, No.3, (April 1991), pp. 267-274, ISSN 0001-5172

Bischoff, S. C., de Weck, A. L. and Dahinden, C. A. (1990). Interleukin 3 and granulocyte/macrophage-colony-stimulating factor render human basophils responsive to low concentrations of complement component C3a. *Proceedings of the*

National Academy of Science of the United States of America, Vol.87, No.17, (September 1990), pp. 6813-6817, ISSN 0027-8424

Bito, L. Z. (1977). Inflammatory effects of endotoxin-like contaminants in commonly used protein preparations. *Science*, Vol.196, No.4285, (April 1977), pp. 83-85, ISSN 0036-8075

Bokisch, V. A. and Muller-Eberhard, H. J. (1970). Anaphylatoxin inactivator of human plasma: its isolation and characterization as a carboxypeptidase. *The Journal of Clinical Investigation*, Vol.49, No.12, (December 1970), pp. 2427-2436, ISSN 0021-9738

Boulay, F., Mery, L., Tardif, M., Brouchon, L. and Vignais, P. (1991). Expression cloning of a receptor for C5a anaphylatoxin on differentiated HL-60 cells. *Biochemistry*, Vol.30, No.12, (March 1991), pp. 2993-2999, ISSN 0006-2960

Bowser, C., Erstein, D. P., Silverberg, J. I., Nowakowski, M. and Joks, R. (2010). Correlation of plasma complement split product levels with allergic respiratory disease activity and relation to allergen immunotherapy. *Annals of Allergy, Asthma & Immunology*, Vol.104, No.1, (January 2010), pp. 42-49, ISSN 1081-1206

Braun, L., Christophe, T. and Boulay, F. (2003). Phosphorylation of key serine residues is required for internalization of the complement 5a (C5a) anaphylatoxin receptor via a beta-arrestin, dynamin, and clathrin-dependent pathway. *Journal of Biological Chemistry*, Vol.278, No.6, (February 2003), pp. 4277-4285, ISSN 0021-9258

Brown, K. M., Kondeatis, E., Vaughan, R. W., Kon, S. P., Farmer, C. K., Taylor, J. D., He, X., Johnston, A., Horsfield, C., Janssen, B. J., Gros, P., Zhou, W., Sacks, S. H. and Sheerin, N. S. (2006). Influence of donor C3 allotype on late renal-transplantation outcome. *The New England Journal of Medicine*, Vol.354, No.19, (May 2006), pp. 2014-2023, ISSN 0028-4793

Bullens, D. M., Truyen, E., Coteur, L., Dilissen, E., Hellings, P. W., Dupont, L. J. and Ceuppens, J. L. (2006). IL-17 mRNA in sputum of asthmatic patients: linking T cell driven inflammation and granulocytic influx?. *Respiratory Research*, Vol.7, (November 2006), pp. 135, ISSN 1465-9921

Burg, M., Martin, U., Bock, D., Rheinheimer, C., Kohl, J., Bautsch, W. and Klos, A. (1996). Differential regulation of the C3a and C5a receptors (CD88) by IFN-gamma and PMA in U937 cells and related myeloblastic cell lines. *Journal of Immunology*, Vol.157, No.12, (December 1996), pp. 5574-5581, ISSN 0022-1767

Busche, M. N. and Stahl, G. L. (2010). Role of the complement components C5 and C3a in a mouse model of myocardial ischemia and reperfusion injury. *German Medical Science*, Vol.8, (September 2010), ISSN 1612-3174

Cain, S. A. and Monk, P. N. (2002). The orphan receptor C5L2 has high affinity binding sites for complement fragments C5a and C5a des-Arg(74). *Journal of Biological Chemistry*, Vol.277, No.9, (March 2002), pp. 7165-7169, ISSN 0021-9258

Castro, F. F., Schmitz-Schumann, M., Rother, U. and Kirschfink, M. (1991). Complement activation by house dust: reduced reactivity of serum complement in patients with bronchial asthma. *International Archives of Allergy and Applied Immunology*, Vol.96, No.4, pp. 305-310, ISSN 0002-5915

Chao, T. H., Ember, J. A., Wang, M., Bayon, Y., Hugli, T. E. and Ye, R. D. (1999). Role of the second extracellular loop of human C3a receptor in agonist binding and receptor function. *Journal of Biological Chemistry*, Vol.274, No.14, (April 1999), pp. 9721-9728, ISSN 0021-9258

Chen, N. J., Mirtsos, C., Suh, D., Lu, Y. C., Lin, W. J., McKerlie, C., Lee, T., Baribault, H., Tian, H. and Yeh, W. C. (2007). C5L2 is critical for the biological activities of the anaphylatoxins C5a and C3a. *Nature*, Vol.446, No.7132, (March 2007), pp. 203-207, ISSN 0028-0836

Christophe, T., Rabiet, M. J., Tardif, M., Milcent, M. D. and Boulay, F. (2000). Human complement 5a (C5a) anaphylatoxin receptor (CD88) phosphorylation sites and their specific role in receptor phosphorylation and attenuation of G protein-mediated responses. Desensitization of C5a receptor controls superoxide production but not receptor sequestration in HL-60 cells. *Journal of Biological Chemistry*, Vol.275, No.3, (January 2000), pp. 1656-1664, ISSN 0021-9258

Cianflone, K., Vu, H., Walsh, M., Baldo, A., and Sniderman, A. (1989). Metabolic response of Acylation Stimulating Protein to an oral fat load. *Journal of Lipid Research*, Vol.30, No.11, (November 1989), pp. 1727-1733, ISSN 0022-2275

Cole, L., Bellomo, R., Hart, G., Journois, D., Davenport, P., Tipping, P. and Ronco, C. (2002). A phase II randomized, controlled trial of continuous hemofiltration in sepsis. *Critical Care Medicine*, Vol.30, No.1, (January 2002), pp. 100-106, ISSN 0090-3493

Crass, T., Raffetseder, U., Martin, U., Grove, M., Klos, A., Kohl, J. and Bautsch, W. (1996). Expression cloning of the human C3a anaphylatoxin receptor (C3aR) from differentiated U-937 cells. *European Journal of Immunology*, Vol.26, No.8, (August 1996), pp. 1944-1950, ISSN 0014-2980

Czermak, B. J., Sarma, V., Pierson, C. L., Warner, R. L., Huber-Lang, M., Bless, N. M., Schmal, H., Friedl, H. P. and Ward, P. A. (1999). Protective effects of C5a blockade in sepsis. *Nature Medicine*, Vol.5, No.7, (July 1999), pp. 788-792, ISSN 1078-8956

D'Ambrosio, A. L., Pinsky, D. J. and Connolly, E. S. (2001). The role of the complement cascade in ischemia/reperfusion injury: implications for neuroprotection. *Molecular Medicine*, Vol.7, No.6, (June 2001), pp. 367-382, ISSN 1757-4684

Daffern, P. J., Pfeifer, P. H., Ember, J. A. and Hugli, T. E. (1995). C3a is a chemotaxin for human eosinophils but not for neutrophils. I. C3a stimulation of neutrophils is secondary to eosinophil activation. *The Journal of Experimental Medicine*, Vol.181, No.6, (June 1995), pp. 2119-2127, ISSN 0022-1007

Davoust, N., Jones, J., Stahel, P. F., Ames, R. S. and Barnum, S. R. (1999). Receptor for the C3a anaphylatoxin is expressed by neurons and glial cells. *Glia*, Vol.26, No.3, (May 1999), pp. 201-211, ISSN 1098-1136

DeMartino, J. A., Van Riper, G., Siciliano, S. J., Molineaux, C. J., Konteatis, Z. D., Rosen, H. and Springer, M. S. (1994). The amino terminus of the human C5a receptor is required for high affinity C5a binding and for receptor activation by C5a but not C5a analogs. *Journal of Biological Chemistry*, Vol.269, No.20, (May 1994), pp. 14446-14450, ISSN 0021-9258

DiScipio, R. G., Daffern, P. J., Jagels, M. A., Broide, D. H. and Sriramarao, P. (1999). A comparison of C3a and C5a-mediated stable adhesion of rolling eosinophils in postcapillary venules and transendothelial migration in vitro and in vivo. *Journal of Immunology*, Vol.162, No.2, (January 1999), pp. 1127-1136, ISSN 0022-1767

Drouin, S. M., Corry, D. B., Kildsgaard, J. and Wetsel, R. A. (2001). Cutting edge: the absence of C3 demonstrates a role for complement in Th2 effector functions in a murine model of pulmonary allergy. *Journal of Immunology*, Vol.167, No.8, (October 2001), pp. 4141-4145, ISSN 0022-1767

Drouin, S. M., Corry, D. B., Hollman, T. J., Kildsgaard, J. and Wetsel, R. A. (2002). Absence of the complement anaphylatoxin C3a receptor suppresses Th2 effector functions in a murine model of pulmonary allergy. *Journal of Immunology*, Vol.169, No.10, (November 2002), pp. 5926-5933, ISSN 0022-1767

Elsner, J., Oppermann, M., Czech, W. and Kapp, A. (1994). C3a activates the respiratory burst in human polymorphonuclear neutrophilic leukocytes via pertussis toxin-sensitive G-proteins. *Blood*, Vol.83, No.11, (June 1994), pp. 3324-3331, ISSN 0006-4971

Eltzschig, H. K. and Collard, C. D. (2004). Vascular ischaemia and reperfusion injury. *British Medical Bulletin*, Vol.70, (October 2004), pp. 71-86, ISSN 0007-1420

Elward, K., Griffiths, M., Mizuno, M., Harris, C. L., Neal, J. W., Morgan, B. P. and Gasque, P. (2005). CD46 plays a key role in tailoring innate immune recognition of apoptotic and necrotic cells. *Journal of Biological Chemistry*, Vol.280, No.43, (October 2005), pp. 36342-36354, ISSN 0021-9258

Ember, J. A. and Hugli, T. E. (1997). Complement factors and their receptors. *Immunopharmacology*, Vol.38, No.1-2, (December 1997), pp. 3-15, ISSN 1567-5769

Ferraresso, M., Macor, P., Valente, M., Della Barbera, M., D'Amelio, F., Borghi, O., Raschi, E., Durigutto, P., Meroni, P. and Tedesco, F. (2008). Posttransplant ischemia-reperfusion injury in transplanted heart is prevented by a minibody to the fifth component of complement. *Transplantation*, Vol.86, No.10, (November 2008), pp. 1445-1451, ISSN 0041-1337

Figueroa, E., Gordon, L. E., Feldhoff, P. W. and Lassiter, H. A. (2005). The administration of cobra venom factor reduces post-ischemic cerebral injury in adult and neonatal rats. *Neuroscience Letters*, Vol.380, No.1-2, (May 2005), pp. 48-53, ISSN 0304-3940

Flierl, M. A., Rittirsch, D., Chen, A. J., Nadeau, B. A., Day, D. E., Sarma, J. V., Huber-Lang, M. S. and Ward, P. A. (2008). The complement anaphylatoxin C5a induces apoptosis in adrenomedullary cells during experimental sepsis. *PLoS One*, Vol.3, No.7, (July 2008), pp. e2560, ISSN 1932-6203

Foreman, K. E., Glovsky, M. M., Warner, R. L., Horvath, S. J. and Ward, P. A. (1996). Comparative effect of C3a and C5a on adhesion molecule expression on neutrophils and endothelial cells. *Inflammation*, Vol.20, No.1, (February 1996), pp. 1-9, ISSN 0360-3997

Fureder, W., Agis, H., Willheim, M., Bankl, H. C., Maier, U., Kishi, K., Muller, M. R., Czerwenka, K., Radaszkiewicz, T., Butterfield, J. H., Klappacher, G. W., Sperr, W. R., Oppermann, M., Lechner, K. and Valent, P. (1995). Differential expression of complement receptors on human basophils and mast cells. Evidence for mast cell heterogeneity and CD88/C5aR expression on skin mast cells. *Journal of Immunology*, Vol.155, No.6, (September 1995), pp. 3152-3160, ISSN 0022-1767

Gaca, J. G., Appel, J. Z., 3rd, Lukes, J. G., Gonzalez-Stawinski, G. V., Lesher, A., Palestrant, D., Logan, J. S., Love, S. D., Holzknecht, Z. E., Platt, J. L., Parker, W. and Davis, R. D. (2006). Effect of an anti-C5a monoclonal antibody indicates a prominent role for anaphylatoxin in pulmonary xenograft dysfunction. *Transplantation*, Vol.81, No.12, (June 2006), pp. 1686-1694, ISSN 0041-1337

Gao, H., Neff, T. A., Guo, R. F., Speyer, C. L., Sarma, J. V., Tomlins, S., Man, Y., Riedemann, N. C., Hoesel, L. M., Younkin, E., Zetoune, F. S. and Ward, P. A. (2005). Evidence for a functional role of the second C5a receptor C5L2. *Faseb Journal*, Vol.19, No.8, (June 2005), pp. 1003-1005, ISSN 0892-6638

Gasque, P., Chan, P., Fontaine, M., Ischenko, A., Lamacz, M., Gotze, O. and Morgan, B. P. (1995). Identification and characterization of the complement C5a anaphylatoxin receptor on human astrocytes. *Journal of Immunology*, Vol.155, No.10, (November 1995), pp. 4882-4889, ISSN 0022-1767

Gasque, P., Singhrao, S. K., Neal, J. W., Gotze, O. and Morgan, B. P. (1997). Expression of the receptor for complement C5a (CD88) is up-regulated on reactive astrocytes, microglia, and endothelial cells in the inflamed human central nervous system. *The American Journal of Pathology*, Vol.150, No.1, (January 1997), pp. 31-41, ISSN 0002-9440

Gasque, P., Singhrao, S. K., Neal, J. W., Wang, P., Sayah, S., Fontaine, M. and Morgan, B. P. (1998). The receptor for complement anaphylatoxin C3a is expressed by myeloid cells and nonmyeloid cells in inflamed human central nervous system: analysis in multiple sclerosis and bacterial meningitis. *Journal of Immunology*, Vol.160, No.7, (April 1998), pp. 3543-3554, ISSN 0022-1767

Gavrilyuk, V., Kalinin, S., Hilbush, B. S., Middlecamp, A., McGuire, S., Pelligrino, D., Weinberg, G. and Feinstein, D. L. (2005). Identification of complement 5a-like receptor (C5L2) from astrocytes: characterization of anti-inflammatory properties. *Journal of Neurochemistry*, Vol.92, No.5, (March 2005), pp. 1140-1149, ISSN 0022-3402

Gerard, C., Bao, L., Orozco, O., Pearson, M., Kunz, D. and Gerard, N. P. (1992). Structural diversity in the extracellular faces of peptidergic G-protein-coupled receptors. Molecular cloning of the mouse C5a anaphylatoxin receptor. *Journal of Immunology*, Vol.149, No.8, (October 1992), pp. 2600-2606, ISSN 0022-1767

Gerard, N. P. and Gerard, C. (1991). The chemotactic receptor for human C5a anaphylatoxin. *Nature*, Vol.349, No.6310, (February 1991), pp. 614-617, ISSN 0028-0836

Gerard, N. P., Bao, L., Xiao-Ping, H., Eddy, R. L., Jr., Shows, T. B. and Gerard, C. (1993). Human chemotaxis receptor genes cluster at 19q13.3-13.4. Characterization of the human C5a receptor gene. *Biochemistry*, Vol.32, No.5, (February 1993), pp. 1243-1250, ISSN

Gerard, N. P., Lu, B., Liu, P., Craig, S., Fujiwara, Y., Okinaga, S. and Gerard, C. (2005). An anti-inflammatory function for the complement anaphylatoxin C5a-binding protein, C5L2. *Journal of Biological Chemistry*, Vol.280, No.48, (December 2005), pp. 39677-39680, ISSN 0021-9258

Gerber, B. O., Meng, E. C., Dotsch, V., Baranski, T. J. and Bourne, H. R. (2001). An activation switch in the ligand binding pocket of the C5a receptor. *Journal of Biological Chemistry*, Vol.276, No.5, (February 2001), pp. 3394-3400, ISSN 0021-9258

GeurtsvanKessel, C. H. and Lambrecht, B. N. (2008). Division of labor between dendritic cell subsets of the lung. *Mucosal Immunology*, Vol.1, No.6, (November 2008), pp. 442-450, ISSN 1933-0219

Giannini, E., Brouchon, L. and Boulay, F. (1995). Identification of the major phosphorylation sites in human C5a anaphylatoxin receptor in vivo. *Journal of Biological Chemistry*, Vol.270, No.32, (August 1995), pp. 19166-19172, ISSN 0021-9258

Gonczi, Z., Varga, L., Hidvegi, T., Schmidt, B., Panya, A., Kokai, M. and Fust, G. (1997). The severity of clinical symptoms in ragweed-allergic patients is related to the extent of ragweed-induced complement activation in their sera. *Allergy*, Vol.52, No.11, (November 1997), pp. 1110-1114, ISSN 0105-4538

Goya, T., Morisaki, T. and Torisu, M. (1994). Immunologic assessment of host defense impairment in patients with septic multiple organ failure: relationship between complement activation and changes in neutrophil function. *Surgery*, Vol.115, No.2, (February 1994), pp. 145-155, ISSN 0039-6060

Groeneveld, A. B., Tacx, A. N., Bossink, A. W., van Mierlo, G. J. and Hack, C. E. (2003). Circulating inflammatory mediators predict shock and mortality in febrile patients with microbial infection. *Clinical Immunology*, Vol.106, No.2, (February 2003), pp. 106-115, ISSN 1521-6616

Gueler, F., Rong, S., Gwinner, W., Mengel, M., Brocker, V., Schon, S., Greten, T. F., Hawlisch, H., Polakowski, T., Schnatbaum, K., Menne, J., Haller, H. and Shushakova, N. (2008). Complement 5a receptor inhibition improves renal allograft survival. *Journal of the American Society of Nephrology*, Vol.19, No.12, (December 2008), pp. 2302-2312, ISSN 1046-6673

Guo, Q., Subramanian, H., Gupta, K. and Ali, H. (2011). Regulation of c3a receptor signaling in human mast cells by g protein coupled receptor kinases. *PLoS One*, Vol.6, No.7, (July 2011), pp. e22559, ISSN 1932-6203

Guo, R. F., Huber-Lang, M., Wang, X., Sarma, V., Padgaonkar, V. A., Craig, R. A., Riedemann, N. C., McClintock, S. D., Hlaing, T., Shi, M. M. and Ward, P. A. (2000). Protective effects of anti-C5a in sepsis-induced thymocyte apoptosis. *The Journal of Clinical Investigation*, Vol.106, No.10, (November 2000), pp. 1271-1280, ISSN 0021-9738

Guo, R. F., Riedemann, N. C., Laudes, I. J., Sarma, V. J., Kunkel, R. G., Dilley, K. A., Paulauskis, J. D. and Ward, P. A. (2002). Altered neutrophil trafficking during sepsis. *Journal of Immunology*, Vol.169, No.1, (July 2002), pp. 307-314, ISSN 0022-1767

Guo, R. F., Riedemann, N. C., Bernacki, K. D., Sarma, V. J., Laudes, I. J., Reuben, J. S., Younkin, E. M., Neff, T. A., Paulauskis, J. D., Zetoune, F. S. and Ward, P. A. (2003). Neutrophil C5a receptor and the outcome in a rat model of sepsis. *Faseb Journal*, Vol.17, No.13, (October 2003), pp. 1889-1891, ISSN 0892-6638

Gutzmer, R., Lisewski, M., Zwirner, J., Mommert, S., Diesel, C., Wittmann, M., Kapp, A. and Werfel, T. (2004). Human monocyte-derived dendritic cells are chemoattracted to C3a after up-regulation of the C3a receptor with interferons. *Immunology*, Vol.111, No.4, (April 2004), pp. 435-443, ISSN 1365-2567

Hack, C. E., Nuijens, J. H., Felt-Bersma, R. J., Schreuder, W. O., Eerenberg-Belmer, A. J., Paardekooper, J., Bronsveld, W. and Thijs, L. G. (1989). Elevated plasma levels of the anaphylatoxins C3a and C4a are associated with a fatal outcome in sepsis. *The American Journal of Medicine*, Vol.86, No.1, (January 1989), pp. 20-26, ISSN 0002-9343

Han, G., Geng, S., Li, Y., Chen, G., Wang, R., Li, X., Ma, Y., Shen, B. and Li, Y. (2011) gammadeltaT-cell function in sepsis is modulated by C5a receptor signalling. *Immunology*, Vol.133, No.3, pp. 340-349, ISSN 1365-2567

Hart, M. L., Walsh, M. C. and Stahl, G. L. (2004). Initiation of complement activation following oxidative stress. In vitro and in vivo observations. *Molecular Immunology*, Vol.41, No.2-3, (June 2004), pp. 165-171, ISSN 0161-5890

Hartmann, K., Henz, B. M., Kruger-Krasagakes, S., Kohl, J., Burger, R., Guhl, S., Haase, I., Lippert, U. and Zuberbier, T. (1997). C3a and C5a stimulate chemotaxis of human mast cells. *Blood*, Vol.89, No.8, (April 1997), pp. 2863-2870, ISSN 0006-4971

Hasegawa, K., Tamari, M., Shao, C., Shimizu, M., Takahashi, N., Mao, X. Q., Yamasaki, A., Kamada, F., Doi, S., Fujiwara, H., Miyatake, A., Fujita, K., Tamura, G., Matsubara, Y., Shirakawa, T. and Suzuki, Y. (2004). Variations in the C3, C3a receptor, and C5 genes affect susceptibility to bronchial asthma. *Human Genetics,* Vol.115, No.4, (September 2004), pp. 295-301, ISSN 0340-6717

Hecke, F., Schmidt, U., Kola, A., Bautsch, W., Klos, A. and Kohl, J. (1997). Circulating complement proteins in multiple trauma patients--correlation with injury severity, development of sepsis, and outcome. *Critical Care Medicine,* Vol.25, No.12, (December 1997), pp. 2015-2024, ISSN 0090-3493

Hellings, P. W., Kasran, A., Liu, Z., Vandekerckhove, P., Wuyts, A., Overbergh, L., Mathieu, C. and Ceuppens, J. L. (2003). Interleukin-17 orchestrates the granulocyte influx into airways after allergen inhalation in a mouse model of allergic asthma. *American Journal of Respiratory Cell and Molecular Biology,* Vol.28, No.1, (January 2003), pp. 42-50, ISSN 1044-1549

Hidvegi, T., Schmidt, B., Varga, L., Dervaderics, M., Lantos, A., Gonczi, Z., Barok, J., Otos, M., Kirschfink, M., Spath, P. and et al. (1995). In vitro complement activation by ragweed allergen extract in the sera of ragweed allergic and non-allergic persons. *Immunology Letters,* Vol.48, No.1, (November 1995), pp. 65-71, ISSN 0165-2478

Hill, J. H. and Ward, P. A. (1971). The phlogistic role of C3 leukotactic fragments in myocardial infarcts of rats. *The Journal of Experimental Medicine,* Vol.133, No.4, (April 1971), pp. 885-900, ISSN 0022-1007

Hollmann, T. J., Haviland, D. L., Kildsgaard, J., Watts, K. and Wetsel, R. A. (1998). Cloning, expression, sequence determination, and chromosome localization of the mouse complement C3a anaphylatoxin receptor gene. *Molecular Immunology,* Vol.35, No.3, (February 1998), pp. 137-148, ISSN 0161-5890

Hopken, U. E., Lu, B., Gerard, N. P. and Gerard, C. (1996). The C5a chemoattractant receptor mediates mucosal defence to infection. *Nature,* Vol.383, No.6595, (September 1996), pp. 86-89, ISSN 0028-0836

Huang, R., Lian, J. P., Robinson, D. and Badwey, J. A. (1998). Neutrophils stimulated with a variety of chemoattractants exhibit rapid activation of p21-activated kinases (Paks): separate signals are required for activation and inactivation of paks. *Molecular and Cell Biology,* Vol.18, No.12, (December 1998), pp. 7130-7138, ISSN 1098-5549

Huber-Lang, M., Sarma, J.V., McGuire, S.R., Lu, K.T., Guo, R.F., Padgaonkar, V.A., Younkin, E.M., Laudes, I.J., Riedmann, N.C., Younger, J.G. and Ward, P.A. (2001). Protective effects of anti-C5a peptide antibodies in experimental sepsis. *Faseb Journal,* Vol.15, No.3, (January 2001), pp. 568-570, ISSN 0892-6638

Huber-Lang, M. S., Younkin, E. M., Sarma, J. V., McGuire, S. R., Lu, K. T., Guo, R. F., Padgaonkar, V. A., Curnutte, J. T., Erickson, R. and Ward, P. A. (2002). Complement-induced impairment of innate immunity during sepsis. *Journal of Immunology,* Vol.169, No.6, (September 2002), pp. 3223-3231, ISSN 0022-1767

Huber-Lang, M. S., Riedeman, N. C., Sarma, J. V., Younkin, E. M., McGuire, S. R., Laudes, I. J., Lu, K. T., Guo, R. F., Neff, T. A., Padgaonkar, V. A., Lambris, J. D., Spruce, L., Mastellos, D., Zetoune, F. S. and Ward, P. A. (2002). Protection of innate immunity by C5aR antagonist in septic mice. *Faseb Journal,* Vol.16, No.12, (October 2002), pp. 1567-1574, ISSN 0892-6638

Huber-Lang, M., Younkin, E. M., Sarma, J. V., Riedemann, N., McGuire, S. R., Lu, K. T., Kunkel, R., Younger, J. G., Zetoune, F. S. and Ward, P. A. (2002). Generation of C5a by phagocytic cells. *American Journal of Pathology,* Vol.161, No.5, (November 2002), pp. 1849-1859, ISSN 0002-9440

Huber-Lang, M. S., Sarma, J. V., McGuire, S. R., Lu, K. T., Padgaonkar, V. A., Younkin, E. M., Guo, R. F., Weber, C. H., Zuiderweg, E. R., Zetoune, F. S. and Ward, P. A. (2003). Structure-function relationships of human C5a and C5aR. *Journal of Immunology* , Vol.170, No.12, (June 2003), pp. 6115-6124, ISSN 0022-1767

Hugli, T. E. (1981). The structural basis for anaphylatoxin and chemotactic functions of C3a, C4a, and C5a. *Critical Reviews in Immunology*, Vol.1, No.4, (February 1981), pp. 321-366, ISSN 1040-8401

Humbles, A. A., Lu, B., Nilsson, C. A., Lilly, C., Israel, E., Fujiwara, Y., Gerard, N. P. and Gerard, C. (2000). A role for the C3a anaphylatoxin receptor in the effector phase of asthma. *Nature*, Vol.406, No.6799, (August 2000), pp. 998-1001, ISSN 0028-0836

Jagels, M. A., Daffern, P. J. and Hugli, T. E. (2000). C3a and C5a enhance granulocyte adhesion to endothelial and epithelial cell monolayers: epithelial and endothelial priming is required for C3a-induced eosinophil adhesion. *Immunopharmacology*, Vol.46, No.3, (March 2000), pp. 209-222, ISSN 1567-5769

Johnson, A. R., Hugli, T. E. and Muller-Eberhard, H. J. (1975). Release of histamine from rat mast cells by the complement peptides C3a and C5a. *Immunology*, Vol.28, No.6, (June 1975), pp. 1067-1080, ISSN 1365-2567

Johswich, K., Martin, M., Thalmann, J., Rheinheimer, C., Monk, P. N. and Klos, A. (2006). Ligand specificity of the anaphylatoxin C5L2 receptor and its regulation on myeloid and epithelial cell lines. *Journal of Biological Chemistry*, Vol.281, No.51, (December 2006), pp. 39088-39095, ISSN 0021-9258

Jordan, J. E., Montalto, M. C. and Stahl, G. L. (2001). Inhibition of mannose-binding lectin reduces postischemic myocardial reperfusion injury. *Circulation*, Vol.104, No.12, (September 2001), pp. 1413-1418, ISSN 0009-7322

Kalant, D., MacLaren, R., Cui, W., Samanta, R., Monk, P. N., Laporte, S. A. and Cianflone, K. (2005). C5L2 is a functional receptor for acylation-stimulating protein. *Journal of Biological Chemistry*, Vol.280, No.25, (June 2005), pp. 23936-23944, ISSN 0021-9258

Kaplan, A. P. (2004). Chronic urticaria: pathogenesis and treatment. *The Journal of Allergy and Clinical Immunology*, Vol.114, No.3, (September 2004), pp. 465-474; quiz 475, ISSN 0091-6749

Karp, C. L., Grupe, A., Schadt, E., Ewart, S. L., Keane-Moore, M., Cuomo, P. J., Kohl, J., Wahl, L., Kuperman, D., Germer, S., Aud, D., Peltz, G. and Wills-Karp, M. (2000). Identification of complement factor 5 as a susceptibility locus for experimental allergic asthma. *Nature Immunology*, Vol.1, No.3, (September 2000), pp. 221-226, ISSN 1529-2908

Karp, D. R. (2005). Complement and systemic lupus erythematosus. *Current Opinions in Rheumatology*, Vol.17, No.5, (September 2005), pp. 538-542, ISSN 1040-8711

Kew, R. R., Ghebrehiwet, B. and Janoff, A. (1987). Characterization of the third component of complement (C3) after activation by cigarette smoke. *Clinical Immunology and Immunopathology*, Vol.44, No.2, (August 1987), pp. 248-258, ISSN 0090-1229

Khirwadkar, K., Zilow, G., Oppermann, M., Kabelitz, D. and Rother, K. (1993). Interleukin-4 augments production of the third complement component by the alveolar epithelial cell line A549. *International Archives of Allergy and Immunology*, Vol.100, No.1, pp. 35-41, ISSN 1018-2438

Kikuchi, Y. and Kaplan, A. P. (2002). A role for C5a in augmenting IgG-dependent histamine release from basophils in chronic urticaria. *The Journal of Allergy and Clinical Immunology*, Vol.109, No.1, (January 2002), pp. 114-118, ISSN 0091-6749

Kohl, J., Baelder, R., Lewkowich, I. P., Pandey, M. K., Hawlisch, H., Wang, L., Best, J., Herman, N. S., Sproles, A. A., Zwirner, J., Whitsett, J. A., Gerard, C., Sfyroera, G., Lambris, J. D. and Wills-Karp, M. (2006). A regulatory role for the C5a anaphylatoxin in type 2 immunity in asthma. *The Journal of Clinical Investigation,* Vol.116, No.3, (March 2006), pp. 783-796, ISSN 0021-9738

Korosec, P., Subic, T., Adamic, K., Silar, M. and Kosnik, M. (2009). C5a-induced in vitro basophil activation in patients with chronic urticaria: a pilot study. *Wien Klin Wochenschr,* Vol.121, No.9-10, pp. 339-343, ISSN 0043-5325

Krug, N., Tschernig, T., Erpenbeck, V. J., Hohlfeld, J. M. and Kohl, J. (2001). Complement factors C3a and C5a are increased in bronchoalveolar lavage fluid after segmental allergen provocation in subjects with asthma. *American Journal of Respiratory and Critical Care Medicine,* Vol.164, No.10 Pt 1, (November 2001), pp. 1841-1843, ISSN 1073-449X

Kuehn, H. S. and Gilfillan, A. M. (2007). G protein-coupled receptors and the modification of FcepsilonRI-mediated mast cell activation. *Immunology Letters,* Vol.113, No.2, (November 2007), pp. 59-69, ISSN 0165-2478

Kupp, L. I., Kosco, M. H., Schenkein, H. A. and Tew, J. G. (1991). Chemotaxis of germinal center B cells in response to C5a. *European Journal of Immunology,* Vol.21, No.11, (November 1991), pp. 2697-2701, ISSN 0022-1767

Kuroki, M. and O'Flaherty, J. T. (1999). Extracellular signal-regulated protein kinase (ERK)-dependent and ERK-independent pathways target STAT3 on serine-727 in human neutrophils stimulated by chemotactic factors and cytokines. *Biochemistry Journal,* Vol.341 (Pt 3), (August 1 1999), pp. 691-696, ISSN 0264-6021

Lacy, M., Jones, J., Whittemore, S. R., Haviland, D. L., Wetsel, R. A. and Barnum, S. R. (1995). Expression of the receptors for the C5a anaphylatoxin, interleukin-8 and FMLP by human astrocytes and microglia. *Journal of Neuroimmunology,* Vol.61, No.1, (August 1995), pp. 71-78, ISSN 0165-5728

Lajoie, S., Lewkowich, I. P., Suzuki, Y., Clark, J. R., Sproles, A. A., Dienger, K., Budelsky, A. L. and Wills-Karp, M. (2010). Complement-mediated regulation of the IL-17A axis is a central genetic determinant of the severity of experimental allergic asthma. *Nature Immunology,* Vol.11, No.10, (October 2010), pp. 928-935, ISSN 1529-2908

Lambrecht, B. N., De Veerman, M., Coyle, A. J., Gutierrez-Ramos, J. C., Thielemans, K. and Pauwels, R. A. (2000). Myeloid dendritic cells induce Th2 responses to inhaled antigen, leading to eosinophilic airway inflammation. *The Journal of Clinical Investigation,* Vol.106, No.4, (August 2000), pp. 551-559, ISSN 0021-9738

Lambrecht, B. N. and Hammad, H. (2009). Biology of lung dendritic cells at the origin of asthma. *Immunity,* Vol.31, No.3, (September 2009), pp. 412-424, ISSN 1074-7613

Langkabel, P., Zwirner, J. and Oppermann, M. (1999). Ligand-induced phosphorylation of anaphylatoxin receptors C3aR and C5aR is mediated by "G protein-coupled receptor kinases. *European Journal of Immunology,* Vol.29, No.9, (September 1999), pp. 3035-3046, ISSN 0014-2980

Laudes, I. J., Chu, J. C., Sikranth, S., Huber-Lang, M., Guo, R. F., Riedemann, N., Sarma, J. V., Schmaier, A. H. and Ward, P. A. (2002). Anti-c5a ameliorates coagulation/fibrinolytic protein changes in a rat model of sepsis. *American Journal of Pathology,* Vol.160, No.5, (May 2002), pp. 1867-1875, ISSN 0002-9440

Lee, D. K., George, S. R., Cheng, R., Nguyen, T., Liu, Y., Brown, M., Lynch, K. R. and O'Dowd, B. F. (2001). Identification of four novel human G protein-coupled receptors expressed in the brain. *Brain Research. Molecular Brain Research*, Vol.86, No.1-2, (January 2001), pp. 13-22

Lee, S. H., Rhim, T., Choi, Y. S., Min, J. W., Kim, S. H., Cho, S. Y., Paik, Y. K. and Park, C. S. (2006). Complement C3a and C4a increased in plasma of patients with aspirin-induced asthma. *American Journal of Respiratory and Critical Care Medicine*, Vol.173, No.4, (February 2006), pp. 370-378, ISSN 0090-3493

Lett-Brown, M. A. and Leonard, E. J. (1977). Histamine-induced inhibition of normal human basophil chemotaxis to C5a. *Journal of Immunology*, Vol.118, No.3, (March 1977), pp. 815-818, ISSN 0022-1767

Lewis, A. G., Kohl, G., Ma, Q., Devarajan, P. and Kohl, J. (2008). Pharmacological targeting of C5a receptors during organ preservation improves kidney graft survival. *Clinical and Experimental Immunology*, Vol.153, No.1, (July 2008), pp. 117-126, ISSN 0009-9104

Lewkowich, I. P., Herman, N. S., Schleifer, K. W., Dance, M. P., Chen, B. L., Dienger, K. M., Sproles, A. A., Shah, J. S., Kohl, J., Belkaid, Y. and Wills-Karp, M. (2005). CD4+CD25+ T cells protect against experimentally induced asthma and alter pulmonary dendritic cell phenotype and function. *Journal of Experimental Medicine*, Vol.202, No.11, (December 2005), pp. 1549-1561, ISSN 0022-1007

Li, K., Anderson, K. J., Peng, Q., Noble, A., Lu, B., Kelly, A. P., Wang, N., Sacks, S. H. and Zhou, W. (2008). Cyclic AMP plays a critical role in C3a-receptor-mediated regulation of dendritic cells in antigen uptake and T-cell stimulation. *Blood*, Vol.112, No.13, (December 2008), pp. 5084-5094, ISSN 0006-4971

Link, C., Hawlisch, H., Meyer zu Vilsendorf, A., Gyleruz, S., Nagel, E. and Kohl, J. (1999). Selection of phage-displayed anti-guinea pig C5 or C5a antibodies and their application in xenotransplantation. *Molecular Immunology*, Vol.36, No.18, (December 1999), pp. 1235-1247, ISSN 0161-5890

Lo, R. K., Wise, H. and Wong, Y. H. (2006). Prostacyclin receptor induces STAT1 and STAT3 phosphorylations in human erythroleukemia cells: a mechanism requiring PTX-insensitive G proteins, ERK and JNK. *Cell Signaling*, Vol.18, No.3, (March 2006), pp. 307-317, ISSN 0898-6568

Lukacs, N. W., Glovsky, M. M. and Ward, P. A. (2001). Complement-dependent immune complex-induced bronchial inflammation and hyperreactivity. *American Journal of Physiology. Lung Cellular and Molecular Physiology*, Vol.280, No.3, (March 2001), pp. L512-518, ISSN 1040-0605

Marc, M. M., Korosec, P., Kosnik, M., Kern, I., Flezar, M., Suskovic, S. and Sorli, J. (2004). Complement factors c3a, c4a, and c5a in chronic obstructive pulmonary disease and asthma. *American Journal of Respiratory Cell and Molecular Biology*, Vol.31, No.2, (August 2004), pp. 216-219, ISSN 1073-449X

Markiewski, M. M., DeAngelis, R. A., Benencia, F., Ricklin-Lichtsteiner, S. K., Koutoulaki, A., Gerard, C., Coukos, G. and Lambris, J. D. (2008). Modulation of the antitumor immune response by complement. *Nature Immunology*, Vol.9, No.11, (November 2008), pp. 1225-1235, ISSN 1529-2908

Maruo, K., Akaike, T., Ono, T., Okamoto, T. and Maeda, H. (1997). Generation of anaphylatoxins through proteolytic processing of C3 and C5 by house dust mite protease. *The Journal of Allergy and Clinical Immunology*, Vol.100, No.2, (August 1997), pp. 253-260, ISSN 0091-6749

Mastellos, D., Germenis, A. E. and Lambris, J. D. (2005). Complement: an inflammatory pathway fulfilling multiple roles at the interface of innate immunity and development. *Current Drug Targets in Inflammation and Allergy*, Vol.4, No.1, (February 2005), pp. 125-127, ISSN 1871-5281

McCarthy, K. and Henson, P. M. (1979). Induction of lysosomal enzyme secretion by alveolar macrophages in response to the purified complement fragments C5a and C5a des-arg. *Journal of Immunology*, Vol.123, No.6, (December 1979), pp. 2511-2517, ISSN 0022-1767

McCloskey M.A., Fan Y and Luther S. (1999). Chemotaxis of rat mast cells toward adenine nucleotides. *Journal of Immunology*, Vol.163, No.2, (July 1999), pp. 970-977, ISSN 0022-1767

McColl, B. W., Allan, S. M. and Rothwell, N. J. (2009). Systemic infection, inflammation and acute ischemic stroke. *Neuroscience*, Vol.158, No.3, (February 2009), pp. 1049-1061, ISSN 0306-4522

McKinley, L., Alcorn, J. F., Peterson, A., Dupont, R. B., Kapadia, S., Logar, A., Henry, A., Irvin, C. G., Piganelli, J. D., Ray, A. and Kolls, J. K. (2008). TH17 cells mediate steroid-resistant airway inflammation and airway hyperresponsiveness in mice. *Journal of Immunology*, Vol.181, No.6, (September 2008), pp. 4089-4097, ISSN 0022-1767

Melendi, G. A., Hoffman, S. J., Karron, R. A., Irusta, P. M., Laham, F. R., Humbles, A., Schofield, B., Pan, C. H., Rabold, R., Thumar, B., Thumar, A., Gerard, N. P., Mitzner, W., Barnum, S. R., Gerard, C., Kleeberger, S. R. and Polack, F. P. (2007). C5 modulates airway hyperreactivity and pulmonary eosinophilia during enhanced respiratory syncytial virus disease by decreasing C3a receptor expression. *Journal of Virology*, Vol.81, No.2, (January 2007), pp. 991-999, ISSN 0022-538X

Mery, L. and Boulay, F. (1993). Evidence that the extracellular N-terminal domain of C5aR contains amino-acid residues crucial for C5a binding. *European Journal of Haematology*, Vol.51, No.5, (November 1993), pp. 282-287, ISSN 0902-4441

Methner, A., Hermey, G., Schinke, B. and Hermans-Borgmeyer, I. (1997). A novel G protein-coupled receptor with homology to neuropeptide and chemoattractant receptors expressed during bone development. *Biochemical and Biophysical Research Communications*, Vol.233, No.2, (April 1997), pp. 336-342, ISSN 0006-291X

Mizutani, N., Nabe, T. and Yoshino, S. (2009). Complement C3a regulates late asthmatic response and airway hyperresponsiveness in mice. *Journal of Immunology*, Vol.183, No.6, (September 2009), pp. 4039-4046, ISSN 0022-1767

Mocco, J., Mack, W. J., Ducruet, A. F., Sosunov, S. A., Sughrue, M. E., Hassid, B. G., Nair, M. N., Laufer, I., Komotar, R. J., Claire, M., Holland, H., Pinsky, D. J. and Connolly, E. S., Jr. (2006). Complement component C3 mediates inflammatory injury following focal cerebral ischemia. *Circulation Research*, Vol.99, No.2, (July 2006), pp. 209-217, ISSN 0009-7330

Monk, P. N. and Partridge, L. J. (1993). Characterization of a complement-fragment-C5a-stimulated calcium-influx mechanism in U937 monocytic cells. *Biochemistry Journal*, Vol.295 (Pt 3), (November 1993), pp. 679-684, ISSN 0264-6021

Monk, P. N., Scola, A. M., Madala, P. and Fairlie, D. P. (2007). Function, structure and therapeutic potential of complement C5a receptors. *British Journal of Pharmacology*, Vol.152, No.4, (October 2007), pp. 429-448, ISSN 1476-5381

Nagata, S. and Glovsky, M. M. (1987). Activation of human serum complement with allergens. I. Generation of C3a, C4a, and C5a and induction of human neutrophil aggregation. *The Journal of Allergy and Clinical Immunology*, Vol.80, No.1, (July 1987), pp. 24-32, ISSN 0091-6749

Nakae, H., Endo, S., Inada, K., Takakuwa, T., Kasai, T. and Yoshida, M. (1994). Serum complement levels and severity of sepsis. *Research Communications in Chemical Pathology and Pharmacology*, Vol.84, No.2, (May 1994), pp. 189-195, ISSN 0034-5164

Nakae, H., Endo, S., Inada, K. and Yoshida, M. (1996). Chronological changes in the complement system in sepsis. *Surgery Today*, Vol.26, No.4, pp. 225-229, ISSN 0941-1291

Nakamura, T., Xi, G., Hua, Y., Schallert, T., Hoff, J. T. and Keep, R. F. (2004). Intracerebral hemorrhage in mice: model characterization and application for genetically modified mice. *Journal of Cerebral Blood Flow and Metabolism*, Vol.24, No.5, (May 2004), pp. 487-494, ISSN 0271-678X

Nataf, S., Davoust, N., Ames, R. S. and Barnum, S. R. (1999). Human T cells express the C5a receptor and are chemoattracted to C5a. *Journal of Immunology*, Vol.162, No.7, (April 1999), pp. 4018-4023, ISSN 0022-1767

Niederbichler, A. D., Hoesel, L. M., Westfall, M. V., Gao, H., Ipaktchi, K. R., Sun, L., Zetoune, F. S., Su, G. L., Arbabi, S., Sarma, J. V., Wang, S. C., Hemmila, M. R. and Ward, P. A. (2006). An essential role for complement C5a in the pathogenesis of septic cardiac dysfunction. *Journal of Experimental Medicine*, Vol.203, No.1, (January 2006), pp. 53-61, ISSN 0022-1007

Nilsson, G., Johnell, M., Hammer, C. H., Tiffany, H. L., Nilsson, K., Metcalfe, D. D., Siegbahn, A. and Murphy, P. M. (1996). C3a and C5a are chemotaxins for human mast cells and act through distinct receptors via a pertussis toxin-sensitive signal transduction pathway. *Journal of Immunology*, Vol.157, No.4, (August 1996), pp. 1693-1698, ISSN 0022-1767

Nishino, H., Czurko, A., Fukuda, A., Hashitani, T., Hida, H., Karadi, Z. and Lenard, L. (1994). Pathophysiological process after transient ischemia of the middle cerebral artery in the rat. *Brain Research Bulletin*, Vol.35, No.1, pp. 51-56, ISSN 0361-9230

Ober, C., Cox, N. J., Abney, M., Di Rienzo, A., Lander, E. S., Changyaleket, B., Gidley, H., Kurtz, B., Lee, J., Nance, M., Pettersson, A., Prescott, J., Richardson, A., Schlenker, E., Summerhill, E., Willadsen, S. and Parry, R. (1998). Genome-wide search for asthma susceptibility loci in a founder population. The Collaborative Study on the Genetics of Asthma. *Human Molecular Genetics*, Vol.7, No.9, (September 1998), pp. 1393-1398, ISSN 0964-6906

Ohno, M., Hirata, T., Enomoto, M., Araki, T., Ishimaru, H. and Takahashi, T. A. (2000). A putative chemoattractant receptor, C5L2, is expressed in granulocyte and immature dendritic cells, but not in mature dendritic cells. *Molecular Immunology*, Vol.37, No.8, (June 2000), pp. 407-412, ISSN 0161-5890

Okinaga, S., Slattery, D., Humbles, A., Zsengeller, Z., Morteau, O., Kinrade, M. B., Brodbeck, R. M., Krause, J. E., Choe, H. R., Gerard, N. P. and Gerard, C. (2003). C5L2, a nonsignaling C5A binding protein. *Biochemistry*, Vol.42, No.31, (August 2003), pp. 9406-9415, ISSN 0006-2960

Palomares, O., Yaman, G., Azkur, A. K., Akkoc, T., Akdis, M. and Akdis, C. A. (2010). Role of Treg in immune regulation of allergic diseases, *European Journal of Immunology*, Vol.40, No.5, (May 2010), pp. 1232-1240, ISSN 0014-2980

Park, J. W., Taube, C., Joetham, A., Takeda, K., Kodama, T., Dakhama, A., McConville, G., Allen, C. B., Sfyroera, G., Shultz, L. D., Lambris, J. D., Giclas, P. C., Holers, V. M. and Gelfand, E. W. (2004). Complement activation is critical to airway hyperresponsiveness after acute ozone exposure. *American Journal of Respiratory Cell and Molecular Biology*, Vol.169, No.6, (March 2004), pp. 726-732, ISSN 1044-1549

Park, K. W., Tofukuji, M., Metais, C., Comunale, M. E., Dai, H. B., Simons, M., Stahl, G. L., Agah, A. and Sellke, F. W. (1999). Attenuation of endothelium-dependent dilation of pig pulmonary arterioles after cardiopulmonary bypass is prevented by monoclonal antibody to complement C5a. *Anesthesia and Analgesia*, Vol.89, No.1, (July 1999), pp. 42-48, ISSN 0003-2999

Pene, J., Chevalier, S., Preisser, L., Venereau, E., Guilleux, M. H., Ghannam, S., Moles, J. P., Danger, Y., Ravon, E., Lesaux, S., Yssel, H. and Gascan, H. (2008). Chronically inflamed human tissues are infiltrated by highly differentiated Th17 lymphocytes. *Journal of Immunology*, Vol.180, No.11, (June 2008), pp. 7423-7430, ISSN 0022-1767

Peng, Q., Li, K., Anderson, K., Farrar, C. A., Lu, B., Smith, R. A., Sacks, S. H. and Zhou, W. (2008). Local production and activation of complement up-regulates the allostimulatory function of dendritic cells through C3a-C3aR interaction. *Blood*, Vol.111, No.4, (February 2008), pp. 2452-2461, ISSN 0006-4971

Peng, Q., Li, K., Patel, H., Sacks, S. H. and Zhou, W. (2006). Dendritic cell synthesis of C3 is required for full T cell activation and development of a Th1 phenotype. *Journal of Immunology*, Vol.176, No.6, (March 2006), pp. 3330-3341, ISSN 0022-1767

Peng, T., Hao, L., Madri, J. A., Su, X., Elias, J. A., Stahl, G. L., Squinto, S. and Wang, Y. (2005). Role of C5 in the development of airway inflammation, airway hyperresponsiveness, and ongoing airway response. *The Journal of Clinical Investigation*, Vol.115, No.6, (June 2005), pp. 1590-1600, ISSN 0021-9738

Perianayagam, M. C., Balakrishnan, V. S., Pereira, B. J. and Jaber, B. L. (2004). C5a delays apoptosis of human neutrophils via an extracellular signal-regulated kinase and Bad-mediated signalling pathway. *European Journal of Clinical Investigation*, Vol.34, No.1, (January 2004), pp. 50-56, ISSN 0021-9738

Perianayagam, M. C., Madias, N. E., Pereira, B. J. and Jaber, B. L. (2006). CREB transcription factor modulates Bcl2 transcription in response to C5a in HL-60-derived neutrophils. *European Journal of Clinical Investigation*, Vol.36, No.5, (May 2006), pp. 353-361, ISSN 0014-2972

Pieters, W. R., Houben, L. A., Koenderman, L. and Raaijmakers, J. A. (1995). C5a-induced migration of human monocytes is primed by dexamethasone. *American Journal of Respiratory Cell and Molecular Biology*, Vol.12, No.6, (June 1995), pp. 691-696, ISSN 1044-1549

Pratt, J. R., Basheer, S. A. and Sacks, S. H. (2002). Local synthesis of complement component C3 regulates acute renal transplant rejection. *Nature Medicine*, Vol.8, No.6, (June 2002), pp. 582-587, ISSN 1078-8956

Premont, R. T. and Gainetdinov, R. R. (2007). Physiological roles of G protein-coupled receptor kinases and arrestins. *Annual Review of Physiology*, Vol.69, pp. 511-534, ISSN 0066-4278

Proctor, L. M., Arumugam, T. V., Shiels, I., Reid, R. C., Fairlie, D. P. and Taylor, S. M. (2004). Comparative anti-inflammatory activities of antagonists to C3a and C5a receptors in a rat model of intestinal ischaemia/reperfusion injury. *British Journal of Pharmacology*, Vol.142, No.4, (June 2004), pp. 756-764, ISSN 1476-5381

Pundir P and Kulka M. (2010). The role of G protein-coupled receptors in mast cell activation by antimicrobial peptides: is there a conneciton? *Immunology & Cell Biology*, Vol.88, No.6, (August 2010), pp. 632-640, ISSN 0818-9641

Rabiet, M. J., Huet, E. and Boulay, F. (2007). The N-formyl peptide receptors and the anaphylatoxin C5a receptors: an overview. *Biochimie*, Vol.89, No.9, (September 2007), pp. 1089-1106, ISSN 0300-9084

Richardson, R. M., Pridgen, B. C., Haribabu, B., Ali, H. and Snyderman, R. (1998). Differential cross-regulation of the human chemokine receptors CXCR1 and CXCR2. Evidence for time-dependent signal generation. *Journal of Biological Chemistry*, Vol.273, No.37, (September 1998), pp. 23830-23836, ISSN 0021-9258

Ricklin, D., Hajishengallis, G., Yang, K. and Lambris, J. D. (2010). Complement: a key system for immune surveillance and homeostasis. *Nature Immunology*, Vol.11, No.9, (September 2010), pp. 785-797, ISSN 1529-2908

Riedemann, N. C., Guo, R. F., Laudes, I. J., Keller, K., Sarma, V. J., Padgaonkar, V., Zetoune, F. S. and Ward, P. A. (2002). C5a receptor and thymocyte apoptosis in sepsis. *Faseb Journal*, Vol.16, No.8, (June 2002), pp. 887-888, ISSN 0892-6638

Riedemann, N. C., Guo, R. F., Neff, T. A., Laudes, I. J., Keller, K. A., Sarma, V. J., Markiewski, M. M., Mastellos, D., Strey, C. W., Pierson, C. L., Lambris, J. D., Zetoune, F. S. and Ward, P. A. (2002). Increased C5a receptor expression in sepsis. *The Journal of Clinical Investigation*, Vol.110, No.1, (July 2002), pp. 101-108, ISSN 0021-9738

Rittirsch, D., Flierl, M. A., Nadeau, B. A., Day, D. E., Huber-Lang, M., Mackay, C. R., Zetoune, F. S., Gerard, N. P., Cianflone, K., Kohl, J., Gerard, C., Sarma, J. V. and Ward, P. A. (2008). Functional roles for C5a receptors in sepsis. *Nature Medicine*, Vol.14, No.5, (May 2008), pp. 551-557, ISSN 1078-8956

Rousseau, S., Dolado, I., Beardmore, V., Shpiro, N., Marquez, R., Nebreda, A. R., Arthur, J. S., Case, L. M., Tessier-Lavigne, M., Gaestel, M., Cuenda, A. and Cohen, P. (2006). CXCL12 and C5a trigger cell migration via a PAK1/2-p38alpha MAPK-MAPKAP-K2-HSP27 pathway. *Cell Signaling*, Vol.18, No.11, (November 2006), pp. 1897-1905, ISSN 0898-6568

Rus, H., Cudrici, C. and Niculescu, F. (2005). C5b-9 complement complex in autoimmune demyelination and multiple sclerosis: dual role in neuroinflammation and neuroprotection. *Annals of Medicine*, Vol.37, No.2, pp. 97-104, ISSN 0785-3890

Rynkowski, M. A., Kim, G. H., Garrett, M. C., Zacharia, B. E., Otten, M. L., Sosunov, S. A., Komotar, R. J., Hassid, B. G., Ducruet, A. F., Lambris, J. D. and Connolly, E. S. (2009). C3a receptor antagonist attenuates brain injury after intracerebral hemorrhage. *Journal of Cereberal Blood Flow and Metabolism*, Vol.29, No.1, (January 2009), pp. 98-107, ISSN 0271-678X

Sachse, C., Wolterink, G. and Pallua, N. (2000). Neutrophil intracellular pH and phagocytosis after thermal trauma. *Clinica Chimica Acta*, Vol.295, No.1-2, (May 2000), pp. 13-26, ISSN 0009-8981

Samson, M., Edinger, A. L., Stordeur, P., Rucker, J., Verhasselt, V., Sharron, M., Govaerts, C., Mollereau, C., Vassart, G., Doms, R. W. and Parmentier, M. (1998). ChemR23, a putative chemoattractant receptor, is expressed in monocyte-derived dendritic cells and macrophages and is a coreceptor for SIV and some primary HIV-1 strains. *European Journal of Immunology*, Vol.28, No.5, (May 1998), pp. 1689-1700, ISSN 0014-2980

Santini, F., Gaidarov, I. and Keen, J. H. (2002). G protein-coupled receptor/arrestin3 modulation of the endocytic machinery. *Journal of Cell Biology*, Vol.156, No.4, (February 2002), pp. 665-676, ISSN 0021-9525

Sarma, J. V. and Ward, P. A. (2011). The complement system. *Cell and Tissue Research*, Vol.343, No.1, (January 2011), pp. 227-235, ISSN 0302-766X

Sayah, S., Patte, C., Gasque, P., Chan, P., Ischenko, A., Vaudry, H. and Fontaine, M. (1997). Characterization of rat C5a anaphylatoxin receptor (C5aR): cloning of rat C5aR cDNA and study of C5aR expression by rat astrocytes. *Brain Research. Molecular Brain Research*, Vol.48, No.2, (September 1997), pp. 215-222

Schindler, R., Gelfand, J. A. and Dinarello, C. A. (1990). Recombinant C5a stimulates transcription rather than translation of interleukin-1 (IL-1) and tumor necrosis factor: translational signal provided by lipopolysaccharide or IL-1 itself. *Blood*, Vol.76, No.8, (October 1990), pp. 1631-1638, ISSN 0006-4971

Schraufstatter, I. U., Trieu, K., Sikora, L., Sriramarao, P. and DiScipio, R. (2002). Complement c3a and c5a induce different signal transduction cascades in endothelial cells. *Journal of Immunology*, Vol.169, No.4, (August 2002), pp. 2102-2110, ISSN 0022-1767

Scola, A. M., Johswich, K. O., Morgan, B. P., Klos, A. and Monk, P. N. (2009). The human complement fragment receptor, C5L2, is a recycling decoy receptor. *Molecular Immunology*, Vol.46, No.6, (March 2009), pp. 1149-1162, ISSN 0161-5890

Scott, M. G., Benmerah, A., Muntaner, O. and Marullo, S. (2002). Recruitment of activated G protein-coupled receptors to pre-existing clathrin-coated pits in living cells. *Journal of Biological Chemistry*, Vol.277, No.5, (February 2002), pp. 3552-3559, ISSN 0021-9258

Selberg, O., Hecker, H., Martin, M., Klos, A., Bautsch, W. and Kohl, J. (2000). Discrimination of sepsis and systemic inflammatory response syndrome by determination of circulating plasma concentrations of procalcitonin, protein complement 3a, and interleukin-6. *Critical Care Medicine*, Vol.28, No.8, (August 2000), pp. 2793-2798, ISSN 0090-3493

Settmacher, B., Bock, D., Saad, H., Gartner, S., Rheinheimer, C., Kohl, J., Bautsch, W. and Klos, A. (1999). Modulation of C3a activity: internalization of the human C3a receptor and its inhibition by C5a. *Journal of Immunology*, Vol.162, No.12, (June 1999), pp. 7409-7416, ISSN 0022-1767

Shima, M. and Adachi, M. (1996). Effects of environmental tobacco smoke on serum levels of acute phase proteins in schoolchildren. *Preventive Medicine*, Vol.25, No.5, (September-October 1996), pp. 617-624, ISSN 0091-7435

Showell, H. J., Glovsky, M. M. and Ward, P. A. (1982). C3a-induced lysosomal enzyme secretion from human neutrophils: lack of inhibition by f met-leu-phe antagonists and inhibition by arachidonic acid antagonists. *International Archives of Allergy and Applied Immunology*, Vol.67, No.3, pp. 227-232, ISSN 0020-5915

Skokowa, J., Ali, S. R., Felda, O., Kumar, V., Konrad, S., Shushakova, N., Schmidt, R. E., Piekorz, R. P., Nurnberg, B., Spicher, K., Birnbaumer, L., Zwirner, J., Claassens, J. W., Verbeek, J. S., van Rooijen, N., Kohl, J. and Gessner, J. E. (2005). Macrophages induce the inflammatory response in the pulmonary Arthus reaction through G alpha i2 activation that controls C5aR and Fc receptor cooperation. *Journal of Immunology*, Vol.174, No.5, (Mach 2005), pp. 3041-3050, ISSN 0022-1767

Smith, J. K., Chi, D. S., Krish, G., Reynolds, S. and Cambron, G. (1990). Effect of exercise on complement activity. *Annals of Allergy*, Vol.65, No.4, (October 1990), pp. 304-310, ISSN 0003-4738

Solomkin, J. S., Jenkins, M. K., Nelson, R. D., Chenoweth, D. and Simmons, R. L. (1981). Neutrophil dysfunction in sepsis. II. Evidence for the role of complement activation products in cellular deactivation. *Surgery*, Vol.90, No.2, (August 1981), pp. 319-327, ISSN 0039-6060

Solomkin, J. S., Cotta, L. A., Satoh, P. S., Hurst, J. M. and Nelson, R. D. (1985). Complement activation and clearance in acute illness and injury: evidence for C5a as a cell-directed mediator of the adult respiratory distress syndrome in man. *Surgery*, Vol.97, No.6, (June 1985), pp. 668-678, ISSN 0039-6060

Soruri, A., Kiafard, Z., Dettmer, C., Riggert, J., Kohl, J. and Zwirner, J. (2003). IL-4 down-regulates anaphylatoxin receptors in monocytes and dendritic cells and impairs anaphylatoxin-induced migration in vivo. *Journal of Immunology*, Vol.170, No.6, (March 2003), pp. 3306-3314, ISSN 0022-1767

Speyer, C. L., Gao, H., Rancilio, N. J., Neff, T. A., Huffnagle, G. B., Sarma, J. V. and Ward, P. A. (2004). Novel chemokine responsiveness and mobilization of neutrophils during sepsis. *Americanl Journal of Pathology*, Vol.165, No.6, (December 2004), pp. 2187-2196, ISSN 0002-9440

Stevens, J. H., O'Hanley, P., Shapiro, J. M., Mihm, F. G., Satoh, P. S., Collins, J. A. and Raffin, T. A. (1986). Effects of anti-C5a antibodies on the adult respiratory distress syndrome in septic primates. *The Journal of Clinical Investigation*, Vol.77, No.6, (June 1986), pp. 1812-1816, ISSN 0021-9738

Stimler, N. P., Bloor, C. M. and Hugli, T. E. (1983). C3a-induced contraction of guinea pig lung parenchyma: role of cyclooxygenase metabolites. *Immunopharmacology*, Vol.5, No.3, (February 1983), pp. 251-257, ISSN 1567-5769

Subramanian, H., Kashem, S. W., Collington, S. J., Qu, H., Lambris, J. D. and Ali, H. (2011). PMX-53 as a dual CD88 antagonist and an agonist for Mas-related gene 2 (MrgX2) in human mast cells. *Molecular Pharmacology*, Vol.79, No.6, (June 2011), pp. 1005-1013, ISSN 0026-895X

Szeplaki, G., Szegedi, R., Hirschberg, K., Gombos, T., Varga, L., Karadi, I., Entz, L., Szeplaki, Z., Garred, P., Prohaszka, Z. and Fust, G. (2009). Strong complement activation after acute ischemic stroke is associated with unfavorable outcomes. *Atherosclerosis*, Vol.204, No.1, (May 2009), pp. 315-320, ISSN 0021-9150

Takafuji, S., Tadokoro, K., Ito, K. and Dahinden, C. A. (1994). Degranulation from human eosinophils stimulated with C3a and C5a. *International Archives of Allergy and Immunology*, Vol.104 Suppl 1, No.1, pp. 27-29, ISSN 1018-2438

Tardif, M., Brouchon, L., Rabiet, M. J. and Boulay, F. (2003). Direct binding of a fragment of the Wiskott-Aldrich syndrome protein to the C-terminal end of the anaphylatoxin C5a receptor. *Biochemistry Journal*, Vol.372, No.Pt 2, (June 2003), pp. 453-463, ISSN 0264-6021

Taube, C., Thurman, J. M., Takeda, K., Joetham, A., Miyahara, N., Carroll, M. C., Dakhama, A., Giclas, P. C., Holers, V. M. and Gelfand, E. W. (2006). Factor B of the alternative complement pathway regulates development of airway hyperresponsiveness and inflammation. *Proceedings of the National Academy of Science of the United States of America*, Vol.103, No.21, (May 2006), pp. 8084-8089, ISSN 0027-8424

Thurman, J. M., Ljubanovic, D., Edelstein, C. L., Gilkeson, G. S. and Holers, V. M. (2003). Lack of a functional alternative complement pathway ameliorates ischemic acute renal failure in mice. *Journal of Immunology*, Vol.170, No.3, (February 2003), pp. 1517-1523, ISSN 0022-1767

Tsang, S. H., Burns, M. E., Calvert, P. D., Gouras, P., Baylor, D. A., Goff, S. P. and Arshavsky, V. Y. (1998). Role for the target enzyme in deactivation of photoreceptor G protein in vivo. *Science*, Vol.282, No.5386, (October 1998), pp. 117-121, ISSN 0036-8705

Urra, X., Cervera, A., Villamor, N., Planas, A. M. and Chamorro, A. (2009). Harms and benefits of lymphocyte subpopulations in patients with acute stroke. *Neuroscience*, Vol.158, No.3, (Feb 6 2009), pp. 1174-1183, ISSN 0306-4522

Utoh, J., Utsunomiya, T., Imamura, T., Katsuya, H., Miyauchi, Y. and Kambara, T. (1989). Complement activation and neutrophil dysfunction in burned patients with sepsis--a study of two cases. *The Japanese Journal of Surgery*, Vol.19, No.4, (July 1989), pp. 462-467, ISSN 0047-1909

Van Beek, J., Bernaudin, M., Petit, E., Gasque, P., Nouvelot, A., MacKenzie, E. T. and Fontaine, M. (2000). Expression of receptors for complement anaphylatoxins C3a and C5a following permanent focal cerebral ischemia in the mouse. *Experimental Neurology*, Vol.161, No.1, (January 2000), pp. 373-382, ISSN 0014-4886

Vasthare, U. S., Barone, F. C., Sarau, H. M., Rosenwasser, R. H., DiMartino, M., Young, W. F. and Tuma, R. F. (1998). Complement depletion improves neurological function in cerebral ischemia. *Brain Research Bulletin*, Vol.45, No.4, pp. 413-419, ISSN 0361-9230

Venkatesha, R. T., Berla Thangam, E., Zaidi, A. K. and Ali, H. (2005). Distinct regulation of C3a-induced MCP-1/CCL2 and RANTES/CCL5 production in human mast cells by extracellular signal regulated kinase and PI3 kinase. *Molecular Immunology*, Vol.42, No.5, (March 2005), pp. 581-587, ISSN 0161-5890

Vibhuti, A., Gupta, K., Subramanian, H., Guo, Q. and Ali, H. (2011). Distinct and shared roles of beta-arrestin-1 and beta-arrestin-2 on the regulation of C3a receptor signaling in human mast cells. *PLoS One*, Vol.6, No.5, (May 2011), pp. e19585, ISSN 1932-6203

Vieyra, M., Leisman, S., Raedler, H., Kwan, W. H., Yang, M., Strainic, M. G., Medof, M. E. and Heeger, P. S. (2011). Complement regulates CD4 T-cell help to CD8 T cells required for murine allograft rejection. *American Journal of Pathology*, Vol.179, No.2, (Aug ust 2011), pp. 766-774, ISSN 0002-9440

Wagner, E. and Frank, M. M. (2010). Therapeutic potential of complement modulation. *Nature Reviews Drug Discovery*, Vol.9, No.1, (January 2010), pp. 43-56, ISSN 1474-1776

Wagner, M. H., Sonntag, J., Strauss, E. and Obladen, M. (1999). Complement and contact activation related to surfactant response in respiratory distress syndrome. *Pediatric Research*, Vol.45, No.1, (January 1999), pp. 14-18, ISSN 0031-3998

Wakashin, H., Hirose, K., Maezawa, Y., Kagami, S., Suto, A., Watanabe, N., Saito, Y., Hatano, M., Tokuhisa, T., Iwakura, Y., Puccetti, P., Iwamoto, I. and Nakajima, H. (2008). IL-23 and Th17 cells enhance Th2-cell-mediated eosinophilic airway inflammation in mice. *American Journal of Respiratory Cell and Molecular Biology*, Vol.178, No.10, (November 2008), pp. 1023-1032, ISSN 1044-1549

Walters, D. M., Breysse, P. N., Schofield, B. and Wills-Karp, M. (2002). Complement factor 3 mediates particulate matter-induced airway hyperresponsiveness. *American Journal of Respiratory Cell and Molecular Biology*, Vol.27, No.4, (October 2002), pp. 413-418, ISSN 1044-1549

Ward, P.A. (2004). The dark side of C5a in sepsis. *Nature Reviews Immunology*, Vol.4, No.2, (February 2004), pp. 133-142, ISSN 1474-1733

Weaver, D. J., Jr., Reis, E. S., Pandey, M. K., Kohl, G., Harris, N., Gerard, C. and Kohl, J. (2010). C5a receptor-deficient dendritic cells promote induction of Treg and Th17 cells. *European Journal of Immunology*, Vol.40, No.3, (March 2010), pp. 710-721, ISSN 0022-1767

Webster, R. O., Zanolari, B. and Henson, P. M. (1980). Neutrophil chemotaxis in response to surface-bound C5A. *Experimental Cell Research*, Vol.129, No.1, (September 1980), pp. 55-62, ISSN 0014-4827

Weinberg, P. F., Matthay, M. A., Webster, R. O., Roskos, K. V., Goldstein, I. M. and Murray, J. F. (1984). Biologically active products of complement and acute lung injury in patients with the sepsis syndrome. *The American Review of Respiratory Disease*, Vol.130, No.5, (November 1984), pp. 791-796, ISSN 0003-0805

Weiser, M. R., Williams, J. P., Moore, F. D., Jr., Kobzik, L., Ma, M., Hechtman, H. B. and Carroll, M. C. (1996). Reperfusion injury of ischemic skeletal muscle is mediated by natural antibody and complement. *Journal of Experimental Medicine*, Vol.183, No.5, (May 1996), pp. 2343-2348, ISSN 0022-1007

Willars, G. B. (2006). Mammalian RGS proteins: multifunctional regulators of cellular signalling. *Seminars in Cell and Developmental Biology*, Vol.17, No.3, (June 2006), pp. 363-376, ISSN 1084-9521

Wills-Karp, M. (2007). Complement activation pathways: a bridge between innate and adaptive immune responses in asthma. *Proceedings of the American Thoracic Society*, Vol.4, No.3, (July 2007), pp. 247-251, ISSN 1546-3222

Wjst, M., Fischer, G., Immervoll, T., Jung, M., Saar, K., Rueschendorf, F., Reis, A., Ulbrecht, M., Gomolka, M., Weiss, E. H., Jaeger, L., Nickel, R., Richter, K., Kjellman, N. I., Griese, M., von Berg, A., Gappa, M., Riedel, F., Boehle, M., van Koningsbruggen, S., Schoberth, P., Szczepanski, R., Dorsch, W., Silbermann, M., Wichmann, H. E. and et al. (1999). A genome-wide search for linkage to asthma. German Asthma Genetics Group. *Genomics*, Vol.58, No.1, (May 1999), pp. 1-8, ISSN 0888-7543

Woodruff, T. M., Arumugam, T. V., Shiels, I. A., Reid, R. C., Fairlie, D. P. and Taylor, S. M. (2004). Protective effects of a potent C5a receptor antagonist on experimental acute limb ischemia-reperfusion in rats. *The Journal of Surgical Research*, Vol.116, No.1, (January 2004), pp. 81-90, ISSN 0022-4804

Wust, S. K., Blumenthal, M. N., Corazalla, E. O., Benson, B. A. and Dalmasso, A. P. (2006). Complement in asthma: sensitivity to activation and generation of C3a and C5a via the different complement pathways. *Translational Research: The Journal of Laboratory and Clincial Medicine*, Vol.148, No.4, (October 2006), pp. 157-163, ISSN 1931-5244

Xu, R., Wang, R., Han, G., Wang, J., Chen, G., Wang, L., Li, X., Guo, R., Shen, B. and Li, Y. (2010). Complement C5a regulates IL-17 by affecting the crosstalk between DC and gammadelta T cells in CLP-induced sepsis. *European Journal of Immunology*, Vol.40, No.4, (April 2010), pp. 1079-1088, ISSN 0022-1767

Yan, J., Allendorf, D. J., Li, B., Yan, R., Hansen, R. and Donev, R. (2008). The role of membrane complement regulatory proteins in cancer immunotherapy. *Advances in Experimental Medicine and Biology*, Vol.632, pp. 159-174, ISSN 0065-2598

Yanamadala, V. and Friedlander, R. M. (2010). Complement in neuroprotection and neurodegeneration. *Trends in Molecular Medicine*, Vol.16, No.2, (February 2010), pp. 69-76, ISSN 1471-4914

Yilmaz, G., Arumugam, T. V., Stokes, K. Y. and Granger, D. N. (2006). Role of T lymphocytes and interferon-gamma in ischemic stroke. *Circulation*, Vol.113, No.17, (May 2006), pp. 2105-2112, ISSN 0009-7322

Zhang, H., Qin, G., Liang, G., Li, J., Barrington, R. A. and Liu, D. X. (2007). C5aR-mediated myocardial ischemia/reperfusion injury. *Biochemical and Biophysical Research Communications*, Vol.357, No.2, (June 2007), pp. 446-452, ISSN 0006-291X

Zheng, X., Zhang, X., Feng, B., Sun, H., Suzuki, M., Ichim, T., Kubo, N., Wong, A., Min, L. R., Budohn, M. E., Garcia, B., Jevnikar, A. M. and Min, W. P. (2008). Gene silencing of complement C5a receptor using siRNA for preventing ischemia/reperfusion injury. *American of Journal Pathology*, Vol.173, No.4, (October 2008), pp. 973-980, ISSN 0002-9440

Zhang, X., Lewkowich, I. P., Kohl, G., Clark, J. R., Wills-Karp, M. and Kohl, J. (2009). A protective role for C5a in the development of allergic asthma associated with altered levels of B7-H1 and B7-DC on plasmacytoid dendritic cells. *Journal of Immunology*, Vol.182, No.8, (April 2009), pp. 5123-5130, ISSN 0022-1767

Zhang, X., Schmudde, I., Laumonnier, Y., Pandey, M. K., Clark, J. R., Konig, P., Gerard, N. P., Gerard, C., Wills-Karp, M. and Kohl, J. (2010). A critical role for C5L2 in the pathogenesis of experimental allergic asthma. *Journal of Immunology*, Vol.185, No.11, (December 2010), pp. 6741-6752, ISSN 0022-1767

Zhou, W., Patel, H., Li, K., Peng, Q., Villiers, M. B. and Sacks, S. H. (2006). Macrophages from C3-deficient mice have impaired potency to stimulate alloreactive T cells. *Blood*, Vol.107, No.6, (March 2006), pp. 2461-2469, ISSN

Zimmermann, T., Laszik, Z., Nagy, S., Kaszaki, J. and Joo, F. (1989). The role of the complement system in the pathogenesis of multiple organ failure in shock. *Progress in Clinical and Biological Research*, Vol.308, (1989), pp. 291-297, ISSN 0361-7742

10

Parasitic Infections and Inflammatory Diseases

Joziana M.P. Barçante[1], Thales A. Barçante[2],
Ana Paula Peconick[1], Luciano J. Pereira[1] and Walter S. Lima[3]
[1]*Departamento de Medicina Veterinária, Universidade Federal de Lavras*
[2]*ICBS, Pontifícia Universidade Católica de Minas Gerais*
[3]*Departamento de Parasitologia, Universidade Federal de Minas Gerais*
Brazil

1. Introduction

The mammalian immune system is continuously exposed to infectious microorganisms as well as innocuous substances in the environment. Depending on the genetic makeup, the innate and adaptive immune responses develop and determine the frequency and the course of infectious diseases. The immune response to an infection is initiated by molecular recognition of damage-associated patterns (DAMPs) by receptors of the innate immunity, that, most of the time, occurs as an inflammatory reaction (Turvey & Broide, 2010).

The inflammation associated to parasite organisms is a complex reaction of the vascular tissues against infection, exposition to toxins or cellular injury involving extravascular accumulation of plasmatic proteins and leukocytes, as well as production of cytokines from the injured tissue. It is an essential component of multifactorial pathogenesis involved in different diseases (Scrivo et al., 2011). The acute inflammation is a common result of innate immune response; however local immune adaptative factors can also promote inflammation (Lukic et al., 2009). The morphologic transformations and functional characteristics of immunological responses and consequently, of the inflammatory processes intend to destroy, to dilute or to isolate the harmful agent. Virtually, all the acute or chronic diseases are lead or modulated by the inflammation. Although the inflammation serves to a protective function in the control of parasitic infections and promotion of tecidual repair, this can also cause injury and illness itself. Schistosomiasis is an exemple of parasitary disease caused predominantly by the host immune response to schistosome eggs (ova) and the granulomatous reaction they evoke (Burke et al., 2009). In some cases, the inflammation can even persist after the removal of the infectious agent, contributing to the chronic inflammation (Vodovotz et al., 2009).

Amongst the various infectious agents, helminth parasites are regarded as master manipulators of the host immune system, often inducing a long-lasting asymptomatic form of infection. Parasitic worms can establish and reproduce in mammalian hosts, switching off the inflammatory immune response and inducing a tolerant response to parasite antigens. The time of duration and the intensity of the inflammatory agent determine different degrees or phases of transformation in tissues (Zaccone et al., 2006).

Chronic infection with high burden of helminths can induce regulatory mechanisms to prevent excessive inflammation. Recent studies regarding immunological interactions between eosinophils and helminthic parasites have made important advances in understanding the innate role of eosinophils in controlling eosinophil-associated tissue inflammation involved in infection by tissue migratory helminthic parasites (Shin et al., 2009). These regulatory mechanisms may also affect the immune responses against other antigens, because it promotes a polarization of the response. The identification of regulatory mechanisms has already helped developing new models to understand helminth infections, which remain among the most prevalent chronic diseases in the world today. Several studies have verified that helminths can downregulate a range of immunopathological conditions, with the regulatory T cell being one of the most common mechanisms in play (Fallon & Mangan, 2007; Maizels & Yazdanbakhsh, 2008).

2. Helminth infection and inflammation

The inflammation involves a set of complex interactions between soluble factors and cells that can appear in any tissue during traumatic, infectious, after-ischemic, toxic or auto-immune injury (Nathan, 2002). It represents an adaptation of the loss of the cellular and tecidual homostasis, with important physiological functions, that include the defense of the organism host, remodelling and tecidual repairing, regulation of the metabolism, amongst others, controlled by transcription of genes (Medzhitov, 2008; Medzhitov & Horng, 2009).

The cellular profile of the acute inflammatory response is constituted basically by lymphocytes, neutrophils, monocytes, eosinophils and mast cells. The most defined subgroups of effective cells of CD4+ cellular ancestry are the Th1 and Th2 cells. These subgroups develop from CD4+ naïve (inactive) precursors and the differentiation pattern is initiated by stimulations at the beginning of the immunological response. INF-γ is the cytokine of signature of the Th1 cells; whereas IL- 4 and IL-5 are the cytokines that define Th2 cells. Th1 and Th2 Cells can also differentiate from the distinguishing expression of molecules of adhesion and receptors of chemokines and other cytokines. It is important to determine if the response to a pathogen will lead to protection of the host or to the evolution of the illness and this can be verified by the balance between Th1 and Th2 response (Jankovic et al., 2001; Yates et al., 2004). It has been also characterized the Th17 sub-group with pro-inflammatory activity, mainly in auto-immune illnesses, and the main cytokine involved is IL-17 (Weaver et al., 2006).

The Th2 cells are involved in the differentiation and proliferation of B lymphocytes, in the production of antibodies and activation of cells of the innate immune system. Therefore, the eosinophils found in subacute inflammations caused by helminthes, are very important cells in the inflammatory response mediated by Th2 cells. The neutrophils have high potential of diapedesis and fast migration speed, present fagocitic action, if deceased, can provoke tecidual necrosis due to the release of its lysosomal enzymes in the interstice. Basophils and mast cells are granular cells that have their number increased in chronic processes. The macrophages, originated from monocytes, are professional mononuclear fagocitc cells and antigen presenters that in the parasitic infection are activated by an alternative form, dependent on Th2 cytokines (Rothenberg & Hogan, 2006).

The vascular and esudative alterations that originate the inflammatory clinical signals (heat, redness, tumor, pain and loss of the function) culminate with the last inflammatory phase, the productive-reparative phase (Lukic et al., 2009).

The chronic response is a tecidual reaction characterized by the increase of the degrees of cells and other tissue elements next to the repairing area, ahead of the permanence of the aggressive agent. The chronic inflammation is always preceded by the acute inflammation. Clinically, in the chronic inflammation, the characteristic cardinal signals of the acute reactions are not observed (Cuzzocrea, 2005).
Although many physiological functions of the inflammatory response are unknown, the pathological aspects of diverse types of inflammation are well described and many are the organisms that serve as models for elucidating those concepts (Medzhitov, 2008).
Infection with helminth parasites induces immune effector responses that are characterized by IgE antibody production, tissue and peripheral blood eosinophilia, and participation of inflammatory mediator-rich tissue mast cells (Klion & Nutman, 2004). In parasitic infections, although these types of responses can certainly induce pathologic reactions, they have also been implicated in mediating protective immunity to the helminth parasites. Helminth infections are associated with a predominant induction of a Th2 type of immune response, that involves the interaction of signals from the T cells receptors, transcription factors like T-bet, STAT-6 and GATA-3 and cellular interactions mediated by cytokines (Jankovic et al., 2001; Yates et al., 2004). The Th2 response is polarized by interleukins: IL-4, IL-5, IL-9 and IL-13 (Fallon & Mangan, 2007). Activated mast cells, eosinophils and basophils infiltrate in the tissue as result of a Th2 exacerbated cellular type reaction that initiates the production of IgE and promote the tecidual eosinophilia and mast cells hyperplasia (Rothenberg & Hogan, 2006). The main points of the anti-helmintic response promoted by the Th2 profile are schematized in figure 1. Helminthes cause chronic stimulation of T cells, mostly without the strong immune natural reaction that is necessary for Th1 differentiation. Thus, Th2 cells can develop in response to the *A. vasorum* that possibly caused persistent or repeated stimulation of the T cells with little inflammation or activation of macrophages.

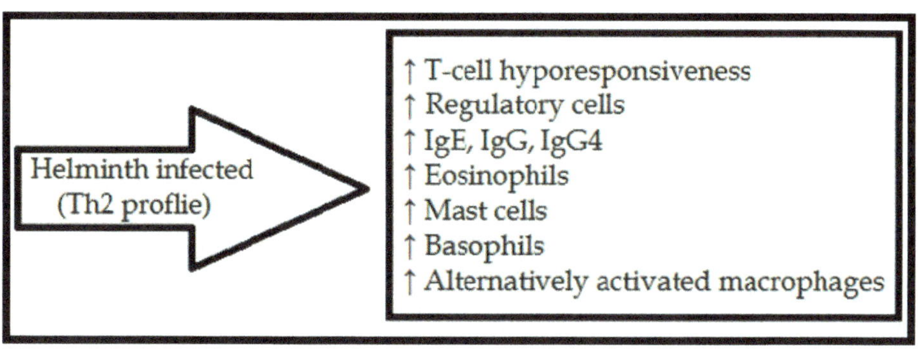

Fig. 1. Imunological alterations of the Th2 profile caused by helminth infections (Adapted from Fallon & Mangan, 2007).

The Th2 type response does not demand the activation of dendritic cells by microbial adjuvants, differently of the Th1 cells. It is reported that the initial production of IL-4 is not elicited by T cells (or at least not conventional T cells) in reaction to a constant infection that was not capable to induce an exacerbated initial inflammatory response by the production of INF-γ (Jankovic et al., 2001).

Helminth infections can modulate allergic processes due to association with the development of the Th2 response. They also stimulate regulatory mechanisms associated to animal suppression of the allergic response in human beings and animal models (Fallon & Mangan, 2007). Previous studies confirm this attractive potential of helminth infections to produce a suppressor reaction to different concomitant processes (Lukic et al., 2009).

3. The parasite model

Angiostrongylus vasorum is a nematode of the Metastrongyloidea superfamily which adult form is found in the right ventricle, pulmonary artery (and its branches) of domestic dogs and wild carnivores. The *A. vasorum* is widely spread in all continents. The infection is highly prevalent in dogs in the southeast of France, the United Kingdom, Ireland and Uganda (Guilhon & Cens 1973; Dodd 1973; Bwagamoi 1974) with several cases reported in the United States, Canada and Brazil (Lima et al. 1985; Lima et al. 1994; Edwards, 1995; Duarte et al., 2007).

Adult worms of *A. vasorum* live in the right ventricle of the heart and the pulmonary artery, where sexual reproduction and oviposture take place. The first-stage larvae (L1) hatch into the alveoli, migrate up the bronchial tree, are swallowed and eliminated to the environment with the host feces. The intermediate host, snails and slugs, either terrestrial or aquatic become infected through invasion or ingestion of L1. Larvae invade mollusks tissues where they undergo first and second molts, reaching the infective third-stage larvae (L3) (Guilhon & Afghahi, 1969; Rosen et al., 1970). Infection of the dog results from ingestion of free L3; ingestion of infective intermediate host or paratenic host (Barçante et al., 2003). Third-stage larvae (L3) invade mesenteric lymph nodes where they undergo third and fourth molt molts. Young adult nematodes migrate to the right side of the heart and pulmonary artery where they develop to sexual maturity.

A determinant factor in the pathology of canine angiostrongylosis seems to be related to the location of the parasite in the definitive host. The presence of the parasite inside the arteries and branches of the host promotes a mechanical and metabolic action on the vessels walls, which may alter its homeostasis, resulting in pneumonia, loss of racing performance, coughing and anemia (Jones et al., 1980). Severely infected dogs may develop cardiac insufficiency, pulmonary fibrosis followed by weight loss, hemorrhagic diatheses and death (Dood, K., 1973. *Angiostrongylus vasorum* (Baillet, 1866) infestation in a greyhound kennels.*Vet. Rec.* 92, p. 195.Dood, 1973; Lombard 1984; Cury & Lima, 1995; Costa & Tafuri, 1997; Oliveira-Jr et al., 2004).

In this context, *Angiostrongylus vasorum* has been used as a model for the study of pulmonary inflammatory diseases. In this series of experiments, we observed that the Bronchoalveolar lavage (BAL) is a valuable diagnostic technique that also provides additional diagnostic information for canine angiostrongylosis. In spite of the fact that the parasitological examination of the feces is considered the main standard for the diagnosis of angiostrongylosis in the patent period of the disease, the occurrence of animals with clinical symptomatology and without eliminating larvae with the feces is not rare (Barçante et al., 2008). The aims of this chapter is to present the results of BAL as a procedure to evaluate the acute and chronic phases of an *Angiostrongylus vasorum* infection for cytological and serological analyses of an pulmonary inflammatory disease caused by a parasitary infection.

3.1 Bronchoalveolar lavage (BAL) procedure

BAL is a procedure that retrieves cells and other elements from the lungs for evaluation, which helps in the diagnosis of many inflammatory and pulmonary diseases. The technique is considered to be a safe procedure performed in dogs to collect samples from the lungs (Clercx & Peeters, 2007, Basso et al., 2008, Hawkins et al., 2008).

BAL has been used to obtain specimens that could represent a development in distal lung, to diagnose viral, bacterial, protozoal and fungal infections, as well as neoplasia and other diseases (Hawkins, 1992). Cytologic and microbiologic evaluation of the fluid can be used to characterize pulmonary and inflammatory diseases in several mammalians species (Hawkins et al., 2008).

In the present work, the BAL procedure was performed through the use of an endotracheal tube on seven *A. vasorum* infected dogs and on five non-infected dogs lined as a control group.

3.2 Animals

Twelve one-year-old mongrel dogs (*C. familiaris*) free from any *A. vasorum* infections were used in this experiment. Following the manufacturer's directions, the dogs were treated 15, 30, 60 and 90 days after their birth with 7.5 mg of praziquantel; 7.5 mg of pyrantel and 37.5 mg of febantel per kg of body weight (Drontal®, Bayer-Saúde Animal, São Paulo, SP, Brazil) in order to eliminate any worm infections caused by other common canine parasites.

The experimentation protocols are in agreement with the Ethical Principles in Animal Experimentation, adopted by the Ethics Committee in Animal Experimentation (CETEA/UFMG), and were approved under number 060/03.

3.3 Parasitic infection

First-stage larvae of *A. vasorum* (L1) were isolated as described by Barçante et al. (2003). Third-stage larvae (L3) were recovered from snails, as described by Barçante (2004), and counted under a stereomicroscope (40×).

Seven dogs were orally inoculated with 100 L3 of *A. vasorum* per kilogram of body weight. Five non-infected animals were kept as control. From 20 days post-infection (dpi) to 330 dpi, fecal samples were collected daily from the cage of each animal of the infected group and submitted to a modified Baermann apparatus (Barçante et al., 2003) to recover the L1 to determine the pre-patent period (PPP).

BAL was performed on days 0, 30, 60, 90, 120, 180, 240 and 330 after the infection with *A. vasorum* L3 as described by Barçante et al. (2008).

3.4 Cellular evaluation of BAL

The viability of the cell population was estimated from 10 µL of total BALF diluted 1/10 in RPMI medium containing 0.4% Trypan Blue (Sigma). Membrane-damaged cells allowed the fast penetration of Trypan Blue, and these blue cells were immediately counted in a Neubauer's chamber and assumed as not viable. In order to quantify the recovered cells, the BALF was separated from the supernatant and cells through centrifugation at 200 × *g* for 10 min at 4 °C. The cell pellet was washed twice with a RPMI-1640 medium (Gibco, Grand Island, NY, USA) and resuspended in complete RPMI (10% fetal calf serum added). Total cell counts were determined by using a Neubauer's chamber. For differential cell counts, aliquots were removed to make a final concentration of 1×10^5 cells/mL and the cytocentrifuge preparations (Cytospin 2, Southern Instruments, UK) were stained with May-Grünwald-Giemsa. The differential cell counts were performed based on the morphological appearance of the cells and on the frequency in which they appear. The total number of cells counted was 200 cells per preparation (Barçante et al., 2008).

The healthy immune system must keep the balance in order to react against infectious agents, to finish the immune response and to support the self-tolerance. The absence of adequate response submits the individual to deleterious effects of the invasion pathogen, since an overreaction can generate harmful inflammatory processes. The recent demonstration of different phenotype of cells, now called T regulatory cells, reintroduced the paradigm that the auto-reactivity and exacerbated responses are also regulated by particular subtypes of lymphocytes (Cruvinel et al., 2008). Characteristically, parasitic helminthes can infect their hosts for years or decades. To achieve such chronic infections, the host's immune system is tolerated to the presence of the parasite through the stimulation of selective immune suppression. Host immune responses limit, and in some instances eliminate nematode infections. There is considerable interest in enhancing these natural processes to achieve the control of infection or disease. Characteristically, parasitic helminths can infect their hosts for years or decades. To achieve such chronic infections, the host's immune system is tolerated to the presence of the parasite through the stimulation of selective immune suppression (Fallon & Mangan, 2007). Host immune responses limit, and in some instances eliminate nematode infections (Yazdanbakhsh et al., 2001). There is considerable interest in enhancing these natural processes to achieve the control of infection or disease.

This work reports that the *A. vasorum* infection resulted in an increase of relative neutrophils and eosinophils counts. In contrast, there was a significant decrease in the alveolar macrophage relative count in infected animals from 60 to 330 dpi. This study showed that the technique allowed retrieving cells and other elements that line the lung surface for cytological and serological evaluation, which provided information about inflammatory diseases, and the diagnosis and prognosis of pulmonary parasites such as *A. vasorum*.

There were no significant differences in the total average cell counts and the differential cell count data for non-infected animals among the seven procedures ($p > 0.05$) (Fig.2). On average, 69% or more of all nucleated cells in all the BALF of non-infected dogs were alveolar macrophages (Fig. 2A). Neutrophils accounted for 12% of the nucleated cells in the BALF from non-infected animals. On average, lymphocytes accounted for 14%, and eosinophils, for 4% of the nucleated cells. Epithelial cells were less than 1% of the total number of nucleated cells. This profile was unaltered during the 330 days of research (Fig. 2).

The differential cell count revealed significant differences between infected and non-infected dogs. Differently from what was observed in non-infected animals, dogs infected with *A. vasorum* showed notable variations in relative differential cell counts during the infection (Fig. 3). Absolute counts of infected animals revealed that alveolar macrophage showed a significant increase in number at 30 and 180 dpi. Relative counts showed that alveolar macrophage accounted for 73.1% of the cell population at day 0. Then there was a significant

decrease to an average of almost 25% of the cell population in infected animals from 60 to 330 dpi. Multinucleated giant cells were also identified (Fig. 4A).
Neutrophils were well preserved and were morphologically similar to those in peripheral blood. Cytoplasm was clear to slightly granular. Nuclear hypersegmentation (more than four distinct nuclear lobes) was seen occasionally. From 30 to 330 dpi, the relative number and absolute number of neutrophils was significantly elevated in the animals in the infected group ($p < 0.05$). Neutrophils comprised the vast majority of all cells seen from 90 to 330 dpi (Fig. 3, Fig. 4B).

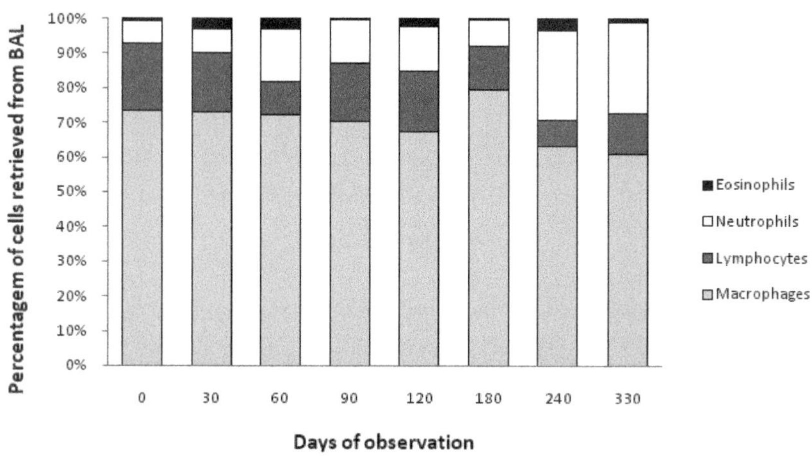

Fig. 2. Differential cell count (%) of the bronchoalveolar lavage fluid of the five non-infected dogs lined as a control group.

Eosinophils were clearly identified in the May-Grünwald-Giemsa stained specimens because of the presence of distinct eosinophlic cytoplasmic granules of various sizes. Nuclei of some eosinophils were lobed and the cells, therefore, resembled the circulating eosinophili of peripheral blood; however, in many eosinophils, the nucleus was spherical or ovoid rather than lobed, and was eccentrically located (Fig.4C). Absolute counts of infected animals revealed that eosinophils showed a significant increase in number from 30 to 330 dpi (Fig. 3). Relative counts showed that the eosinophils accounted for 2.8% of the cell population at day 0, and had a remarkable increase during the infection. Eosinophils predominated, accounting for 50.6% at 30 dpi and 37.1% at 60 dpi. From 30 to 330 dpi, the number of eosinophils in the BALF was significantly greater than in the non-infected animals or the normal values described in current literature.
The lymphocytes appeared as small round cells. The nuclei were round with dense chromatin patterns. Absolute counts of infected animals revealed that alveolar lymphocytes showed a significant increase in number at 30, 60 and 120 dpi. Relative counts showed that this type was increased in infected dogs from 30 to 120 dpi ($p < 0.05$) (Fig. 3). The lymphocytes accounted for 13.4% of the cell population at day zero and had a slight decrease during the infection with no statistical significance ($p > 0.05$).

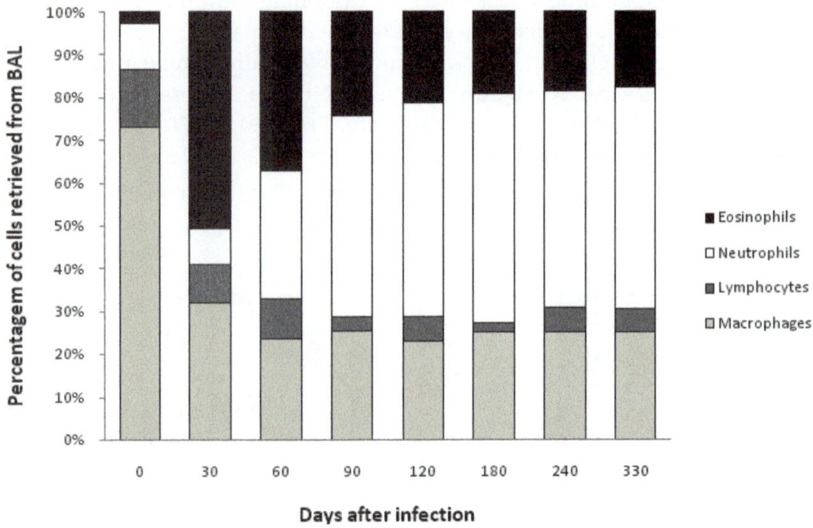

Fig. 3. Differential cell count (%) of the bronchoalveolar lavage fluid of the seven dogs infected with 100 third stage larva of Angiostrongylus vasorum/kg body weight.

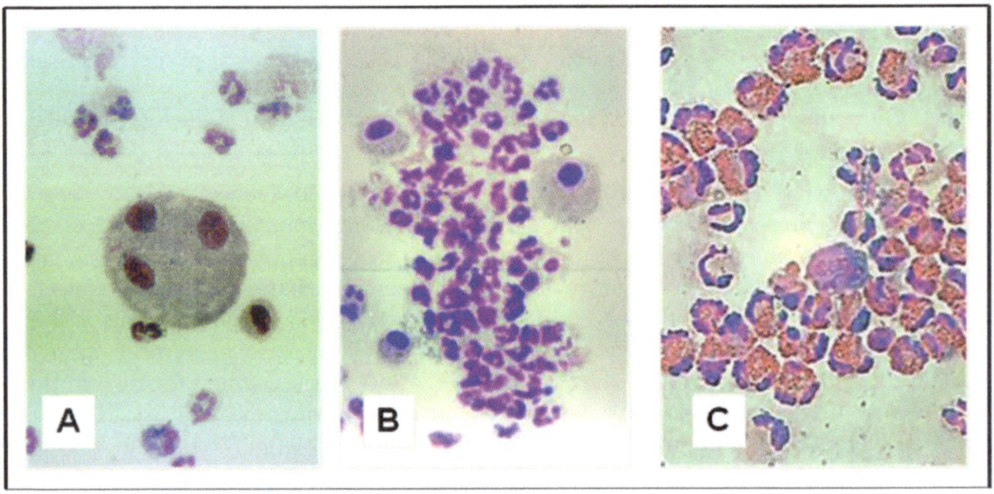

Fig. 4. Cytocentrifuged preparation of bronchoalveolar lavage fluid (BALF) from infected and non-infected dogs. May-Grünwald-Giemsa's stain. (A) BALF of a dog with chronical angiostrongylosis (120 dpi). The field contains a multinucleated giant cell (arrow) surrounded by neutrophils (40X objective). (B) BALF of a dog with chronical angiostrongylosis (120 dpi). The field contains a large amount of neutrophils. (C) BALF of a dog with acute angiostrongylosis (30 dpi). The predominant cells are eosinophils with presence of distinct eosinophlic cytoplasmic granules of various sizes.

4. Eosinophil response to parasitary infection

Profound blood and tissue eosinophilia are among the hallmark features of parasitic helminth infection, observed in response to activation of $CD4^{+}$ TH2 lymphocyte at specific stage of parasite life cycle (Rothenberg & Hogan, 2006). Despite of this, the kinetics of eosinophilia after infection with any parasitic infection have been difficult to define because the time of initial infection can be defined only rarely (Klion & Nutman, 2004). However, in the present study we described an experimental animal infection with the initiation of the eosinophilia and its natural regulation.

The eosinophils were proven to play a major role in the immune response to helminthic infections. Eosinophilia has been pointed out as a key factor in many helminthic infections, which demonstrated that eosinophils and neutrophils can be attracted and activated by host mediators or antigens excreted or secreted (E/S) by *Onchocerca volvulus*. Therefore, we can correlate the eosinophils and also the neutrophils influx in the lungs of infected dogs with the biology of the lifecycle of the parasite involved. Furthermore, larva growth and its products of secretion and excretion are known to induce an increase in pulmonary cellularity. In this context, transendothelial migration is essential for eosinophil recruitment from blood vessels into inflammatory tissues. The selective homing of Th2 cells in certain sites of inflammation is different from the Th1. The Th2 cells recruitment is dependent of particular chemokines that are highly expressed in places of helminthic infection, particularly in mucous tissues. At the inflammatory site, further interaction with invading parasites occurs via adherence with subsequent larval damage mediated by releases of eosinophil toxic granular effector molecules.

In this series of experiments, it was observed that the high pulmonary cellularity is inversely proportional to the larval output in dog feces. The larva migration from the vessels to the alveoli seems to be difficult because of the inflammatory process of the mucosal system, which consists of a mechanical and immunological barrier to larvae. The immune response that develops during this time often proceeds to cause pathologic changes that must be the primary cause of disease, since eosinophils exert a functional duality, participating in protective immune responses during parasitary infections as well as in the induction of cell and tissue damage. As results of the cell and tissue damage the larva spreads to different organs and tissues of the dog because of this mechanical barrier. The presence of larvae in sites different from those described in the natural route of the parasite lifecycle generally leads to animal death or lesions that can change the normal organ function. In this way, during chronic *A. vasorum* infection, the cellular infiltration typically observed is constituted predominantly of eosinophils and neutrophils. The eosinophils recruited into worm-infected tissues are further activated by various inflammatory stimuli, which may contribute to related eosinophil-mediated tissue inflammatory responses (Shin et al., 2009).

Despite major changes in the pulmonary cellularity following immunodulation that takes place during the chronic infection, the eosinophils may play an important role in the innate immune response of chronic infection. The activated eosinophils secrete the content of its granules, including main basic and cationic proteins, which are capable to destroy even the resistant tegument of helminthes, as it represents a relevant protective mechanism. These proteins perform various biological activities. Cytotoxic granules injure both the host tissue and the parasite (Brushi et al., 2008). It has been suggested that the immunoglobulins IgG and IgA are able to trigger eosinophils degranulation (Hogan et al., 2008). However, the presence of IgE receptors on eosinophils remains controversial. Recently, T cell has also been shown to have a role in eosinophil degranulation. Knockout mice that lacked T and B cells were infected with *Nippostrongylus brasiliensis*, and IL-4- expressing eosinophils were recruited to pulmonary tissues but failed to degranulate. Reconstruction with CD-4$^+$ T cells promoted the accumulation of degranulated IL-4-expressing eosinophils, but only if the T cells were stimulated with a cognate antigen. These facts indicate that T-helper cells confer antigen specificity on eosinophils cytotoxicity but not on the cytokine responses (Brushi et al., 2008).

In the present work, we demonstrated that a peak eosinophil levels occurs 30-60 days after infection, which is consistent with the pre-patent period and initial larvae release. At the inflammatory site, it was observed larval damage mediated by releases of eosinophil toxic granular effector molecules. More interesting was a spontaneous decrease in eosinophil numbers in the absence of treatment, suggesting active downregulation of the eosinophlia. This active and spontaneous modulation of eosinophilia generally occurs when infections became patent (sexually mature adults began egg laying and larval release) (Klion & Nutman, 2004).

5. Mast cells – Eosinophils interaction

As one of the most highly cationic proteins synthesized by eosinophils, MBP (major basic protein) is a small protein that is expressed as two different homologs (MBP1 e MBP2). A substantial body of literature has emerged demonstrating that eosinophils have the capacity to regulate mast cell function (Rothenberg & Hogan, 2006). Several studies have shown that MBP induces mast cell activation. Interestingly, activation of eosinophils with the mast cell protease chymase promotes production of eosinophil-derived stem cell factor, a crictical mast cell growth factor (Rothenberg & Hogan, 2006). Eosinophils also produce nerve growth factor (NGF), a cytokine involved in survival, functional maintenance of sympathetic neurons and also in immune regulation. This cytokine is performed in eosinophil which promotes mast cell survival and activation and acts in an autocrine fashion by activating release of eosinophil peroxidase (EPO). EPO activates rat peritoneal muscles to release histamine, suggesting a role of eosinophil-derived NGF in mast cell-eosinophil interactions. Thus, eosinophil and mast cells communicate in a bidirectional fashion (Rothenberg & Hogan, 2006).

6. Antihelmintic therapy

In a recent article published by Morgan and Shaw (2010) it was reported that three antihelmintic drugs have been employed for the treatment of *A. vasorum* infection in dogs: Fenbendazole (off label use - Panacur, Intervet-Schering Plough Animal Health - 25-50 mg/kg orally once daily for 7-21 days); Milbemycin oxime (Milbemax, Novartis Animal Health 0.5 mg/kg orally once weekly for 4 weeks) and Moxidectin (Advocate, Bayer Animal Health Minimum 2.5 mg/kg topically - 0.1 ml/kg of 2.5% spot-on, single dose). Mebendazole (50-100 mg/kg orally two times daily over five to 10 days) was also considered effective elsewhere (Bolt et al., 1994).

Antihelmintic drugs are told to reduce adult worm burdens in experimental infected dogs (Milbemycin oxime) and also prevent establishment of adult parasites (Moxidectin) (Conboy, 2004; Schnyder et al., 2009). It is reported that antigens released during therapy (anaphylactic shock) and dead adult stages (emboli) can cause side effects (Staebler et al.,

2006).Corticosteroids can be used to prevent adverse reactions to killed worm antigen and to reduce fibrosis in recuperating lungs. The significance of these effects has not yet been recognized. Treatment is more likely to be successful with early antihelmintic therapy, which, given the low sensitivity of larval recognition, should not necessarily be delayed until an ultimate diagnosis is reached (Morgan & Shaw; 2010).

7. Conclusion

In this review, we emphasize two points. The first is that the BAL technique allowed the retrieval of cells and other elements that line the lung surface (airway) for cytological evaluation, providing information about inflammatory diseases and possible diagnosis and prognosis of pulmonary parasites like *A. vasorum*. The second is that in angiostrongyliasis, tissue-migratory phase has evolved to attenuate eosinophil-mediated tissue inflammatory responses for their survival in hosts.

We can conclude that BAL is an accurate technique for the diagnosis of canine angiostrongylosis, especially in situations when fecal exams are parasitologically negative and the clinical symptomatology matches the infection.

In this sense, the present chapter meant to point out that BAL is an important instrument for the differential diagnosis of occult infections and an auxiliary method for *A. vasorum* infection follow-up. In addition, an important model for the study of Th2 immune response and object of study to think of immune system modulation.

8. References

Barçante, J.M., Barçante, T.A., Ribeiro, V.M., Oliveira-Jr, S.D., Dias, S.R.C., Negrão-Corrêa, D., Lima, W.S. (2008). Cytological and parasitological analysis of bronchoalveolar lavage fluid for the diagnosis of Angiostrongylus vasorum infection in dogs, *Veterinary Parasitology* Vol. 158: 93-102.

Barçante, J.M.P. (2004). Aspectos clínicos, parasitológicos e imunológicos de cães experimentalmente infectados por Angiostrongylus vasorum, *Rev. Bras. Parasitol. Vet.* Vol. 13: 96–99.

Barçante, J.M.P., Barçante, T.A., Dias, S.R.C., Vieira, L.Q., Lima,W.S., Negrão-Corrêa, D.A. (2003). A method to obtain Angiostrongylus vasorum first-stage larvae from dog feces. *Parasitol. Res.* Vol. 89: 89–93.

Basso, P.C., Barcellos, H.H.A., Brun,M.V., Rodrigues, L.B., Bortolini, C.E., Melatti, L., Neto, J.F.S., Bastiani, P.V., Valle, S.F., Santos, L.R. (2008). Tracheobronchic washing in dogs by means of rigid endoscopy or endotracheal tube. Cienc. Rural 38: 723–728.

Bolt, G., Monrad, J., Koch, J., Jensen, A.L. (1994). Canine angiostrongylosis: a review. Vet. Rec. Vol. 135:447-52.

Bruschi, F., Korenaga, M., Watanabe, N. (2008) Eosinophils and Trichinella infection: toxic for the parasite and the host? *Trends in Parasitology*, Vol. 24: 462-467.

Burke, M.L., Jones, M.K., Gobert, G.N., Li, Y.S., Ellis, M.K., McManus, D.P. (2009). Immunopathogenesis of human schistosomiasis, *Parasite Immunol.* Vol. 31(4): 163-76.

Bwangamoi, O. (1974). Renal Lymphoyd and pulmonary lesion in naturally acquired canine angiostrongylosis in Uganda, *Bull. Epizoot. Dis. Afr.* Vol. 22: 55-68.

Clercx, C., Peeters, D. (2007). Canine eosinophilic bronchopneumopath., *Vet. Clin. N. Am. Small Anim. Pract.* Vol. 37: 917–935.

Conboy, G. (2004). Natural infections of *Crenosoma vulpis* and *Angiostrongylus vasorum* in dogs in Atlantic Canada and their treatment with milbemycin oxime, *Veterinary Record* Vol. 155, 16-18.

Costa, J.O., Tafuri, W.L. (1997). Estudo anátomo-patológico de cães infectados experimentalmente pelo Angiostrongylus vasorum (Baillet, 1866) Kamenski 1905, *Arq. Bras. Med. Vet. Zootec.*Vol. 49: 389–407.

Cruvinel, W.M., Mesquita, Jr D., Araújo, J.A.P., Salmazi, K.C., Kallas, E.G., Andrade, L.E.C. (2008). Células T Regulatórias Naturais (TREGS) em Doenças Reumáticas, *Rev Bras Reumatol* Vol. 48(6): 342-355.

Cury, M.C., Lima, W.S. (1995). Aspectos clínicos de cães infectados experimentalmente com Angiostrongylus vasorum, *Arq. Bras. Med. Vet. Zootec.*Vol. 48: 27–34.

Cuzzocrea, S. (2005). Shock, inflammation and PARP, *Pharmacological Research* Vol. 52:72–82.

Dodd, K. (1973). *Angiostrongylus vasorum* (Baillet, 1866) infestation in a greyhound Kennels, *Vet. Rec.* Vol. 92: 195-197.

Fallon, P.G., Mangan, N.E. (2007). Suppression of TH2-type allergic reactions by helminth infection, *Nature Rev.*Vol. 7:220-230.

Guilhon, J., Cens, B. (1973). Angiostrongylus vasorum (Baillet, 1866) Etude biologique et morfologique. *Ann. Parasitol.* Vol. 48: 567–596.

Hawkins, E.C. (1992). Diagnostic tests for the lower respiratory tract. In: Nelson, R.W., Couto, G.C. (Eds.), Essentials of Small Animal Internal Medicine. Mosby, Philadelphia, p. 185.

Hawkins, E.C., DeNicola, D.B., Kuehn, N.F. (2008). Bronchoalveolar lavage in the evaluation of pulmonary disease in the dog and cat, *J. Vet. Intern. Med.* Vol. 4: 267–274.

Hogan, S.P. *et al.* (2008.) Eosinophils: biological properties and role in health and disease, *Clin. Exp. Allergy* Vol. 38: 709–750.

Jankovic, D., Liu, Z., Gause, W.C. (2001). Th1- and Th2-cell commitment during infectious disease: asymmetry in divergent pathways, *Trends Immunol.* Vol. 22(8): 450-457.

Jones, G.W., Neal, C., Turner, G.R.J. 1980. Angiostrongylus vasorum infection in dogs in Cornwall, Vet. Rec. Vol. 26: 83.

Khatami, M. 2005. Developmental phases of inflammation induced massive lymphoid hyperplasia and extensive changes in epithelium in an experimental model of allergy. Implications for a direct link between inflammation and carcinogenesis, *American Journal of Therapeutics*. Vol. 12: 117–126.

Khatami, M. 2006. Focusing on promotion of innate immune response system for therapy, diagnosis and prevention of tumor/ cancer (abstract). In 4th annual cytokine and inflammation conference (pp. 30–31). San Diego, CA.

Khatami, M. 2007. Standardizing cancer biomarkers criteria: Data elements as a foundation for a database. Inflammatory mediator/M-CSF as model marker, *Cell Biochemistry and Biophysics*. Vol. 47: 187–198.

Khatami, M. 2008. "Yin and Yang" in inflammation: Duality in innate immune cell function and tumorigenesis, *Expert Opinion on Biological Therapy*. Vol. 8: 1461–1472.

Khatami, M. 2009. Inflammation, Aging, and Cancer: Tumoricidal Versus Tumorigenesis of Immunity, *Cell Biochem Biophys.* Vol. 55: 55-79.

Klion, A.D., Nutman, T.B. (2004). The role of eosinophil in host defense against helminth parasites, *J Allergy Clin Immunol.* Vol. 113:30-37.

Lima, W.S.; Costa, H.M.A.; Guimarães, M.P.; Leite, A.C.R. (1985). *Angiostrongylus vasorum* (Baillet, 1866) Nematoda: Prothostrongylidae em cães de Minas Gerais, Brasil, *Mem. Inst. Oswaldo Cruz* Vol.80: 233-235.

Lima, W.S.; Guimarães, M.P.; Lemos, I.S. (1994). Occurrence of *Angiostrongylus vasorum* in the lungs of Brasilian fox *Dusicyon vetulus, J. Helminthol.* Vol.68: 87.

Lukic, M.L., Arsenijevic, N., Mitchison, N.A. (2009). Inflammation at the interface of Innate and Acquired Immunity, *Molecular Immunology* Vol. 47: 1–2.

Maizels, R.M., Yazdanbakhsh, M. (2008) T-cell regulation in helminth parasite infections: implications for inflammatory diseases, *Chem Immunol Allergy* Vol. 94:112-23.

Medzhitov, R. (2008). Origin and physiological roles of inflammation, *Nature* Vol. 454: 428-435.

Medzhitov, R., Horng, T. (2009). Transcriptional control of the inflammatory response. *Nature Rev.* Vol. 9:692-703.

Morgan, E., Shaw, S. (2010). Angiostrongylus vasorum infection in dogs: continuing spread and developments in diagnosis and treatment, *J. Small Anim Pract.* Vol. 51(12): 616-21.

Nathan, C. (2002). Points of control in inflammation, *Nature* Vol. 420: 846–852.

Oliveira-Jr, S.D., Barçante, J.M.P., Barçante, T.A., Ribeiro, V.M., Lima, W.S. (2004). Ectopic location of adult worms and first-stage larvae of Angiostrongylus vasorum in an infected dog, *Vet. Parasitol.* Vol. 121: 293–296.

Pinsker, K.L., Norin, A.J., Kamholz, S.L., Montefusco, C., Schreiber, K., Hagstrom, J.W.C., Veith, F.J. (1980). Cell content in repetitive canine bronchoalveolar lavage, *Acta Cytol.* Vol. 24: 558–563.

Rothenberg, M.E., Hogan, S.P. (2006) The eosinphil, Annu Rev. Immunol. Vol. 24: 147-174.

Schnyder, M., Fahrion, A., Ossent, P., Kohler, L., Webster, P., Heine, J., Deplazes, P. (2009). Larvicidal effect of imidacloprid / moxidectin spot-on solution in dogs experimentally infected with Angiostrongylus vasorum, *Veterinary Parasitology* Vol. 166: 326-332.

Scrivo, R., Vasile, M., Bartosiewicz, I., Valesini, G. (2011). Inflammation as "common soil" of the multifactorial diseases, *Autoimmunoty Reviews* Vol. 10: 369-374.

Shin, M.H., Lee, Y.A., Min, D. (2009). Eosinophil-mediated tissue inflammatory responses in helminth infection, *Korean J Parasitol.* Vol. 47: 125-131.

Staebler, S., Ochs, H., Steffen, F., Naegeli, F., Borel, N., Sieber-Ruckstuhl, N., Deplazes, P. (2006). Autochthonous infections with Angiostrongylus vasorum in dogs in Switzerland and Germany. *EJCAP* Vol. 16(1):95-99.

Turvey, S.E., Broide, D.H. (2010) Innate immunity *J. Allergy and Clinical Immunology* Vol. 125(2): 524-532.

Vodovotz, Y., Constantine, G., Rubin, J., Csete, M., Voit, E.O., An, G. (2009). Mechanistic simulations of inflammation: Current state and future prospects, *Mathematical Biosciences* Vol. 217: 1–10.

Weaver, C.T., Harrington, L.E., Mangan, P.R., Gavrieli, M., Murphy, K.M. (2006) Th17: an effector CD4 T cell lineage with regulatory T cell ties, *Immunity* Vol. 24: 677–688.

Yates, A., Callar, R., Stark, J. (2004). Combining cytokine signalling with T-bet and GATA-3 regulation in Th1 and Th2 differentiation: a model for cellular decision-making, *J. Theoretical Biology* Vol. 231: 181–196.

Yazdanbakhsh, M., Biggelaar, A., Maizels, R.M. (2001). The responses with atopy: immunoregulation in chronic helminth infections and reduced allergic disease, *Trends Immunol.* Vol. 22: 372–377.

Zaccone, P., Fehervari, Z., Phillips, J.M., Dunne, D.W., Cooke, A. (2006) Parasitic worms and inflammatory diseases, *Parasite Immunol.* Vol. 28(10): 515-523.

11

Involvement of Microglial Cathepsin B in Pro-Interleukin-1β Processing and Persistent Pain

Hiroshi Nakanishi
Department of Aging Science and Pharmacology, Faculty of Dental Science, Kyushu University, Fukuoka
Japan Science and Technology Agency, CREST, 5, Sanbancho, Chiyoda-ku, Tokyo
Japan

1. Introduction

A group of proteases in the endosomal/lysosomal proteolytic system have been designated as cathepsins, which is derived from the Greek term meaning "to digest". Considering that cathepsins can irreversibly cleave peptide bonds, the primary function of cathepsins has been believed to be their "disintegration action". However, there is increasing evidence that cathepsins can also exert "modulator actions" by which substrates are activated after limited cleavage. There is substantial evidence that cathepsin B (EC 3.4.22.1), a typical cysteine lysosomal protease, is markedly upregulated in activated microglia that accumulate in pathological sites of the brain. Beyond its bulk proteolysis in the endosomal/lysosomal system, cathepsin B can be secreted from activated microglia in its mature form to induce neuronal apoptosis and degrade Aβ peptides that accumulate in the brain. Furthermore, cathepsin B is also leaked into the cytosol, where it plays an essential role in the inflammatory response initiated by activated microglia in the brain.

Recently, the leakage of cathepsin B from the lysosomes has been suggested to trigger the activation of the NOD-like receptor (NLR) family, pyrin domain-containing 3 (NLRP3) inflammasome in microglia/macrophages after phagocytosis of various molecules including fibrillar Aβ42 and silica crystals. After activation, the NLRP3 inflammasome can mediate pro-caspase-1 activation to promote the processing and secretion of proinflammatory cytokines, such as interleukin-1 β (IL-1 β) and IL-18. However, the precise role of leaked cathepsin B in the activation of the NLRP3 inflammasome remains to be determined. Furthermore, there is still evidence suggesting that cathepsin B is associated with the maturation of pro-IL-1β in the endosomal/lysosomal system, because cathepsin B can effectively cleave pro-caspase-1 in a cell-free system only at an acidic pH. I herein review our current understanding of the mechanism and roles of cathepsin B in the processing and secretion of IL-1β and IL-18. Further, i also discuss a possible involvement of cathepsin B in the induction of persistent pain.

2. Cathepsin B and neuronal death

2.1 Neuronal death induced by cathepsin B-secreted from microglia

Microglia are known to release a number of soluble molecules that can influence neuronal signaling and survival. Kingham and Pocock (2001) focused on cathepsin B, which increased in the culture medium of microglia following stimulation with chromogranin A (CGA), a glycophosphoprotein secreted by degenerating neurons. They demonstrated that cathepsin B is a major causative factor for CGA-activated microglia-induced neuronal apoptosis using neutralizing anti-cathepsin B antibodies. Gan et al. (2004) found that freshly sonicated Aβ42 did not cause neuronal death when added directly to neuron, but activated BV2 microglial cells to release toxic factors that caused significant neuronal death. To determine the toxic molecules secreted from Aβ42-stimulated microglia, they conducted a large scale expression profiling analyses using filter-based cDNA arrays made from BV2 cDNA libraries enriched for Aβ42-activated microglial genes. Cathepsin B was identified to be one of the 554 genes transcriptionally induced by freshly sonicated Aβ42. Furthermore, specific inhibition of cathepsin B using either siRNA-mediated gene silencing or a specific cathepsin B inhibitor completely abolished the neurotoxicity mediated by Aβ42-activated BV2 microglial cells, suggesting that cathepsin B plays a crucial role in neuronal death mediated by Aβ-activated inflammatory responses. However, further studies will be needed to identify the mechanism of secretion of cathepsin B and its extracellular substrates.

2.2 Involvement of intracellular cathepsin B in microglia-induced neuronal death

Wendt et al. (2009) analyzed the neurotoxicity of conditioned medium from lipopolysaccharide (LPS)-activated microglia. Experiments with membrane-permeable and membrane-impermeable cathepsin B inhibitors suggested that blocking extracellular cathepsin B had no effect on LPS-stimulated microglia-mediated neuronal death. In contrast, intracellular cathepsin B may trigger the release of neurotoxic factors from activated microglia. In fact, it has been reported that cathepsin B is involved in the trafficking of tumor necrosis factor-α-containing vesicles to the plasma membrane of macrophages (Ha et al., 2008).

3. Cathepsin B and Aβ

To determine the role of cathepsin B in the processing of amyloid precursor protein and Aβ metabolism in vivo, Mueller-Steiner et al. (2006) crossed cathepsin B-deficient mice with transgenic mice that overexpressed human amyloid precursor protein (hAPP mice). Cathepsin B ablation in hAPP mice did not affect the levels of the C-terminal fragments of hAPP, suggesting that cathepsin B dose not significantly affect the processing of hAPP. In contrast, cathepsin B ablation significantly increased the plaque deposition and Aβ42 levels in the hippocampaus. On the other hand, the injection of Lenti-cathepsin B into the hippocampus significantly reduced Aβ deposition in aged hAPP mice. These observations strongly suggest that cathepsin B is secreted from microglia accumulated around the senile plaques, and is involved in the degradation of Aβ42 and reduction of established plaques.

4. Cathepsin B and inflammation

4.1 The "lysosomal rupture model" and "reactive oxygen species (ROS) model" of activation of the NLRP3 inflammasome

Two different models, the "lysosomal rupture model" proposed by Latz's group (University of Bonn) and the "ROS model" proposed by Tschopp's group (University of Lausanne), have recently been proposed to account for perturbations in phagocytic processes that activate the NLRP3 inflammasome. According to the lysosomal rupture model, phagocytosis of fibrillar Aβ42 or silica crystals by LPS-primed microglia/macrophages causes phagosomal destabilization and lysosomal rupture. The subsequent secretion of cathepsin B into the cytoplasm triggers the activation of the NLRP3 inflammasome directly or indirectly, leading to the production and secretion of mature IL-1β (Hornung et al., 2008; Halle et al., 2008).

Activator	Phagocyte	Cathepsin B-dependency	NLRP3-dependency	Disease	Reference
Fibrillar Aβ	Microglia	+ (cytosol)	+	Altzheimer's disease	Halle et al.
CGA	Microglia	+ (phagolysosome)	?	Inflammatory pain	Terada et al.
Silica crystal	Macrophage	+ (cytosol)	+	Silicosis	Hornung et al.
Choresterol crystal	Macrophage	+ (cytosol)	+	Atherosclerosis	Duewell et al.
IAPP	Dendritic cell	+ (?)	+	Type 2 Diabetes	Masters et al.
MSU	Macrophage	?	+	Gout	Dostert et al.
Asbestos fiber	Macrophage	?	+	Asbestosis	Dostert et al.

CGA: chromogranin A; IAPP: islet amyloid peptide; MSU: monosodium urate crystal

Table 1. IL-1β production pathways and diseases

This model is supported by observations that a specific inhibitor of cathepsin B, CA074Me, significantly inhibited the IL-1β secretion from LPS-primed microglia and macrophages after phagocytosis of fibrillar Aβ and silica crystal, respectively (Hornung et al., 2008; Halle et al., 2008). Furthermore, the mean level of IL-1β secreted from cathepsin B-deficient macrophages following the phagocytosis of fibrillar Aβ was significantly lower than that from wild-type macrophages (Halle et al., 2008). Interestingly, CA074Me had no effect on the amount of IL-1β secreted from LPS-primed microglia following treatment with ATP (Table 1). Furthermore, a direct disruption of lysosomes by treatment with hypotonic media or L-leucyl-L-leucil methyl ester was shown to be sufficient for the activation of NLRP3 (Hornung et al., 2008). On the other hand, according to the ROS model, particulate activators of the NLRP3 inflammasome including asbestos fibers and silica crystals trigger the generation of short-lived ROS, and treatment with various ROS scavengers blocks the activation of the NLRP3 inflammasome in response to these particulate activators (Dostert et al., 2008) . Various danger signals stimulate phagocytes to induce various IL-1β production pathways, which are associated with various diseases (Table 1).

More recently, however, reports opposing both of these models have appeared. Dostert et al. (2009) demonstrate that cathepsin B-deficient macrophages exhibited a normal NLRP3 inflammasome-dependent IL-1β production in response to silica crystals, urea crystals or aluminum salts, which raises questions about the specificity of CA074Me. Lysosomal rupture is associated with the release of numerous other enzymes, therefore CA074Me might inhibit other released proteases that acts as the essential signal to activate the NLRP3 inflammasome (Montaser et al., 2002). In fact, cathepsin L-deficient macrophages were also used to show that cholesterol crystals led to a diminished release of IL-1β in comparison with wild-type cells (Duewell et al., 2010). However, the dependence of cholesterol crystal-induced IL-1β release on cathepsin B or L was less pronounced at higher concentrations, thus suggesting the functional redundancy of cathepsin B/L, or the potential presence of additional proteases. Furthermore, Masters et al. (2010) showed that the secretion of IL-1β from bone marrow-derived dendritic cells after phagocytosis of islet amyloid polypeptide, a unique polypeptide constituent of amyloid found in pancreatic islet, was significantly inhibited by a specific inhibitor of either cathepsin B or ROS. Proving the importance of the lysosomal rupture model will require identification of the putative cathepsin B substrate(s) that activate the NLRP3 inflammasome. Detailed analyses are also needed to clarify the involvement of cathepsins other than cathepsin B for activation of the NLRP3 inflammasome. On the other hand, proving the importance of the ROS model will require that the source of the ROS that activate the NLRP3 inflammasome be clarified. Phagocytosed particulates that are too large to be efficiently cleared are likely to induce the production of ROS on their way to lysosomes. Therefore, the lysosomal rupture model could be viewed as forming part of a more general ROS pathway. It is likely that the activation of the NLRP3 is more complex and may require a combination of factors, including both enzymatic activities of cathepsins and ROS activity.

4.2 Alternative mechanisms underlying the cathepsin B-dependent activation of pro-caspase-1

There is still evidence suggesting that cathepsin B is directly associated with the proteolytic cleavage of pro-IL-1β in the endosomal/lysosomal system. Cathepsin B can efficiently cleave pro-caspase-11 in a cell-free system even at a neutral pH, but it cleaves pro-caspase-1 only at an acidic pH (Vancompernolle et al., 1998). Furthermore, Hentze et al. (2003) found that cathepsin B is directly involved in the proteolytic cleavage of pro-casapase-1 in THP-1 monocytic cells after stimulation with the microbial toxin nigericin. However, the size of the cleaved fragments of pro-caspase-1 generated by cathepsin B (37 and 40 kDa) is different from the active fragments that are produced by caspase-1 self-processing (10 and 20 kDa). It is possible that the fragments of pro-caspase-1 resulting from the cleavage by cathepsin B may be further cleaved to the active fragments by self-processing. It should also be considered whether cathepsin B is indirectly involved in the activation of pro-caspase-1 though its direct activation of pro-caspase-11, because caspase-11 is known to be play a crucial role in the activation of pro-caspase-1 (Kang et al., 2000).

During the course of experiments to examine the role of cathepsin B in microglial apoptosis, we found that cathepsin B-deficiency abrogated the secretion of IL-1β from microglia following treatment with CGA (Terada et al., 2010). Detailed analyses revealed that cathepsin B-deficiency and CA074Me significantly inhibited the proteolytic processing of pro-IL-1β and secretion of mature IL-1β from microglia following treatment with CGA without affecting the increased production of pro-IL-1β. Furthermore, there was no sign of any leakage of cathepsin B in microglia following treatment with CGA. The typical size of the primary lysosomes is below 1 μm in diameter, whereas the mean diameter of cathepsin B-containing enlarged lysosomes in CGA-stimulated microglia was 4.2 μm. Furthermore, cathepsin B-positive enlarged lysosomes were found to be acidic compartments. These findings are consistent with previous observations that IL-1β and cathepsin D are colocalized within endolysosome-related vesicles, and that the secretion of IL-1β involves the exocytosis of these vesicles in LPS-activated human monocytes (Andrei et al., 1999).

Interestingly, CGA is known to activate microglia through scavenger receptor class-A (SR-A; Hooper et al., 2009). Cathepsin B-containing enlarged lysosomes are considered to be phagolysosomes formed by a fusion of SR-A-mediated phagosomes and primary lysosomes. Therefore, pro-caspase-1 and pro-IL-1β in the cytoplasm may be trapped in these cathepsin B-containing phagolysosomes during their formation triggered by a binding of CGA to SR-A. Furthermore, cathepsin B activates pro-caspase-1 and caspase-1 subsequently proteolytically cleaves pro-IL-1β and pro-IL-18 to their mature forms. Finally, mature IL-1β and IL-18 are secreted extracellulary by exocytosis (Figure 1).

5. Cathepsin B and Inflammatory pain

Cathepsin B deficiency or treatment with a specific inhibitor of cathepsin B, CA074Me, was found to abrogate CGA-induced activation of pro-caspase-1 and subsequent processing of the inactive forms of IL-1β and IL-18 to their mature forms in microglia. Furthermore, the existence of multiple pathways that can induce the proteolytic cleavage of pro-IL-1β and pro-IL-18 in microglia was further demonstrated, probably indicating that there is a backup system for generating these cytokines. CGA activates cathepsin B-dependent but NLRP3-independent pathways for the processing of both IL-1β and IL-18, whereas ATP activates NLRP3-dependent but cathepsin B-independent pathways for their processing. These *in vitro* observations using cultured microglia prompted us to further investigate the role of cathepsin B in chronic pain generation, because both IL-1β and IL-18 are involved in the initiation of inflammatory and pain hypersensitivity (Samad et al., 2001; Sweitzer et al., 2001; Kawasaki et al., 2008; Miyoshi et al., 2008). Furthermore, Inoue's group (Kyushu University) introduced the concept that signals derived from spinal microglia after spinal nerve injury are the core mechanisms underlying neuropathic pain (Tsuda et al., 2003; Coull et al., 2005; Scholz & Woolf, 2007). Following intra-plantar injection of complete Freund's adjuvant (CFA), both hyperalgesia (an augmented pain response to noxious stimulation) and allodynia (a pain produced by normally non-painful stimulation) develop in the injected paw. As expected, cathepsin B deficiency or the intrathecal administration of a specific cathepsin B inhibitor significantly inhibited both CFA-induced mechanical allodynia and thermal hyperalgesia without affecting peripheral inflammation. In contrast, cathepsin B-deficiency had no significant effect on spinal nerve injury-induced mechanical allodynia. At the same time, mature IL-1β and IL-18 were expressed in the spinal microglia of cathepsin B-deficient mice following spinal nerve-transection, but not after CFA treatment. Treatment with minocycline, a microglial activation inhibitor, completely prevented the development of CFA-induced mechanical allodynia and thermal hyperalgesia, thus suggesting that microglial activation and inflammatory immune responses in the spinal cord are involved in CFA-induced mechanical allodynia and thermal hyperalgesia (Shan et al., 2007). Therefore, it is considered that peripheral CFA-treatment triggers cathepsin B-dependent caspase-1 activation pathways for the processing of both IL-1β and IL-18 in spinal microglia, leading to pain hypersensitivity (Figure 1). On the other hand, spinal nerve-injury activates cathepsin B-independent pathways for the processing of both IL-1β and IL-18 in spinal microglia. A MMP-9-dependent mechanism has been proposed as an alternative pathway for the proteolytic cleavage of pro-IL-1β in the spinal cord following nerve injury (Kawasaki et al., 2008).

Following the peripheral inflammation, IL-1β and IL-18 are secreted from activated spinal microglia in a cathepsin B-dependent manner. IL-1β and IL-18 subsequently induce COX-2 in spinal neurons, leading to the production of prostaglandin E_2 (PGE_2). PGE_2 activates protein kinase A (PKA) through increase in cAMP levels by binding to PGE_2 receptors of the

EP2 subtype. PKA then causes phosphorylation and inhibition of glycine receptors containing the α3 subunits (GlyRα3). This disinhibition induces hypersensitivity of pain. IL-1β and IL-18 are also known to directly enhance responses mediated by NMDA receptors.

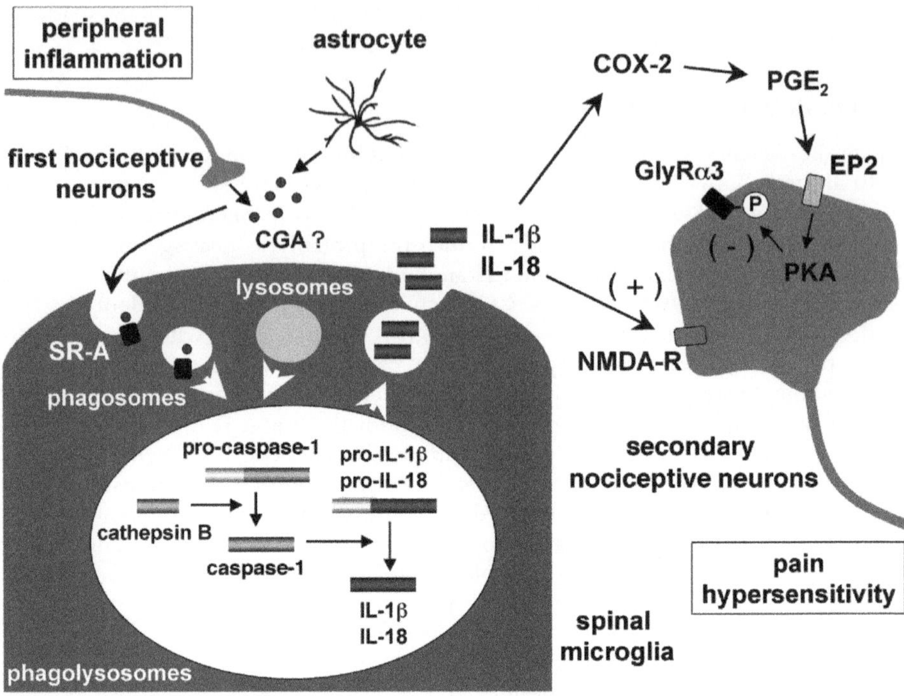

Fig. 1. Schematic representation of the role of cathepsin B in the initiation of inflammatory pain.

6. Conclusion

The lysosomal rupture and subsequent leakage of cathepsin B has been proposed as the common molecular basis underlying apoptosis and inflammation. Although a lysosomal rupture has pathological significance, we have demonstrated that cathepsin B is involved in the proteolytic processing of pro-caspase-1 to its active form in the phagolysosomes of microglia, even in the absence of leakage. Therefore, it is considered that cathepsin B-dependency and the mechanism of action depend on the activator or stimulus. The growing understanding of the proteolytic systems of cathepsins in the central nervous system could contribute to the development of protease inhibitors as therapeutic interventions against chronic inflammation-related diseases including chronic pain.

7. Acknowledgment

This study was supported by Japan and the Technology Agency, CREST, and Grants-in-Aid from the Ministry of Education, Culture, Sports, Science, and Technology, Japan.

8. References

Andrei, C., Dazzi, C., Lotti, L., Torrisi, M.R., Chimini, G. & Rubartelli, A. (1999). The secretory route of the leaderless protein interleukin 1β involves exocytosis of endosome-related vesicles, *Molecular Biology of the Cell* Vol. 10 (No. 5): 1463-1475.

Coull, J.A.M., Beggs, S., Boudreau, D., Boivin, D., Tsuda, M., Inoue, K., Gravel, C., Salter, M.W. & De Koninck, Y. (2005). BDNF from microglia causes the shift in neuronal anion gradient underlying neuropathic pain, *Nature* Vol. 438 (No. 7070): 1017-1021.

Dostert, C., Pétrilli, V., Van Bruggen, Steele, C., Mossman, B.T. & Tscopp, J. (2008). Innate Immune activation through Nalp3 inflammasome sensing of asbestos and silica, *Science* Vol. 320 (No. 5876): 674-677.

Dostert, C., Guarda, G., Romero, J.K., Menu, P., Gross, O., Tardivel, A., Suva, M.-L., Stehle, J.-C., Kopf, M., Stamenkovic, I., Corradin, G. & Tschopp, J. (2009). Malarial hemozoin is a Nalp3 inflammasome activating danger signal, *PLoS One* Vol. 4 (No. 8): e6510.

Duewell, P., Kono, H., Rayner, K.J., Sirois, C.M., Vladimer, G., Bauernfeind, F.G., Abela, G.S., Franchi, L., Nuňez, G., Schnurr, M., Espevik, T., Lien, E., Fitzgerald, K.A., Rock, K.L., Moore, K.J., Wright, S.D., Hornung, V. & Latz, E. (2010). NLRP3 inflammasomes are required for atherogenesis and activated by cholesterol crystals, *Nature* Vol. 464 (No. 7293): 1357-1362.

Gan, L., Ye, S., Chu, A., Anton, K., Yi, S., Vincent, V.A., von Schack, D., Chin, D., Murray, J., Lohr, S., Patthy, L., Gonzalez-Zulueta, M., Nikolich, K & Urfer, R. (2004) Identification of cathepsin B as a mediator of neuronal death induced by Aβ-activated microglial cells using a functional genomic approach, *Journal of Biological Chemistry* Vol. 279 (No. 7): 5565-5572.

Ha, S.-D., Martins, A., Khazaie, K., Han, J., Chann, B.M.C. & Kim, S.O. (2008). Cathepsin B is involved in the trafficking of TNF-α-containing vesicles to the plasma membrane in macrophages, *Journal of Immunology* Vol. 181 (No. 1): 690-697.

Halle, A., Hornung, V., Petzold, G.C., Stewart, C.R., Monks, B.G., Reinheckel, T., Fitzgerald, K.A., Latz, E., Moore, K.J. & Golenbock, D.T. (2008) The NALP3 inflammasome is involved in the innate immune response to amyloid-β, *Nature Immunology* Vol. 9 (No. 8): 857-865.

Hornung, V., Bauernfeind, F., Halle, A., Samstad, E.O., Kono, H., Rock, K.L., Fitzgerald, K.A. & Latz, E. (2008). Silica crystals and aluminum salts activate the NALP3 inflammasome through phagosomal destabilizatiuon, *Nature Immunology* Vol. 9 (No. 8): 847-856.

Hentze, H., Lin, X.Y., Choi, M.S.K., Porter, A.G. (2003). Critical role for cathepsin B in Mediating caspase-1-dependent interleukin-18 maturation and caspase-1 - independent necrosis triggered by the microbial toxin nigericin, *Cell Death and Differenciation* Vol. 10 (No. 9): 956-968.

Hooper, C., Fry, V.A.H., Sevastou, I.G. & Pocock, J.M. (2009). Scavenger receptor control of chromogranin A-induced microglial stress and neurotoxic cascades, *FEBS Letters* Vol. 583 (No. 21): 3461-3466.

Kang, S.-J., Wang, S., Hara, H., Peterson, E.P., Namura, S., Amin-Hanjani, S., Huang, Z., Srinivasan, A., Tomaselli, K.J., Tornberry, N.A., Moskowitz, M. & Yuang, J. (2000). Dual role of caspase-11 in mediating activation of caspase-1 and caspase-3 under pathological conditions, *Journal of Cell Biology* Vol. 149 (No. 3): 613-622.

Kawasaki,Y., Xu, Z.-Z., Wang, X., Park, J.Y., Zhuang, Z.-Y., Tan, P.-H., Gao, Y.-J., Roy, G., Corfas, G., Lo, E.H. & Ji, R.-R. (2008). Distinct roles of matrix metalloproteases in the early- and late-phase development of neuropathic pain. *Nature Medicine* Vol.14 (No. 3): 331-336.

Kingham, P.J. & Pocock J.M. (2001) . Microglial secreted cathepsin B induces neuronal apoptosis, *Journal of Neurochemistry* Vol. 76 (No. 5): 1475-1484.

Masters, S.L., Dunne, A., Subramanian, S.I., Hull, R.L., Tannahill, G.M., Sharp, F.A., Becker, C., Franchi, L., Yoshihara, E., Chen, Z., Mullooly, N., Mielke L.A., Harris, J., Coll, R.C., Mills, K.H.G., Mok, K.H., Newsholme, P., Nuňez, G., Yodoi, J., Kahn, S.E., Lavelle, E.D. & O'Neill L.A.J. (2010). Activation of the NLRP3 inflammasome by islet amyloid polypeptide provides a mechanism for enhanced IL-1β in type 2 diabetes, *Nature Immunology* Vol. 11 (No. 10): 897-904.

Miyoshi, K., Obata, K., Kondo, T., Okamura, H. & Noguchi, K. (2008). Interleukin-18 -mediated microglia/astrocyte interaction in the spinal cord enhances neuropathic pain procesng after nerve injury, Journal of Neuroscience Vol. 28 (No. 48): 12775-12787.

Montaser, M., Lalmanach, G. & Mach, L. (2002). CA-074, but not its methyl ester CA-074Me, is a selective inhibitor of cathepsin B within living cells, *Biological Chemistry* Vol. 383 (No. 7-8): 1305-1308.

Mueller-Steiner, S., Zhou, Y., Arai, H., Roberson, E.D., Sun, B., Chen, J., Wang, X., Yu, G., Esposito, L., Mucke, L. & Gan, L. (2006). Antiamyloidogenic and neuroprotective functions of cathepsin B: Implications for Alzheimer's disease, *Neuron* Vol. 51 (No. 6): 703-714.

Samad, T.A., Moore, K.A., Sapirstein, A., Billet, S., Allchorne, A., Poole, S., Bonventre, J.V., Woolf, C.J. (2001). Interleukin-1β-mediated induction of cox-2 in the CNS contributes to inflammatory pain hypersensitivity, Nature Vol. 410 (No. 6827): 471-475.

Scholz, J. & Woolf, C.J. (2007). The neuropathic pain triad: neurons, immune cells and glia, *Nature Neuroscience* Vol. 10 (No. 11): 1361-1368.

Shan, S., Qi-Liang, M.-Y., Hong, C., Tingting, L., Mei, H., Haili, P., Yan-Qing, W., Zhi-Qi, Z., Yu-Qiu, Z. (2007). Is functional state of spinal microglia involved in the anti-allodynic and anti-hyperalgesic effects of electroacupuncture in rat model of monoarthritis? *Neurobiology of Disease* Vol. 26 (No. 3): 558-568.

Sweitzer, S., Martin, D. & Deleo, J.A. (2001). Intratechal interleukin-1 receptor antagonist in Combination with soluble tumor necrosis factor recepyor exhibits an anti- allodynic action in a rat model of neuropathic pain. *Neuroscience* Vol. 103 (No. 2): 529-539.

Terada, K., Yamada, J., Hayashi, Y., Wu, Z. & Nakanishi, H. (2010). Involvement of cathepsin B in the processing and secretion of interlukin-1-β in chromogranin A -stimulated microglia, *Glia* Vol. 58 (No. 1): 114-124.

Tsuda, M., Shigemoto-Mogami, Y., Koizumi, S., Mizokoshi, A., Kohsaka, S., Salter, M.W. & Inoue, K. (2003). $P2X_4$ receptors induced in spinal microglia gate tactile allodynia after nerve injury, *Nature* Vol. 424 (No. 6950): 778-783.

Vancompernolle, K., Van Herreweghe, F., Pynaert, G., Van de Craen, M., De Vos, K., Totty, N., Sterling, A., Fiers, W., Vandenabeele, P. & Grooten, J. (1998). Atractyloside -induced release of cathepsin B, a protease with caspase-processing activity, *FEBS Letters* Vol. 438 (No. 3): 150-158.

Wendt, W., Schulten, R., Stichel, C.C. & Lübbert, H. (2009). Intra- versus extracellular effects of microglia-derived cysteine proteases in a conditioned medium transfer model, *Journal of Neurochemistry* Vol. 110 (No. 6): 1931-1941.

12

"Suppressor of Cytokine Signalling" Molecules in Infection and Inflammation

Berit Carow and Martin E. Rottenberg
Dept. of Microbiology, Tumor and Cell Biology, Karolinska Institutet, Stockholm
Sweden

1. Introduction

Cytokines are messengers that coordinate the development and function of leukocytes and therefore are indispensable for the initiation, maintenance and termination of all types of immune responses. A tight control of cytokine functions is crucial for both, the control of infections and the prevention of infection-associated immunopathology. Different intracellular mechanisms of cytokine signal inhibition are involved in the regulation of innate and adaptive immune responses. Among these, the family of suppressor of cytokine signalling (SOCS) proteins identified more than a decade ago (Endo *et al.* 1997; Naka *et al.* 1997; Starr *et al.* 1997) are non-redundant negative feedback inhibitors of both pro-inflammatory but also of anti-inflammatory cytokine responses (Kubo *et al.* 2003; Yoshimura *et al.* 2007).

Type I and type II cytokine receptors do not possess a cytoplasmic kinase activity and therefore are dependent on associated Janus kinases (JAKs). JAKs conduct the signal of many cytokines including many interleukins (IL), all interferons (IFN) and hemopoietins. Activated JAKs cross-phosphorylate themselves and phosphorylate the associated cytokine receptor creating binding sites for proteins that contain phosphotyrosine binding SH2 domains. The SH2 domain of signal transducers and activators of transcription (STATs) then binds to the phosphorylated receptors. Recruited STATs get phosphorylated by the adjacent JAKs, and act as binding sites for the SH2 domain of another STATs, which also will be phosphorylated. The STAT dimer translocates into the nucleus where it acts as a transcription factor activating the transcription of specific genes. The diversity of STAT-mediated intracellular pathways is due to the presence of 7 STATs, activated by different receptors. Moreover, activated STAT dimers act as homo- or heterodimers, which increases the diversity of target promoters and thereby of gene patterns that can be activated.

The JAK-STAT pathway can be negatively regulated at different stages: protein tyrosine phosphatases remove phosphates from cytokine receptors and activated STATs, whereas PIAS (protein inhibitors of activated STATs) act in the nucleus (Leonard & O'Shea 1998; Krebs & Hilton 2001; Hebenstreit *et al.* 2005; Shuai 2006). In this chapter we will focus on the role of another inhibitor of the JAK-STAT pathway, the SOCS proteins. The importance of these proteins is evidenced by the fact that mice deficient for some of the SOCS proteins demonstrated a non-redundant role of SOCS proteins in regulating the immune system (Alexander 2002).

SOCS proteins play a role in balancing immune functions at different levels, including the differentiation of immune cell populations and their activation by environmental stimuli. Both deletion and over-expression of SOCS proteins in animal models provided insights into their importance of regulating the responsiveness to cytokines. Accumulated today's knowledge on the immunobiology of SOCS proteins convert them into new potential targets for treatment of inflammatory diseases but might also help to improve infection control.

2. SOCS at the molecular level

The family of SOCS proteins consists of 8 members (cytokine inducible SH2 protein, CIS, SOCS1-7), which share a central modulator organization with a SH2 domain, a C-terminal SOCS box and an amino-terminal domain of variable length (fig. 1). The SOCS-box was shown to interact with elongin A and B, cullin 5 and ring box. This complex acts as an E3 ubiquitin ligase, initiating ubiquitination in other words the covalent binding of ubiquitin to target proteins, which is followed by the proteosomal degradation of bound signalling complexes as JAKs and cytokine receptors (Verdier *et al.* 1998; Kamura *et al.* 2004; Piessevaux *et al.* 2008). The SH2 domain of SOCS proteins determines the specificity of the SOCS and CIS proteins for the respective cytokine receptors (Endo *et al.* 1997; Nicholson *et al.* 2000).

So far, SOCS1 and SOCS3 are the most studied SOCS proteins. They both contain a N-terminal kinase inhibitory region (KIR) that is absent in other SOCS proteins (fig. 1). The KIRs of SOCS1 and SOCS3 can directly inhibit JAK tyrosine kinase activity, acting as pseudo-substrates, and by that can block the interaction of JAKs with their substrate STAT molecules. JAK inhibition by SOCS1 and 3 takes place even in the absence of the SOCS box (Yasukawa *et al.* 1999; Zhang *et al.* 2001). SOCS1 can bind to the catalytic domain of JAK2 and to Tyk2 a molecule of the JAK family that mediates IFN-α/β signalling. SOCS1 has also been shown to bind directly to type I IFN receptors (IFNar1) (Fenner *et al.* 2006) and to the IFN-γ receptor inhibiting efficiently STAT1-mediated signalling (Kubo *et al.* 2003; Qing *et al.* 2005; Fenner *et al.* 2006). Furthermore, SOCS1 can bind to the insulin receptor (Mooney *et al.* 2001; Rui *et al.* 2002) and to the glucocorticoid receptor via its SH2 domain (Haffner *et al.* 2008). Besides JAK2, SOCS3 binds to a variety of receptors as the common IL-6 family co-receptor gp130 at the phosphorylated tyrosine 757, erythropoietin receptor, granulocyte colony stimulating factor (GCSF) receptor, growth hormone receptor (Hansen *et al.* 1999;

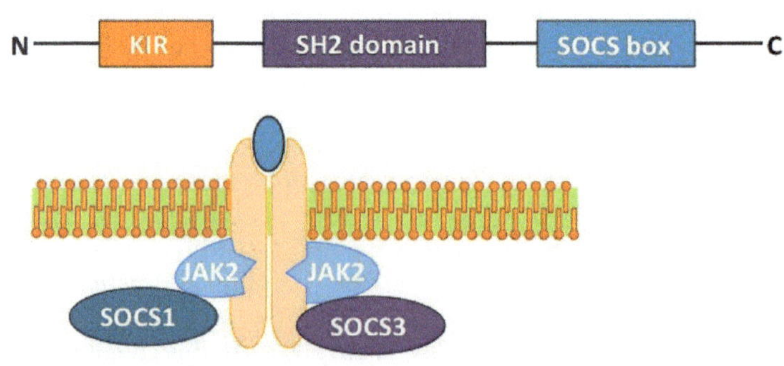

Fig. 1. Schematic structure of SOCS1 and SOCS3 proteins shown in upper panel, SOCS1 and SOCS3 as negative regulators of JAK/STAT signalling in lower panel. SOCS1 preferably binds directly to the JAK activation loop while the SH2 domain of SOCS3 binds to the cytokine receptor.

Nicholson *et al.* 2000; Sasaki *et al.* 2000; Hortner *et al.* 2002a; Hortner *et al.* 2002b) and cytokine receptors IL2Rβ and IL-12Rβ1(Cohney *et al.* 1999; Yamamoto *et al.* 2003). Possible interactions of SOCS1 and SOCS3 with Toll-like Receptor (TLR) signalling have been described and will be discussed later.

3. SOCS1

SOCS1 is expressed constitutively in the thymus, spleen, lung and testes of mice. SOCS1 mRNA expression can be rapidly induced by many cytokines, especially IFNs, and serves as a classical feed back loop inhibiting its inducing pathway (Naka *et al.* 1997; Starr *et al.* 1997). Importantly, SOCS1 mRNA expression increases even in response to microbial molecules such as LPS, Pam_3Cys and CpG oligonucleotides that signal via TLR (Dalpke *et al.* 2001; Alexander 2002; Fujimoto & Naka 2003; Dennis *et al.* 2006). Furthermore, hormones like insulin (Emanuelli *et al.* 2000), cardiotrophin (Hamanaka *et al.* 2001) or glucocorticoids (Bhattacharyya *et al.* 2011) have been shown to stimulate SOCS1 expression.
$SOCS1^{-/-}$ animals die within 3 weeks after birth due to fatty degeneration and necrosis of the liver (Naka *et al.* 1998; Starr *et al.* 1998). These mice show retarded growth, lymphopenia and multi-organ haematopoietic infiltrates. At least in part, the spontaneous inflammatory disease is thought to be due to IFN-γ hyper-responsiveness of SOCS1-deficient tissue, because $SOCS1^{-/-}IFN\text{-}\gamma^{-/-}$ as well as $SOCS1^{-/-}STAT1^{-/-}$ mice survive healthy until adulthood (Alexander *et al.* 1999; Marine *et al.* 1999b). The importance of IFN-γ was further apparent in mice heterozygous for IFN-γ and lacking SOCS1 that survived until 5 month of age before succumbing with myocardis and polymyositis (Metcalf *et al.* 2000). SOCS1 mice, treated with neutralizing antibodies from birth, died of the same phenotype reaching adulthood (Bullen *et al.* 2001). A similar expected protection from lethality was observed in $SOCS1^{-/-}$ crossed with $IFN\text{-}\gamma R^{-/-}$ and $STAT1^{-/-}$ mice. Furthermore, $RAG2^{-/-}SOCS1^{-/-}$ are healthy to at least 3 month of age, implicating that IFN-γ secreted by T and/ or NKT cells might be responsible for the tremendous inflammation observed (Marine *et al.* 1999b). In fact, depletion of NKT cell by antibody-treatment significantly increased the survival of mice. Surprisingly, mice with a conditional knock down for SOCS1 in T and NKT cells did not display any of the $SOCS1^{-/-}$ pathologies, indicating that a deletion of SOCS1 in T and NKT cells is not sufficient for the hyper-inflammation but that this was due an uncontrolled response of myeloid cells together with an excessive neonatal IFN-γ release (Chong *et al.* 2003). The fact that myeloid cells are involved was demonstrated by the lethality of chimeric mice, which received $SOCS1^{-/-}$ bone marrow after irradiation (Metcalf *et al.* 2003). On the other hand, T cells were also required for SOCS1-mediated lethality since $SOCS1^{-/-}$ mice with a SOCS1 transgene expressed only by T cells survived. Interestingly, the survival of $SOCS1^{-/-}$ mice also increased when back-crossed to $IFNar1^{-/-}$ mice (lacking one of the IFN-α/β R subunits) indicating that even type I IFNs in part contribute to the lethal inflammation of SOCS1 deficient animals. Altogether, SOCS1 lethality is mainly due to both an exacerbated secretion of IFN-γ by T and NKT cells during the neonatal period and to a hyper-response of myeloid cells to IFN-γ, but IFN-γ-independent immune responses such as type I IFN and others discussed below are also likely to contribute to it.
The use of conditional knock down mice, as well as in vitro experiments with different cell populations allowed a more precise definition of the role of SOCS1 in different cell lineages. A combination of SOCS1 conditional knock downs in hematopoetic cells using the cre-lox technology confirmed that SOCS1 deficiency in both T cells and macrophages

is critical to result in lethal inflammation (Chong *et al.* 2005). SOCS1$^{fl/-}$ LysM-cre mice deficient for SOCS1 in myeloid cells showed signs of morbidity starting from 50 days of age with splenomegaly as the most prominent feature. Moribund SOCS1$^{lox/-}$ LysM-cre mice showed aberrantly activated T cells and elevated serum levels of IFN-γ, TNF-α and IL-12 p40. SOCS1$^{fl/fl}$ Lck-cre mice, deleted for SOCS1 in T- and NKT-cell compartment did not develop lethal multi-organ inflammation but developed multiple lymphoid abnormalities, including enhanced differentiation of thymocytes toward CD8 T cells and very high percentages of peripheral CD8 T cells with a memory phenotype (Chong *et al.* 2005).

SOCS1$^{-/-}$ mice could also be partially protected from neonatal lethality when crossed with STAT1$^{-/-}$, STAT4$^{-/-}$ or STAT6$^{-/-}$ mice but nevertheless showed a chronic inflammation with aberrant T cell activation (Metcalf *et al.* 2000; Naka *et al.* 2001; Eyles *et al.* 2002). STAT6 and STAT4 are two STAT family members that specifically mediate signals that emanate from the IL-4/ IL-13 and IL-12 receptors, respectively (Wurster *et al.* 2000). IL-4/ IL-13 and IL-12 are cytokines that are important regulators of the proliferation, differentiation and functional capacity of lymphocytes. Although the impact of genetic deletion of STAT4 and STAT6 genes in the survival of SOCS1 deficient animals is lower than that of STAT1, this demonstrates that SOCS1 also regulates IL-4 and IL-12 signalling. Uncontrolled responses to IL-12, an inflammatory cytokine, could contribute to increased IFN-γ secretion by T cells production and, as indicated above, to the development of inflammatory disease in SOCS1$^{-/-}$ mice (Eyles *et al.* 2002). IL-4, like IFN-γ, induces de novo expression of SOCS-1 in primary macrophages. Induction of SOCS1 gene expression by IL-4 is STAT6-dependent and SOCS1 feedback inhibits expression of STAT6-responsive genes. Upon binding to their ligand the IL-4 and IL-12 receptors induce tyrosine phosphorylation of the JAK2 protein kinase (Wurster *et al.* 2000). In relation, SOCS1 deletion in T cells resulted in an elevated production of both IFN-γ and IL-4, which might indicate an enhanced function of Th2 populations in addition to Th1 cells. Overexpression of SOCS1 in Th2 cells has been shown to repress STAT6 activation and inhibit IL-4-induced proliferation, while depletion of SOCS1 by an anti-sense SOCS1 enhanced cell proliferation and induced activation of STAT6 in Th2 cells (Yu *et al.* 2004). On the other hand, the role of SOCS1 in a Th2 skewed immune responses has been suggested (Lee *et al.* 2009), in relation to the fact that SOCS1 expression is 5-fold higher in Th1 than in Th2 cells (Egwuagu *et al.* 2002).

Dendritic cells (DCs) play a critical role in initiating and regulating adaptive immune responses. Silencing of SOCS1 in DCs broke self-tolerance to tumor antigens and increased the magnitude of antigen-presentation (Shen *et al.* 2004; Evel-Kabler *et al.* 2006). Moreover, the increased responses of SOCS1$^{-/-}$ T and NK cells to IL-12 (Eyles *et al.* 2002), and the IFN-γ-mediated inflammatory disease in mice deficient for SOCS1 in regulatory T (Treg) cells (Lu *et al.* 2009; Lu *et al.* 2010) showed a SOCS1-mediated control of Treg cell function, but also highlights the relevance of SOCS1 as target molecule in these diseases. In Treg cells specific microRNA regulated SOCS1 expression.

SOCS1 has also been shown to inhibit B cell proliferation in vitro and autoantibody production in vivo, through suppression of BAFF/BLyS a B cell growth and differentiation factor, that has been implicated in systemic autoimmune diseases (Hanada *et al.* 2003).

Taken together, several findings indicate that SOCS1 is involved in the regulation of Th1 responses by modulating the responses of different immune cells, such as macrophages, DCs, Th1 and Treg cells.

3.1 Role of SOCS1 in infectious diseases and inflammation

SOCS1 deficient mice are hypersensitive to LPS-induced endotoxic shock, associated with increased levels of IL-12 and TNF-α (Kinjyo *et al.* 2002). Surprisingly, even though IFN-γ$R^{-/-}$ mice are very resistant to endotoxic shock (Car *et al.* 1994), additional knock-out of IFN-γ or STAT1 did not rescue SOCS1$^{-/-}$ mice from lethal LPS injection, demonstrating that SOCS1 attenuates IFN-independent mechanisms that mediate septic lethal shock (Car *et al.* 1994; Kinjyo *et al.* 2002; Nakagawa *et al.* 2002). Furthermore, elevated sensitivity to endotoxin shock was observed in SOCS1$^{fl/fl}$ LysM-cre mice lacking SOCS1 in macrophages and neutrophils (Hashimoto *et al.* 2009b). Another contributing factor to the elevated sensitivity might be that SOCS1 mediates the protective effect of cardiotrophin-1 in sepsis-induced cardiomyocyte depression (Tanimoto *et al.* 2005).

These findings suggest an interaction of SOCS1 with components of TLR signalling underlying the role of SOCS1 in protection against septic shock. In fact, binding of SOCS1 to IRAK1 and the p65 subunit of NFκB has been shown to destabilize and limit NFκB activation (Kinjyo *et al.* 2002; Nakagawa *et al.* 2002; Ryo *et al.* 2003; Maine *et al.* 2007). Others demonstrated that SOCS1 might also bind to apoptosis signal-regulating kinase 1 (ASK1) and regulate mitogen-activated protein kinases JNK and p38 (He *et al.* 2006). Furthermore, SOCS1 was shown to mediate the degradation of the adaptor protein Mal, involved in TLR2 and TLR4 signalling (Mansell *et al.* 2006). However, results from other investigators could not confirm a direct effect of SOCS1 on TLR signalling (Baetz *et al.* 2004; Gingras *et al.* 2004) . SOCS1 over-expression did not affect TLR signalling, instead the inhibition of IFN-α/β-mediated STAT1 activation by SOCS1 has been suggested to account for the observed sensitivity to LPS in IFN-$\gamma^{-/-}$/SOCS1$^{-/-}$ mice (Baetz *et al.* 2004; Gingras *et al.* 2004). Thus, further work is required to clarify whether SOCS1 is directly involved in the regulation of TLR signalling.

A wide range of pathogens including parasites, bacteria and viruses are potent stimulators of SOCS1 expression in the host. Despite obvious differences in the immunobiology and in the type of protective or deleterious immune responses elicited, for most intracellular infections studied, SOCS1 expression is apparently facilitating pathogen replication. But by hampering inflammatory reactions SOCS1 may also improve the pathological outcome of infections and thereby reduce morbidity. In this respect, manipulation of the immune system by SOCS1 conveys an adaptive advantage to pathogens. Microbes replicating in macrophages can be thought of hijacking the host SOCS system as an immune evasion mechanism.

To unravel the role of SOCS1 different infection models knock out and conditional knock down mouse strains have been applied. Other tools, such as lentiviruses encoding SOCS1 siRNA and treatment with small molecules inhibiting or mimicking SOCS1 action have also been used. Altogether, targeting SOCS1 may serve as a tool to improve the control of different infections and their pathological outcomes.

3.1.1 Viral infections

Several viruses including Herpes Simplex Virus (HSV)(Frey *et al.* 2009), human respiratory syncytial virus (RSV) (Hashimoto *et al.* 2009a), hepatitis C (HCV)(Yao *et al.* 2011), Ebola (Okumura *et al.* 2010) and human-immunodeficiency (HIV)(Yadav *et al.* 2009) virus were found to up regulate SOCS1 (Yang *et al.* 2008; Frey *et al.* 2009; Hashimoto *et al.* 2009a;

Hashimoto *et al.* 2009b; Okumura *et al.* 2010; Yao *et al.* 2011). Since SOCS1 is interfering with the type I IFN signalling, a role for SOCS1 in incrementing susceptibility to viral infection could be expected.

SOCS1$^{-/-}$/IFN-$\gamma^{-/-}$ mice outlived Semliki Forest virus (SFV)-infected control mice substantially (Alexander *et al.* 1999). Even though serum levels of IFN-α/β were lower in infected SOCS1$^{-/-}$ mice than in controls, an increased sensitivity to IFN-α/β was associated to resistance. The IFN-ar1 chain of the IFN-α/β receptor was shown to interact with SOCS1 and therefore inhibited efficient host responses (Fenner *et al.* 2006).

In another model, human T cell lymphotropic virus (HTLV) replication in peripheral blood mononuclear cells correlated with induction of SOCS1 and inhibition of IFN-α/β and IFN-stimulated gene expression (Oliere *et al.* 2010). These authors also showed that HTLV infection-induced SOCS1 mediated proteosomal degradation of IRF3, the blockade of IFN-gene expression and enhanced viral load. Of importance, SOCS1 did not only inhibit type I IFN-mediated viral defences but was found to impair efficient IFN-α stimulated anti-tumoral defences in mice (Zitzmann *et al.* 2007).

In vivo, injection of dnSOCS1 construct into the hearts of coxsackievirus-infected mice attenuated both virus replication and cardiomyocyte damage, protecting the heart from viral infection, suggesting that SOCS1 is a relevant therapeutic target (Yasukawa *et al.* 2003b).

Recently, specific microRNAs were found to regulate IFN-α/β responses. Infection with vesicular stromatitis virus (VSV), was shown to stimulate miR-155 expression that, by inhibition of SOCS1, positively regulated host antiviral innate immune response by promoting IFN-α/β responses (Wang *et al.* 2010). Thus, while SOCS1 is up-regulated during inflammatory IFN-mediated responses, miRNA might be a new mechanism by which the host can fine-tune its antiviral state.

Besides type I IFNs, responses to IFN-γ can be an essential component of control of some viral infections. The HSV-infection in keratinocytes, stimulated SOCS1 expression and made them refractory to IFN-γ, whereas HSV infected fibroblasts did not increase SOCS1 levels and developed an antiviral state after IFN-γ stimulation (Frey *et al.* 2009). Treatment of cells with a SOCS1 antagonist peptide as well as silencing SOCS1 with siRNA protected keratinocytes from HSV-1 infection and restored responsiveness to IFN-γ.

In contrast to suppression of IFN-mediated protective responses by SOCS1, in other virus infections unrestrained immune responses can cause damaging immunopathology. In these cases impairment of cytokine responses with SOCS1 may prevent inflammatory damage. Thus, in a vaccinia virus infection model, the administration of a small tyrosine inhibitor peptide that binds to JAK2 and inhibits STAT1 phosphorylation as well as a peptide mimicking the SOCS1 KIR region protected mice against lethal virus infection (Ahmed *et al.* 2009).

Clinical studies showed T cell exhaustion in chronically HCV-infected individuals. Interestingly, the expression of programmed death receptor 1 (PD1) and SOCS1 was increased in T cells and macrophages (Frazier *et al.* 2010; Zhang *et al.* 2011). In both cell types, blocking of PD1 signalling reduced SOCS1 expression and led to improved T cell proliferation and IL-12 secretion by macrophages respectively.

Studies on HIV progressor patients showed that SOCS1 expression was elevated in CD4 T cells displaying reduced IRF1 expression after IFN-γ stimulation in comparison to healthy controls (Yadav *et al.* 2009). Furthermore, SOCS1 was found to bind to HIV gag protein

improving production and stability of HIV-1 particles (Ryo et al. 2008). In a HIV vaccination model in mice, silencing of SOCS1 in DC using siRNA increased the secretion of IL-12 and other pro-inflammatory cytokines resulting in enhanced memory humoral and cellular immune responses (Song *et al.* 2006). Recently, it was shown that treatment of DCs from HIV patients with SOCS1 siRNA augmented the frequency of polyfunctional cytotoxic T cells (T cells secreting IL-2, TNF-α and IFN-γ are associated with protection)(Subramanya *et al.* 2010), suggesting that silencing SOCS1 in DCs may contribute to improved HIV-vaccination.
Taken together, SOCS1 induction is a successful tool of various viruses to diminish antiviral IFN responses, leading in many of the infections to impaired control of infection.

3.1.2 Bacterial infections

Studies on the role of SOCS1 have been focussed on intracellular bacterial infections in which IFN-γ usually plays a major protective role. Research from our laboratory showed that *Chlamydia pneumoniae* infection of macrophages induced SOCS1 expression in a STAT-1 and IFN-α/β dependent manner (Yang *et al.* 2008). Infected SOCS1$^{-/-}$ macrophages displayed lower bacterial titers and higher levels of IFN-regulated genes as iNOS (inducible nitric oxide synthase) and IDO (indoleamine dioxygenase), that participate in the control of intracellular bacteria. RAG1$^{-/-}$/SOCS1$^{-/-}$ mice showed 10-fold lower bacteria numbers in lungs than controls 6 days after infection. However, RAG1$^{-/-}$/SOCS1$^{-/-}$ mice died within seven days after infection with *C. pneumoniae* showing a severe pulmonary inflammation, whereas RAG1$^{-/-}$ mice survived for more than 60 days. Thus, SOCS1 has a crucial role in preventing lethal inflammation in *C. pneumoniae* infection.
Tuberculosis is another disease in which IFN-γ plays a critical role in containing bacterial levels and in the maintenance of the latent asymptomatic disease in infected individuals. Infection with different mycobacterial species such as *Mycobacterium bovis* (Imai *et al.* 2003), *M. avium* (Vazquez *et al.* 2006) and *M. tuberculosis* have been shown to stimulate SOCS1 in macrophages (Imai *et al.* 2003; Vazquez *et al.* 2006; Srivastava *et al.* 2009; Carow *et al.* 2011). Different innate immune receptors including TLR, NLR and DC-SIGN were found to mediate SOCS1 stimulation in mycobacterial infected myeloid cells (Srivastava *et al.* 2009).
Experiments from our laboratory and others, showed improved *M. tuberculosis* control in SOCS1 deficient macrophages and DCs (Srivastava *et al.* 2009; Carow *et al.* 2011). SOCS1$^{-/-}$ infected macrophages expressed higher levels of IFN-γ-responsive genes but also higher levels of IFN-γ itself than infected control cells. In agreement, SOCS1$^{-/-}$ macrophages secreted higher amounts of IFN-γ in response to IL-12, and although levels of IL-12 were not altered, SOCS1$^{-/-}$ macrophages displayed increased IL-12Rβ1 expression (Fig. 2). Of importance, the improved control of *M. tuberculosis* or *M. bovis* BCG by SOCS1$^{-/-}$ was lost in IFN-γ$^{-/-}$/SOCS1$^{-/-}$ macrophages, indicating that IFN-γ secretion mediates the improved mycobacterial control by SOCS1$^{-/-}$ macrophages. Moreover, despite SOCS1 expression, *M. tuberculosis*-infected macrophages were unimpaired in their response to IFN-γ. Altogether, as depicted in fig. 2, this suggests that SOCS1 regulates the secretion of rather than the response to IFN-γ, via controlling responses to IL-12 and that this causes mycobacterial resistance of macrophages. As stated above, SOCS1 regulates STAT4 activation in response to IL-12, which probably accounts for this mechanism (Eyles *et al.* 2002) (Fig. 2).

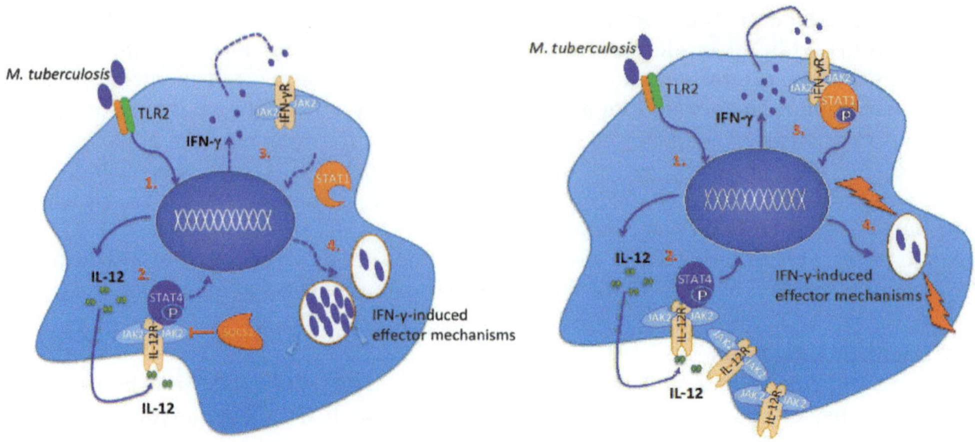

Fig. 2. SOCS1 in *M. tuberculosis*-infected macrophages

Macrophage responses and control of *M. tuberculosis* infection in absence (left panel) or presence (right panel) of SOCS1 regulating IFN-γ mediated genes.

RAG1-/-SOCS1-/- as well as SOCS1fl/fl LysM-cre mice displayed lower bacterial loads in the lungs early after aerosol infection with *M. tuberculosis*, indicating that SOCS1 expression by macrophages facilitates *M. tuberculosis* infection. However, RAG1-/-/SOCS1-/- and IFN-γ-/-/SOCS1-/- mice showed a dramatic pulmonary inflammation from 3 weeks after *M. tuberculosis* infection without reduced bacteria numbers in different organs. This inflammatory response was caused by SOCS1-deficiency in non-macrophage cells, since it was not observed in *M. tuberculosis*-infected SOCS1fl/fl LysM-cre mice. Overall, *M. tuberculosis* infection induces SOCS1 that by diminishing IL-12 responses impairs IFN-γ secretion by macrophages. This results in lower levels of IFN-γ-regulated genes and in increased pulmonary bacterial levels at early time points. Later during infection, SOCS1 in non-macrophages cells protects mice from severe inflammation. At these later time points, macrophages containing bacteria are able to respond to IFN-γ and reduce bacterial levels, despite SOCS1 expression. Thus, SOCS1 does not mediate resistance to infection at late time points (fig. 3).

A role of SOCS1 in T cells during *M. tuberculosis* has been envisaged (Srivastava *et al.* 2011). However, SOCS1fl/fl Lck-cre mice deficient for SOCS1 in T cells showed no reduction in *M. tuberculosis* numbers in the lung (unpublished observation).

We have also analysed the expression of SOCS1 in tuberculosis patients. We found higher SOCS1 mRNA levels in blood samples from pulmonary tuberculosis patients than in endemic controls (Srivastava *et al.* 2009; Masood *et al.* submitted). Furthermore, SOCS1 transcripts were raised in T cells of patients with far advanced as compared with those showing a moderately advanced disease (Masood *et al.* submitted). This confirmed studies describing an over-representation of SOCS1 (as well as other interferon-induced genes) in active tuberculosis patients compared to latent patients (Berry *et al.* 2010).

In summary, SOCS1 possesses two roles during infection: on the one hand it suppresses protective immune responses but on the other hand also prevents the development of detrimental inflammation. Therefore, it clearly depends on the stage of infection, but also on the type of the infection and the genetics of the host whether SOCS1 improves or worsens the outcome of infection.

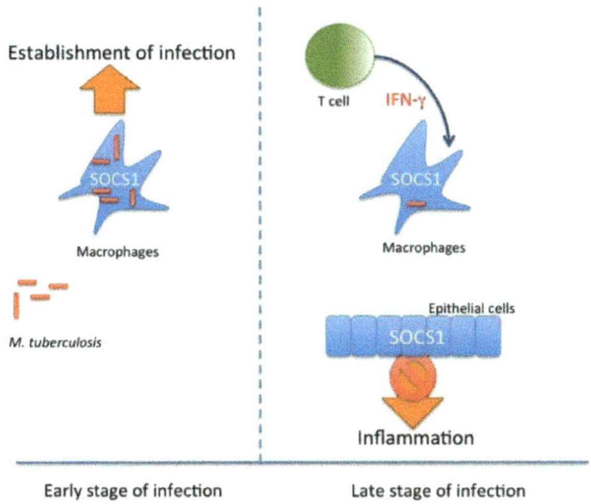

Fig. 3. Role of SOCS1 during different stages of M. tuberculosis infection

3.1.3 Parasite infections

The role of SOCS1 was also studied in a limited number of infections with parasites. SOCS1$^{-/-}$ mice were resistant to development of cerebral malaria after infection with *Plasmodium berghei*. This is surprising since IFN-γ mediates cerebral malaria in this model (Bullen *et al.* 2003b). However, the underlying mechanisms were not revealed.

SOCS1$^{-/-}$ macrophages were capable of killing *Leishmania major* at a 100-fold lower IFN-γ concentration than WT macrophages (Alexander *et al.* 1999). However, SOCS1$^{+/-}$ *L. major*-infected mice showed a worsened infection immunopathology, with larger dermal lesions but without reduction of parasites (Bullen *et al.* 2003a).

Another parasite, *Toxoplasma gondii* induced *SOCS1* expression in macrophages. SOCS1 over-expressing macrophages were unable to control parasite growth in response to IFN-γ whereas SOCS1$^{-/-}$ macrophages were restored in their ability to induce IFN-γ responsive genes after *T. gondii* infection (Zimmermann *et al.* 2006).

Moreover, recent data show that implantation of the parasite *Brugia malayi*, a causative agent of lymphatic filariasis, generated Th2 responses associated with development of M2 macrophages in mice. Expression of SOCS1 not only controlled the secretion of pro-inflammatory cytokines in M1 macrophages but was involved in maintaining M2 differentiation (Whyte *et al.* 2011). In line, patients with filariasis showed increased Th2 and impaired Th1 antigen-specific responses, which was associated with increased T cell expression by SOCS1 (Babu *et al.* 2005). Altogether, the function of SOCS1 during infections with parasites resembles that in bacterial infections, balancing anti-pathogen responses and the severity of inflammation.

4. SOCS3

SOCS3 is an important endogenous inhibitor of STAT3-mediated cytokine signalling. SOCS3 has been shown to be induced by different hormones including ciliary neutrophilic factor, leptin, prolactin and growth hormones (Adams *et al.* 1998; Bjorbaek *et al.* 1998; Bjorbaek *et al.* 1999; Pezet *et al.* 1999) and cytokines like leukemia inhibitory factor, IL-11, IL-10, IL-2, IL-27 and IL-6 (Starr *et al.* 1997; Auernhammer & Melmed 1999; Bousquet *et al.* 1999; Cassatella *et al.* 1999; Cohney *et al.* 1999) but also by microbial molecular patterns as LPS or CpG (Stoiber *et al.* 1999; Dalpke *et al.* 2001).

Among these, the role SOCS3 in regulation of IL-6 responses has been studied in detail. IL-6 is a pro-inflammatory cytokine that has been found to play a role in many inflammatory diseases, while IL-10 is a potent anti-inflammatory cytokine, which suppresses gene activation through TLR signalling pathways, but can also inhibit Th1 responses at different levels. While it is known that STAT3 is essential for the biological actions of both IL-6 and IL-10, it was unclear for many years how these two cytokines could have exactly opposing functions.

Interestingly, an inhibitory role for SOCS3 could only be shown for cytokines binding to the IL-6 receptor whereas the signalling of IL-10 that also stimulates STAT3-activation was unaffected by SOCS3 (Song & Shuai 1998; Lang *et al.* 2003; Yasukawa *et al.* 2003a; Kimura *et al.* 2004; Shuai 2006). This is explained by the ability of SOCS3 to bind to the IL-6 receptor subunit gp130 (Tyr 759) but not to the IL-10 receptor (Nicholson *et al.* 2000; Lehmann *et al.* 2003; Yasukawa *et al.* 2003a). STAT3 activation in response to IL-6 is prolonged in absence of SOCS3. It has been proposed that the sustained activation of STAT3 is essential for the anti-inflammatory effect, while transient activation of STAT3 promotes inflammation (Yasukawa *et al.* 2003a).

Gp130 is a promiscuous cytokine receptor subunit that mediates signalling by IL-6 and other cytokines such as IL-11, IL-27, leukemia inhibitory factor (LIF) and cardiotrophin-1 (Taga & Kishimoto 1997). Gp130 is present on hematopoietic and nonhematopoietic cells, and its expression can vary depending on the cell's activation status (Andersson *et al.* 1978). Gp130 itself does not bind to cytokines but acts as a co-receptor. When the cytokine (for example IL-6) binds to the IL-6Ra, it triggers a heterodimeric association with gp130 to form a signalling complex (Silver & Hunter 2010). SOCS3 also modulates signalling of gp-130-dependent cytokines. Moreover, the mutation of SOCS3 binding site on the gp130 receptor increased STAT3 activation in response to IL-6 and stimulated IL-10-like anti-inflammatory responses (Ohtani *et al.* 2000; Croker *et al.* 2003; Lang *et al.* 2003; Yasukawa *et al.* 2003a). Such anti-inflammatory responses are abolished when the gp130 Y759 mutated mice possessed a monoallelic deletion of STAT3 (McLoughlin *et al.* 2005; Yoshimura *et al.* 2007). As already mentioned above, SOCS3 inhibits also signalling via non gp130 containing cytokine and hormone receptors such as GCSF, leptin, IL-12 and even IFNs (Song & Shuai 1998; Bousquet *et al.* 1999; Bjorbak *et al.* 2000; Shen *et al.* 2000; Hortner *et al.* 2002b).

SOCS3 knock out mice die during embryonic life due to placental defects (Marine *et al.* 1999a; Roberts *et al.* 2001). The early death is caused by enhanced LIF signalling, since SOCS3$^{-/-}$ mice showed altered trophoblast differentiation. Animals, in which the SOCS3 deletion in the placenta was rescued by a tetraploid rescue method, showed extended embryonic life. However, rescued SOCS3$^{-/-}$ embryos died due to cardiac hypertrophy (Takahashi *et al.* 2003).

4.1 SOCS3 in myeloid cells/granulopoiesis

Mice with a conditional knock down of SOCS3 in myeloid cells demonstrated the role of SOCS3 in suppression of IL-6/gp130 signalling. SOCS3-deficient macrophages stimulated with IL-6 displayed an increased magnitude and duration of STAT1 and STAT3 activation in comparison to controls (Croker *et al.* 2003; Lang *et al.* 2003; Yasukawa *et al.* 2003a).

Mice deficient for SOCS3 in myeloid cells are resistant to LPS-induced endotoxic shock whereas STAT3 deficient mice are highly sensitive (Takeda *et al.* 1999; Yasukawa *et al.* 2003a). Thus, STAT3 activation mediates anti-inflammatory IL-10 signalling and in the absence of SOCS3, similar anti-inflammatory properties in response to IL-6 (Johnston & O'Shea 2003). Furthermore, macrophages lacking SOCS3 were shown to secrete reduced levels of TNF-α and IL-12 after IL-6 and LPS stimulation (Yasukawa *et al.* 2003a).
In a similar manner, DCs deficient for STAT3 contributed to T cell hyper-activation while in the absence of SOCS3, DCs induced a selective expansion of regulatory T cells (Cheng *et al.* 2003; Matsumura *et al.* 2007). An overexpression of SOCS3 in DCs resulted a reduction of expression of co-stimulatory molecules and IL-12. Moreover, SOCS3-deficient and overexpressing DCs had the capacity to suppress EAE development (Li *et al.* 2006; Matsumura *et al.* 2007).
Croker et al. (2003) and Lang et al (2003) on the other hand, using SOCS3 deficient macrophages found an increased STAT1 activation and elevated levels of IFN-γ-regulated genes in response to IL-6.

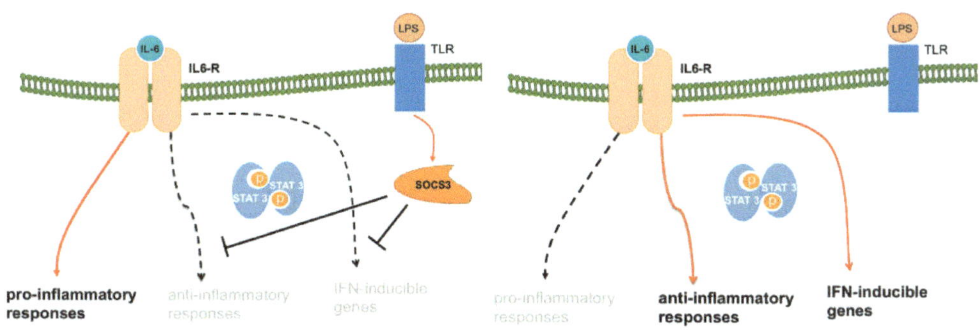

Fig. 4. SOCS3 inhibits anti-inflammatory and IFN-inducible genes in response to IL-6. Adapted from (Johnston & O'Shea 2003)

Other molecular targets of SOCS3 have been reported: SOCS3 inhibited the activation of TNF-receptor-associated factor 6 (TRAF6) and TGF-β-activated kinase 1 (TAK1), essential for both TLR- and IL-1-induced responses (Frobose *et al.* 2006). Prele et al. (2006) found no differences in LPS responses of SOCS3 transfected human macrophages. Thus, further studies are required to determine whether there is a direct role for SOCS3 in TLR signalling.
Upon over-expression, SOCS3 was found to bind to the GCSF receptor and reduced STAT3 activation in response to GCSF (Hortner *et al.* 2002b; Hermans *et al.* 2003). In agreement, deletion of SOCS3 in the myeloid or hematopoietic cells increased numbers of neutrophils, which showed increased survival and proliferative capacity (Croker *et al.* 2004; Kimura *et al.* 2004). Following GCSF injection SOCS3-deficient mice developed neutrophilia, and a spectrum of inflammatory pathologies, characterised by neutrophil infiltration in multiples tissues (Croker *et al.* 2008). Overall, SOCS3 regulates survival, growth and activation of neutrophils and an inhibition of SOCS3 may enhance the essential neutrophil recovery after chemotherapy or neutropenia.

4.1.1 SOCS3 in T cells

T cell development in the thymus is unaffected by SOCS3 (Chen *et al.* 2006). However, SOCS3 might play an active role in T cell proliferation and differentiation.

The proliferation of T cells was found to be regulated by SOCS3. T cells overexpressing SOCS3 showed reduced proliferation to mitogens and anti-CD28 (Banerjee *et al.* 2002; Matsumoto *et al.* 2003). On the other hand, SOCS3-deficient CD8 T cells also showed enhanced anti-CD3-induced proliferation. Neutralization of IL-27 also limited T cell proliferation indicating that IL-27 responses are impaired by SOCS3 and account for diminished T cell proliferation (Brender *et al.* 2007).

There is a reciprocal relation between SOCS1 and SOCS3 expression levels in T cells, with high SOCS1 and low SOCS3 expression in Th1 cells whereas high SOCS3 and low SOCS1 expression was found in Th2 cells (Egwuagu *et al.* 2002; Seki *et al.* 2003). However, there are conflicting results whether levels of SOCS3 actively influences the Th1/Th2 balance. Overexpression of SOCS3 in murine T cells resulted in elevated Th2 and decreased Th1 responses during allergy. Furthermore, a reduced Th2 response characterized by decreased IL-4 and increased IFN-γ production was shown in $SOCS3^{+/-}$ mice (Seki *et al.* 2003). A SOCS3 mediated regulation of STAT5 activation was reported to account for the altered Th1/Th2 balance. Another explanation for reduced Th2 responses was suggested by Kinjyo et al. (2006) using Lck $SOCS3^{fl/fl}$ mice, in which Th3-like T cells with higher IL-10 and TGF-β levels were found. These cytokines may then suppress Th1 responses accounting for the decreased Th1/Th2 ratio in SOCS3 deficient mice. However this observation was not confirmed by others: mice with a specific deletion of SOCS3 in the lymphoid cells were reported to have an unaltered Th1 and Th2 cell differentiation (Chen *et al.* 2006). Instead, loss of SOCS3 resulted in enhanced Th17 generation and enhanced STAT3 activation in response to IL-23. Th17 is a T cell subset that produces IL-17 and plays a key role in different autoimmune diseases and in the defense against fungal infections. STAT3 interacted with the *IL17A* and *IL-17F* promoter (Kinjyo *et al.* 2006). TGF-β-mediated the inhibition of SOCS3 expression and therefore prolonged STAT3 activation promoting Th17 development (Qin *et al.* 2009).

The importance of SOCS3 in impairing Th17 development was further confirmed in a study of an atherosclerosis model in mice with a T cell specific SOCS3 knock down and in a rheumatoid arthritis model in mice lacking SOCS3 in hematopoietic and endothelial cells (Wong *et al.* 2006; Taleb *et al.* 2009).

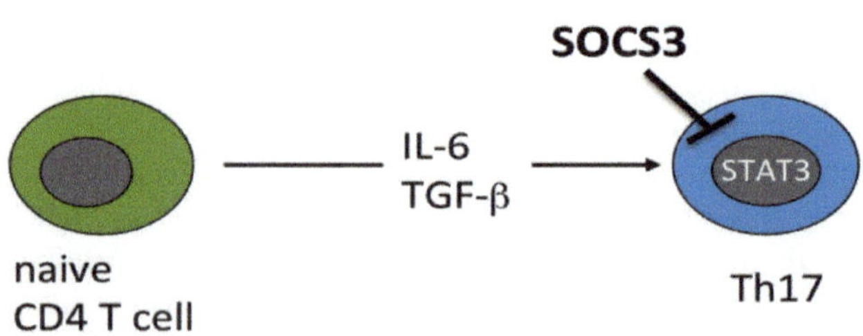

Fig. 5. SOCS3 hampers Th17 cell development

Regulatory T cells, a subset of CD4 T cells that suppress T cell-mediated immune responses and maintain tolerance to self-antigens, were found to be deficient for SOCS3 protein expression (Pillemer *et al.* 2007). Over-expression of SOCS3 in T regs impaired their

proliferation and suppressive function. The role of SOCS3 on T cell differentiation is still not completely understood but it seems likely that SOCS3 impedes both T reg function (and thereby increasing immune responses) and Th17 differentiation (impairing inflammatory responses, fig. 5).
SOCS3 has also been shown to modulate B cell development by affecting the lodging of precursor B cells to the bone marrow, via the regulation of responses to CXCL12 (Le *et al.* 2007).

4.1.2 SOCS3 in leptin and insulin resistance

Infections are accompanied by tissue insulin resistance, as manifested by worsening of metabolic control in diabetic patients and decreased glucose tolerance in non-diabetic subjects. A propensity towards glucose intolerance and diabetes has been documented in patients with chronic HCV infection. Diabetes patients are more susceptible to infections such as tuberculosis or candidiasis. These associated diseases could be linked to SOCS expressin. As stated below pathogen molecules can stimulate SOCS3 expression. SOCS3 binds to the leptin and insulin receptor and inhibits STAT3 activation in response to leptin and insulin respectively (Clement *et al.* 1998; Bjorbak *et al.* 2000; Emanuelli *et al.* 2000; Eyckerman *et al.* 2000; Chen *et al.* 2006). Leptin is an adipocyte-derived hormone that regulates food intake and energy homeostasis (Flier 2004). Leptin-resistance, common in human obesity and in acquired obesity in rodents, may be regulated by SOCS3 (Bjorbaek *et al.* 1998). High fat diet fed SOCS3$^{+/-}$ mice as well as neural cell-specific SOCS3- knock-down mice showed reduced diet-induced obesity, together with increased leptin and insulin sensitivity (Howard *et al.* 2004; Mori *et al.* 2004; Kievit *et al.* 2006). Furthermore, SOCS3 deficient adipocytes were protected from TNF-α-induced insulin resistance (Shi *et al.* 2004). However, mice with a knock down of SOCS3 in hepatocytes displayed increased insulin sensitivity in the liver but developed obesity and systemic insulin resistance with age (Torisu *et al.* 2007). This insulin resistance was accounted by increased inflammatory responses due to the lack of SOCS3. Accordingly, overexpression of SOCS3 in the liver of mice induced insulin resistance, whereas silencing of SOCS3 with antisense oligonucleotides in obese diabetic mice improved insulin sensitivity (Ueki *et al.* 2004a; Ueki *et al.* 2004b). The consistency of the effect of SOCS3 in different approaches on both leptin and insulin resistance indicates SOCS3 as a unique mediator of both obesity and insulin resistance.

4.2 Role of SOCS3 in infectious diseases and inflammation

Similar to SOCS1, SOCS3 expression can be stimulated by both cytokines but also TLR agonists. Additionally, several pathogens including viruses, bacteria and parasites have been shown to stimulate SOCS3 expression. But due to multiple binding partners of SOCS3, it is hard to predict the role of SOCS3 in different infections.

4.2.1 Viral infections

SOCS3 was found to inhibit type I IFN signalling although SOCS3 was less effective than SOCS1 (Song & Shuai 1998; Shen *et al.* 2000). Infection with several viruses induced SOCS3 expression that correlated with reduced STAT1 activation in response to IFN-α/β. HSV stimulated SOCS3 in different human cell lines but not in the B-cell line AKATA. In contrast to SOCS3-expressing cell lines, infected AKATA cells showed no impaired IFN-α/β mediated STAT1 activation during HSV infection. Silencing of SOCS3 using anti-sense nucleotides significantly hampered replication of HSV (Yokota *et al.* 2005). Similar observations were done during Influenza A, HCV and Epstein Barr virus infections indicating that SOCS3 expression facilitates viral infections (Bode *et al.* 2003; Le Goffic *et al.* 2007; Pothlichet *et al.* 2008; Michaud *et al.* 2010).

Interestingly, mice with a T cell-specific SOCS3 deletion showed increased T cell activation and viral clearance without development of immunopathology during the infection with lymphocytic chriomeningitis virus (LCMV) (Pellegrini *et al.* 2011). Treatment of LCMV-infected mice with IL-7 repressed SOCS3 expression and promoted IL-6 production resulting in enhanced T cell effector functions, numbers and viral clearance. However, the deletion of SOCS3 in all hematopoietic cells induced neutrophilia and early lethality in LCMV-infected mice (Pellegrini *et al.* 2011).

Patients with genotype 1 HCV infection tend to have higher levels of SOCS3 expression, providing a rationale for their propensity toward a lack of therapeutic response (Kim *et al.* 2009). Moreover, one SOCS3 genotype (-4874 AA) expressed SOCS3 at elevated levels and showed a poorer response to therapy (Persico *et al.* 2008).

4.2.2 Bacterial infections

The infection of macrophages with *Salmonella enterica* has been shown to increment SOCS3 but not SOCS1 expression (Uchiya & Nikai 2005). SOCS3 stimulation was dependent on the *Salmonella* pathogenicity island 2 important for bacterial virulence. Infected macrophages showed impaired STAT1 and STAT3 activation in response to IL-6 or IFN-γ respectively, which might prevent effective bacterial killing.

Infection of macrophages with *Mycobacterium avium* or *M. bovis* raised SOCS1 and SOCS3 levels in a TLR2-NOTCH1 dependent pathway (Imai *et al.* 2003; Vazquez *et al.* 2006; Narayana & Balaji 2008).

Patients with active tuberculosis were found to have higher SOCS3 expression levels in whole blood and T cells in comparison to latently infected controls or to patients after chemotherapy (Mistry *et al.* 2007; Jacobsen *et al.* 2010). We observed that SOCS3 expression in blood non-T cells from patients with TB was negatively associated with severity of disease (Masood *et al*, 2011). Atogether the role of SOCS3 in bacterial infections is far from clear.

4.2.3 Parasites

Little is known about the role of SOCS3 in parasites. Infection of macrophages with the parasite *Leishmania dovani* was shown to stimulate SOCS3 expression. SOCS3 levels associated with reduced STAT1 activation after IFN-γ stimulation and therefore with reduced protection (Bertholet *et al.* 2003).

On the contrary, mice lacking SOCS3 in T cells were more susceptible to *Leishmania major* infections. SOCS3-deficiency in T cells led to increased anti-inflammatory TGF-β and IL-10 secretion by T cells and reduced immunoglobulin levels (Kinjyo *et al.* 2006).

Mice bearing a mutation in the SOCS3 binding site of the gp130 receptor displayed increased susceptibility to *Toxoplasma gondii*. A decreased IL-12 production by DCs resulted in reduced IFN-γ secretion by NK cells of these mice. Addition of IL-12 as well as neutralization of IL-6 could restore the wild type phenotype indicating that an altered IL-6 signalling was responsible for increased susceptibility (Silver *et al.* 2011).

	pathogen	mechanism	pathology	pathogen control
SOCS1	SFV	↓ IFN-α/β signalling		worsened
	HTLV-1	↓ IFN-α/β signalling.		worsened
	VSV	↓ IFN-α/β signalling.		worsened
	HSV-1	↓ IFN-γ signalling.		worsened
	Vaccinia Virus	↓immune responses	improved	improved
	HIV-1	Ubiquitination of HIVgag		worsened
	C. pneumoniae	↓IFN-γ signalling	improved	worsened
	M. tuberculosis - *M. bovis* BCG	↓ IL-12 signalling	improved	worsened
	P. berghi ANKA	???	worsened	worsened
	L. major	↓ IFN-γ signalling	improved	worsened
	T. gondii	↓ IFN-γ signalling		worsened
	B. malayi	Th1/Th2 ratio		worsened
SOCS3	HSV-1	↓IFN-α/β signalling.		worsened
	RSV	↓IFN-α/β signalling.		
	HIV-1	↓IFN-α/β signalling		
	Influenza A Virus	↓IFN-α/β signalling		worsened
	LCMV	↓T cell activation	worsened	worsened
	L. major	↓TGF-β IL-10 production by T cells	?	improved
	T. gondii (gp130 mutation)	↑IL-12 induction in dendritic cells	improved	improved

Table 1. Role of SOCS molecules during microbial infections.

5. Conclusion

SOCS expression is tightly regulated to prevent inflammation while maintaining protective anti-microbial responses. Pathogens are able to potently stimulate SOCS1 and 3 protein expression following infection and hijack SOCS function promoting their survival. In most infections studied, the stimulation of SOCS1 and SOCS3 expression by infectious agents resulted in a worsened pathogen control even though the nature of immune inhibition by the SOCS proteins differed. Thus, SOCS proteins can be manipulated to increase innate immune mechanisms, but also the triggering and the magnitude of adaptive immune responses. This converts SOCS proteins into very attractive therapeutic targets. However manipulation of SOCS levels always bears the risk of increased inflammatory responses. A better understanding of the role of SOCS in infections is required to better gauge SOCS manipulation leading to potentially new therapies.

6. References

Adams, T.E., Hansen, J.A., Starr, R., Nicola, N.A., Hilton, D.J. & Billestrup, N. (1998) Growth hormone preferentially induces the rapid, transient expression of SOCS-3, a novel inhibitor of cytokine receptor signaling. *The Journal of Biological Chemistry* 273, 1285-1287.

Ahmed, C.M., Dabelic, R., Waiboci, L.W., Jager, L.D., Heron, L.L. & Johnson, H.M. (2009) SOCS-1 mimetics protect mice against lethal poxvirus infection: identification of a novel endogenous antiviral system. *Journal of Virology* 83, 1402-1415.

Alexander, W.S. (2002) Suppressors of cytokine signalling (SOCS) in the immune system. *Nature Reviews. Immunology* 2, 410-416.

Alexander, W.S., Starr, R., Fenner, J.E., Scott, C.L., Handman, E., Sprigg, N.S., Corbin, J.E., Cornish, A.L., Darwiche, R., Owczarek, C.M., Kay, T.W., Nicola, N.A., Hertzog, P.J., Metcalf, D. & Hilton, D.J. (1999) SOCS1 is a critical inhibitor of interferon gamma signaling and prevents the potentially fatal neonatal actions of this cytokine. *Cell* 98, 597-608.

Andersson, L.C., Gahmberg, C.G., Kimura, A.K. & Wigzell, H. (1978) Activated human T lymphocytes display new surface glycoproteins. *Proceedings of the National Academy of Sciences of The United States of America* 75, 3455-3458.

Auernhammer, C.J. & Melmed, S. (1999) Interleukin-11 stimulates proopiomelanocortin gene expression and adrenocorticotropin secretion in corticotroph cells: evidence for a redundant cytokine network in the hypothalamo-pituitary-adrenal axis. *Endocrinology* 140, 1559-1566.

Babu, S., Kumaraswami, V. & Nutman, T.B. (2005) Transcriptional control of impaired Th1 responses in patent lymphatic filariasis by T-box expressed in T cells and suppressor of cytokine signaling genes. *Infection and Immunity* 73, 3394-3401.

Baetz, A., Frey, M., Heeg, K. & Dalpke, A.H. (2004) Suppressor of cytokine signaling (SOCS) proteins indirectly regulate toll-like receptor signaling in innate immune cells. *The Journal Of Biological Chemistry* 279, 54708-54715.

Banerjee, A., Banks, A.S., Nawijn, M.C., Chen, X.P. & Rothman, P.B. (2002) Cutting edge: Suppressor of cytokine signaling 3 inhibits activation of NFATp. *Journal Of Immunology* 168, 4277-4281.

Berry, M.P., Graham, C.M., McNab, F.W. *Et Al.* (2010) An interferon-inducible neutrophil-driven blood transcriptional signature in human tuberculosis. *Nature* 466, 973-977.

Bertholet, S., Dickensheets, H.L., Sheikh, F., Gam, A.A., Donnelly, R.P. & Kenney, R.T. (2003) Leishmania donovani-induced expression of suppressor of cytokine signaling 3 in human macrophages: a novel mechanism for intracellular parasite suppression of activation. *Infection and Immunity* 71, 2095-2101.

Bhattacharyya, S., Zhao, Y., Kay, T.W. & Muglia, L.J. (2011) Glucocorticoids target suppressor of cytokine signaling 1 (SOCS1) and type 1 interferons to regulate Toll-like receptor-induced STAT1 activation. *Proceedings Of The National Academy of Sciences of the United States of America* 108, 9554-9559.

Bjorbaek, C., Elmquist, J.K., El-Haschimi, K., Kelly, J., Ahima, R.S., Hileman, S. & Flier, J.S. (1999) Activation of SOCS-3 messenger ribonucleic acid in the hypothalamus by ciliary neurotrophic factor. *Endocrinology* 140, 2035-2043.

Bjorbaek, C., Elmquist, J.K., Frantz, J.D., Shoelson, S.E. & Flier, J.S. (1998) Identification of SOCS-3 as a potential mediator of central leptin resistance. *Molecular Cell* 1, 619-625.

Bjorbak, C., Lavery, H.J., Bates, S.H., Olson, R.K., Davis, S.M., Flier, J.S. & Myers, M.G., Jr. (2000) SOCS3 mediates feedback inhibition of the leptin receptor via Tyr985. *The Journal of Biological Chemistry* 275, 40649-40657.

Bode, J.G., Ludwig, S., Ehrhardt, C., Albrecht, U., Erhardt, A., Schaper, F., Heinrich, P.C. & Haussinger, D. (2003) IFN-alpha antagonistic activity of HCV core protein involves induction of suppressor of cytokine signaling-3. *The FASEB Journal : Official Publication of the Federation of American Societies for Experimental Biology* 17, 488-490.

Bousquet, C., Susini, C. & Melmed, S. (1999) Inhibitory roles for SHP-1 and SOCS-3 following pituitary proopiomelanocortin induction by leukemia inhibitory factor. *The Journal of Clinical Investigation* 104, 1277-1285.

Brender, C., Tannahill, G.M., Jenkins, B.J., Fletcher, J., Columbus, R., Saris, C.J., Ernst, M., Nicola, N.A., Hilton, D.J., Alexander, W.S. & Starr, R. (2007) Suppressor of cytokine signaling 3 regulates CD8 T-cell proliferation by inhibition of interleukins 6 and 27. *Blood* 110, 2528-2536.

Bullen, D.V., Baldwin, T.M., Curtis, J.M., Alexander, W.S. & Handman, E. (2003a) Persistence of lesions in suppressor of cytokine signaling-1-deficient mice infected with Leishmania major. *Journal of Immunology* 170, 4267-4272.

Bullen, D.V., Darwiche, R., Metcalf, D., Handman, E. & Alexander, W.S. (2001) Neutralization of interferon-gamma in neonatal SOCS1-/- mice prevents fatty degeneration of the liver but not subsequent fatal inflammatory disease. *Immunology* 104, 92-98.

Bullen, D.V., Hansen, D.S., Siomos, M.A., Schofield, L., Alexander, W.S. & Handman, E. (2003b) The lack of suppressor of cytokine signalling-1 (SOCS1) protects mice from the development of cerebral malaria caused by Plasmodium berghei ANKA. *Parasite Immunology* 25, 113-118.

Car, B.D., Eng, V.M., Schnyder, B., Ozmen, L., Huang, S., Gallay, P., Heumann, D., Aguet, M. & Ryffel, B. (1994) Interferon gamma receptor deficient mice are resistant to endotoxic shock. *The Journal of Experimental Medicine* 179, 1437-1444.

Carow, B., X. Qun Ye, D. Gavier-Widen, S. Bhuju, W. Oehlmann, M. Singh, M. Skold, L. Ignatowicz, A. Yoshimura, H. Wigzell, and M. E. Rottenberg. 2011. Silencing Suppressor of Cytokine Signaling-1 (SOCS1) in macrophages improves *Mycobacterium tuberculosis* Control in an Interferon-γ–dependent manner. *The Journal of Biological Chemistry* 286:26873-26887.

Cassatella, M.A., Gasperini, S., Bovolenta, C., Calzetti, F., Vollebregt, M., Scapini, P., Marchi, M., Suzuki, R., Suzuki, A. & Yoshimura, A. (1999) Interleukin-10 (IL-10) selectively enhances CIS3/SOCS3 mRNA expression in human neutrophils: evidence for an IL-10-induced pathway that is independent of STAT protein activation. *Blood* 94, 2880-2889.

Chen, Z., Laurence, A., Kanno, Y., Pacher-Zavisin, M., Zhu, B.M., Tato, C., Yoshimura, A., Hennighausen, L. & O'Shea, J.J. (2006) Selective regulatory function of Socs3 in the formation of IL-17-secreting T cells. *Proceedings of the National Academy of Sciences Of the United States of America* 103, 8137-8142.

Cheng, F., Wang, H.W., Cuenca, A., Huang, M., Ghansah, T., Brayer, J., Kerr, W.G., Takeda, K., Akira, S., Schoenberger, S.P., Yu, H., Jove, R. & Sotomayor, E.M. (2003) A critical role for Stat3 signaling in immune tolerance. *Immunity* 19, 425-436.

Chong, M.M., Cornish, A.L., Darwiche, R., Stanley, E.G., Purton, J.F., Godfrey, D.I., Hilton, D.J., Starr, R., Alexander, W.S. & Kay, T.W. (2003) Suppressor of cytokine signaling-1 is a critical regulator of interleukin-7-dependent CD8+ T cell differentiation. *Immunity* 18, 475-487.

Chong, M.M., Metcalf, D., Jamieson, E., Alexander, W.S. & Kay, T.W. (2005) Suppressor of cytokine signaling-1 in T cells and macrophages is critical for preventing lethal inflammation. *Blood* 106, 1668-1675.

Clement, K., Vaisse, C., Lahlou, N., Cabrol, S., Pelloux, V., Cassuto, D., Gourmelen, M., Dina, C., Chambaz, J., Lacorte, J.M., Basdevant, A., Bougneres, P., Lebouc, Y., Froguel, P. & Guy-Grand, B. (1998) A mutation in the human leptin receptor gene causes obesity and pituitary dysfunction. *Nature* 392, 398-401.

Cohney, S.J., Sanden, D., Cacalano, N.A., Yoshimura, A., Mui, A., Migone, T.S. & Johnston, J.A. (1999) SOCS-3 is tyrosine phosphorylated in response to interleukin-2 and suppresses STAT5 phosphorylation and lymphocyte proliferation. *Molecular and Cellular Biology* 19, 4980-4988.

Croker, B.A., Krebs, D.L., Zhang, J.G., Wormald, S., Willson, T.A., Stanley, E.G., Robb, L., Greenhalgh, C.J., Forster, I., Clausen, B.E., Nicola, N.A., Metcalf, D., Hilton, D.J., Roberts, A.W. & Alexander, W.S. (2003) SOCS3 negatively regulates IL-6 signaling in vivo. *Nature Immunology* 4, 540-545.

Croker, B.A., Metcalf, D., Robb, L., Wei, W., Mifsud, S., DiRago, L., Cluse, L.A., Sutherland, K.D., Hartley, L., Williams, E., Zhang, J.G., Hilton, D.J., Nicola, N.A., Alexander, W.S. & Roberts, A.W. (2004) SOCS3 is a critical physiological negative regulator of G-CSF signaling and emergency granulopoiesis. *Immunity* 20, 153-165.

Croker, B.A., Mielke, L.A., Wormald, S., Metcalf, D., Kiu, H., Alexander, W.S., Hilton, D.J. & Roberts, A.W. (2008) Socs3 maintains the specificity of biological responses to cytokine signals during granulocyte and macrophage differentiation. *Experimental Hematology* 36, 786-798.

Dalpke, A.H., Opper, S., Zimmermann, S. & Heeg, K. (2001) Suppressors of cytokine signaling (SOCS)-1 and SOCS-3 are induced by CpG-DNA and modulate cytokine responses in APCs. *Journal of Immunology* 166, 7082-7089.

Dennis, V.A., Jefferson, A., Singh, S.R., Ganapamo, F. & Philipp, M.T. (2006) Interleukin-10 anti-inflammatory response to Borrelia burgdorferi, the agent of Lyme disease: a possible role for suppressors of cytokine signaling 1 and 3. *Infection and Immunity* 74, 5780-5789.

Egwuagu, C.E., Yu, C.R., Zhang, M., Mahdi, R.M., Kim, S.J. & Gery, I. (2002) Suppressors of cytokine signaling proteins are differentially expressed in Th1 and Th2 cells: implications for Th cell lineage commitment and maintenance. *Journal of Immunology* 168, 3181-3187.

Emanuelli, B., Peraldi, P., Filloux, C., Sawka-Verhelle, D., Hilton, D. & Van Obberghen, E. (2000) SOCS-3 is an insulin-induced negative regulator of insulin signaling. *The Journal of Biological Chemistry* 275, 15985-15991.

Endo, T.A., Masuhara, M., Yokouchi, M. *Et Al.* (1997) A new protein containing an SH2 domain that inhibits JAK kinases. *Nature* 387, 921-924.

Evel-Kabler, K., Song, X.T., Aldrich, M., Huang, X.F. & Chen, S.Y. (2006) SOCS1 restricts dendritic cells' ability to break self tolerance and induce antitumor immunity by regulating IL-12 production and signaling. *The Journal of Clinical Investigation* 116, 90-100.

Eyckerman, S., Broekaert, D., Verhee, A., Vandekerckhove, J. & Tavernier, J. (2000) Identification of the Y985 and Y1077 motifs as SOCS3 recruitment sites in the murine leptin receptor. *FEBS Letters* 486, 33-37.

Eyles, J.L., Metcalf, D., Grusby, M.J., Hilton, D.J. & Starr, R. (2002) Negative regulation of interleukin-12 signaling by suppressor of cytokine signaling-1. *The Journal of Biological Chemistry* 277, 43735-43740.

Fenner, J.E., Starr, R., Cornish, A.L., Zhang, J.G., Metcalf, D., Schreiber, R.D., Sheehan, K., Hilton, D.J., Alexander, W.S. & Hertzog, P.J. (2006) Suppressor of cytokine signaling 1 regulates the immune response to infection by a unique inhibition of type I interferon activity. *Nature Immunology* 7, 33-39.

Flier, J.S. (2004) Obesity wars: molecular progress confronts an expanding epidemic. *Cell* 116, 337-350.

Frazier, A.D., Zhang, C.L., Ni, L., Ma, C.J., Zhang, Y., Wu, X.Y., Atia, A.N., Yao, Z.Q. & Moorman, J.P. (2010) Programmed death-1 affects suppressor of cytokine signaling-1 expression in T cells during hepatitis C infection. *Viral Immunology* 23, 487-495.

Frey, K.G., Ahmed, C.M., Dabelic, R., Jager, L.D., Noon-Song, E.N., Haider, S.M., Johnson, H.M. & Bigley, N.J. (2009) HSV-1-induced SOCS-1 expression in keratinocytes: use of a SOCS-1 antagonist to block a novel mechanism of viral immune evasion. *Journal of Immunology* 183, 1253-1262.

Frobose, H., Ronn, S.G., Heding, P.E., Mendoza, H., Cohen, P., Mandrup-Poulsen, T. & Billestrup, N. (2006) Suppressor of cytokine Signaling-3 inhibits interleukin-1 signaling by targeting the TRAF-6/TAK1 complex. *Molecular Endocrinology* 20, 1587-1596.

Fujimoto, M. & Naka, T. (2003) Regulation of cytokine signaling by SOCS family molecules. *Trends in Immunology* 24, 659-666.

Gingras, S., Parganas, E., de Pauw, A., Ihle, J.N. & Murray, P.J. (2004) Re-examination of the role of suppressor of cytokine signaling 1 (SOCS1) in the regulation of toll-like receptor signaling. *The Journal of Biological Chemistry* 279, 54702-54707.

Haffner, M.C., Jurgeit, A., Berlato, C., Geley, S., Parajuli, N., Yoshimura, A. & Doppler, W. (2008) Interaction and functional interference of glucocorticoid receptor and SOCS1. *The Journal of Biological Chemistry* 283, 22089-22096.

Hamanaka, I., Saito, Y., Yasukawa, H., Kishimoto, I., Kuwahara, K., Miyamoto, Y., Harada, M., Ogawa, E., Kajiyama, N., Takahashi, N., Izumi, T., Kawakami, R., Masuda, I., Yoshimura, A. & Nakao, K. (2001) Induction of JAB/SOCS-1/SSI-1 and CIS3/SOCS-3/SSI-3 is involved in gp130 resistance in cardiovascular system in rat treated with cardiotrophin-1 in vivo. *Circulation Research* 88, 727-732.

Hanada, T., Yoshida, H., Kato, S., Tanaka, K., Masutani, K., Tsukada, J., Nomura, Y., Mimata, H., Kubo, M. & Yoshimura, A. (2003) Suppressor of cytokine signaling-1 is essential for suppressing dendritic cell activation and systemic autoimmunity. *Immunity* 19, 437-450.

Hansen, J.A., Lindberg, K., Hilton, D.J., Nielsen, J.H. & Billestrup, N. (1999) Mechanism of inhibition of growth hormone receptor signaling by suppressor of cytokine signaling proteins. *Molecular Endocrinology* 13, 1832-1843.

Hashimoto, K., Ishibashi, K., Ishioka, K., Zhao, D., Sato, M., Ohara, S., Abe, Y., Kawasaki, Y., Sato, Y., Yokota, S., Fujii, N., Peebles, R.S., Jr., Hosoya, M. & Suzutani, T. (2009a) RSV replication is attenuated by counteracting expression of the suppressor of cytokine signaling (SOCS) molecules. *Virology* 391, 162-170.

Hashimoto, M., Ayada, T., Kinjyo, I., Hiwatashi, K., Yoshida, H., Okada, Y., Kobayashi, T. & Yoshimura, A. (2009b) Silencing of SOCS1 in macrophages suppresses tumor development by enhancing antitumor inflammation. *Cancer Science* 100, 730-736.

He, Y., Zhang, W., Zhang, R., Zhang, H. & Min, W. (2006) SOCS1 inhibits tumor necrosis factor-induced activation of ASK1-JNK inflammatory signaling by mediating ASK1 degradation. *The Journal of Biological Chemistry* 281, 5559-5566.

Hebenstreit, D., Luft, P., Schmiedlechner, A., Duschl, A. & Horejs-Hoeck, J. (2005) SOCS-1 and SOCS-3 inhibit IL-4 and IL-13 induced activation of Eotaxin-3/CCL26 gene expression in HEK293 cells. *Molecular Immunology* 42, 295-303.

Hermans, M.H., van de Geijn, G.J., Antonissen, C., Gits, J., van Leeuwen, D., Ward, A.C. & Touw, I.P. (2003) Signaling mechanisms coupled to tyrosines in the granulocyte colony-stimulating factor receptor orchestrate G-CSF-induced expansion of myeloid progenitor cells. *Blood* 101, 2584-2590.

Hortner, M., Nielsch, U., Mayr, L.M., Heinrich, P.C. & Haan, S. (2002a) A new high affinity binding site for suppressor of cytokine signaling-3 on the erythropoietin receptor. *European Journal of Biochemistry / FEBS* 269, 2516-2526.

Hortner, M., Nielsch, U., Mayr, L.M., Johnston, J.A., Heinrich, P.C. & Haan, S. (2002b) Suppressor of cytokine signaling-3 is recruited to the activated granulocyte-colony stimulating factor receptor and modulates its signal transduction. *Journal of Immunology* 169, 1219-1227.

Howard, J.K., Cave, B.J., Oksanen, L.J., Tzameli, I., Bjorbaek, C. & Flier, J.S. (2004) Enhanced leptin sensitivity and attenuation of diet-induced obesity in mice with haploinsufficiency of Socs3. *Nature Medicine* 10, 734-738.

Imai, K., Kurita-Ochiai, T. & Ochiai, K. (2003) Mycobacterium bovis bacillus Calmette-Guerin infection promotes SOCS induction and inhibits IFN-gamma-stimulated JAK/STAT signaling in J774 macrophages. *FEMS Immunology and Medical Microbiology* 39, 173-180.

Jacobsen, M., Repsilber, D., Kleinsteuber, K., Gutschmidt, A., Schommer-Leitner, S., Black, G., Walzl, G. & Kaufmann, S.H. (2010) Suppressor of cytokine signaling-3 is affected in T-cells from tuberculosisTB patients. *Clinical Microbiology and Infection : the Official Publication of the European Society of Clinical Microbiology and Infectious Diseases.*

Johnston, J.A. & O'Shea, J.J. (2003) Matching SOCS with function. *Nature Immunology* 4, 507-509.

Kamura, T., Maenaka, K., Kotoshiba, S., Matsumoto, M., Kohda, D., Conaway, R.C., Conaway, J.W. & Nakayama, K.I. (2004) VHL-box and SOCS-box domains determine binding specificity for Cul2-Rbx1 and Cul5-Rbx2 modules of ubiquitin ligases. *Genes & Development* 18, 3055-3065.

Kievit, P., Howard, J.K., Badman, M.K., Balthasar, N., Coppari, R., Mori, H., Lee, C.E., Elmquist, J.K., Yoshimura, A. & Flier, J.S. (2006) Enhanced leptin sensitivity and improved glucose homeostasis in mice lacking suppressor of cytokine signaling-3 in POMC-expressing cells. *Cell Metabolism* 4, 123-132.

Kim, K.A., Lin, W., Tai, A.W., Shao, R.X., Weinberg, E., De Sa Borges, C.B., Bhan, A.K., Zheng, H., Kamegaya, Y. & Chung, R.T. (2009) Hepatic SOCS3 expression is strongly associated with non-response to therapy and race in HCV and HCV/HIV infection. *J Hepatol* 50, 705-711.

Kimura, A., Kinjyo, I., Matsumura, Y., Mori, H., Mashima, R., Harada, M., Chien, K.R., Yasukawa, H. & Yoshimura, A. (2004) SOCS3 is a physiological negative regulator for granulopoiesis and granulocyte colony-stimulating factor receptor signaling. *The Journal of Biological Chemistry* 279, 6905-6910.

Kinjyo, I., Hanada, T., Inagaki-Ohara, K., Mori, H., Aki, D., Ohishi, M., Yoshida, H., Kubo, M. & Yoshimura, A. (2002) SOCS1/JAB is a negative regulator of LPS-induced macrophage activation. *Immunity* 17, 583-591.

Kinjyo, I., Inoue, H., Hamano, S., Fukuyama, S., Yoshimura, T., Koga, K., Takaki, H., Himeno, K., Takaesu, G., Kobayashi, T. & Yoshimura, A. (2006) Loss of SOCS3 in T helper cells resulted in reduced immune responses and hyperproduction of interleukin 10 and transforming growth factor-beta 1. *The Journal of Experimental Medicine* 203, 1021-1031.

Krebs, D.L. & Hilton, D.J. (2001) SOCS proteins: negative regulators of cytokine signaling. *Stem Cells* 19, 378-387.

Kubo, M., Hanada, T. & Yoshimura, A. (2003) Suppressors of cytokine signaling and immunity. *Nature Immunology* 4, 1169-1176.

Lang, R., Pauleau, A.L., Parganas, E., Takahashi, Y., Mages, J., Ihle, J.N., Rutschman, R. & Murray, P.J. (2003) SOCS3 regulates the plasticity of gp130 signaling. *Nature Immunology* 4, 546-550.

Le Goffic, R., Pothlichet, J., Vitour, D., Fujita, T., Meurs, E., Chignard, M. & Si-Tahar, M. (2007) Cutting Edge: Influenza A virus activates TLR3-dependent inflammatory and RIG-I-dependent antiviral responses in human lung epithelial cells. *Journal Of Immunology* 178, 3368-3372.

Le, Y., Zhu, B.M., Harley, B., Park, S.Y., Kobayashi, T., Manis, J.P., Luo, H.R., Yoshimura, A., Hennighausen, L. & Silberstein, L.E. (2007) SOCS3 protein developmentally regulates the chemokine receptor CXCR4-FAK signaling pathway during B lymphopoiesis. *Immunity* 27, 811-823.

Lee, C., Kolesnik, T.B., Caminschi, I., Chakravorty, A., Carter, W., Alexander, W.S., Jones, J., Anderson, G.P. & Nicholson, S.E. (2009) Suppressor of cytokine signalling 1 (SOCS1) is a physiological regulator of the asthma response. *Clin Exp Allergy* 39, 897-907.

Lehmann, U., Schmitz, J., Weissenbach, M., Sobota, R.M., Hortner, M., Friederichs, K., Behrmann, I., Tsiaris, W., Sasaki, A., Schneider-Mergener, J., Yoshimura, A., Neel, B.G., Heinrich, P.C. & Schaper, F. (2003) SHP2 and SOCS3 contribute to Tyr-759-dependent attenuation of interleukin-6 signaling through gp130. *The Journal of Biological Chemistry* 278, 661-671.

Leonard, W.J. & O'Shea, J.J. (1998) Jaks and STATs: biological implications. *Annual Review of Immunology* 16, 293-322.

Li, Y., Chu, N., Rostami, A. & Zhang, G.X. (2006) Dendritic cells transduced with SOCS-3 exhibit a tolerogenic/DC2 phenotype that directs type 2 Th cell differentiation in vitro and in vivo. *Journal of Immunology* 177, 1679-1688.

Lu, L.F., Boldin, M.P., Chaudhry, A., Lin, L.L., Taganov, K.D., Hanada, T., Yoshimura, A., Baltimore, D. & Rudensky, A.Y. (2010) Function of miR-146a in controlling Treg cell-mediated regulation of Th1 responses. *Cell* 142, 914-929.

Lu, L.F., Thai, T.H., Calado, D.P., Chaudhry, A., Kubo, M., Tanaka, K., Loeb, G.B., Lee, H., Yoshimura, A., Rajewsky, K. & Rudensky, A.Y. (2009) Foxp3-dependent microRNA155 confers competitive fitness to regulatory T cells by targeting SOCS1 protein. *Immunity* 30, 80-91.

Maine, G.N., Mao, X., Komarck, C.M. & Burstein, E. (2007) COMMD1 promotes the ubiquitination of NF-kappaB subunits through a cullin-containing ubiquitin ligase. *The EMBO Journal* 26, 436-447.

Mansell, A., Smith, R., Doyle, S.L., Gray, P., Fenner, J.E., Crack, P.J., Nicholson, S.E., Hilton, D.J., O'Neill, L.A. & Hertzog, P.J. (2006) Suppressor of cytokine signaling 1 negatively regulates Toll-like receptor signaling by mediating Mal degradation. *Nature Immunology* 7, 148-155.

Marine, J.C., McKay, C., Wang, D., Topham, D.J., Parganas, E., Nakajima, H., Pendeville, H., Yasukawa, H., Sasaki, A., Yoshimura, A. & Ihle, J.N. (1999a) SOCS3 is essential in the regulation of fetal liver erythropoiesis. *Cell* 98, 617-627.

Marine, J.C., Topham, D.J., McKay, C., Wang, D., Parganas, E., Stravopodis, D., Yoshimura, A. & Ihle, J.N. (1999b) SOCS1 deficiency causes a lymphocyte-dependent perinatal lethality. *Cell* 98, 609-616.

Masood, K.I., Rottenberg, M.E., Carow, B., Rao, N., Ashraf, M., Hussain, R. & Hasan, Z. (submitted) Differential expression of Suppressor of Cytokine Signaling molecules 1 and 3 in association with severity in tuberculosis.

Matsumoto, A., Seki, Y., Watanabe, R., Hayashi, K., Johnston, J.A., Harada, Y., Abe, R., Yoshimura, A. & Kubo, M. (2003) A role of suppressor of cytokine signaling 3 (SOCS3/CIS3/SSI3) in CD28-mediated interleukin 2 production. *The Journal of Experimental Medicine* 197, 425-436.

Matsumura, Y., Kobayashi, T., Ichiyama, K., Yoshida, R., Hashimoto, M., Takimoto, T., Tanaka, K., Chinen, T., Shichita, T., Wyss-Coray, T., Sato, K. & Yoshimura, A. (2007) Selective expansion of foxp3-positive regulatory T cells and immunosuppression by suppressors of cytokine signaling 3-deficient dendritic cells. *Journal of Immunology* 179, 2170-2179.

McLoughlin, R.M., Jenkins, B.J., Grail, D., Williams, A.S., Fielding, C.A., Parker, C.R., Ernst, M., Topley, N. & Jones, S.A. (2005) IL-6 trans-signaling via STAT3 directs T cell infiltration in acute inflammation. *Proceedings of the National Academy of Sciences of the United States of America* 102, 9589-9594.

Metcalf, D., Di Rago, L., Mifsud, S., Hartley, L. & Alexander, W.S. (2000) The development of fatal myocarditis and polymyositis in mice heterozygous for IFN-gamma and lacking the SOCS-1 gene. *Proceedings of the National Academy of Sciences of the United States of America* 97, 9174-9179.

Metcalf, D., Mifsud, S., Di Rago, L. & Alexander, W.S. (2003) The lethal effects of transplantation of Socs1-/- bone marrow cells into irradiated adult syngeneic recipients. *Proceedings of the National Academy of Sciences of the United States of America* 100, 8436-8441.

Michaud, F., Coulombe, F., Gaudreault, E., Paquet-Bouchard, C., Rola-Pleszczynski, M. & Gosselin, J. (2010) Epstein-Barr virus interferes with the amplification of IFNalpha secretion by activating suppressor of cytokine signaling 3 in primary human monocytes. *Plos One* 5, e11908.

Mistry, R., Cliff, J.M., Clayton, C.L., Beyers, N., Mohamed, Y.S., Wilson, P.A., Dockrell, H.M., Wallace, D.M., van Helden, P.D., Duncan, K. & Lukey, P.T. (2007) Gene-expression patterns in whole blood identify subjects at risk for recurrent tuberculosis. *The Journal of Infectious Diseases* 195, 357-365.

Mooney, R.A., Senn, J., Cameron, S., Inamdar, N., Boivin, L.M., Shang, Y. & Furlanetto, R.W. (2001) Suppressors of cytokine signaling-1 and -6 associate with and inhibit the insulin receptor. A potential mechanism for cytokine-mediated insulin resistance. *The Journal of Biological Chemistry* 276, 25889-25893.

Mori, H., Hanada, R., Hanada, T., Aki, D., Mashima, R., Nishinakamura, H., Torisu, T., Chien, K.R., Yasukawa, H. & Yoshimura, A. (2004) Socs3 deficiency in the brain elevates leptin sensitivity and confers resistance to diet-induced obesity. *Nature Medicine* 10, 739-743.

Naka, T., Matsumoto, T., Narazaki, M., Fujimoto, M., Morita, Y., Ohsawa, Y., Saito, H., Nagasawa, T., Uchiyama, Y. & Kishimoto, T. (1998) Accelerated apoptosis of lymphocytes by augmented induction of Bax in SSI-1 (STAT-induced STAT inhibitor-1) deficient mice. *Proceedings of the National Academy of Sciences of the United States of America* 95, 15577-15582.

Naka, T., Narazaki, M., Hirata, M., Matsumoto, T., Minamoto, S., Aono, A., Nishimoto, N., Kajita, T., Taga, T., Yoshizaki, K., Akira, S. & Kishimoto, T. (1997) Structure and function of a new STAT-induced STAT inhibitor. *Nature* 387, 924-929.

Naka, T., Tsutsui, H., Fujimoto, M., Kawazoe, Y., Kohzaki, H., Morita, Y., Nakagawa, R., Narazaki, M., Adachi, K., Yoshimoto, T., Nakanishi, K. & Kishimoto, T. (2001) SOCS-1/SSI-1-deficient NKT cells participate in severe hepatitis through dysregulated cross-talk inhibition of IFN-gamma and IL-4 signaling in vivo. *Immunity* 14, 535-545.

Nakagawa, R., Naka, T., Tsutsui, H., Fujimoto, M., Kimura, A., Abe, T., Seki, E., Sato, S., Takeuchi, O., Takeda, K., Akira, S., Yamanishi, K., Kawase, I., Nakanishi, K. & Kishimoto, T. (2002) SOCS-1 participates in negative regulation of LPS responses. *Immunity* 17, 677-687.

Narayana, Y. & Balaji, K.N. (2008) NOTCH1 up-regulation and signaling involved in Mycobacterium bovis BCG-induced SOCS3 expression in macrophages. *The Journal of Biological Chemistry* 283, 12501-12511.

Nicholson, S.E., De Souza, D., Fabri, L.J., Corbin, J., Willson, T.A., Zhang, J.G., Silva, A., Asimakis, M., Farley, A., Nash, A.D., Metcalf, D., Hilton, D.J., Nicola, N.A. & Baca, M. (2000) Suppressor of cytokine signaling-3 preferentially binds to the SHP-2-binding site on the shared cytokine receptor subunit gp130. *Proceedings of the National Academy of Sciences of the United States of America* 97, 6493-6498.

Ohtani, T., Ishihara, K., Atsumi, T., Nishida, K., Kaneko, Y., Miyata, T., Itoh, S., Narimatsu, M., Maeda, H., Fukada, T., Itoh, M., Okano, H., Hibi, M. & Hirano, T. (2000) Dissection of signaling cascades through gp130 in vivo: reciprocal roles for STAT3- and SHP2-mediated signals in immune responses. *Immunity* 12, 95-105.

Okumura, A., Pitha, P.M., Yoshimura, A. & Harty, R.N. (2010) Interaction between Ebola virus glycoprotein and host toll-like receptor 4 leads to induction of proinflammatory cytokines and SOCS1. *Journal of Virology* 84, 27-33.

Oliere, S., Hernandez, E., Lezin, A., Arguello, M., Douville, R., Nguyen, T.L., Olindo, S., Panelatti, G., Kazanji, M., Wilkinson, P., Sekaly, R.P., Cesaire, R. & Hiscott, J. (2010) HTLV-1 evades type I interferon antiviral signaling by inducing the suppressor of cytokine signaling 1 (SOCS1). *Plos Pathogens* 6, e1001177.

Pellegrini, M., Calzascia, T., Toe, J.G. *Et Al.* (2011) IL-7 engages multiple mechanisms to overcome chronic viral infection and limit organ pathology. *Cell* 144, 601-613.

Persico, M., Capasso, M., Russo, R., Persico, E., Croce, L., Tiribelli, C. & Iolascon, A. (2008) Elevated expression and polymorphisms of SOCS3 influence patient response to antiviral therapy in chronic hepatitis C. *Gut* 57, 507-515.

Pezet, A., Favre, H., Kelly, P.A. & Edery, M. (1999) Inhibition and restoration of prolactin signal transduction by suppressors of cytokine signaling. *The Journal of Biological Chemistry* 274, 24497-24502.

Piessevaux, J., Lavens, D., Peelman, F. & Tavernier, J. (2008) The many faces of the SOCS box. *Cytokine & Growth Factor Reviews* 19, 371-381.

Pillemer, B.B., Xu, H., Oriss, T.B., Qi, Z. & Ray, A. (2007) Deficient SOCS3 expression in CD4+CD25+FoxP3+ regulatory T cells and SOCS3-mediated suppression of Treg function. *European Journal of Immunology* 37, 2082-2089.

Pothlichet, J., Chignard, M. & Si-Tahar, M. (2008) Cutting edge: innate immune response triggered by influenza A virus is negatively regulated by SOCS1 and SOCS3 through a RIG-I/IFNAR1-dependent pathway. *Journal of Immunology* 180, 2034-2038.

Qin, H., Wang, L., Feng, T., Elson, C.O., Niyongere, S.A., Lee, S.J., Reynolds, S.L., Weaver, C.T., Roarty, K., Serra, R., Benveniste, E.N. & Cong, Y. (2009) TGF-beta promotes Th17 cell development through inhibition of SOCS3. *Journal of Immunology* 183, 97-105.

Qing, Y., Costa-Pereira, A.P., Watling, D. & Stark, G.R. (2005) Role of tyrosine 441 of interferon-gamma receptor subunit 1 in SOCS-1-mediated attenuation of STAT1 activation. *The Journal of Biological Chemistry* 280, 1849-1853.

Roberts, A.W., Robb, L., Rakar, S., Hartley, L., Cluse, L., Nicola, N.A., Metcalf, D., Hilton, D.J. & Alexander, W.S. (2001) Placental defects and embryonic lethality in mice lacking suppressor of cytokine signaling 3. *Proceedings of the National Academy of Sciences of the United States of America* 98, 9324-9329.

Rui, L., Yuan, M., Frantz, D., Shoelson, S. & White, M.F. (2002) SOCS-1 and SOCS-3 block insulin signaling by ubiquitin-mediated degradation of IRS1 and IRS2. *The Journal of Biological Chemistry* 277, 42394-42398.

Ryo, A., Suizu, F., Yoshida, Y., Perrem, K., Liou, Y.C., Wulf, G., Rottapel, R., Yamaoka, S. & Lu, K.P. (2003) Regulation of NF-kappaB signaling by Pin1-dependent prolyl isomerization and ubiquitin-mediated proteolysis of p65/RelA. *Molecular Cell* 12, 1413-1426.

Ryo, A., Tsurutani, N., Ohba, K. et al. (2008) SOCS1 is an inducible host factor during HIV-1 infection and regulates the intracellular trafficking and stability of HIV-1 Gag. *Proceedings Of the National Academy of Sciences of the United States of America* 105, 294-299.

Sasaki, A., Yasukawa, H., Shouda, T., Kitamura, T., Dikic, I. & Yoshimura, A. (2000) CIS3/SOCS-3 suppresses erythropoietin (EPO) signaling by binding the EPO receptor and JAK2. *The Journal of Biological Chemistry* 275, 29338-29347.

Seki, Y., Inoue, H., Nagata, N. *Et Al.* (2003) SOCS-3 regulates onset and maintenance of T(H)2-mediated allergic responses. *Nature Medicine* 9, 1047-1054.

Shen, L., Evel-Kabler, K., Strube, R. & Chen, S.Y. (2004) Silencing of SOCS1 enhances antigen presentation by dendritic cells and antigen-specific anti-tumor immunity. *Nature Biotechnology* 22, 1546-1553.

Shen, X., Hong, F., Nguyen, V.A. & Gao, B. (2000) IL-10 attenuates IFN-alpha-activated STAT1 in the liver: involvement of SOCS2 and SOCS3. *FEBS Letters* 480, 132-136.

Shi, H., Tzameli, I., Bjorbaek, C. & Flier, J.S. (2004) Suppressor of cytokine signaling 3 is a physiological regulator of adipocyte insulin signaling. *The Journal of Biological Chemistry* 279, 34733-34740.

Shuai, K. (2006) Regulation of cytokine signaling pathways by PIAS proteins. *Cell Research* 16, 196-202.

Silver, J.S. & Hunter, C.A. (2010) gp130 at the nexus of inflammation, autoimmunity, and cancer. *Journal of Leukocyte Biology* 88, 1145-1156.

Silver, J.S., Stumhofer, J.S., Passos, S., Ernst, M. & Hunter, C.A. (2011) IL-6 Mediates the Susceptibility of Glycoprotein 130 Hypermorphs to Toxoplasma gondii. *Journal of Immunology*.

Song, M.M. & Shuai, K. (1998) The suppressor of cytokine signaling (SOCS) 1 and SOCS3 but not SOCS2 proteins inhibit interferon-mediated antiviral and antiproliferative activities. *The Journal of Biological Chemistry* 273, 35056-35062.

Song, X.T., Evel-Kabler, K., Rollins, L., Aldrich, M., Gao, F., Huang, X.F. & Chen, S.Y. (2006) An alternative and effective HIV vaccination approach based on inhibition of antigen presentation attenuators in dendritic cells. *Plos Medicine* 3, e11.

Srivastava, V., Manchanda, M., Gupta, S., Singla, R., Behera, D., Das, G. & Natarajan, K. (2009) Toll-like receptor 2 and DC-SIGNR1 differentially regulate suppressors of cytokine signaling 1 in dendritic cells during Mycobacterium tuberculosis infection. *The Journal of Biological Chemistry* 284, 25532-25541.

Srivastava, V., Vashishta, M., Gupta, S., Singla, R., Singla, N., Behera, D. & Natarajan, K. (2011) Suppressors of cytokine signaling inhibit effector T cell responses during Mycobacterium tuberculosis Infection. *Immunology and Cell Biology*.

Starr, R., Metcalf, D., Elefanty, A.G., Brysha, M., Willson, T.A., Nicola, N.A., Hilton, D.J. & Alexander, W.S. (1998) Liver degeneration and lymphoid deficiencies in mice lacking suppressor of cytokine signaling-1. *Proceedings of the National Academy of Sciences of the United States of America* 95, 14395-14399.

Starr, R., Willson, T.A., Viney, E.M., Murray, L.J., Rayner, J.R., Jenkins, B.J., Gonda, T.J., Alexander, W.S., Metcalf, D., Nicola, N.A. & Hilton, D.J. (1997) A family of cytokine-inducible inhibitors of signalling. *Nature* 387, 917-921.

Stoiber, D., Kovarik, P., Cohney, S., Johnston, J.A., Steinlein, P. & Decker, T. (1999) Lipopolysaccharide induces in macrophages the synthesis of the suppressor of cytokine signaling 3 and suppresses signal transduction in response to the activating factor IFN-gamma. *Journal of Immunology* 163, 2640-2647.

Subramanya, S., Armant, M., Salkowitz, J.R., Nyakeriga, A.M., Haridas, V., Hasan, M., Bansal, A., Goepfert, P.A., Wynn, K.K., Ladell, K., Price, D.A., N, M., Kan-Mitchell, J. & Shankar, P. (2010) Enhanced induction of HIV-specific cytotoxic T lymphocytes by dendritic cell-targeted delivery of SOCS-1 siRNA. *Molecular Therapy : The Journal of the American Society of Gene Therapy* 18, 2028-2037.

Taga, T. & Kishimoto, T. (1997) Gp130 and the interleukin-6 family of cytokines. *Annual Review of Immunology* 15, 797-819.

Takahashi, Y., Carpino, N., Cross, J.C., Torres, M., Parganas, E. & Ihle, J.N. (2003) SOCS3: an essential regulator of LIF receptor signaling in trophoblast giant cell differentiation. *The EMBO Journal* 22, 372-384.

Takeda, K., Clausen, B.E., Kaisho, T., Tsujimura, T., Terada, N., Forster, I. & Akira, S. (1999) Enhanced Th1 activity and development of chronic enterocolitis in mice devoid of Stat3 in macrophages and neutrophils. *Immunity* 10, 39-49.

Taleb, S., Romain, M., Ramkhelawon, B., Uyttenhove, C., Pasterkamp, G., Herbin, O., Esposito, B., Perez, N., Yasukawa, H., Van Snick, J., Yoshimura, A., Tedgui, A. & Mallat, Z. (2009) Loss of SOCS3 expression in T cells reveals a regulatory role for interleukin-17 in atherosclerosis. *The Journal of Experimental Medicine* 206, 2067-2077.

Tanimoto, K., Saito, Y., Hamanaka, I., Kuwahara, K., Harada, M., Takahashi, N., Kawakami, R., Nakagawa, Y., Nakanishi, M., Adachi, Y., Shirakami, G., Fukuda, K., Yoshimura, A. & Nakao, K. (2005) SOCS1/JAB likely mediates the protective effect of cardiotrophin-1 against lipopolysaccharide-induced left ventricular dysfunction in vivo. *Circulation Journal : Official Journal of the Japanese Circulation Society* 69, 1412-1417.

Torisu, T., Sato, N., Yoshiga, D., Kobayashi, T., Yoshioka, T., Mori, H., Iida, M. & Yoshimura, A. (2007) The dual function of hepatic SOCS3 in insulin resistance in vivo. *Genes to Cells : Devoted to Molecular & Cellular Mechanisms* 12, 143-154.

Uchiya, K. & Nikai, T. (2005) Salmonella pathogenicity island 2-dependent expression of suppressor of cytokine signaling 3 in macrophages. *Infection and Immunity* 73, 5587-5594.

Ueki, K., Kondo, T. & Kahn, C.R. (2004a) Suppressor of cytokine signaling 1 (SOCS-1) and SOCS-3 cause insulin resistance through inhibition of tyrosine phosphorylation of insulin receptor substrate proteins by discrete mechanisms. *Molecular and Cellular Biology* 24, 5434-5446.

Ueki, K., Kondo, T., Tseng, Y.H. & Kahn, C.R. (2004b) Central role of suppressors of cytokine signaling proteins in hepatic steatosis, insulin resistance, and the metabolic syndrome in the mouse. *Proceedings of the National Academy of Sciences of The United States of America* 101, 10422-10427.

Vazquez, N., Greenwell-Wild, T., Rekka, S., Orenstein, J.M. & Wahl, S.M. (2006) Mycobacterium avium-induced SOCS contributes to resistance to IFN-gamma-mediated mycobactericidal activity in human macrophages. *Journal of Leukocyte Biology* 80, 1136-1144.

Verdier, F., Chretien, S., Muller, O., Varlet, P., Yoshimura, A., Gisselbrecht, S., Lacombe, C. & Mayeux, P. (1998) Proteasomes regulate erythropoietin receptor and signal transducer and activator of transcription 5 (STAT5) activation. Possible involvement of the ubiquitinated Cis protein. *The Journal of Biological Chemistry* 273, 28185-28190.

Wang, P., Hou, J., Lin, L., Wang, C., Liu, X., Li, D., Ma, F., Wang, Z. & Cao, X. (2010) Inducible microRNA-155 feedback promotes type I IFN signaling in antiviral innate immunity by targeting suppressor of cytokine signaling 1. *Journal of Immunology* 185, 6226-6233.

Whyte, C.S., Bishop, E.T., Ruckerl, D., Gaspar-Pereira, S., Barker, R.N., Allen, J.E., Rees, A.J. & Wilson, H.M. (2011) Suppressor of cytokine signaling (SOCS)1 is a key determinant of differential macrophage activation and function. *Journal of Leukocyte Biology*.

Wong, P.K., Egan, P.J., Croker, B.A., O'Donnell, K., Sims, N.A., Drake, S., Kiu, H., McManus, E.J., Alexander, W.S., Roberts, A.W. & Wicks, I.P. (2006) SOCS-3 negatively regulates innate and adaptive immune mechanisms in acute IL-1-dependent inflammatory arthritis. *The Journal of Clinical Investigation* 116, 1571-1581.

Wurster, A.L., Tanaka, T. & Grusby, M.J. (2000) The biology of Stat4 and Stat6. *Oncogene* 19, 2577-2584.

Yadav, A., Fitzgerald, P., Sajadi, M.M., Gilliam, B., Lafferty, M.K., Redfield, R. & Reid, W. (2009) Increased expression of suppressor of cytokine signaling-1 (SOCS-1): A mechanism for dysregulated T helper-1 responses in HIV-1 disease. *Virology* 385, 126-133.

Yamamoto, K., Yamaguchi, M., Miyasaka, N. & Miura, O. (2003) SOCS-3 inhibits IL-12-induced STAT4 activation by binding through its SH2 domain to the STAT4 docking site in the IL-12 receptor beta2 subunit. *Biochemical and Biophysical Research Communications* 310, 1188-1193.

Yang, T., Stark, P., Janik, K., Wigzell, H. & Rottenberg, M.E. (2008) SOCS-1 protects against Chlamydia pneumoniae-induced lethal inflammation but hampers effective bacterial clearance. *Journal of Immunology* 180, 4040-4049.

Yao, Z.Q., Ni, L., Zhang, Y., Ma, C.J., Zhang, C.L., Dong, Z.P., Frazier, A.D., Wu, X.Y., Thayer, P., Borthwick, T., Chen, X.Y. & Moorman, J.P. (2011) Differential regulation of T and B lymphocytes by PD-1 and SOCS-1 signaling in hepatitis C virus-associated non-Hodgkin's lymphoma. *Immunological Investigations* 40, 243-264.

Yasukawa, H., Misawa, H., Sakamoto, H., Masuhara, M., Sasaki, A., Wakioka, T., Ohtsuka, S., Imaizumi, T., Matsuda, T., Ihle, J.N. & Yoshimura, A. (1999) The JAK-binding protein JAB inhibits Janus tyrosine kinase activity through binding in the activation loop. *The EMBO Journal* 18, 1309-1320.

Yasukawa, H., Ohishi, M., Mori, H., Murakami, M., Chinen, T., Aki, D., Hanada, T., Takeda, K., Akira, S., Hoshijima, M., Hirano, T., Chien, K.R. & Yoshimura, A. (2003a) IL-6 induces an anti-inflammatory response in the absence of SOCS3 in macrophages. *Nature Immunology* 4, 551-556.

Yasukawa, H., Yajima, T., Duplain, H., Iwatate, M., Kido, M., Hoshijima, M., Weitzman, M.D., Nakamura, T., Woodard, S., Xiong, D., Yoshimura, A., Chien, K.R. & Knowlton, K.U. (2003b) The suppressor of cytokine signaling-1 (SOCS1) is a novel therapeutic target for enterovirus-induced cardiac injury. *The Journal of Clinical Investigation* 111, 469-478.

Yokota, S., Yokosawa, N., Okabayashi, T., Suzutani, T. & Fujii, N. (2005) Induction of suppressor of cytokine signaling-3 by herpes simplex virus type 1 confers efficient viral replication. *Virology* 338, 173-181.

Yoshimura, A., Naka, T. & Kubo, M. (2007) SOCS proteins, cytokine signalling and immune regulation. *Nature Reviews. Immunology* 7, 454-465.

Yu, C.R., Mahdi, R.M., Ebong, S., Vistica, B.P., Chen, J., Guo, Y., Gery, I. & Egwuagu, C.E. (2004) Cell proliferation and STAT6 pathways are negatively regulated in T cells by STAT1 and suppressors of cytokine signaling. *Journal of Immunology* 173, 737-746.

Zhang, J.G., Metcalf, D., Rakar, S., Asimakis, M., Greenhalgh, C.J., Willson, T.A., Starr, R., Nicholson, S.E., Carter, W., Alexander, W.S., Hilton, D.J. & Nicola, N.A. (2001) The

SOCS box of suppressor of cytokine signaling-1 is important for inhibition of cytokine action in vivo. *Proceedings of the National Academy of Sciences of the United States of America* 98, 13261-13265.

Zhang, Y., Ma, C.J., Ni, L., Zhang, C.L., Wu, X.Y., Kumaraguru, U., Li, C.F., Moorman, J.P. & Yao, Z.Q. (2011) Cross-talk between programmed death-1 and suppressor of cytokine signaling-1 in inhibition of IL-12 production by monocytes/macrophages in hepatitis C virus infection. *Journal of Immunology* 186, 3093-3103.

Zimmermann, S., Murray, P.J., Heeg, K. & Dalpke, A.H. (2006) Induction of suppressor of cytokine signaling-1 by Toxoplasma gondii contributes to immune evasion in macrophages by blocking IFN-gamma signaling. *Journal of Immunology* 176, 1840-1847.

Zitzmann, K., Brand, S., De Toni, E.N., Baehs, S., Goke, B., Meinecke, J., Spottl, G., Meyer, H.H. & Auernhammer, C.J. (2007) SOCS1 silencing enhances antitumor activity of type I IFNs by regulating apoptosis in neuroendocrine tumor cells. *Cancer Research* 67, 5025-5032.

13

Review of Cytomegalovirus Anterior Uveitis

C. E. Pang
Singapore National Eye Centre
Singapore

1. Introduction

Cytomegalovirus (CMV), a member of the herpes family which includes herpes simplex virus (HSV) 1 and 2, varicella zoster virus (VZV), and Epstein-Barr virus (EBV), is ubiquitous worldwide. About 85% of persons above the age of 40 in the general community are seropositive.[1] CMV infections manifest more usually in immunocompromised individuals especially in patients with acquired immune deficiency syndrome (AIDS); however more recently, CMV infections have been reported in the immunocompetent person, manifesting as corneal endotheliitis as well as anterior uveitis associated with elevated intraocular pressure (IOP; hypertensive anterior uveitis).[2-8] This chapter aims to review the ocular features and treatment of CMV anterior uveitis in the immunocompetent person.

2. Pathophysiology

Viruses are increasingly being implicated as a cause of what was previously considered to be idiopathic ocular inflammations in immunocompetent patients. CMV and HSV have been associated with Possner-Schlossman Syndrome (PSS)[4,9,10] and rubella and HSV have been associated with Fuchs Heterochromic Iridocyclitis (FHI).[11-13] In various studies, the presence of CMV deoxyribonucleic acid (DNA) has been identified in 41.7% of FHI and 52.8% of PSS eyes.[14]

The overlap between the different viruses and the variability in clinical presentations do suggest that ocular manifestations of viral diseases in immunocompetent patients may not be specific to a particular virus but rather a response to the viral infection based on the individual's genetic make-up and immune status.[14]

These viruses share common characteristics. The core contains a linear double-stranded DNA, which is surrounded by a capsid and an envelope. The envelope is a derivative of the core membrane of the infected cells and consists of lipids with inserted viral glycoprotein. There are specific receptors of the glycoproteins of the envelope that recognize complementary receptors on the host cell membrane and bind to them by adsorption. The envelope and the cell membrane fuse while the viral nucleocapsid enters the cell. The viral proteins are then produced in a cascade. The synthesis of DNA and assembly of capsid take place in the nucleus while the production of infected particles in the cytoplasm leads to destruction of the host cell.[15-16] Viral DNA has been detected in monocytes, dendritic cells, megakaryocytes, and myeloid progenitor cells in the bone marrow.

Herpetic viruses are well known for their ability to cause keratitis, anterior uveitis, scleritis, and retinitis.[17-19] Anterior uveitis is unilateral and typically has a chronic and/or recurrent character. Intraocular pressure (IOP) elevation, keratitis, endotheliitis, and stromal iris atrophy commonly accompany it. The iris stroma is infiltrated with lymphocytes, and an increase in IOP is typically seen on activation of the uveitis, probably due to an outflow obstruction. This outflow obstruction can be explained by both a viral trabeculitis with swelling of the trabecular cells and an obstruction of the trabecular meshwork by inflammatory debris.[18-19]

The pathogenesis of CMV uveitis, although not completely understood, is believed to include various mechanisms such as viral replication, ischemic vasculitis, lymphocytic infiltration of the iris stroma or intraocular nerves. In addition, persistent and recurrent viral infection may cause an inflammatory reaction manifested as uveitis, or can trigger the immune system itself against viral antigens, eventually causing tissue and organ inflammation and damage.[20-24]

3. Ocular features

CMV in the anterior segment is a newly described entity that occurs even in people who are not infected with the human immunodeficiency virus (HIV).

CMV infection can cause a spectrum of ocular manifestations, varying in severity from a mild self-limiting iritis with sector iris atrophy,[6] to features of PSS,[4-9] to the more chronic form resembling FHI, or even corneal endotheliitis.[7] Two common features seen in these eyes with CMV uveitis are elevated IOP and iris atrophy. These features are consistent with the finding of CMV in the smooth muscle cells of the iris, the ciliary body, and the endothelial cells of the Schlemm canal.[17]

In an analysis of published studies of non-HIV, CMV-associated anterior uveitis in immunocompetent patients, researchers found clinical presentations including endotheliitis, recurrent acute anterior uveitis and ocular hypertension, and chronic anterior uveitis.[12] Eyes with such CMV-associated anterior uveitis usually have no corneal scars, no posterior synechiae, no flare or fibrin and no posterior segment involvement.

Corneal endotheliitis may be unilateral or bilateral, typically causes blurred vision and is associated with corneal edema, Descemet's folds, as well as fine and medium keratic precipitates that may be pigmented. Other associated clinical signs include iris atrophy, mild anterior chamber activity, reduced endothelial cell count, elevated IOP, coin-like lesions and the "owl eye sign" on confocal microscopy, representing inclusion bodies and macrophages.

As mentioned, CMV can present clinically as PSS or FHI. PSS and FHI are 2 separate clinical entities that are similar in some aspects, but yet have important distinguishing features. Both have elevated intraocular pressures during the episodes of acute iritis (hypertensive anterior uveitis). Both have only a mild non-granulomatous anterior chamber activity with no posterior synechiae formation. However, PSS is an acute, intermittent, recurrent glaucomatocyclitic crisis with few keratic precipitates, while FHI is a chronic iridocyclitis with diffuse, fine, stellate keratic precipitates and may have vitritis. Exact aetiology of both conditions is still arguable although the consensus is that they are attributable to viruses including CMV as mentioned above.

PSS is usually unilateral, with symptoms of redness, blurring, haloes and unilateral headache. Clinical features include elevated IOP, anterior chamber cells (grades ½ to 2+)

and fine to medium keratic precipitates either in a ring or linear pattern. Diffuse and patchy iris stromal atrophy is common.

FHI may be unilateral or bilateral. The main symptom is blurred vision. Clinical features include elevated IOP, anterior chamber cells (grades 1 to 2+), fine feathery, diffuse keratic precipitates and diffuse "moth-eaten" iris atrophy.

From literature data to date, 110 eyes of 106 non-HIV positive patients with CMV anterior segment infection have been described[4-9] of which 27 eyes of 24 patients had endotheliitis, 57 eyes had acute recurrent anterior uveitis and the remaining had chronic anterior uveitis. All the 83 anterior uveitis eyes and 24 of the endotheliitis eyes had ocular hypertension.

4. Diagnosis

The usefulness of aqueous humor sampling has been established in both anterior uveitis and posterior uveitis. A number of recent studies have shown the benefit of aqueous humor polymerase chain reaction (PCR) for the diagnosis of infectious uveitis and revealed a good degree of concordance between intraocular antibody and real-time PCR. Testing for DNA tends to be positive at the outset (and/or early at reactivation) and antibody testing can be positive at any point in time.[25] A positive test result indicates at the most that the virus may be involved, but is by no means conclusive. A negative test does not exclude the herpes virus as a cause of the uveitis either.

A minimum of 100 μl aqueous should be obtained via a diagnostic anterior chamber paracentesis and the samples must be delivered to the laboratory at 18 to 25 degrees Celsius within one hour or stored and transported at 2 to 4 degrees Celsius within 24 hours. The samples should be aliquoted immediately on arrival at the laboratory and used for DNA extraction immediately or kept at −20 degrees Celsius and used for DNA extraction within one week.

Diagnostic anterior chamber paracentesis should involve the use of a 27-gauge needle inserted into the temporal, perilimbal, inferior one-third of the cornea; directed downwards while avoiding the lens. This has been shown to be a simple and safe office procedure.[26] Identification of the CMV virus makes it possible to institute the appropriate antiviral medication.

5. Treatment

Management of CMV anterior uveitis may involve the use of topical non-steroidal anti-inflammatory agents, topical steroids, topical anti-glaucoma medications and topical or systemic antivirals. Patients should also be co-managed by the infectious disease physician to exclude systemic cytomegalovirus infections and other forms of immunocompromised states.

Topical non-steroidal anti-inflammatory agents have been employed in the immediate setting to reduce ocular inflammation and treat the patient symptomatically. This is especially useful when the use of topical steroids is delayed intentionally till after the diagnostic anterior chamber paracentesis to allow better yield of viral DNA load when performing aqueous sampling.

Topical steroids alone may be able to reduce the inflammation and IOP in a minority of cases. More commonly, combination with anti-glaucoma medication will give rise to more

effective lowering of IOP. However, steroids may cause steroid-induced glaucoma as a side effect. This is especially seen in patients who are on steroids for a long duration.
Glaucoma therapy can be initiated in a stepwise manner in the following order, unless there are any contraindications to the medication: β-blocker, α-2 agonists, topical acetazolamide, and lastly, prostaglandin analogs. If the IOP exceeds 40 mm Hg, systemic acetazolamide can be considered. The medications when tailed down should be reduced in a stepwise manner as well, but in reverse order.
Mydriatics or cycloplegics can be used as an adjunct to relieve any ciliary spasm, stabilize the blood aqueous barrier and assist in fundal evaluation.
The main mode of antiviral therapy in these eyes has been systemic ganciclovir or valganciclovir.[5-8,14,27-28] Some authors have also used intravitreal injections of ganciclovir[28] or ganciclovir gel[14] with variable outcomes. In many cases, the inflammation resolved with therapy, only to recur on cessation of treatment.[5-7] Although there is no consensus as to which route of administration is most suitable, topical ganciclovir gel has been shown to produce less number of recurrences as compared to systemic gangciclovir.[29]
Response to therapy in eyes with chronic anterior uveitis can be defined as the clinical resolution of anterior chamber cells and keratic precipitates and good IOP control with or without glaucoma medications while on treatment. In eyes with acute recurrent anterior uveitis, response can be defined as absence of recurrence of inflammation and normalisation of IOP without glaucoma medications other than that given during the acute episode while on treatment.
All treated eyes responded to therapy, in terms of the severity of the inflammation and IOP control, to the initial antiviral treatment. However, 77.7% relapsed within eight months after stopping treatment, according to the experience of some authors.[6,29] This indicates that CMV anterior uveitis may require a longer period of treatment, perhaps similar to that of herpetic uveitis or even other methods of treatment.

6. References

[1] Yoser SL, Forster DJ and Rao NA. Systemic viral infections and their retinal and choroidal manifestations, Surv Ophthalmol 1993; 37: 313–352.
[2] Koizumi N, Suzuki T, Uno T, et al. Cytomegalovirus as an etiologic factor in corneal endotheliitis. Ophthalmology. 2008 ; 115(2): 292-297.
[3] Teoh SB, Thean L and Koay E. Cytomegalovirus in aetiology of Posner-Schlossman syndrome: evidence from quantitative polymerase chain reaction, Eye 2005; 19: 1338–1340.
[4] Bloch-Michel E, Dussaix E, Cerqueti P, et al. Possible role of cytomegalovirus infection in the etiology of the Posner-Schlossmann syndrome, Int Ophthalmol 1987; 11: 95–96.
[5] De Schryver I, Rozenberg F, Cassoux N, et al., Diagnosis and treatment of cytomegalovirus iridocyclitis without retinal necrosis, Br J Ophthalmol 2006; 90: 852–855.
[6] Markomichelakis NN, Canakis C, Zafirakis P, et al. Cytomegalovirus as a cause of anterior uveitis with sectoral iris atrophy, Ophthalmology 2002; 109: 879–882.
[7] Van Boxtel LA, van der Lelij A, van der Meer J. Cytomegalovirus as a cause of anterior uveitis in immunocompetent patients, Ophthalmology 2007: 114: 1358–1362.
[8] Chee SP, Bascal K, Jap A, et al. Corneal endotheliitis associated with evidence of cytomegalovirus infection, Ophthalmology 2007; 114: 798–803.

[9] Teoh SB, Thean L, Koay E. Cytomegalovirus in aetiology of Posner-Schlossman syndrome: evidence from quantitative polymerase chain reaction. Eye 2005; 19: 1338-1340.
[10] Yamamoto S, Pavan-Langston D, Tada R, et al. Possible role of herpes simplex virus in the origin of Posner-Schlossman syndrome. Am J Ophthalmol 1995; 119: 796-798.
[11] Baraquet IS, Li Q, Wang Y, O'Brien TP, et al. Herpes simplex virus DNA identification from aqueous fluid in Fuchs heterochromic iridocyclitis. Am J Ophthalmol 2000;129:672-673.
[12] Quentin CD, Reiber H. Fuchs heterochromic cyclitis: rubella virus antibodies ans genome in aqueous humor. Am J Ophthalmol 2004; 138: 46-54.
[13] de Groot-Mijnes JDF, de Visser L, Rothova A, et al. Rubella virus is associated with Fuchs heterochromic iridocyclitis. Am J Ophthalmol 2006; 141: 212-214.
[14] Chee SP, Bascal K, Jap A, et al. Clinical features of cytomegalovirus in anterior uveitis in immunocompetent patients. Am J Ophthalmol 2008; 145: 834-40.
[15] Roizman B: Herpesviridae. In: Fields BN, Knipe DM, Howley PM, eds: Virology, 3rd ed. Philadelphia, Lippincott-Raven, 1996.
[16] Spring SB, Roizman B: Herpes Simplex Virus products in productive and abortive infection. III. Differentiation of infectious virus derived from nucleus and cytoplasm with respect to stability and size. J Virol 1968; 2: 979.
[17] B. Daicker,B. Cytomegalovirus panuveitis with infection of corneo-trabecular endothelium in AIDS, Ophthalmologica 1988; 197: 169–175.
[18] Heiligenhaus A, Helbig H, Fiedler M. Herpesviruses. In: C.S. Foster and A.T. Vitale, Editors, Diagnosis and Treatment of Uveitis, W.B. Saunders, Philadelphia 2002: 315–332.
[19] Holland EJ, Mozayeni RM, Schwartz GS. Herpes simplex keratitis. In: J.H. Krachmer, M.J. Mannis and E.J. Holland, Editors, Cornea. Vol. 2. Cornea and External Disease: Clinical Diagnosis and Management, Mosby, St. Louis 1997: 1191–1223.
[20] Liesegang TJ: Ocular herpes simplex infection: pathogenesis and current therapy. Mayo Clin Proc 1988; 63:1092.
[21] Sundmacher R and Neumann-Haefelin D: Herpes simplex virus isolations from the aqueous of patients suffering from local iritis, endotheliitis, and prolonged disciform keratitis with glaucoma. Klin Monatsbl Augenheilkd 1979; 175: 488-501.
[22] Pavan-Langston D: Herpes Zoster Ophthalmicus: Medical and surgical management. In Spaeth G, Katz L, Parker KW (eds): Current therapy in ophthalmic surgery. Philadelphia: BC Decker, 1989: 99.
[23] Liesegang TJ: Corneal complications from herpes zoster ophthalmicus. Ophthalmology 1985; 92: 316-24.
[24] Kijlstra A: The value of laboratory testing in uveitis. Eye 1990; 4: 732-736.
[25] De Groot-Mijnes J, Rothova A, van Loon AM et al., Polymerase chain reaction and Goldmann-Witmer coefficient analysis are complimentary for the diagnosis of infectious uveitis, Am J Ophthalmol 2006; 141: 313–318.
[26] Van der Lelij A, Rothova A, Diagnostic anterior chamber paracentesis in uveitis; a safe procedure?, Br J Ophthalmol 1997; 81: 976–979.
[27] Sira M, Murray PI. Treatment of cytomegalovirus anterior uveitis with oral valaciclovir. Ocul Immunol Inflamm 2007; 15: 31–2.

[28] Chung RS, Chua CN. Intravitreal ganciclovir injections in aqueous cytomegalovirus DNA positive hypertensive iritis. Eye 2006; 20: 1080.
[29] Chee SP, Jap A. Cytomegalovirus anterior uveitis: outcome of treatment. Br J Ophthalmol. 2010; 94:1648-52.

14

Role of the Neutrophil NADPH Oxidase and S100A8/A9 in the Pathophysiology of Chronic Inflammation

Sabrina Bréchard, Véronique Schenten and Eric J. Tschirhart
University of Luxembourg
Luxembourg

1. Introduction

Reactive oxygen species (ROS) are low-molecular-weight inorganic and highly reactive compounds that are produced during normal aerobic cell metabolism. At low level, ROS have a transient mode of action and important physiological roles in maintaining intracellular cell redox status, physical-chemical properties of membranes, protein kinase and transcriptional factor activities. They participate in the regulation of many aspects of fundamental cellular function, including growth-specific and migration-related signalling pathways, gene expression, GTPase-dependent cytoskeletal rearrangements, cell proliferation and apoptosis. Multiple endogenous macromolecules, participating in cellular signalling networks, bear redox-active moieties (e.g., methionine, cysteine, guanine) at functional regions that render them sensitive to ROS. Consequently, ROS emerge, not only as second messengers, but also as diffusible modulators able to produce stable secondary signalling molecules.

A major source of ROS are phagocytic cells such as polymorphonuclear neutrophils that are found activated and adherent to the endothelium or migrating through the extravascular tissue matrix. ROS produced by neutrophils are designed to kill the invading pathogens and have an important role in priming the immune system. The phagocyte NADPH oxidase, also referred as NOX2, is composed of several membane-bound and cytosolic subunits that assemble rapidly in the phagosomal or plasma membrane (Fig. 1). This allows the concentrated release of ROS at sites of inflammation where the pathogen is located (Ohno et al., 1982) and diffusion over short distances, enabling these second messengers to act on adjacent neighbouring targets. Since many years, it is known that ROS interactions with lipids contribute to disturbances in cell structure (Thaw et al., 1983) and alterations of functional activities (Bellomo et al., 1982; Poot et al., 1988) enhancing the ability of the phagocytes to kill invading microorganisms (Quinn et al., 1995).

Under physiological conditions, ROS are eliminated by several defence mechanisms (e.g., antioxidant enzymes) to maintain a normal intracellular redox environment and control the signalling cascades.

However, when these protective mechanisms are overwhelmed by excessive amounts of ROS, due to inappropriate activation of phagocytes or alterations of the antioxidant defence system, a situation of oxidative stress can occur resulting in abnormal physiological responses. During a prolonged period, focal regions of the endothelium can be exposed to aberrant levels of ROS, which in turn cause the destruction of healthy tissue. Indeed, at high concentrations and continued exposure, ROS can damage all types of biomolecules including DNA, lipids, carbohydrates and proteins.

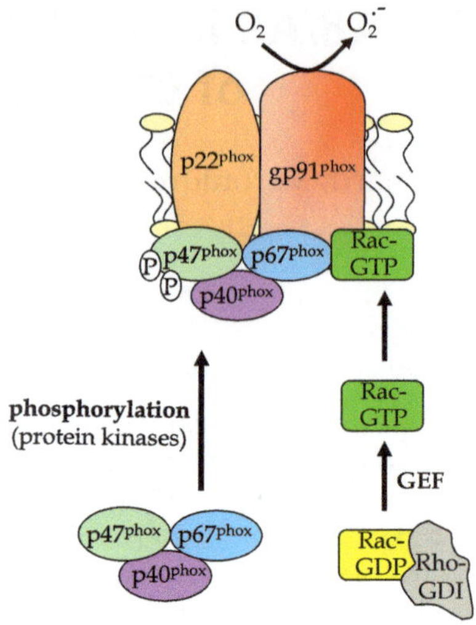

Fig. 1. Assembly and activation of the phagocyte NADPH oxidase, NOX2 (for reviews, see Babior et al., 2002; Sheppard et al., 2005). NOX2 activation is mediated by the assembly of cytosolic subunits ($p40^{phox}$, $p47^{phox}$, and $p67^{phox}$) with the membrane subunits ($p22^{phox}$ and $gp91^{phox}$ constituting the flavocytochrome b_{558}). Phosphorylation of $p47^{phox}$, by protein kinases, is notably required for translocation of $p47^{phox}$ to the membrane and binding to $p22^{phox}$. The guanine nucleotide exchange factor (GEF) triggers GTP binding to Rac promoting the membrane translocation and the binding to $p67^{phox}$ necessary to the assembly of active NOX2 and superoxide anion production.

2. Toxicity of neutrophil NADPH oxidase (NOX2)-mediated release of ROS: Pathophysiological roles

2.1 Molecular damage caused by ROS

Irreversible oxidative modification of macromolecules including proteins, lipids, DNA and carbohydrates are typically viewed as the primary cellular targets of ROS and contribute to cell injury. Consequently, oxidized biomolecules are linked to the pathophysiology of multiple chronic human diseases and are the most commonly used biomarkers of oxidative damage isolated from tissues and biological fluids (for review, see Dalle-Donne et al., 2006).

2.1.1 Lipid peroxidation

Lipid peroxidation is a complex process in which oxidants, generated by NADPH oxidase of activated neutrophils, react the most abundantly with polyunsaturated fatty acids (e.g., linoleic acid and arachidonic acid) to form a variety of products including aldehydes, lipid radicals and hydrocarbons. Peroxidation of lipids can disrupt the organization of the membrane modifying its physical properties and causing changes in fluidity and permeability, inhibition of metabolic processes, and alterations of ion transport (Nigam & Schewe, 2000).

Polyunsaturated fatty acid residues of phospholipids nearby membrane were found to be extremely sensitive to oxidation by the highly reactive hydroxyl radical (Siems et al., 1995). The initial reaction of hydroxyl radical with polyunsaturated fatty acids produces an alkyl radical, which in turn reacts with molecular oxygen to form a peroxyl radical in a perpetuating chain reaction. Once formed, peroxyl radicals can undergo subsequent cyclization to generate endoperoxides, which leads to the final production of malondialdehyde (Mao et al., 1999; Marnett, 2002). Malondialdehyde reacts with DNA, predominantly with deoxyguanosine, to form exocyclic adducts most of which are mutagenic in mammalian cells.

The major aldehyde product of lipid peroxidation other than malondialdehyde is 4-hydroxy-2-nonenal (4-HNE) that is a weakly mutagenic metabolite but with a high cytotoxicity. The cytotoxic effects are thought to be due to the ability of 4-HNE to react readily with sulfhydryl groups by a Michael addition mechanism to form stable thioether derivatives (Esterbauer et al., 1975; Esterbauer et al., 1991). 4-HNE is a potent inhibitor of sulfhydryl enzymes, such as the glycolytic enzyme glyceraldehyde-3-phosphate dehydrogenase (GAPDH) via modification of the cysteine residue (Cys-149) at the catalytic site (Uchida & Stadtman, 1993). Later, it was suggested that 4-HNE inactivation of GAPDH is not due to the modification of the catalytic center but to the sequential and selective modification of amino acids (His-164, Cys-281, Cys-244, His-327 and Lys-331) primarily located in the surface of the GAPDH molecule (Ishii et al., 2003).

4-HNE reacts also with selective histidine residues of proteins including insulin (which lacks cysteine) contributing to the cytotoxic action of 4-HNE (Uchida & Stadtman, 1992). In certain proteins, lysine c-amino groups, but not histidine, is the major target amino acid of 4-HNE. Lysine modification in glucose-6-phosphate dehydrogenase via Schiff-base formation is associated with a loss of enzyme activity (Sweda et al., 1993) and 4-HNE modification on low density lipoproteins have been implicated in the pathophysiology of atherosclerosis (Jessup et al., 1986; Vindis et al., 2007).

2.1.2 Protein oxidation

Many different types of oxidative modification of proteins can be induced by ROS. Cysteine and methionine residues of proteins are highly susceptible to oxidation by various forms of ROS. Oxidation of cysteine residues can lead to the formation of a mixed disulphide between protein thiol groups and low molecular weight thiol compounds (reversible S-glutathiolation). Carbonyl groups are major products of ROS-mediated oxidation proteins and the concentration of these derivatives is an adapted marker of protein oxidation (Berlett et al., 1997; Chevion et al., 2000). Protein modifications elicited by oxidative attack on lysine, arginine, proline or threonine, or by secondary reaction of cysteine, histidine or lysine residues with carbonyl compounds can result in the formation of protein derivatives possessing highly reactive carbonyl groups such as aldehydes and ketones (Berlett et al., 1997). Oxidation of some critical methionine residues causes a complete inhibition of actin polymerization and destabilization of the structure of actin filaments (Dalle-Donne et al., 2002).

Oxidative modification of proteins by ROS is implicated in the etiology and/or progression of a broad variety of age-related degenerative pathologies, atherosclerosis, muscular dystrophy, rheumatoid arthritis (Chevion et al., 2000; Moreira et al., 2010; Stadtman &

Berlett, 1997). Various human diseases have been associated with carbonylated proteins (Table 1): acute respiratory distress syndrome, Alzheimer's disease, rheumatoid arthritis, chronic lung disease, and diabetes (for review, see Dalle-Donne et al., 2003).

2.1.3 Nucleic acid oxidation

Permanent genetic material damage due to oxidative stress can represent the first step to mutagenesis, carcinogenesis, and ageing. ROS are known to react with all components of the DNA molecule and impair DNA repair mechanisms. DNA modification can affect both the purine and pyrimidine bases and also the deoxyribose backbone (Aruoma et al., 1989). DNA modification has been reported to accumulate over the life span of the cell participating to ageing (von Zglinicki et al., 1995). Telomere DNA is deficient in the repair of single-strand breaks produced by hydroxyl radicals affecting telomere length and hence active cell division (Oikawa et al., 2001; Petersen et al., 1998; Saretzki et al., 1999). The most extensively studied DNA lesion is the formation of 8-oxo-7-hydro-deoxyguanosine (8-OH-guanine) generated by the reaction of hydroxyl radicals with guanine repeats. 8-OH-guanine is particularly mutagenic and cytotoxic. It is elevated in leukocytes and sera of patients with rheumatoid arthritis (Table 1) and probably participates in joint inflammation by activating immune cells, which in turn produce excessive pro-inflammatory cytokines (Hajizadeh et al., 2003).

2.1.4 Carbohydrate oxidation

Glycosaminoglycans (GAGs) are major components of extracellular matrix and their increased synthesis and degradation are hallmarks of chronic inflammation and tissue fibrosis. GAGs determine the structure, viscosity and permeability of the ground substance in connective tissue and play a critical role in ion transport, nutrient diffusion, water homeostasis, intercellular signalling and collagen synthesis. GAG oxidation is known to have important biological consequences in particular on endothelial cell adhesion and proliferation (Underwood et al., 1998; Vissers et al., 1991) that are involved in atherogenesis. Chondroitin sulphates and hyaluronic acid, which contain glucosamine and glucuronic acid, are critical GAGs present in synovial joints that have been shown to be fragmented by ROS (Rees et al., 2004). The hypochlorite-mediated depolymerization of GAGs has been shown to produce polymer-derived chloramide, the major species formed due to the reaction of hypochlorite with glucosamine or galactosamine residues (Hawkins & Davis, 1998; Rees et al., 2003). Lower molecular weight hyaluronic acid fragments accumulate during inflammation and may have a role in the activation of phagocytes through the stimulation of interleukin-1β and TNF-α expression (Noble et al., 1993) resulting in an exacerbation of the inflammatory process and tissue damage.

2.2 NOX2-derived ROS and inflammatory diseases

Chronic inflammation was hypothesized as the loss of balance between apoptosis and wound healing leading to disruption of protective mechanisms of immune system (Khatami, 2005, 2008, 2009). Unresolved inflammation-induced excessive expression of pro- and anti-inflammatory mediators causes erosion of tissue integrity initiating the development of chronic inflammatory diseases or cancer (Khatami, 2011).

Molecular alterations, induced by exaggerated ROS generation during oxidative stress, represent an important cause of injury in many inflammatory diseases (Table 1). ROS production is a prominent feature in various cardiovascular-related diseases such as hypertension, atherosclerosis, and ischemic heart diseases. Moreover, it was suggested that ROS play a role in a variety of age-related diseases such as some neurological diseases like Alzheimer's disease, type 2 diabetes or even reproductive disorders (for reviews, see Kukreja & Hess, 1992; Reddy et al., 2009; Valko et al., 2007). Among this pleiad of diseases, ROS derived from the neutrophil NADPH oxidase complex (NOX2) have notably been implicated in the pathophysiology of rheumatoid arthritis, atherosclerosis, chronic obstructive inflammatory disease and inflammation-associated cancer.

2.2.1 Chronic inflammatory diseases

Rheumatoid arthritis is the most common type of rheumatological disorder with a prevalence of 0.4% to 0.7% worldwide (Alamanos et al., 2006; Englund et al., 2010). Rheumatoid arthritis is a chronic, destructive, autoimmune joint disease resulting in enormous pathologic sequelae including pain, stiffness, deformity, swelling, as well as systemic effects associated with inflammation limiting activities of daily living. Rheumatoid arthritis principally affects peripheral synovial joints but additionally extra-articular complications, including atherosclerotic vascular disease and premature mortality, can be associated to the disease (Carroll et al., 2006). Indeed, cardiovascular complications are the leading cause of death (42%) among patients with rheumatoid arthritis (Callahan et al., 1995). The pathogenesis of rheumatoid arthritis is a complex process with several distinguishing features involving macrophage-like synoviocytes and fibroblast-like synoviocytes proliferation, pannus formation, cartilage and bone erosion.

The presence of abundant numbers of neutrophils in the synovial fluid of patients with rheumatoid arthritis participate to joint damage via the release of potent effectors of cartilage destruction such as proteases and NOX2-mediated ROS production. The pathogenesis of rheumatoid arthritis is predominantly linked to the formation of ROS to the site of inflammation and tissue lesions caused by elevated ROS concentration participate to the perpetuation of inflammation. These oxidative derivatives may depolymerize hyaluronic acid and inactivate endogenous inhibitors of proteases (Chatham et al., 1993; Edwards & Hallett, 1997; Larbre et al., 1994; Robinson et al., 1992). Rheumatoid arthritis fluids can also contain large quantities of immune complexes and their deposition has been considered to be a major determinant of neutrophil-mediated destructive joint process which is characteristic of rheumatoid arthritis. Indeed, neutrophils primed and isolated from the synovial fluid of patients with rheumatoid arthritis can secrete substantial quantities of ROS in response to immune complexes (Ottonello et al., 2002).

Neutrophils have also been found at sites of atherosclerotic plaque rupture where they appear to be functionally active to generate ROS. Infiltrated neutrophils into atherosclerotic plaque underline the fact that these pro-inflammatory cells contribute to plaque vulnerability and erosion (Hosokawa et al., 2011).

The inflammatory processes in the lung are characterized by an influx of neutrophils into the airways. Increased levels of NOX2-derived ROS produced by inflammatory cells of the airways in the lung have been recognized to contribute importantly in the pathogenesis of asthma and chronic obstructive pulmonary disease (Rahman, 2002). The enhanced expression of surface adhesion molecule Mac-1, which favours the recruitment of neutrophils to the inflammatory site, is coupled with an increase of NOX2 activity. It augments the potential of ROS to induce lung injury, contributing to the development of chronic obstructive pulmonary disease (Noguera et al., 2001). Oxidative stress can reduce the histone deacetylase activity allowing the access of transcription factors as NF-κB, AP-1 and Nrf2 to the DNA and leading to enhanced pro-inflammatory or reduced antioxidant gene expression in various lung cells (Ito et al., 2001; Kersul et al., 2001; Mercado et al., 2011). Moreover, ROS may play a role in enhancing the mucus secretion through the modulation of enzymatic activities such as src homology 2-containing protein tyrosine phosphatase, p38 MAPK or receptor tyrosine kinases (epidermal growth factor receptor) (Jang et al., 2010; Kohri et al., 2002; Meng et al., 2002).

2.2.2 Cancer-associated inflammation

Persistent chronic inflammation contributes to increase the risk of cancer and promote cancer development and progression. The inflammatory response triggered by infection is involved in the pathogenesis of approximately 20% of human tumors (e.g., Helicobacter pylori infection is associated with gastric cancer). Cancer-related inflammation is characterized by the presence of infiltrating immune and inflammatory cells (notably T-lymphocytes, tumor-associated macrophages and neutrophils) in the microenvironment of the tumor increasing generation of ROS and angiogenic factors, matrix-degrading enzyme and growth factor activities, and altering cytokine and chemokine expression. Accumulating evidence shows that chronic inflammation can promote an environment that is favourable to all the stages of human tumors. Six hallmarks have been proposed by Hanahan & Weinberg (Hanahan & Weinberg, 2011) to characterize the multistep of thè carcinogenesis including sustaining proliferative signalling, evading growth suppressors, resisting cell death, enabling replicative immortality, inducing angiogenesis, and activating invasion and metastasis. It has been proposed that the genome instability leading to cancer-related inflammation represents the seventh hallmark of tumorigenesis (Allavena et al., 2008; Mantovani, 2010).

The link between chronic inflammation and cancer has been suggested by the enhanced colorectal cancer susceptibility of persons with inflammatory bowel disease (e.g., ulcerative colitis and Crohn's disease). Repeated injury and repair triggered by chronic inflammation may increase cell turnover and permanent changes in the genome leading ultimately to tumorigenesis. It is generally accepted that cancer initiation may be a pathological consequence of ROS-induced DNA lesions that in turn result in mutations activating oncogenes or inactivating tumor-suppressor genes (Klaunig & Kamendulis, 2004). Chronic exposure to ROS may also alter normal cellular and molecular signalling pathways. ROS have been shown to activate transcription factors such NF-κB, AP-1 and STATs. NF-κB is known to be constitutively activated in a variety of malignancies (Brar et al., 2003) contributing to abnormal malignant cell division through enhanced expression of anti-apoptotic factors (Bcl-2), and proliferative factors, such as cyclin D1 (Brar et al., 2003). The interest in the role of neutrophils in the inflammatory origin of cancer (Table 1) is recent and has considerably increased over the last years. In addition of its function in host defence, a critical role for NOX2-mediated ROS production has been pointed in the induction and development of malignant cells. Human neutrophils can directly damage DNA and can induce malignant transformation, which suggest that phagocytic cells are carcinogenic (Brar et al., 2003; Knaapen et al., 1999). The leukotriene LTB-4 and cytokine IL-8 are recognized to play a crucial role in neutrophil recruitment into airways during lung cancer in particular when progressing to the next stage of cancer (Carpagnano et al., 2011).

Source	Targets/alterations	
ROS	Nucleic acid oxidation Hyaluronic acid depolymerization Protease inhibitor inactivation	Rheumatoid arthritis
ROS	Lipid peroxidation Atherosclerotic plaque erosion	Atherosclerosis
ROS	Histone deacetylase activity reduction p38 MAPK, EGFR, SHP2 modulation	Chronic obstructive pulmonary disease
ROS	DNA lesions Transcription factor activation	Lung cancer
ROS	Carbonylated proteins	Diabetes, Alzheimer's disease
S100A8/A9	NF-κB, p38 MAPK activation	Rheumatoid arthritis
S100A8/A9	Myeloid-derived suppressor cell accumulation p38 MAPK, p44/42 kinase activation	Cancer

Table 1. Some human inflammatory diseases associated with ROS and S100A8/A9

3. Description of the signal transduction pathways regulating NOX2 with emphasis on the role of Ca^{2+} mobilization

Ca^{2+} is a ubiquitous second messenger that functions over a wide and defined spatio-temporal range. Normal cytosolic free Ca^{2+} concentration ($[Ca^{2+}]_c$) in resting mammalian cells is maintained to low levels, in a range of 50-150 nM, compared to an endoplasmic reticulum and extracellular Ca^{2+} concentration of ~500 μM and ~2000 μM, respectively. When Ca^{2+} channels are opened in the plasma membrane, Ca^{2+} can rapidly flows into the cytosol and reach a concentration of 1 μM in a few seconds. Alternatively, Ca^{2+} influx can be delivered to low sustained Ca^{2+} levels to control appropriate cellular activities. A broad class of Ca^{2+} channels, differing for regulatory mechanisms and intracellular distribution, can be activated allowing the control by adapted Ca^{2+}-signalling systems of many divergent cellular processes (exocytosis, muscle contraction, gene transcription, fertilization, meiosis, immune response, muscle contraction) with the right frequency and intensity. Fluctuations in $[Ca^{2+}]_c$ are initiated at a localized site and diffuse inside the cell in the form of intracellular Ca^{2+} waves. In this view, neutrophils show irregular $[Ca^{2+}]_c$ spikes during phagocytosis and after stimulation by the bacterial chemopeptide fMLF (Dewitt et al., 2006; Jaconi et al., 1988).

3.1 Store-operated Ca^{2+} entry mechanism

The receptor-mediated Ca^{2+} influx required for NOX2 activation in neutrophils is predominantly the result of the activation of the so-called store-operated Ca^{2+} entry (SOCE), which is initiated by a fall in intracellular Ca^{2+} store content. The store depletion is coupled to the opening of store-operated Ca^{2+} channels (SOCs) localized in the plasma membrane, giving rise to a substantial Ca^{2+} influx. The SOCE mechanism involves G-protein-coupled receptors (e.g., N-formylpeptide receptor, FPR) that are associated to phospholipase C activation. This enzyme generates inositol 1,4,5 trisphosphate, which in turn mediates the depletion of Ca^{2+} from endoplasmic reticulum (Fig. 2). The fall of Ca^{2+} within the stores is sensed by the stromal interaction molecule protein 1 (STIM1) that translocates through the endoplasmic reticulum membrane to aggregate with SOCs (for review, see Putney, 2007). Activation of SOCs results in a Ca^{2+} influx into the cell and subsequent $[Ca^{2+}]_c$ elevation.

Direct evidence in support of SOCE has been provided by the electrophysiological demonstration of Ca^{2+} currents evoked by depleting intracellular Ca^{2+} stores (Hoth & Penner, 1992). This current was termed Ca^{2+} release-activated Ca^{2+} current (I_{crac}). Icrac is a non-voltage activated, an inwardly rectifying and a highly selective current for Ca^{2+} with a very positive reversal potential level (greater than + 60 mV) (Parekh & Penner, 1997). I_{crac} is not the only store-operated Ca^{2+} current, and it is now apparent that SOCE encompasses a family of Ca^{2+}-permeable channels as judged by their diverse biophysical properties in different cell types. This disparity indicates that SOCs are likely to possess different molecular structures (for review, see Salido et al., 2011). Recent advances in the understanding of the potential molecular composition of SOCs has been the discovery of two families of transmembrane proteins, STIM and Orai (Peinelt et al., 2006; Prakriya et al., 2006; Soboloff et al., 2006). The selective Crac channel pore is formed by a tetrameric arrangement of Orai1 dimers, which is induced by the interaction with the C-terminus of STIM (Penna et al., 2009). STIM1 acts as a Ca^{2+} sensor/activator of Orai1 and Orai1 constitutes the pore-forming component of Crac channels (Mercer et al., 2006). However, SOC currents that display distinct properties from I_{crac} may involve channels composed of transient receptor potential canonical (TRPC) subunits. In this sense, novel insights into the molecular components and the regulation of SOCs have been provided. TRPC1 and Orai1 could constitute distinct Ca^{2+} and I_{crac} channels, respectively, both of which are gated by STIM1 in response to store depletion and contribute to SOCE (Cheng et al., 2011).

3.2 Non-store-operated Ca^{2+} entry mechanism

SOCE is not the only pathway for Ca^{2+} influx in non-excitable cells; it can be supplied by alternative pathways dependent on the generation of second messengers but unrelated to store depletion. Constitutive STIM1 in the plasma membrane could regulate the activity of the arachidonic-acid-regulated Ca^{2+}-selective channels (ARC channels) (Mignen et al., 2007), whose activation is entirely independent of store depletion. The molecular structure of functional ARC channels is formed by a pentameric assembly of Orai1 and Orai3 subunits; these latter subunits determine the selectivity of ARC channels for arachidonic acid (Mignen et al., 2009). Beside ARC channels, other Ca^{2+} channels are activated by a variety of second messengers. Accumulating evidence show that members of TRPC could be activated by diacylglycerol (Bréchard et al., 2008; Hofmann et al., 1999). In addition, cyclic adenosine diphosphoribose, via its hydrolysis product (adenosine diphosphoribose), could support Ca^{2+} entry through the activation of TRPM2, a member of transient receptor potential family (Heiner et al., 2006; Howard et al., 1993; Lange et al., 2008).

3.3 Ca^{2+} dependence of NOX2 activation

It is well-known that, among complex transductional networks, Ca^{2+} mobilization acts a primordial role in receptor-mediated activation of NOX2 by neutrophils (Bréchard et al.,

2008; Foyouzi-Youssefi et al., 1997). Knock-down of putative constituents of SOCE mechanism (Orai1, STIM1) by specific siRNA or decrease of SOC activity by pharmacological inhibitors (MRS1845, SK&F96365 or 2-APB) led to a diminished NOX2 activity in the plasma membrane (Bréchard et al., 2008, 2009; Lee et al., 2005) underlining the preponderant function of SOCE in the regulation of NOX2. Activation of Ca^{2+} signal is reported as an on-switch for NOX2 activity not directly correlated with spiking activity in cytosolic Ca^{2+} (Brasen et al., 2011).

Extracellular Ca^{2+} entry is also required for intraphagosomal oxidative activation and has been temporally correlated with NOX2 activity (Dewitt et al., 2002). Ca^{2+} influx appears to be necessary for an optimal intraphagosomal oxidative activity but not sufficient to initiate oxidative activation (Dewitt et al., 2002). Orai1 and STIM1 contribute to the regulation of phagosomal NOX2 activity through the activation of store depletion-regulated Ca^{2+} influx (Braun et al., 2009; Steinckwich et al., 2011).

On the other hand, Itagaki et al. (Itagaki et al., 2005) suggest that Ca^{2+} influx occurring through a mechanism other than SOCE could be a relevant event to activate NOX2. In addition, the TRP channel, TRPC3, appears to be involved in non-SOCE-dependent regulation of NOX2 (Bréchard et al., 2008).

Taken together, these results provide strong evidence for the involvement of two separate Ca^{2+} signalling pathways in NOX2 regulation but no direct correlation between non-SOCE or SOCE and NOX2 has been yet formally established.

3.4 Ca^{2+} targets for the regulation of NOX2 activity

3.4.1 Protein kinase C (PKC)

Activation of protein kinase C (PKCs), a phospholipid-dependent family of serine-threonine protein kinases, is one of the earliest events in multiple signal transduction pathways that control a variety of cellular responses (secretion, gene expression, proliferation and muscle contraction) including NOX2 activity. The PKC family is categorized into three classes on the basis of structure and activation requirements. At least eleven different PKC isoforms have been characterized so far and these isoforms can be grouped into the following three subgroups based on Ca^{2+} dependency, activators and molecular structure. Conventional (classical) PKCs (α, βI, βII, and γ) are Ca^{2+}-dependent via their C2 domains while novel (δ, ε, μ, θ and η) and atypical (ζ and τ/λ) PKCs are Ca^{2+}-independent. Both conventional and novel PKCs are directly activated by phosphatidylserine, diacylglycerol and phorbol esters (such as PMA) through their cysteine-rich C1 domains while atypical isoforms are insensitive to phorbol esters (Hug et al., 1993; Newton 1995; Sargeant & McPhail, 1997). Atypical PKCs, unlike classical and novel PKCs, feature a C1-like domain which does not bind to either diacylglycerol or phorbol esters.

In addition of Ca^{2+}-independent PKCs, conventional PKCs (α and β isoforms) have been found to regulate NOX2 activity (Fig. 2) as shown by studies using antisense strategy or pharmacological inhibitors. Down-regulation of PKCβ and PKCα activity affect superoxide anion production in neutrophil-like HL-60 cells underlying the importance of these two enzymes for a full activation of NOX2 (Korchak et al., 2007).

Since it is known that NOX2 activation is critically dependent on $p47^{phox}$ phosphorylation, a lot of effort has been put into identifying PKCs responsible of this downstream event. The role of PKCα, PKCβ, and PKCβII in the direct phosphorylation and subsequent membrane translocation of $p47^{phox}$ has been pointed by several studies (Fontayne et al., 2002).

Consistent with these assumptions, Brasen et al. (Brasen et al., 2011) postulated that Ca^{2+}-dependent phosphorylation of NOX2 by PKCs may be in accordance with a slower intermediary step between $[Ca^{2+}]_c$ elevation and increases in NOX2 activity.

3.4.2 Monomeric G protein Rac

Rac is a member of the Rho subfamily of small GTPases that is essential in NOX2 regulation (for review, see Bockoch & Diebold, 2002). Three isoforms of Rac are known but only Rac1 and Rac2 are found in neutrophils. In the cytosol, Rac is maintained in an inactive GDP-bound form in a complex with RhoGDI, which regulates Rac targeting to the plasma membrane. RhoGDI must dissociate to allow Rac to translocate to the membrane and interact with its downstream effectors. The guanine nucleotide exchange factors (GEF) induce activation by exchanging GDP for GTP, whereas GTPase activating proteins enhance the intrinsic rate of hydrolysis of bound GTP to GDP, resulting in Rac inactivation. Rac translocation is correlated with its activation (Fleming et al., 1996), but both events are probably regulated independently.
Because Ras-GRF exchange factors harbor a Ca^{2+}-calmodulin binding site (Farnsworth et al., 1995) and Tiam1 exchange factor is phosphorylated by Ca^{2+}-calmodulin-dependent protein kinase II (Fleming et al., 1999), changes in $[Ca^{2+}]_c$ has been proposed to regulate GDP/GTP exchange on Rac1. PKCα and Ca^{2+}/calmodulin-dependent protein kinase II phosphorylate the Rac1-specific exchange factor Tiam1 but only Ca^{2+}/calmodulin-dependent protein kinase II regulates the activity of this exchange factor toward Rac1 (Fleming et al., 1999). Later, it was reported that PKCα, activated by thrombin, can phosphorylate RhoGDI and regulates the dissociation of Rac/RhoGDI complex catalyzing the release of bound GTPases, and subsequent Rac translocation to the plasma membrane (Mehta et al., 2001). Consistent with these findings, Valentin et al. (Valentin et al., 2001) determined that Ca^{2+} influx plays a primordial role in the plasma membrane translocation of Rac1 in neutrophil-like HL-60 cells (Fig. 2). Price et al. (Price et al., 2001) proposed a mechanism whereby $[Ca^{2+}]_c$ elevation triggers conventional PKC dependent Rho-GDI phosphorylation. This event leads to Rac dissociation from the Rac-RhoGDI complex followed by the membrane translocation of Rac and its activation by guanine exchange factors.

3.4.3 Cytosolic PLA_2 ($_cPLA_2$)

$cPLA_2$ causes the release of arachidonic acid from membrane phospholipids via the hydrolysis of fatty acids at the sn-2 position (Marshall et al., 2000). Several studies put forward that $cPLA_2$ is recruited at the plasma membrane in a Ca^{2+}-dependent pathway and PKCα is required for $cPLA_2$ activity (Li et al., 1999; Schievella et al., 1995; Shmelzer et al., 2003). Although underlying mechanisms need to be investigated further, $cPLA_2$ has been associated with the regulation of NOX2. $cPLA_2$ is not required for the membrane translocation of cytosolic NOX2 subunits but appears to have a critical role in NOX2 activation after its assembly (Dana el al., 1998). Indeed, arachidonic acid has been described as a cofactor enhancing the affinity of the assembled NOX2 for NADPH (Shmelzer et al., 2003).

3.4.4 Ca^{2+}-binding protein S100A8 and S100A9

In recent years, members of the large S100 family of proteins containing two EF-hand Ca^{2+}-binding motifs have been involved in the regulation of NOX2. S100A8/A9 have been described as the molecular switch between the receptor-activated, Ca^{2+}-dependent signalling cascade and NOX2 activation.

4. Intracellular functions of S100A8 and S100A9 with particular attention to their role in NOX2 activation

The phagocyte-specific Ca^{2+}-binding proteins S100A8 and S100A9 are largely expressed in the cytoplasm of phagocytes where they exert an intracellular function. The formation of S100A8/A9 heterocomplexes is probably a pre-requisite for their biological activities (Leukert et al., 2006). S100A8 and S100A9 are known to interact with NOX2 subunits (Berthier et al., 2003) and have been proposed as regulators of NOX2 activity. The relevant role for S100A8/A9 complex in oxidative response is probably mediated via their Ca^{2+}-and phosphorylation-dependent translocation upon complex formation at the plasma membrane (Lominadze et al., 2005; Roth et al., 1993; Schenten et al., 2010, 2011) where NOX2 is activated.

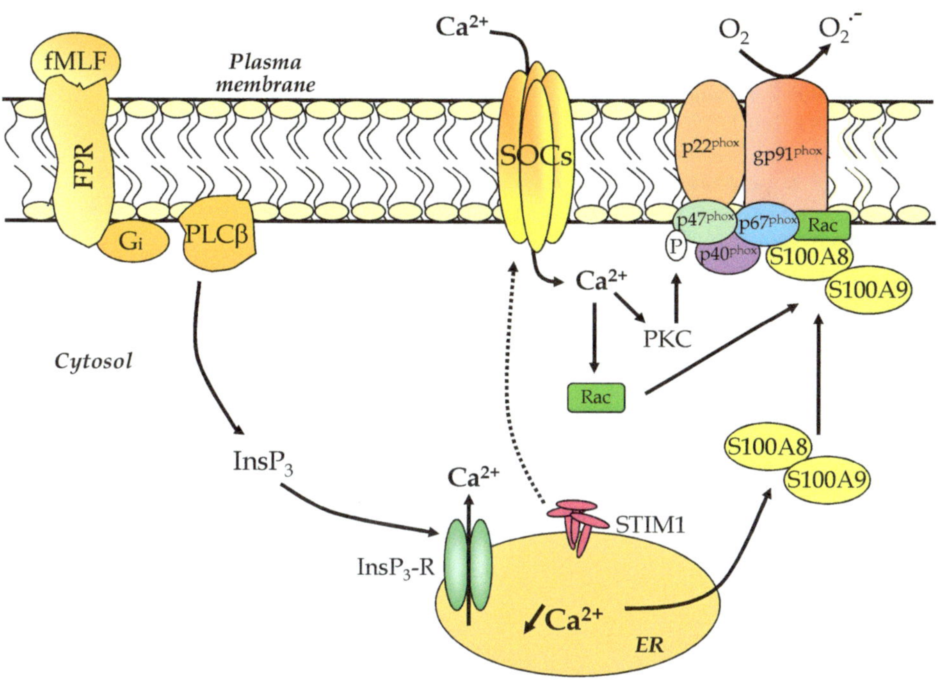

Fig. 2. Model depicting the Ca^{2+}-dependent regulation of NOX2 activity in neutrophils. Binding of the bacterial chemopeptide fMLF to its G-protein-coupled receptor (FPR) leads to the production of inositol 1,4,5-trisphosphate ($InsP_3$) via phospholipase C (PLC) activation. $InsP_3$ interacts with its specific receptor-channel ($InsP_3$-R) on the surface of the endoplasmic reticulum (ER) triggering intracellular Ca^{2+} store depletion and subsequent elevation of $[Ca^{2+}]_c$. The fall of Ca^{2+} within the ER is sensed by the stromal interaction molecule protein 1 (STIM1) resulting in the activation of store-operated Ca^{2+} channels (SOCs) at the plasma membrane and extracellular Ca^{2+} entry. Intracellular Ca^{2+} store depletion participates to the membrane translocation of S100A8/A9 and subsequent NOX2 activation. Elevation of $[Ca^{2+}]_c$ induced by extracellular Ca^{2+} entry mediates the membrane translocation of Rac and stimulates PKC activity involved in the phosphorylation of cytosolic phox proteins.

4.1 Translocation of S100A8/A9 complex to the plasma membrane

An elevation of $[Ca^{2+}]_c$ is necessary for S100A8/A9 relocalization to the plasma membrane. Intracellular Ca^{2+} store depletion appears to be partly responsible for this phenomenon (Schenten et al., 2010) (Fig. 2) but, a supplementary signal for S100A8/A9 translocation is probably required. In this view, it was established that recruitment of S100A8/A9 to the plasma membrane is dependent on S100A9 phosphorylation and subsequently intervene in the regulation of NOX2 activity. This phosphorylation is mediated by p38 MAPK (Vogl et al., 2004) on threonine 113. It has been shown to be regulated by sphingosine kinase activation, which depends on the depletion of intracellular Ca^{2+} stores (Schenten et al., 2011). Furthermore, it has been hypothesized that PKCs plays a role in the regulation of S100A8/A9 by phosphorylating sphingosine kinases. On the other hand, PKCs could modulate S100A8/A9 translocation within cellular compartments by phosphorylating S100A8 (Guignard et al., 1996).

4.2 Interactions between S100A8/A9 and NOX2

To clarify NOX2 regulation processes a method, to isolate the reconstituted assembled NOX2 complex, has been developed, through the purification of neutrophil cytochrome b_{558}. (Berthier et al., 2003; Doussière et al., 2002). The isolated NOX2 complex was able to produce constitutively superoxide anion in absence of any stimulus. NOX2 turnover was only dependent on the source of cytosol (Paclet et al., 2007). The addition of Ca^{2+}-loaded S100A8/A9 to NOX2 complex prepared with neutrophil cytochrome b_{558} and B lymphocyte cytosol, increased the constitutive activity of cytochrome b_{558} to reach a maximum NOX2 turnover ~120 s^{-1}. Moreover, cytochrome b_{558} bound to the heparin-agarose matrix, was also activated by using recombinant S100A8/S100A9, instead of cytosolic factors and without any stimulus.

During the activation process of NOX2, it was shown that S100A8/A9 proteins enhance or induce a transition from an inactive to an active state of cytochrome b_{558}. This change of structural conformation was illustrated by atomic force microscopy (Berthier et al., 2003). The data suggest a specific interaction between S100A8/A9 and cytochrome b_{558}. Moreover, S100A8/A9 complex, which enhances the affinity of $p67^{phox}$ for cytochrome b_{558}, was introduced as a positive allosteric effector of NOX2 activity. Upon translocation, Ca^{2+}-loaded S100A8/S100A9 complex appears to interact preferentially with $p67^{phox}$ that might favour the organization of a scaffold oxidase complex at the membrane level. However, preincubation of S100A8/S100A9 in the absence of Ca^{2+} led to an interaction of this complex with cytochrome b_{558} but not to its conformational change resulting in ROS production. It supports the fact that the role of S100A8/A9 in NOX2 activation is dependent on Ca^{2+} (Berthier et al., 2009).

5. Pro-inflammatory roles of secreted S100A8/A9: Involvement in pathophysiology

Beside their intracellular functions, S100A8 and S100A9 have been introduced as important pro-inflammatory factors of innate immunity secreted by phagocytes and are considered as damage-associated molecular pattern molecules (Foell & Roth, 2004; Loser, et al., 2010). S100A and S100A9 are known to have antimicrobial effects, transport arachidonic acid to endothelial cells and activate expression of endothelial cell adhesion molecules. Furthermore, the role of S100A8/S100A9 on degranulation (Simard et al., 2010) and on

neutrophil migration (Vandal et al., 2003) has been suggested. S100A8 was recently identified as an endogenous ligand of Toll-like receptor 4 (TLR4), amplifying phagocyte activation during inflammation upstream of TNF-α-dependent effects.
A new inflammatory syndrome characterized by an extraordinary high expression of S100A8/A9 proteins has been described by Sampson et al. (Sampson et al., 2002), which underlines the particular relevance of these two proteins for inflammatory pathologies. This disease is hallmarked by recurrent infections, systemic inflammation, hepatosplenomegaly, hyperzincaemia and hypercalprotectinaemia.
The S100A8/S100A9 complex is found in high concentrations at local sites of inflammation or in the serum of patients with inflammatory diseases. Since S100A8/S100A9 are dramatically up-regulated in rheumatoid arthritis synovial fluid (Baillet et al., 2010; Berntzen et al., 1991; Frosch et al., 2000); they are considered as inflammation biomarkers providing more important and sensitive information about the extent of local inflammation in the affected joints than conventional parameters (such as C-reactive protein) of systemic inflammation (Foell, & Roth, 2004). S100A8/A9 may amplify pro-inflammatory cytokine responses through activation of NF-κB and p38 MAPK pathways in rheumatoid arthritis (Sunahori et al., 2006). Indeed, the receptor for advanced glycation end products (RAGE), able to bind S100 proteins (Hofmann et al., 1999), has been implicated in the pathogenesis of rheumatoid arthritis and atherosclerosis through its ability to amplify inflammatory pathways via the recruitment of p38 MAPK and downstream activation of NF-κB (Ehlermann et al., 2006). S100A8 and S100A9 proteins are likely involved in chronic recurrent disorders by modulating activity of matrix metalloproteinases and inducing the pseudotumoral transformation of the synoviocytes (Hiratsuka et al., 2006; Yong et al., 2007).
High expression of S100A8/A9 was described in various other chronic inflammatory diseases, such as cystic fibrosis, inflammatory bowel disease Crohn's disease, giant cell arteritis, cystic fibrosis, Sjogren's syndrome, systemic lupus erythematosus, and progressive systemic sclerosis (for reviews, see Foell et Roth., 2004; Gebhardt et al., 2006). In addition, overexpression of these proteins has also been seen in many tumor-infiltrating cells (Gebhardt et al., 2006; McKiernan et al.; 2011; Su et al., 2010) underlining the fact S100A8/A9 levels may serve as a potential marker for metastatic progression in certain type of cancers. Human chromosome 1q21, where S100A8 and S100A9 are clustered, is frequently rearranged in human epithelial tumors and tumors of soft tissues, suggesting a link between S100 proteins and tumor formation and metastasis (for reviews, see Gebhardt et al., 2006; Heizmann et al., 2007). The strong up-regulation of S100A8/A9 both in inflammation and in cancer suggests these proteins may play an important role in cancer-associated inflammation by enhancing inflammatory responses. S100A8 and S100A9 promote tumorigenesis by inducing the accumulation of myeloid-derived suppressor cells in the tumor microenvironment and thereby repress host-mediated tumor immunity (Sinha et al., 2008). S100A8/A9 can also promote tumorigenesis by activating pro-tumorigenic signalling pathways. S100A8/A9 have been shown to promote cell growth via p38 MAPK and p44/42 kinase activation in tumor cells in a RAGE-dependent manner (Ghavami et al., 2008).
Taken together with the pro-inflammatory properties described above, the role of S100A8/S100A9 as protective mechanisms in inflammation should also be considered. They are more sensitive to oxidation than low-density lipoproteins and S100A8 is a key target of oxidation by peroxide, hypochlorite and nitric oxide. Thus, post-translational modifications of S100A8/S100A9 proteins induced by ROS may switch their biological properties from a pro-inflammatory towards an anti-inflammatory pattern preventing exaggerated tissue damage by scavenging oxidants (McCormick et al., 2005).

6. Conclusion

Despite many decades of intensive research, the etiology of most chronic inflammatory diseases remains elusive. Current anti-inflammatory therapy focuses on the management of the symptom rather on the maintenance of the function. Substantial increases in the cost of chronic inflammatory diseases are expected in the coming years due to the ageing of the population. For these reasons, there is growing interest in identifying biomarkers and attractive targets for novel anti-inflammatory therapies. Neutrophil NADPH oxidase and S100A8/A9 proteins have pro-inflammatory functions and play a fundamental role in host defence but also have the potential for pathological outcomes. Although physiological responses of neutrophils have been solidly documented, perturbations in S100A8/A9 signalling pathways and regulation of the NADPH oxidase activity have not yet been adequately explored. Given their importance in the pathophysiology of various chronic diseases, global understanding of NADPH oxidase and S100A8/A9 roles is likely to become of major importance over the coming years. It bears the potential to valid novel therapies and diagnostic markers for disease development and risk assessment.

7. References

Alamanos, Y., Voulgari, P.V. & Drosos, A.A. 2006. Incidence and prevalence of rheumatoid arthritis, based on the 1987 American College of Rheumatology criteria: a systematic review. *Seminars in arthritis and rheumatism.*, Dec, 36 (3): 182-188

Allavena, P., Garlanda, C., Borrello, M.G., Sica, A. & Mantovani, A. 2008. Pathways connecting inflammation and cancer. *Curr. Opin. Genet. Dev.*, Feb, 18 (1): 3-10

Aruoma, O.I., Halliwell, B., Gajewski, E. & Dizdaroglu, M. 1989. Damage to the bases in DNA induced by hydrogen peroxide and ferric ion chelates. *J. Biol. Chem.*, Dec 5, 264 (34): 20509-20512

Babior, B.M., Lambeth, J.D. & Nauseef, W. 2002. The neutrophil NADPH oxidase. *Arch. Biochem. Biophys.*, Jan 15, 397 (2): 342-344

Baillet, A., Trocme, C., Berthier, S., Arlotto, M., Grange, L., Chenau, J., Quétant, S., Sève, M., Berger, S., Juvin, R., Morel, F. & Gaudin, P. 2010. Synovial fluid proteomic fingerprint: S100A8, S100A9 and S100A12 proteins discriminate rheumatoid arthritis from other inflammatory joint diseases. *Rheumatology* (Oxford), Apr, 49 (4): 671-682

Bellomo, G., Jewell, S.A., Thor, H. & Orrenius, S. 1982. Regulation of intracellular calcium compartmentation: studies with isolated hepatocytes and t-butyl hydroperoxide. *Proc. Natl. Acad. Sci. USA*, Nov, 79 (22): 6842-6846

Berntzen, H.B., Olmez, U., Fagerhol, M.K. & Munthe, E. 1991. The leukocyte protein L1 in plasma and synovial fluid from patients with rheumatoid arthritis and osteoarthritis. *Scand. J. Rheumatol.*, 20 (2): 74-82

Berlett, B.S. & Stadtman, E.R. 1997. Protein oxidation in aging, disease, and oxidative stress. *J. Biol. Chem.*, Aug 15, 272 (33): 20313-20316

Berthier, S., Paclet, M.H., Lerouge, S., Roux, F., Vergnaud, S., Coleman A.W. & Morel, F. 2003. Changing the conformation state of cytochrome b_{558} initiates NADPH oxidase activation: MRP8/MRP14 regulation. *J. Biol. Chem.*, Jul 11, 278 (28): 25499-25508

Berthier, S, Baillet, A, Paclet, MH, Gaudin, P & Morel, F. 2009. How important are S100A8/S100A9 calcium binding proteins for the activation of phagocyte NADPH oxidase, Nox2. *AIAAMC*, 8: 282-284

Bockoch, G.M. & Diebold, B.A. 2002. Current molecular models for NADPH oxidase regulation by Rac GTPase. *Blood*, Oct 15, 100 (8): 2692-2696

Brar, S.S., Kennedy, T.P., Quinn, M. & Hoidal, J.R. 2003. Redox signaling of NF-κB by membrane NAD(P)H oxidases in normal and malignant cells. *Protoplasma*, May, 221 (1-2): 117–127

Brasen, J.C., Olsen, L.F. & Hallett, M.B. 2011. Extracellular ATP induces spikes in cytosolic free Ca(2+) but not in NADPH oxidase activity in neutrophils. *Biochim. Biophys. Acta*, Aug, 1813 (8): 1446-1452

Braun, A., Gessner, J.E., Varga-Szabo, D., Syed, S.N., Konrad, S., Stegner, D., Vögtle, T., Schmidt, R.E. & Nieswandt, B. 2009. STIM1 is essential for Fcgamma receptor activation and autoimmune inflammation. *Blood*, Jan 29, 113 (5): 1097-1104

Bréchard, S., Melchior, C., Plançon, S., Schenten, V. & Tschirhart, E.J. 2008. Store-operated Ca^{2+} channels formed by TRPC1, TRPC6 and Orai1 and non-store-operated channels formed by TRPC3 are involved in the regulation of NADPH oxidase in HL-60 granulocytes. *Cell Calcium*, Nov, 44 (5): 492-506

Bréchard, S., Plançon, S., Melchior, C. & Tschirhart, E.J. 2009. STIM1 but not STIM2 is an essential regulator of Ca^{2+} influx-mediated NADPH oxidase activity in neutrophil-like HL-60 cells. *Biochem. Pharmacol.*, Sep 1, 78 (5): 504-513

Callahan, L.F. & Pincus, T. 1995. Mortality in the rheumatic diseases. *Arthritis Care Res.*, Dec, 8 (4): 229-241

Carpagnano, G.E., Palladino, G.P., Lacedonia, D., Koutelou, A., Orlando, S. & Foschino-Barbaro, M.P. 2011. Neutrophilic airways inflammation in lung cancer: the role of exhaled LTB-4 and IL-8. *BMC Cancer*, Jun 7, 11: 226

Carroll, L., Hannawi, S., Marwick, T. & Thomas, R. 2006. Rheumatoid arthritis: links with cardiovascular disease and the receptor for advanced glycation end products. *Wien Med. Wochenschr.*, Jan, 156 (1-2): 42-52

Chatham, W.W., Swaim, R., Frohsin, H. Jr., Heck, L.W., Miller, E.J. & Blackburn, W.D. Jr. 1993. Degradation of human articular cartilage by neutrophils in synovial fluid. *Arthritis Rheum.* Janv, 36 (1): 51-58

Cheng, K.T., Liu, X., Ong, H.L., Swaim, W. & Ambudkar, I.S. 2011. Local Ca^{2}+ entry via Orai1 regulates plasma membrane recruitment of TRPC1 and controls cytosolic Ca^{2}+ signals required for specific cell functions. *PLoS Biol.*, Mar, 9 (3): e1001025

Cheng, P., Corzo, C.A., Luetteke, N., Yu, B., Nagaraj, S., Bui, M.M., Ortiz, M., Nacken, W., Sorg, C., Vogl, T., Roth, J. & Gabrilovich, D.I. 2008. Inhibition of dendritic cell differentiation and accumulation of myeloid-derived suppressor cells in cancer is regulated by S100A9 protein. *J. Exp. Med.*, Sep 29, 205 (10): 2235-224

Chevion, M., Berenshtein, E. & & Stadtman, E.R. 2000. Human studies related to protein oxidation: protein carbonyl content as a marker of damage. *Free Radic. Res.*, Nov, 33: S99-S108

Dalle-Donne, I., Rossi, R., Giustarini, D., Gagliano, N., Di Simplicio, P., Colombo, R. & Milzani, A. 2002. Methionine oxidation as a major cause of the functional impairment of oxidized actin. *Free Radic. Biol. Med.*, May 1, 32 (9): 927-937

Dalle-Donne, I., Rossi, R., Giustarini, D., Milzani, A. & Colombo, R. 2003. Protein carbonyl groups as biomarkers of oxidative stress. *Clin. Chim. Acta*, Mar, 329 (1-2): 23-38

Dalle-Donne, I., Rossi, R., Colombo, R., Giustarini, D. & Milzani, A. 2006. Biomarkers of oxidative damage in human disease. *Clin. Chem.*, Apr 52 (4): 601-623

Dana, R., Leto, T.L., Malech, H.L. & Levy, R. 1998. Essential requirement of cytosolic phospholipase A_2 for activation of the phagocyte NADPH oxidase. *J. Biol. Chem.*, Jan 2, 273 (1): 441-445

Dewitt, S. & Hallett, M.B. 2002. Cytosolic free Ca(2+) changes and calpain activation are required for beta integrin-accelerated phagocytosis by human neutrophils. *J. Cell Biol.*, Oct 14, 159 (1): 181-189

Dewitt, S., Tian, W. & Hallett, M.B. 2006. Localised PtdIns(3,4,5)P3 or PtdIns(3,4)P2 at the phagocytic cup is required for both phagosome closure and Ca2+ signalling in HL60 neutrophils. *J. Cell Sci.*, Feb 1, 119 (Pt 3): 443-451

Doussière J., Bouzidi F. & Vignais P.V. 2002. The S100A8/A9 protein as a partner for the cytosolic factors of NADPH oxidase activation in neutrophils. *Eur. J. Biochem.*, Jul, 269 (13): 3246-3255

Edwards, S.W. & Hallett, M.B. 1997. Seeing the wood for the trees: the forgotten role of neutrophils in rheumatoid arthritis. *Immunol. Today*, Jul, 18 (7): 320-324

Ehlermann, P., Eggers, K., Bierhaus, A., Most, P., Weichenhan, D., Greten, J., Nawroth, P.P., Katus, H.A. & Remppis, A. 2006. Increased proinflammatory endothelial response to S100A8/A9 after preactivation through advanced glycation end products. *Cardiovasc . Diabetol.*, Mar 30, 5: 6

Englund, M., Joud, A., Geborek, P., Felson, D.T., Jacobsson, L.T. & Petersson, I.F. 2010. Prevalence and incidence of rheumatoid arthritis in southern Sweden 2008 and their relation to prescribed biologics. *Rheumatology* (Oxford, England), Aug, 2010, 49 (8): 1563-1569

Esterbauer, H., Zollner, H. & Scholz, N. 1975. Reaction of glutathione with conjugated carbonyls. *Z. Naturforsch C.*, Jul-Aug, 30 (4): 466-473

Esterbauer, H., Schaur, R.J. & Zollner, H. 1991. Chemistry and biochemistry of 4-hydroxynonenal, malonaldehyde and related aldehydes. *Free Radic. Biol. Med.*, 11 (1): 81-128

Farnsworth, C.L., Freshney, N.W., Rosen, L.B., Ghosh, A., Greenberg, M.E. & Feig, L.A. 1995. Calcium activation of Ras mediated by neuronal exchange factor Ras-GRF. *Nature*, Aug 10, 376 (6540), 524-527

Fleming, I.N., Elliott, C.M. & Exton, J.H. 1996. Differential translocation of rho family GTPases by lysophosphatidic acid, endothelin-1, and platelet-derived growth factor. *J. Biol. Chem.*, Dec 20, 271 (51), 33067-33073

Fleming, I.N., Elliott, C.M., Buchanan, F.G., Downes, C.P. & Exton, J.H. 1999 . Ca2+/calmodulin-dependent protein kinase II regulates Tiam1 by reversible protein phosphorylation. *J. Biol. Chem.*, Apr 30, 274 (18): 12753-12758

Foell, D. & Roth, J. 2004. Proinflammatory S100 proteins in arthritis and autoimmune disease. *Arthritis Rheum.*, Dec, 50 (12), 3762-3771

Fontayne, A., Dang, P.M., Gougerot-Pocidalo, M.A. & el Benna, J. 2002. Phosphorylation of $p47^{phox}$ sites by PKC α, β II, δ, and ζ: effect on binding to $p22^{phox}$ and on NADPH oxidase activation. *Biochemistry*, Jun 18, 41 (24): 7743-7750

Foyouzi-Youssefi, R., Petersson, F., Lew, D.P., Krause, K.H. & Nusse, O. 1997. Chemoattractant-induced respiratory burst: increases in cytosolic Ca^{2+} concentrations are essential and synergize with a kinetically distinct second signal. *Biochem. J.*, Mar 15, 322 (Pt 3): 709-718

Frosch, M., Strey, A., Vogl, T., Wulffraat, N.M., Kuis, W., Sunderkotter, C., Harms, E., Sorg, C. & Roth, J. 2000. Myeloid-related proteins 8 and 14 are specifically secreted during interaction of phagocytes and activated endothelium and are useful markers for monitoring disease activity in pauciarticular-onset juvenile rheumatoid arthritis. *Arthritis Rheum.*, Mar, 43 (3), 628-637

Gebhardt, C., Németh, J., Angel, P. & Hess, J. 2006. S100A8 and S100A9 in inflammation and cancer. *Biochem. Pharmacol.*, Nov 30, 72 (11): 1622-1631

Ghavami, S., Rashedi, I., Dattilo, B.M., Eshraghi, M., Chazin, W.J., Hashemi, M., Wesselborg, S., Kerkhoff, C. & Los, M. 2008. S100A8/A9 at low concentration promotes tumor cell growth via RAGE ligation and MAP kinase-dependent pathway. *J. Leukoc. Biol.*, Jun, 83 (6): 1484-1492

Guignard, F., Mauel, J. & Markert, M. 1996. Phosphorylation of myeloid-related proteins MRP-14 and MRP-8 during human neutrophil activation. Eur. J. Biochem., Oct 1, 241 (1): 265-271

Hajizadeh, S., DeGroot, J., TeKoppele, J.M., Tarkowski, A. & Collins, L.V. 2003. Extracellular mitochondrial DNA and oxidatively damaged DNA in synovial fluid of patients with rheumatoid arthritis. *Arthritis Res. Ther.*, 5 (5): R234-240

Hanahan, D. & Weinberg, R.A. 2011. Hallmarks of cancer: the next generation. *Cell*, Mar 4, 144 (5): 646-674

Hawkins, C.L. & Davies, M.J. 1998. Degradation of hyaluronic acid, poly- and monosaccharides, and model compounds by hypochlorite: evidence for radical intermediates and fragmentation. *Free Radic. Biol. Med.*, Jun, 24, 1396–1410

Heiner, I., Eisfeld, J., Warnstedt, M. Radukina, N., Jüngling, E. & Lückhoff, A. 2006. Endogenous ADP-ribose enables calcium-regulated cation currents through TRPM2 channels in neutrophil granulocytes. *Biochem. J.*, 2006, Sep 1, 398 (2): 225-232

Heizmann, C.W., Ackermann, G.E. & Galichet, A. 2007. Pathologies involving the S100 proteins and RAGE. *Subcell. Biochem.*, 45: 93-138

Hiratsuka, S., Watanabe, A., Aburatani, H. & Maru, Y. 2006. Tumour-mediated upregulation of chemoattractants and recruitment of myeloid cells predetermines lung metastasis. *Nat. Cell Biol.*, Dec 8 (12): 1369-1375

Hofmann, M.A., Drury, S., Fu, C., Qu, W., Taguchi, A., Lu, Y., Avila, C., Kambham, N., Bierhaus, A., Nawroth, P., Neurath, M.F., Slattery, T., Beach, D., McClary, J., Nagashima, M., Morser, J., Stern, D. & Schmidt, A.M. 1999. RAGE mediates a novel proinflammatory axis: a central cell surface receptor for S100/calgranulin polypeptides. *Cell*, Jun 25, 97 (7): 889-901

Hofmann, T., Obukhov, A.G., Schaefer, M., Harteneck, C., Gudermann, T. & Schultz, G. 1999. Direct activation of human TRPC6 and TRPC3 channels by diacylglycerol. *Nature*, Jan 21, 397 (6716): 259-263

Hosokawa, T., Kumon, Y., Kobayashi, T., Enzan, H., Nishioka, Y., Yuri, K., Wakiguchi, H. & Sugiura, T. 2011. Neutrophil infiltration and oxidant-production in human atherosclerotic carotid plaques. *Histol. Histopathol.*, Jan, 26 (1): 1-11

Hoth, M. & Penner, R. 1992. Depletion of intracellular calcium stores activates a calcium current in mast cells. *Nature*, Jan 23, 355 (6358): 353-356

Howard, M., Grimaldi, J.C., Bazan, J.F. Lund, F.E., Santos-Argumedo, L., Parkhouse, R.M., Walseth, T.F., Lee, H.C. 1993. Formation and hydrolysis of cyclic ADP-ribose catalyzed by lymphocyte antigen CD38. *Science*, Nov 12, 262 (5136): 1056-1059

Hug, H. & Sarre, T.F. 1993. Protein kinase C isoenzymes: divergence in signal transduction? *Biochem. J.*, Apr 15, 291 (Pt 2): 29-343

Ishii, T., Tatsuda, E., Kumazawa, S., Nakayama, T. & Uchida, K. 2003. Molecular basis of enzyme inactivation by an endogenous electrophile 4-hydroxy-2-nonenal: identification of modification sites in glyceraldehyde-3-phosphate dehydrogenase. *Biochemistry*, Apr 1, 42 (12): 3474-3480

Itagaki, K., Kannan, K.B. & Hauser, C.J. 2005. Lysophosphatidic acid triggers calcium entry through a non-store-operated pathway in human neutrophils. *J. Leukoc. Biol.*, Feb, 77 (2): 181-189

Ito, K., Lim, S., Caramori, G., Chung, K.F., Barnes, P.J. & Adcock, I.M. 2001. Cigarette smoking reduces histone deacetylase 2 expression, enhances cytokine expression, and inhibits glucocorticoid actions in alveolar macrophages. *FASEB J.*, Apr, 15 (6): 1110-1112

Jaconi, M.E., Rivest, R.W., Schlegel, W., Wollheim, C.B., Pittet, D. & Lew, PD. 1988 . Spontaneous and chemoattractant-induced oscillations of cytosolic free calcium in single adherent human neutrophils. *J. Biol. Chem.*, Aug 5, 263 (22): 10557-10560

Jang, M.K., Kim, S.H., Lee, K.Y., Kim, T.B., Moon, K.A., Park, C.S., Bae, Y.J., Zhu, Z., Moon, H.B. & Cho, Y.S. 2010. The tyrosine phosphatase, SHP-1, is involved in bronchial mucin production during oxidative stress. *Biochem. Biophys. Res. Commun.*, Feb 26, 393 (1): 137-143

Jessup, W., Jurgens, G., Lang, J., Esterbauer, H. & Dean, R.T. 1986. Interaction of 4-hydroxynonenal-modified low-density lipoproteins with the fibroblast apolipoprotein B/E receptor. *Biochem. J.*, Feb 15, 234 (1): 245-248

Kersul, A.L., Iglesias, A., Ríos, Á., Noguera, A., Forteza, A., Serra, E., Agustí, A. & Cosío, B.G. 2011. Molecular mechanisms of inflammation during exacerbations of chronic obstructive pulmonary disease. *Arch. Bronconeumol.*, Apr, 47 (4): 176-83

Khatami, M. 2005. Developmental phases of inflammation-induced massive lymphoid hyperplasia and extensive changes in epithelium in an experimental model of allergy: implications for a direct link between inflammation and carcinogenesis. *Am. J. Ther.*, Mar-Apr, 12 (2): 117-126

Khatami, M. 2008. 'Yin and Yang' in inflammation: duality in innate immune cell function and tumorigenesis. *Expert Opin. Biol. Ther.*, Oct, 8 (10): 1461-1472

Khatami, M. 2009. Inflammation, aging, and cancer: tumoricidal versus tumorigenesis of immunity: a common denominator mapping chronic diseases. *Cell Biochem. Biophys.*, 55 (2): 55-79

Khatami, M. 2011. Unresolved inflammation: 'immune tsunami' or erosion of integrity in immune-privileged and immune-responsive tissues and acute and chronic inflammatory diseases or cancer. *Expert Opin. Biol. Ther.*, Jun 11 [Epub ahead of print]

Klaunig, J.E. & Kamendulis, L.M. 2004. The role of oxidative stress in carcinogenesis. *Annu. Rev. Pharmacol. Toxicol.*, 44: 239-267

Knaapen, A.M., Seiler, F., Schilderman, P.A., Nehls, P., Bruch, J., Schins, R.P. & Borm, P.J. 1999. Neutrophils cause oxidative DNA damage in alveolar epithelial cells. *Free Radical Biol. Med.*, Jul, 27 (1-2), 234-240

Kohri, K., Ueki, I.F. & Nadel, J.A. 2002. Neutrophil elastase induces mucin production by ligand-dependent epidermal growth factor receptor activation. *Am. J. Physiol. Lung Cell. Mol. Physiol.*, Sept, 283 (3): L531–L540

Korchak, H.M., Dorsey, L.B., Li, H., Mackie, D. & Kilpatrick, L.E. 2007. Selective roles for α-PKC in positive signalling for O_2^- generation and calcium mobilization but not elastase release in differentiated HL60 cells. *Biochim. Biophys. Acta*, Mar, 1773 (3): 440-449

Kukreja, R.C. & Hess, M.L. 1992. The oxygen free radical system: from equations through membrane-protein interactions to cardiovascular injury and protection. *Cardiovasc. Res.*, Jul, 26 (7): 641-655

Lange, I., Penner, R., Fleig, A. & Beck, A. 2008. Synergistic regulation of endogenous TRPM2 channels by adenine dinucleotides in primary human neutrophils. *Cell Calcium*, Dec, 44 (6): 604-615

Larbre, J.P., Moore, A.R., Da Silva, J.A., Iwamura, H., Ioannou, Y. & Willoughby, D.A. 1994. Direct degradation of articular cartilage by rheumatoid synovial fluid: contribution of proteolytic enzymes. *J. Rheumatol.*, Oct, 21 (10): 1796-1801

Lee, C., Xu, D.-Z., Feketeova, E., Kannan, K.B., Fekete, Z., Deitch, E.A., Livingston & D.H., Hauser, C.J. 2005. Store-operated calcium channel inhibition attenuates neutrophil function and postshock acute lung injury. *J. Trauma*, Jul, 59 (1): 56-63

Leukert, N., Vogl, T., Strupat, K., Reichelt, R., Sorg, C. & Roth, J. 2006. Calcium-dependent tetramer formation of S100A8 and S100A9 is essential for biological activity. *J. Mol. Biol.*, Jun 16, 359 (4): 961-972

Li, Q., Subbulakshmi, V., Fields, A.P., Murray, N.R. & Cathcart, M.K. 1999. Protein kinase C alpha regulate human monocytes O_2^- production and low density lipoprotein lipid oxidation. *J. Biol. Chem.*, Feb 5, 274 (6), 3764-3771

Lominadze, G., Rane, M.J., Merchant, M., Cai, J., Ward R.A. & McLeish, K.R. 2005. Myeloid-related protein-14 is a p38 MAPK substrate in human neutrophils. *J. Immunol.*, Jun 1, 174 (11): 7257-7267

Loser, K., Vogl, T., Voskort, M., Lueken, A., Kupas, V., Nacken, W., Klenner, L., Kuhn, A., Foell, D., Sorokin, L., Luger, TA., Roth, J. & Beissert, S. 2010. The Toll-like receptor 4 ligands Mrp8 and Mrp14 are crucial in the development of autoreactive CD8+ T cells. *Nat. Med.*, Jun, 16 (6): 713-717

Mantovani, A. 2010. Molecular pathways linking inflammation and cancer. *Curr. Mol. Med.*, Jun, 10 (4): 369-373

Mao, H., Schnetz-Boutaud, N.C., Weisenseel, J.P., Marnett, L.J. & Stone, M.P. 1999. Duplex DNA catalyzes the chemical rearrangement of a malondialdehyde deoxyguanosine adduct. *Proc. Natl. Acad. Sci. USA*, Jun 8, 96 (12): 6615-6620

Marshall, J., Krump, E., Lindsay, T., Downey, G., Ford, D.A., Zhu, P., Walker, P. & Rubin, B. 2000. Involvement of cytosolic phospholipase A_2 and secretory phospholipase A_2 in arachidonic acid release from human neutrophils. *J. Immunol.*, Feb 15 164 (4): 2084-2091

Marnett, L.J . 2002. Oxy radicals, lipid peroxidation and DNA damage. *Toxicology*, Dec 27, 181-182: 219-222

McCormick, M.M., Rahimi, F., Bobryshev, Y.V., Gaus, K., Zreiqat, H., Cai, H., Lord, R.S. & Geczy, C.L. 2005. S100A8 and S100A9 in human arterial wall. Implications for atherogenesis. *J. Biol. Chem.*, Dec 16, 280 (50): 41521-41529

McKiernan, E., McDermott, E.W., Evoy, D., Crown, J. & Duffy, M.J. 2011. The role of S100 genes in breast cancer progression. *Tumour Biol.*, Jun, 32 (3): 441-450

Mehta, D., Rahman, A. & Malik, A.B. 2001. Protein kinase C-alpha signals rho-guanine nucleotide dissociation inhibitor phosphorylation and rho activation and regulates the endothelial cell barrier function. *J. Biol. Chem.*, Jun 22, 276 (25): 22614-22620

Meng, T.C., Fukada, T. & Tonks, N.K. 2002. Reversible oxidation and inactivation of protein tyrosine phosphatases in vivo. *Mol. Cell*, Feb, 9 (2) 387-399

Mercado, N., Thimmulappa, R., Thomas, C.M., Fenwick, P.S., Chana, K.K., Donnelly, L.E., Biswal, S., Ito, K. & Barnes, P.J. 2011. Decreased histone deacetylase 2 impairs Nrf2 activation by oxidative stress. *Biochem. Biophys. Res. Commun.*, Mar 11, 406 (2): 292-298

Mercer, J.C., Dehaven, W.I., Smyth, J.T., Wedel, B., Boyles, R.R., Bird, G.S. & Putney, J.W. Jr. 2006. Large-store operated calcium selective currents due to co-expression of Orai1 or Orai2 with the intracellular calcium sensor, Stim1. *J. Biol. Chem.*, Aug 25, 281 (34): 24979-24990

Mignen, O., Thompson, J.L. & Shuttleworth, T.J. 2007. STIM1 regulates Ca2+ entry via arachidonate-regulated Ca2+-selective (ARC) channels without store depletion or translocation to the plasma membrane. *J. Physiol.*, Mar 15, 579 (Pt 3): 703-715

Mignen, O., Thompson, J.L. & Shuttleworth, T.J. 2009. The molecular architecture of the arachidonate-regulated Ca2+-selective ARC channel is a pentameric assembly of Orai1 and Orai3 subunits. *J. Physiol.*, Sep 1, 587 (Pt 17): 4181-4197

Moreira, P.I, Sayre, L.M., Zhu, X., Nunomura, A., Smith, M.A. & Perry, G. 2010. Detection and localization of markers of oxidative stress by in situ methods: application in the study of Alzheimer disease. *Methods Mol. Biol.*, 610: 419-34

Newton, A.C. 1995. Protein kinase C: structure, function, and regulation. *J. Biol. Chem.*, Dec 1, 270 (48): 28495-28498

Nigam, S. & Schewe, T. 2000. Phospholipase A(2)s and lipid peroxidation. *Biochim. Biophys. Acta*, Oct 3, 1488 (1-2): 167-181

Noble, P.W., Lake, F.R., Henson, P.M. & Riches, D.W. 1993. Hyaluronate activation of CD44 induces insulin-like growth factor-1 expression by a tumor necrosis factor-alpha-dependent mechanism in murine macrophages. *J. Clin. Invest.*, Jun, 91 (6): 2368-2377

Noguera, A., Batle, S., Miralles, C., Iglesias, J., Busquets, X., MacNee, W. & Agustí, A.G. 2001. Enhanced neutrophil response in chronic obstructive pulmonary disease. *Thorax*, Jun, 56 (6): 432-437

Ohno, Y.I., Hirai, K.I, Kanoh, T., Uchino, H. & Ogawa, K. *1982*. Subcellular localization of hydrogen peroxide production in human polymorphonuclear leukocytes stimulated with lectins, phorbol myristate acetate, and digitonin: an electron microscopic study using CeCl3. *Blood*, Nov, 60 (5): 1195-1202

Oikawa, S., Tada-Oikawa, S. & Kawanishi, S. 2001. Site-specific DNA damage at the GGG sequence by UVA involves acceleration of telomere shortening. *Biochemistry*, Apr 17, 40: 4763-4768

Ottonello, L., Cutolo, M., Frumento, G., Arduino, N., Bertolotto, M., Mancini, M., Sottofattori, E. & Dallegri, F. 2002. Synovial fluid from patients with rheumatoid arthritis inhibits neutrophil apoptosis: role of adenosine and proinflammatory cytokines. *Rheumatology* (Oxford, England) Nov, 41 (11): 1249-1260

Paclet, M.H., Berthier, S., Khun, L., Garin, J. & Morel, F. 2007. Regulation of phagocyte NADPH oxidase activity: identification of two cytochrome b_{558} activation states. *FASEB J.*, Apr, 21(4): 1244-1255

Parekh, A.B. & Penner, R. 1997. Store depletion and calcium influx. *Physiol. Rev.*, Oct, 77 (4): 901-930

Peinelt, C., Vig, M., Koomoa, D.L., Beck, A., Nadler, M.J., Koblan-Huberson M., Lis, A., Fleig, A., Penner, R. & Kinet, J.P. 2006. Amplification of CRAC current by STIM1 and CRACM1 (Orai1). *Nat. Cell Biol.*, Jul, 8 (7): 771-773

Penna, A., Demuro, A., Yeromin, A.V., Zhang, S.L., Safrina, O., Parker, I. & Cahalan, M.D. 2008. The CRAC channel consists of a tetramer formed by Stim-induced dimerization of Orai dimers. *Nature,* Nov 6, 456 (7218): 116-120

Petersen, S., Saretzki, G. & von Zglinicki, T. 1998. Preferential accumulation of single-stranded regions in telomeres of human fibroblasts. *Exp. Cell Res.*, Feb 25, 239: 152-160

Poot, M., Verkerk, A., Koster, J.F., Esterbauer, H. & Jongkind, J.F. 1988. Reversible inhibition of DNA and protein synthesis by cumene hydroperoxide and 4-hydroxy-nonenal. *Mech. Ageing Dev.*, Apr, 43 (1): 1-9

Prakriya, M., Feske, S., Gwack, Y., Srikanth, S., Rao, A. & Hogan, P.G. 2006. Orai1 is an essential pore subunit of the CRAC channel. *Nature*, Sep 14, 443 (7108): 230-233

Putney, J.W. Jr. 2007. New molecular players in capacitative Ca^{2+} entry. *J. Cell Sci.*, Jun 15, 120 (Pt 12): 1959-1965

Price, L.S., Langeslag, M., ten Klooster, J.P., Hordijk, P.L., Jalink, K. & Collard, J.G. 2003 . Calcium signaling regulates translocation and activation of Rac. *J. Biol. Chem.*, Oct 10, 278 (41): 39413-39421

Quinn, M.T., Linner, J.G., Siemsen, D., Dratz, E.A., Buescher, E.S. & Jesaitis, A.J. 1995. Immunocytochemical detection of lipid peroxidation in phagosomes of human neutrophils: correlation with expression of flavocytochrome b. *J. Leukoc. Biol.*, Mar, 57 (3): 415-421

Rahman, I. 2002. Oxidative stress and gene transcription in asthma and chronic obstructive pulmonary disease: antioxidant therapeutic targets. *Curr. Drug Targets Inflamm. Allergy*, Sep, 1 (3): 291-315

Reddy, V.P., Zhu, X., Perry, G. & Smith, M.A. 2009. Oxidative stress in diabetes and Alzheimer's disease. *J. Alzheimers Dis.*, 16 (4): 763-774

Rees, M.D., Hawkins, C.L. & Davies, M. J. 2003. Hypochlorite-mediated fragmentation of glycosaminoglycans and related N-acetyl glycosamines: evidence for chloramide formation, free radical transfer reactions and site-specific fragmentation. *J. Am. Chem. Soc.*, Nov 12, 125, 13719–13733

Rees, M.D., Hawkins, C.L. & Davies, M.J. 2004. Hypochlorite and superoxide radicals can act synergistically to induce fragmentation of hyaluronan and chondroitin sulfates. *Biochem. J.*, Jul 1, 381: 175-184

Robinson, J., Watson, F., Bucknall, R.C. & Edwards, S.W. 1992. Activation of neutrophil reactive-oxidant production by synovial fluid from patients with inflammatory joint disease. Soluble and insoluble immunoglobulin aggregates activate different pathways in primed and unprimed cells. *Biochem. J.*, Sept 1, 286 (Pt 2): 345-351

Roth, J., Burwinkel, F., van den Bos, C., Goebeler, M., Vollmer, E. & Sorg, C. 1993. MRP8 and MRP14, S-100-like proteins associated with myeloid differentiation, are translocated to plasma membrane and intermediate filaments in a calcium-dependent manner. *Blood*, Sep 15, 82 (6): 1875-1883

Salido, G.M., Jardín, I. & Rosado, J.A. 2011. The TRPC ion channels: association with Orai1 and STIM1 proteins and participation in capacitative and non-capacitative calcium entry. *Adv. Exp. Med. Biol.*, 704: 413-433

Sampson, B., Fagerhol, K., Sunderkötter, C., Golden, B.E., Richmond, P., Klein, N., Kovar, I.Z., Beattie, J.H., Wolska-Kusnierz, B., Saito, Y. & Roth, J. 2002. Hyperzincaemia and hypercalprotectinaemia: a new disorder of zinc metabolism. *Lancet*, Nov 30, 360 (9347): 1742-1745

Saretzki, G., Sitte, N., Merkel, U., Wurm, R.E. & von Zglinicki, T. 1999. Telomere shortening triggers a p53-dependent cell cycle arrest via accumulation of G-rich single stranded DNA fragments. *Oncogene*, Sept 16, 18: 5148-5158

Sargeant, S. & McPhail, L.C. 1997. Opsonized zymosan stimulates the redistribution of protein kinase C isoforms in human neutrophils. *J. Immunol.*, Sept 15, 159 (6): 2877-2885

Schenten, V., Bréchard, S., Plançon, S., Melchior, C., Frippiat, J.P. & Tschirhart, E.J. 2010. iPLA(2), a novel determinant in Ca(2+)- and phosphorylation-dependent S100A8/A9 regulated NOX2 activity. *Biochim. Biophys. Acta*, Jul, 1803 (7): 840-847

Schenten, V., Melchior, C., Steinckwich, N., Tschirhart, E.J. & Brechard, S. 2011. Sphingosine kinases regulate NOX2 activity via p38 MAPK-dependent translocation of S100A8/A9. *J. Biol. Leukoc.*, Apr, 89 (4): 587-596

Schievella, A.R., Regier, M.K., Smith, W.L. & Lin, L.L. 1995. Calcium-mediated translocation of cytosolic phospholipase A_2 to the nuclear envelope and endoplasmic reticulum. *J. Biol. Chem.*, Dec 22, 270 (51), 30749-30754

Sheppard, F.R., Kelher, M.R., Moore, E.E., McLaughlin, N.J., Banerjee, A. & Silliman C.C. 2005. Structural organization of the neutrophil NADPH oxidase: phosphorylation and translocation during priming and activation. *J. Leukoc. Biol.*, Nov, 78 (5): 1025-1042

Shmelzer, Z., Haddad, N., Admon, E., Pessach, I., Leto, T.L., Eitan-Hazan, Z., Hershfinkel, M. & Levy, R. 2003. Unique targeting of cytosolic phospholipase A_2 to plasma membranes mediated by the NADPH oxidase in phagocytes. *J. Cell Biol.*, Aug 18, 162 (4): 683-692

Siems, W.G., Grune, T. & Esterbauer, H. 1995. 4-Hydroxynonenal formation during ischemia and reperfusion of rat small intestine. *Life Sci.*, 57 (8): 785-789

Simard, J.C., Girard, D. & Tessier, P.A. 2010. Induction of neutrophil degranulation by S100A9 via a MAPK-dependent mechanism. *J. Leukoc. Biol.*, May 87 (5): 905-914

Sinha, P., Okoro, C., Foell, D., Freeze, H.H., Ostrand-Rosenberg, S. & Srikrishna, G. 2008. Proinflammatory S100 proteins regulate the accumulation of myeloid-derived suppressor cells. *J. Immunol.*, Oct 1, 181 (7): 4666-4675

Soboloff, J., Spassova, M.A., Tang, X.D., Hewavitharana, T., Xu, W. & Gill, D.L. 2006. Orai1 and STIM reconstitute store-operated calcium channel function. *J. Biol. Chem.*, Jul 28, 281 (30): 20661-20665

Stadtman, E.R. & Berlett, B.S. 1997. Reactive oxygen-mediated protein oxidation in aging and disease. *Chem. Res. Toxicol.*, May, 10 (5): 485-494

Steinckwich, N., Schenten, V., Melchior, C., Bréchard, S. & Tschirhart, E.J. 2011. An essential role of STIM1, Orai1, and S100A8-A9 proteins for Ca2+ signaling and FcγR-mediated phagosomal oxidative activity. *J. Immunol.*, Feb 15, 186 (4): 2182-2191

Su, Y.J., Xu, F., Yu, J.P., Yue, D.S., Ren, X.B. & Wang, C.L. 2010. Up-regulation of the expression of S100A8 and S100A9 in lung adenocarcinoma and its correlation with inflammation and other clinical features. *Chin. Med. J. (Engl),* Aug, 123 (16): 2215-22120

Sunahori, K., Yamamura, M., Yamana, J., Takasugi, K., Kawashima, M., Yamamoto, H., Chazin, W.J., Nakatani, Y., Yui, S. & Makino, H. 2006. The S100A8/A9 heterodimer amplifies proinflammatory cytokine production by macrophages via activation of nuclear factor kappa B and p38 mitogen-activated protein kinase in rheumatoid arthritis. *Arthritis Res. Ther.*, 8 (3): R69

Szweda, L.I., Uchida, K., Tsai, L. & Stadtman, E.R. 1993. Inactivation of glucose-6-phosphate dehydrogenase by 4-hydroxy-2-nonenal. Selective modification of an active-site lysine. *J. Biol. Chem.*, Feb 15, 268 (5): 3342-3347

Thaw, H.H., Hamberg, H. & Brunk, U.T. 1983. Acute and irreversible injury following exposure of cultured cells to reactive oxygen metabolites. *Eur. J. Cell Biol.*, Jul, 31 (1): 46-54

Uchida, K. & Stadtman, E.R. 1992. Modification of histidine residues in proteins by reaction with 4-hydroxynonenal. *Proc. Natl. Acad. Sci. USA*, May 15, 89 (10): 4544-4548

Uchida, K. & Stadtman, E.R. 1993. Covalent attachment of 4-hydroxynonenal to glyceraldehyde-3-phosphate dehydrogenase. A possible involvement of intra- and intermolecular cross-linking reaction. *J. Biol. Chem.*, Mar 25, 268 (9): 6388-6393

Underwood, P.A., Mitchell, S.M. & Whitelock, J.M. 1998. Heparin fails to inhibit the proliferation of human vascular smooth muscle cells in the presence of human serum. *J. Vasc. Res.*, Nov-Dec, 35: 449-460

Valko, M., Leibfritz, D., Moncol, J., Cronin, M.T., Mazur, M. & Telser, J. 2007. Free radicals and antioxidants in normal physiological functions and human disease. *Int. J. Biochem. Cell Biol.* 39 (1), 44-84

Valentin, F., Bueb, J., Capdeville-Atkinson, C. & Tschirhart, E. 2001. Rac-1-mediated O2-secretion requires Ca2+ influx in neutrophil-like HL-60 cells. *Cell Calcium*, Jun, 29 (6): 409-415

Vandal, K., Rouleau, P., Boivin, A., Ryckman, C., Talbot, M. & Tessier, PA. 2003. Blockade of S100A8 and S100A9 suppresses neutrophil migration in response to lipopolysaccharide. *J. Immunol.*, Sep 1, 171 (5): 2602-2609

Vindis, C., Escargueil-Blanc, I., Uchida, K., Elbaz, M., Salvayre, R. & Negre-Salvayre, A. 2007. Lipid oxidation products and oxidized low-density lipoproteins impair platelet-derived growth factor receptor activity in smooth muscle cells: implication in atherosclerosis. *Redox Rep.*, 12 (1): 96-100

Vissers, M.C.M. & Winterbourn, C.C. 1991. Oxidative damage to fibronectin. 1. The effects of the neutrophil myeloperoxidase system and HOCl. *Arch. Biochem. Biophys.*, Feb 15, 285: 53-59

Vogl, T., Ludwig, S., Goebeler, M., Strey, A., Thorey, I.S., Reichelt, R., Foell, D., Gerke, V., Manitz, M.P., Nacken, W., Werner, S., Sorg, C. & Roth, J. 2004. MRP8 and MRP14 control microtubule reorganization during transendothelial migration of phagocytes. *Blood*, Dec 15, 104 (13): 4260-4268 von Zglinicki, T., Saretzki, G., Docke, W. & Lotze, C. 1995. Mild hyperoxiashortens telomeres and inhibits proliferation of fibroblasts: a model forsenescence? *Exp. Cell Res.*, Sept, 220 (1), 186-193

Yong, H.Y. & Moon, A. 2007. Roles of calcium-binding proteins. S100A8 and S100A9, in invasive phenotype of human gastric cancer cells. *Arch. Pharm. Res.*, Jan 30 (1): 75-81

Part 2

Medical and Pharmacological Aspects of Inflammatory Diseases

15

Malnutrition and Inflammation

Jorge R. Mujico, Fátima Pérez-de-Heredia,
Sonia Gómez-Martínez and Ascensión Marcos
Institute of Food Science, Technology and Nutrition (ICTAN-CSIC)
Spain

1. Introduction

The relationship between nutrition and immune function is being widely recognized, although its study is relatively recent. The 1968 *World Health Organisation* monograph about "Interactions between Nutrition and Infection" presented the mechanisms linking infection and poor nutritional status. Following the development of immunology as a science, increasing evidence was obtained as well to show how undernutrition impaired resistance to infections and the immune response. It was initially recognized that deficits in certain micronutrients (like vitamins and minerals) had a direct impact on immune function. But the relationship between immune function and nutrition extends far beyond that, and the term immunonutrition has been coined. We are now aware of many conditions of nutritional imbalance (not all necessarily linked to nutritional deficiencies) that lead to impaired immune response. For instance, it is currently believed that nutrition is a key factor in the onset and development of many types of cancer, or that the dietary component of atherosclerosis risk can directly influence immune cells and the inflammatory response; certain nutrients, like seed and fish oils have been shown to respectively induce the release of pro- and anti-inflammatory mediators. Accordingly, the idea of undernutrition has been replaced by that of malnutrition, meaning that inappropriate nutrition or nutritional imbalance *per se*, whether it implies a nutrient deficit or not, influences immune function. That is the reason why overnutrition, or an excessive energy intake, is also now considered as malnutrition.

In this chapter we will discuss three paradigmatic cases of malnutrition that have a strong immune and inflammatory impact: anorexia *nervosa* (AN) and bulimia *nervosa* (BN), as examples of severe undernutrition; obesity, also referred to as overnutrition; and celiac disease (CD), a pathological reaction of the body to a particular type of nutrients that leads to malnutrition. Although these nutrition-related diseases have different origins (psychological for eating disorders, modifiable lifestyle factors for obesity and autoimmune for CD), they all have in common to present an important inflammatory component and to have nutritional treatment as the main therapeutic approach.

2. Eating disorders

Anorexia *nervosa* (AN) and bulimia *nervosa* (BN) are states of malnutrition of psychiatric origin. Although conventionally AN has been described among adolescents, the prevalence of this syndrome is now increasing in prepubertal girls. Since AN starts at very early stages of life, and often implies a chronic and disabling course, severe consequences on somatic and mental health may be developed in adulthood (Marcos et al., 2003). Besides a reduced growth, diminished reproduction rate and an increased risk of osteoporosis, a prolonged course of the disorder may impact on the development of the anorexic patients' brain function, probably due to hormonal dysfunctions coming from the corticoid and gonadal systems, and to severe changes in neuropeptides, all these alterations promoting hence disturbance of the immune system of these patients (Table 1).

Biomarker	Alteration	Reference
Adiponectin	Increased	Leoni et al., 2010
$CD4^+$:$CD8^+$	Decreased	Marcos et al., 1993
C3 (complement)	Decreased	Flierl et al., 2011
Ghrelin	Increased	Terashi, 2011
IL-1	Increased	Allende et al., 1998
IL-6	Increased	Nova & Marcos, 2006
Lymphocytes	Decreased	Marcos et al., 1993
Resistin	Decreased	Leoni et al., 2010
TNF-α	Increased	Nova & Marcos, 2006

Table 1. Inflammation-related blood biomarkers altered in eating disorders

Despite the seriously malnourished state of patients with AN and BN, controversial findings have been published regarding some aspects of the immune system that are otherwise impaired in more typical types of malnutrition, such as protein-energy malnutrition (Nova & Marcos, 2006). In this respect, it should be noted that recent neurobiological insights into this gut-brain crosstalk have revealed a complex, bidirectional communication system that not only ensures the proper maintenance of gastrointestinal homeostasis and digestion but is likely to have multiple effects on affect, motivation and higher cognitive functions, including intuitive decision making. Moreover, disturbances of this system have been involved in a wide range of disorders, including functional and inflammatory gastrointestinal disorders, obesity and eating disorders (Mayer, 2011).

2.1 Altered immunity in eating disorders

Anemia, leukopenia and thrombocytopenia are frequent complications of AN (Cleary et al., 2010) together with relative lymphocytosis (Marcos et al., 1993). Anemia tends to be normocytic and normochromic. Leukopenia manifests as a deficiency of lymphocytes or neutrophils. Thrombocytopenia, if severe, may confer a bleeding risk. However, cell-mediated immunity is usually altered in AN and BN as reflected by lymphocyte subset counts and the response to delayed hypersensitivity tests. Regarding the helper/cytotoxic T cell ratio ($CD4^+$:$CD8^+$), an immunological marker of the nutritional status, the results of our studies on AN and BN patients showed that the duration of the eating disorder and the time when appropriate treatment is achieved are likely contributors to the alteration of this ratio. Immune-competent cell line deficiencies related solely to AN often resolve with nutritional rehabilitation.

The association between lymphocyte subsets and several psychopathological variables which had proved to be able to affect immune cell count in other conditions was investigated in BN patients. A negative correlation between impulsivity and T helper cells ($CD4^+$) was found in controls. In the BN group, the patients with higher anxiety had the lower lymphocyte count, and anxiety and hostility were negatively related to $CD4^+$ count. In addition, helper/cytotoxic T cell ratio negatively correlated in this group with impulsivity, hostility, and depression. In the light of these results, the potential influence of psychopathology on lymphocyte subset counts seems to be specific in BN patients, and more relevant than in healthy controls (Vaz-Leal et al., 2010).

Moreover, the complement cascade, a major component of innate immunity, represents a driving force in the pathophysiology of multiple inflammatory disorders. The role of complement in AN remains poorly understood. Serum C3 levels were significantly lower in patients with AN than in controls. There was a strong correlation between index C3 levels and BMI. Therefore, the C3 complement factor serum levels may represent a sensitive new biomarker for monitoring the severity of disease in AN (Flierl et al., 2011).

2.2 Relationship between eating disorders and the neuroendocrine/immune systems

Immune impairments in AN are less severe than would be expected considering the highly deficient nutritional status of these patients, and also, they seem to be surprisingly free of infectious complications or even common viral infections, at least until the most advanced stages of debilitation (Marcos, 2000). Hypothetically, some of the complex interactions occurring between cytokines and the endocrine system and the central nervous system could provide some compensatory mechanisms to adapt to the limited nutrient supply and possibly result in the perceived lack of infection symptoms. A dysregulated cytokine production and the altered acute-phase response to infection, as well as cortisol and leptin, are considered to be potential factors involved in the adaptation processes occurring in these syndromes (Nova et al., 2002).

Productions of cytokines [interferon (IFN)-γ, interleukin (IL)-2, tumor necrosis factor (TNF)-α, IL-6, and IL-1β] involved in the regulation of the immune response are dysregulated in AN patients. In the context of inflammation, pro-inflammatory cytokines can access the central nervous system and interact with a cytokine network in the brain to influence virtually every aspect of brain function relevant to behaviour, including neurotransmitter metabolism, neuroendocrine function, synaptic plasticity, and neurocircuits that regulate mood, motor activity, motivation, anxiety, and alarm.

TNF-α and IL-6 are two pro-inflammatory cytokines that are involved as mediators of cancer associated cachexia. Similarly, an association has been postulated between elevated plasma levels of pro-inflammatory cytokines in AN and the manifestations of anorexia, cachexia and osteoporosis in these patients. These hypothesis conceive of cytokines as the fundamental regulators of body metabolism in AN and BN. However, it is evident that not all AN patients display the same changes in immune function and cytokine production (Nova & Marcos, 2006). A variable lymphocyte proliferative response to different mitogens has been reported in anorectic subjects (Polack et al., 1993). Different results for cytokine production by peripheral blood mononuclear cells (PBMCs) have also been reported. For instance, a higher spontaneous production of IL-1 by PBMCs has been reported in AN patients in comparison with a control group (Allende et al., 1998), while no differences were observed under similar conditions in other studies (Bessler et al., 1993; Vaisman et al., 1996).

Since complex interactions occur between cytokines and the central nervous system, differences in the capacity of AN patients to evoke a compensatory mechanism through either the neuroendocrine system or the autonomic nervous system could explain the variability of the results found (Nova et al., 2002).
In fact, there is a study that shows specific adipocytokines profiles depending on the subtype of AN: restrictive versus binge/purge and hyperactive versus non-hyperactive forms. These biological signatures have been suggested to interfere with the outcome of the disease (Nogueira et al., 2010). The changes in neuropeptides and in the hypothalamic axis that mediate these changes also receive input from neuroendocrine signals sensitive to satiety and food intake and in turn may be poised to provide significant energy conservation. In fact, leptin is a key hormone in the regulation of food intake, energy expenditure, and neuroendocrine, and alters the immune function. Leptin is also related with obesity and its metabolic disorders; starvation-induced depletion of fat stores is accompanied by alterations of circulating adipocytokines that may have potential repercussions in the pathophysiology of AN. Adiponectin enhances insulin sensitivity, controls body weight, prevents atherosclerosis and negatively regulates immune functions. Plasma adiponectin relates inversely to adiposity and reflects the sequelae of accumulation of excess adiposity. Resistin is a protein hormone produced both by adipocytes and immunocompetent cells that affect fuel homeostasis and insulin action. Plasma resistin levels are decreased in AN, while plasma adiponectin levels are increased. Visfatin seems to correlate with visceral fat mass in patients with obesity. Its possible role in patients with AN is unknown (Leoni et al., 2010). Plasma ghrelin levels present opposite changes in obesity and AN, suggesting that ghrelin is a good marker of nutritional status. This molecule, increased in subjects with restrictive AN, is normalized after refeeding (Terashi et al., 2011).

3. Obesity

Obesity is characterized by the hypertrophy of the adipose tissue, which has its roots in a positive energy balance. It has been long regarded as a mere state of overnutrition -an esthetical issue rather than a real disease. However, obesity appears often linked to metabolic disturbances, like insulin resistance, type 2 diabetes, non-alcoholic fatty liver disease, or coronary events. The underlying cause of these relationships appears to be an inflammatory response initiating in adipose tissue. Indeed, obesity is a state of low-grade chronic systemic inflammation and is associated as well to an altered immune function (Table 2).

3.1 Adipose tissue as an immune organ

There are various histological and functional connections between adipose tissue and the immune system, starting with the fact that immune cells -mainly macrophages and lymphocytes- are normally found in the non-adipose fraction of the tissue (Caspar-Bauguil et al., 2005). In addition, white adipocytes have been suggested to share embryonic origin with immune cells, and characterization of adipose tissue-resident lymphocytes led to the notion that it was an ancestral immune organ (Caspar-Bauguil et al. 2005; Saely et al. 2010). Recently, immature hematopoietic cells have been found in adipose tissue, so that it has been proposed as a site for formation and maturation of immune cell precursors (Poglio et al. 2010).

Biomarker	Source	Alteration	Reference
Adiponectin	Blood	Decreased circulating values	Arita et al. 1999, as cited in Tilg & Moschen 2006.
Leptin	Blood	Increased circulating values	Bulló et al. 2003, as cited in Trayhurn & Wood 2004
M-CSFR	Adipose tissue macrophages	Increased gene expression (in mice)	Weisberg et al. 2003
CD68	Adipose tissue macrophages	Increased gene expression (in mice)	Weisberg et al. 2003
TNF-α	Adipose tissue macrophages, adipocytes	Increased gene expression (in rodents and humans)	Reviewed in Wellen & Hotamisligil 2005
TNF-Rs	Blood	Increased circulating values	Bulló et al. 2003, as cited in Trayhurn & Wood 2004
IL-6	Adipose tissue macrophages, adipocytes	Increased gene expression (in mice)	Reviewed in Wellen & Hotamisligil 2005
IL-6	Blood	Increased circulating values	Bulló et al. 2003, as cited in Trayhurn & Wood 2004
IL-8	Adipose tissue macrophages, adipocytes	Increased gene expression (in mice)	Reviewed in Wellen & Hotamisligil 2005
MCP-1	Adipocytes	Increased gene expression (in mice)	Reviewed in Wellen & Hotamisligil 2005
CRP	Adipocytes	Increased gene expression (in mice)	Reviewed in Wellen & Hotamisligil 2005
CRP	Blood	Increased circulating values	Wärnberg et al. 2006 Bulló et al. 2003, as cited in Trayhurn & Wood 2004
C3, C4	Blood	Increased circulating values	Wärnberg et al. 2006

Table 2. Inflammation-related biomarkers known to be altered in obesity

In the early 2000s, studies in mice showed that the adipose tissue of obese animals was more densely macrophage-infiltrated than that belonging to lean mice. Those macrophages appeared as crown-shaped aggregates, larger with increasing degrees of obesity, and similar to those observed in known inflammatory situations, like rheumatoid arthritis. This finding led to the idea that immune function could be impaired in obesity, and the formation of macrophage aggregates could partially explain the related inflammatory state (Weisberg et al. 2003). Later, two different adipose tissue macrophage phenotypes have been described: the M1 or "classically activated", which acts as pro-inflammatory, and the M2 or "alternatively activated", which acts as anti-inflammatory. Obesity is associated with a phenotypic switch from M2 to M1 polarization (Lumeng et al. 2007). Furthermore, specific deletion of M1 macrophages may improve insulin sensitivity and reduce inflammatory markers (Patsouris et al., 2008, as cited in Nicholls et al., 2011), while absence of the M2 phenotype has been associated with higher susceptibility to obesity, inflammation, and insulin resistance (Odegaard et al., 2007, as cited in Nicholls et al., 2011).

3.2 Obesity, adipokines and cytokines

Adipose tissue secretes a great number of bioactive molecules of different nature, collectively termed adipokines, many of which have immunomodulatory actions. This is the case for the two paradigmatic adipokines, leptin and adiponectin. Leptin, the first adipokine to be discovered, is known to regulate immune function on various levels: it can stimulate monocyte proliferation and differentiation into macrophages, modulate activation of natural killer lymphocytes, and induce the production of pro-inflammatory cytokines, such as TNF-α, IL-6, or IL-12 (Tilg & Moschen, 2006). Adiponectin, considered as an anti-inflammatory and insulin-sensitizing hormone, exerts opposite actions. It inhibits the phagocytic activity and production of TNF-α in macrophages, the differentiation of monocyte precursors, the synthesis of endothelial adhesion molecules, and the formation of foam cells (Koerner et al., 2005), and stimulates the release of anti-inflammatory interleukins, like IL-10 or IL-1ra (Tilg & Moschen, 2006). In obesity, circulating leptin levels are increased, in parallel with body fat mass; on the contrary, adiponectin concentrations correlate inversely with body weight. These changes may contribute to the onset and maintenance of the systemic inflammation present in obesity.

Obese subjects also show elevated circulating levels of various inflammation-related molecules, like C-reactive protein (CRP), haptoglobin, TNF-α, IL-6, or components of the complement system, and this event is linked to the concomitant development of insulin resistance, metabolic disorders, or the increased cardiovascular risk seen in obesity (Wärnberg et al. 2006; Hotamisligil 2006). The raise of inflammatory markers has its roots in the enlargement of body fat mass, and it is explained largely, but not completely, by the infiltrated macrophage-dependent production of cytokines and chemokines. Adipocytes and macrophages share certain phenotypic features, including the capacity to produce and release cytokines. Fat cells secrete, amongst others, TNF-α, IL-6, monocyte chemotactic protein (MCP)-1, TGF-β, or acute phase proteins (revised in Trayhurn & Wood, 2004). Consequently, dysfunction of adipose tissue plays a key role in the development of the obesity-associated systemic inflammation and related pathologies.

Lifestyle-aimed interventions seem to be useful to improve the inflammatory condition in obese subjects. Environmental factors such as physical activity may counteract the consequences of excessive body fat. Cardiorespiratory fitness has been inversely associated with serum levels of inflammatory markers such as CRP and complement factors C3 and C4, all of which were positively associated with body fat (Martínez-Gómez et al., 2010). An intervention programme carried out on overweight/obese adolescents (aged 13-16 years) to promote a healthy lifestyle and lose weight (the EVASYON study), resulted in decreased serum levels of leptin and several cytokines (IL-8, IL-10 and TNF-α), without affecting those of adiponectin, total peptide YY, or even insulin, and these changes seemed to depend on physical activity and fitness (Romeo et al., 2011).

3.3 Proposed mechanisms linking obesity and inflammation in adipose tissue

3.3.1 Fatty acid-induced inflammation

Abnormally elevated blood lipid levels, including free fatty acids, are a common feature in obesity. There are different explanations for this increase. One is known as the "adipose tissue expandability" hypothesis (Virtue & Vidal-Puig, 2010, as cited in Pietiläinen et al., 2011). According to this hypothesis, the adipose tissue has a limited capacity to expand and to store energy. When this limit is exceeded, it leads to enhanced lipolysis within the adipocyte and the subsequent release of free fatty acids into the bloodstream, reaching other tissues and organs, in which they exert toxic effects -a phenomenon known as lipotoxicity. Other studies have demonstrated that inflammatory cytokines increase free fatty acid levels (Grunfeld & Feingold, 1991, as cited in Mei et al., 2011). Finally, recent observations suggest that chronic systemic inflammation stimulates lipolysis and decreases lipogenesis in adipose tissue, while increasing lipid synthesis in skeletal muscle and liver (Mei et al., 2011).

The chemical nature of fatty acids is also relevant in triggering the inflammatory response. Studies with weight-discordant twins have shown that obese individuals, who exhibited signs of insulin resistance and elevated inflammatory and immune response pathways in the adipose tissue when compared to their lean twins, also showed significant differences in adipose tissue fatty acid composition (Pietiläinen et al., 2011). There seems to be a positive feedback loop involving saturated fatty acids (SFA) from adipocytes and cytokines from macrophages, which accelerates the inflammatory change in the adipose tissue in obesity. SFA can increase the production of TNF-α in macrophages, and in turn the latter induce lipolysis in adipocytes (Suganami et al., 2007).

Fatty acids have been suggested to modulate adipokine production and/or secretion. Likewise in macrophages, SFA may stimulate TNF-α and IL-6 expression and release in adipocytes (reviewed in Stryjecki & Mutch, 2011). Adiponectin levels also seem to be associated with fatty acids, being this correlation negative with SFA, palmitoleic (16:1n7) or γ-linolenic (18:3n6) fatty acids, and positive with oleic acid, or total n-6 and n-3 poly-unsaturated fatty acids (PUFA) (Fernandez-Real et al., 2005; Pérez de Heredia et al., 2009).

Alternatively, fatty acids may directly elicit the inflammatory response, through activation of cell receptors. For instance, they are natural ligands for peroxisome proliferator-activated receptors (PPARs); these transcription factors, apart from regulating cell metabolism and adipocyte formation, can suppress the activity of the nuclear factor kappa B (NF-κB), a crucial transcription factor in the initiation of the inflammatory response, and they seem to be involved in the aforementioned phenotypic switch of adipose tissue-resident macrophages (reviewed in Coll et al., 2010). On the other hand, recent evidence has suggested that fatty acids, especially SFA, could also act through the toll-like receptors (TLRs), the activation of which induces the synthesis of inflammatory markers in macrophages and aggravates insulin resistance (Fessler et al., 2009, as cited in Stryjecki & Mutch 2011).

3.3.2 Endoplasmic reticulum stress

The excessive adipose tissue growth has further consequences at the cellular and subcellular levels, and a role has been suggested for endoplasmic reticulum stress in the origin of adipocyte dysfunction in obesity. The endoplasmic reticulum (ER) is a primary site for protein synthesis and triglyceride droplet formation. Under conditions of cellular stress, ER function becomes progressively impaired and this triggers a security mechanism known as the "unfolded protein response" (UPR). The increased demand for protein and triglyceride droplet formation under nutrient excess and cell expansion in obesity may as well induce ER stress and the UPR. Additionally, nutrients themselves may serve as signals leading to ER stress; in relation to the previous section, free fatty acids have been shown to induce the UPR in various cell types. The UPR is linked to the production of reactive oxygen species (ROS) and the activation of inflammatory pathways, with increased expression of cytokines, including IL-8, IL-6, MCP-1, and TNF-α. Paradoxically, glucose deprivation could contribute to ER stress in obesity; this could happen as a result of insulin resistance developing within the adipose tissue. Finally, closing a positive feed-back loop, the inflammatory condition in the obese adipose tissue induces the UPR and enhances ER stress (reviewed in Gregor & Hotamisligil, 2007).

3.3.3 Hypoxia in adipose tissue

The capacity of adipose tissue to change size surpasses that of other organs and tissues. Therefore, adipose tissue expansion in obesity eventually reaches a point where the development of local vasculature is insufficient and cannot meet the oxygen and nutrient demands of distant and enlarged adipocytes. It was hypothesized that hypoxic adipocytes would then produce inflammatory signals in order to stimulate angiogenesis, and later studies in animal and culture models have confirmed this hypothesis (reviewed in Trayhurn et al., 2010). The key element in the initiation of the cellular response to hypoxia is the hypoxia-inducible factor 1 (HIF-1), a transcription factor highly unstable under normal normoxic conditions, but which becomes stabilized when oxygen availability is low. Once stabilized, HIF-1 regulates the expression of a great number of genes involved in different functions that include angiogenesis, inflammation and energy metabolism; some of these genes are leptin, PAI-1 (plasminogen activator inhibitor 1), or MIF (macrophage migration inhibitory factor), which become up-regulated, or adiponectin, which becomes down-regulated (Trayhurn et al., 2010). Hypoxia has in addition important consequences for adipocyte metabolism, as it forces the adipocyte to switch to anaerobic glycolysis to obtain energy from glucose. This results in increased production and release of lactate from adipocytes (Pérez de Heredia et al., 2010a). Lactate has been shown to stimulate inflammatory pathways in macrophages (Samuvel et al. 2009, as cited in Pérez de Heredia et al., 2010a) and seems to enhance lipopolysaccharide (LPS)-induced inflammatory response in preadipocytes (Pérez de Heredia et al., 2010b, as cited in Pérez de Heredia et al., 2010a).

Other cell types present in adipose tissue are responsive to hypoxia, too. Resident macrophages accumulate around hypoxic areas, probably recruited by chemotactic signals released from adipocytes, and respond to hypoxia in a similar manner to adipocytes, by producing pro-inflammatory cytokines. Preadipocytes are also sensitive to the lack of oxygen, although their response is milder than that of mature adipocytes (Trayhurn et al., 2010).

It is apparent that the hypoxia response and HIF-1 activation fail to achieve the expected effect of increasing adipose tissue vascularization, but lead instead to a situation of local fibrosis which initiates adipose tissue dysfunction (Halberg et al., 2009, as cited in Trayhurn et al., 2010). In line with this, hypoxia has been found to induce the UPR in cultured adipocytes (Gregor & Hotamisligil, 2007).

3.4 The influence of the adipose depot in obesity-related inflammation

Most characteristics of adipose tissue vary according to its anatomical localization, and these differences make the visceral depots more clinically relevant than the subcutaneous depot, in relation to the development of metabolic disturbances, insulin resistance or cardiovascular risk. With regards to inflammation, there are several features that render visceral fat more detrimental than subcutaneous one. Firstly, adiponectin gene expression has been found to be lower in visceral than in subcutaneous adipose tissue (Hernández-Morante et al., 2006). Secondly, infiltration of macrophages seems to be greater in visceral than in subcutaneous adipose tissue in obesity (Cancello et al., 2006, as cited in Villaret et al., 2010). And more recently, it has been observed that, in obese subjects, endothelial cells isolated from visceral (omental) fat show a higher expression of genes related to angiogenesis and inflammation than endothelial cells from subcutaneous adipose tissue (Villaret et al., 2010). In addition, the expression of hypoxia-related genes seems to be greater in the visceral adipose tissue, even when it could not be attributed to poorer vascularization in this depot, as compared to the subcutaneous one. Moreover, the cells from visceral fat show more evident signs of cellular senescence than those from subcutaneous fat (Villaret et al., 2010).

In conclusion, obesity-associated chronic systemic inflammation has its origin in adipose tissue dysfunction, and various plausible explanations have been proposed for the phenomenon, although more research is needed to confirm the precise mechanisms for adipose tissue inflammatory response.

4. Celiac disease

Celiac disease (CD) is defined as a permanent intolerance to gluten proteins of wheat, barley and rye. The only treatment for this chronic disease is a lifelong and strict gluten-free diet (GFD) (Mujico et al., 2011). Although CD has been considered a primary gastrointestinal disease, this disease can affect other systemic organs, including the skin, blood (hematologic system) and bone. Recent evidence indicates that both innate and adaptive immune responses are necessary for the phenotypic expression and pathologic changes characteristic of CD (De Nitto et al., 2009). In genetically predisposed individuals, the adaptive response, mediated by the activation of antigen-specific T lymphocytes, drives a pro-inflammatory response, which ends in an immune-mediated enteropathy characterized by villous atrophy, crypt hyperplasia, recruitment of intraepithelial lymphocytes (IELs), and increase of numerous inflammation-related biomarkers (Table 3). In addition, some gluten peptides are able to induce an innate immune response in intestinal mucosa. There is evidence of a direct toxic effect of some gluten peptides in several biological models. However, the failure to control the inflammatory response may be one of the factors underlying gluten intolerance in these individuals (Garrote et al., 2008).

Biomarker	Source	Reference
IFN-α	Intestinal mucosa cultures	Monteleone et al., 2001, as cited in De Nitto et al., 2009
IFN-γ	Intestinal mucosa cultures	Nielsen et al., 1995 & 1998; as cited in De Nitto et al., 2009
	$CD8^+$ αβIELs	Forsberg et al., 2007
	Serum[a]	Manavalan et al., 2010
IL-1α	Serum[b]	Manavalan et al., 2010
IL-1β	Serum[b]	Manavalan et al., 2010
IL-2	Serum[a]	Manavalan et al., 2010
IL-4	Serum[a,b,c]	Manavalan et al., 2010
IL-6	Serum[c,d]	Manavalan et al., 2010 Fornari et al., 1998; Romaldini et al., 2002; as cited in Manavalan et al., 2010
IL-8	Serum[b,c,e]	Manavalan et al., 2010
IL-10	$CD4^+$ and $CD8^+$ αβIELs	Forsberg et al., 2007
	Serum[a,b]	Manavalan et al., 2010 Cataldo et al., 2003, as cited in Manavalan et al., 2010
IL-15	Lamina propria and intestinal epithelium[c]	Di Sabatino et al., 2006 Maiuri et al., 2000; Mention et al., 2003; as cited in De Nitto et al., 2009
	Lamina propria macrophages and dendritic cells	Maiuri et al., 2003, as cited in De Nitto et al., 2009
IL-15Rα	IELs	Di Sabatino et al., 2006
IL-18	Crypts of intestinal mucosa cultures	León et al., 2006
IL-21	Intestinal mucosa cultures	Fina et al., 2008, as cited in De Nitto et al., 2009
TNF-α	$CD4^+$ αβIELs	Forsberg et al., 2007
	Serum	Manavalan et al., 2010
Zonulin	Intestinal tissue lysates	Fasano et al., 2000, as cited in Visser et al., 2009
	Intestinal cell lines	Clemente et al., 2003; Drago et al., 2006; as cited in Visser et al., 2009
	Serum[d]	Fasano et al., 2000, as cited in Visser et al., 2009

[a] Patients on GFD for less than 1 year had significantly higher levels of these biomarkers compared with the patients on GFD for more than 1 year.
[b] Levels of these biomarkers correlated with the TTG IgA levels.
[c] Levels of these biomarkers correlated with the degree of mucosal damage.
[d] Levels of these biomarkers decreased following a GFD.
[e] Levels of these biomarkers remained elevated despite a GFD and remained so even after a year of gluten exclusion.

Table 3. Increased inflammation-related biomarkers in celiac disease

4.1 Link between gliadin, zonulin, and increased intestinal permeability in CD

The intestinal epithelium is the largest mucosal surface and provides an interface between the external environment and the mammalian host. Healthy and mature gut mucosa with its intact tight junctions (TJ) serves as the main barrier to the passage of macromolecules (Visser et al., 2009). In a physiological state, quantitatively small but immunologically active antigens may cross the mucosal barrier. When the integrity of the gut barrier is compromised (TJ disassembly), an immune response to environmental antigens that crossed the gut mucosa may be developed, leading to autoimmune diseases or food allergies (Fasano, 2001b; Mowat, 2003; as cited in Visser et al., 2009).

Several autoimmune diseases are characterized by loss of intestinal barrier function (Fasano, 2001a, as cited in Visser et al., 2009). Quantitative immunoblotting of intestinal tissue lysates from active CD (ACD) patients confirmed the increase in zonulin protein (a human intestinal homolog of zonula occludens toxin, an enterotoxin that reversibly opens the TJ) compared to control tissues. The zonulin upregulation during the acute phase of CD was confirmed by measuring zonulin concentration in sera of 189 CD patients using a sandwich enzyme-linked immunosorbent assay (ELISA). Compared to healthy controls, CD subjects showed significantly higher zonulin serum concentrations during the acute phase of the disease that decreased following a GFD (Fasano et al., 2000, as cited in Visser et al., 2009).

Intestinal cell lines exposed to gliadin released zonulin in the cell medium with subsequent zonulin binding to the cell surface, rearrangement of the cell cytoskeleton, loss of occludin-ZO1 protein–protein interaction, and increased monolayer permeability. Pre-treatment with the zonulin antagonist AT1001 blocked these changes without affecting zonulin release. When exposed to luminal gliadin, intestinal biopsies from celiac patients in remission expressed a sustained luminal zonulin release and increase in intestinal permeability. Conversely, biopsies from non-CD patients demonstrated a limited, transient zonulin release, which was paralleled by a reduction in intestinal permeability that never reached the level of permeability seen in CD tissues. Interestingly, when gliadin was added to the basolateral side of either cell lines or intestinal biopsies, no zonulin release was detected (Clemente et al., 2003; Drago et al., 2006; as cited in Visser et al., 2009). It has been postulated that gliadin binds to the chemokine receptor CXCR3, expressed in human and mouse intestinal epithelium and lamina propria, and leads to activation of the zonulin pathway and increased intestinal permeability in a MyD88-dependent fashion (Lammers et al., 2008, as cited in Visser et al., 2009).

4.2 The mucosal cytokine network involved in CD

Although the pathogenesis of CD is not fully understood, it is known that gluten peptides are deamidated by tissue transglutaminase and presented by $DQ2^+$ or $DQ8^+$ antigen-presenting cells to lamina propria $CD4^+$ T cells (Di Sabatino & Corazza, 2009; Sjöström et al., 1998; as cited in De Nitto et al., 2009). Upon activation, $CD4^+$ T cells polarize along the T helper (Th)1-type pathway, as substantiated by their ability to produce large amounts of IFN-γ, the signature cytokine of Th1 responses. In CD patients on a GFD, IFN-γ production is as low as in healthy controls but it can be stimulated *in vitro* by gluten to reach levels of ACD patients. In these mucosal cultures, neutralization of IFN-γ prevents gliadin-mediated morphological changes thus supporting the role of the adaptive immune response and IFN-γ in CD immunopathology (Nielsen et al., 1995 & 1998; as cited in De Nitto et al., 2009).

ACD is also characterized by a prominent cytokine response of IELs to gluten-containing diet. $CD8^+$ αβIELs retrieved from small intestinal biopsies of children with ACD showed a significant increase in expression levels of both IFN-γ and IL-10, the latter also increased in $CD4^+$ αβIELs. Production of IL-10 may be a common feature of IELs producing pro-inflammatory cytokines, attempting to limit inflammation in an autocrine fashion (Forsberg et al., 2007). TNF-α levels were increased in $CD4^+$ αβIELs, which also showed the highest expression level per cell and constituted the major source of this cytokine. Cytokine levels were low in γδIELs (Forsberg et al., 2007).

Some gluten peptides can induce mucosal damage by directly activating innate immune mechanisms. In particular, it was shown that the p31-43 peptide elicits the production of IL-15 by lamina propria macrophages and dendritic cells in *ex vivo* organ cultures of CD biopsies, thus triggering a sequence of events that culminates in epithelial damage (Maiuri et al., 2003, as cited in De Nitto et al., 2009). These findings correlate well with the demonstration that IL-15 is over-expressed in both the lamina propria and intestinal epithelium of patients with ACD as compared with normal controls or GFD treated CD patients (Maiuri et al., 2000; Mention et al., 2003; as cited in De Nitto et al., 2009). The levels of IL-15 also correlate with the degree of mucosal damage (Di Sabatino et al., 2006).

Epithelium derived IL-15, signalling via IL-15Rα, is critical for the development, activation, and survival of IELs. The IELs of ACD, characterised by higher IL-15Rα expression, showed increased proliferation, production of IFN-γ and TNF-α, and perforin/granzyme dependent cytotoxicity, and a decreased propensity to apoptosis in response to IL-15 (Di Sabatino et al., 2006). These findings suggest that IL-15 plays a crucial role in the generation of epithelial damage in active CD. Blocking IL-15, by suppressing uncontrolled IEL activation and survival, has the potential to provide new therapeutic tools to prevent tissue damage and lymphomagenesis in CD (Di Sabatino et al., 2006).

Biopsies taken from CD patients on a GFD over-expressed IL-21 when challenged *in vitro* with gluten peptides. Interestingly, neutralization of IL-21 activity in *ex vivo* organ cultures of CD biopsies reduced IFN-γ production (Fina et al., 2008, as cited in De Nitto et al., 2009). IFN-α, which is up-regulated in the mucosa of active CD patients and contributes to intensifying IFN-γ production, enhanced the mRNA expression of IL-21 in activated human T cells, thus suggesting a role for IFN-α in the positive control of IL-21 in CD (Monteleone et al., 2001; Strengell et al., 2004; as cited in De Nitto et al., 2009). It is tempting to speculate that IL-21 is part of a positive feedback loop that helps amplify and stabilize the committed Th1 cell phenotype in CD (De Nitto et al., 2009).

Both the active and inactive forms of IL-18 protein have been found in all samples from ACD, and protein expression was only localized within the crypts (León et al., 2006). In ACD, the early response following gluten intake characterized by high IFN-γ levels is driven by IL-18, and probably IL-15, and this alternates with periods of long-standing inflammation with moderate IFN-γ levels, maintained by IL-18 alone (León et al., 2006).

All these observations collectively underline the complexity of the pathogenic mechanism in CD and suggest that the CD-associated mucosal damage relies on the activation of multiple rather than single cell pathways (De Nitto et al., 2009).

4.3 Serum cytokine levels in CD

Since the identification of tissue transglutaminase (TTG) as the autoantigen of CD, detection of anti-TTG IgA antibodies in the serum of CD patients has become an essential tool for the diagnosis of this disorder. Patients with ACD and those on a GFD with positive TTG IgA antibodies had significantly higher serum levels of pro-inflammatory cytokines, such as IFN-γ, IL-1β, TNF-α, IL-6 and IL-8, and also Th2 cytokines such as IL-4 and IL-10, compared with normal controls and patients on GFD without antibodies (Manavalan et al., 2010). There are also data documenting elevated serum levels of IL-10 in CD patients with underlying IgA deficiency (Cataldo et al., 2003, as cited in Manavalan et al., 2010) and high serum levels of IFN-γ in other autoimmune diseases, some of which are associated with CD (Stepniak & Koning, 2006, as cited in Manavalan et al., 2010).

Patients on GFD for less than 1 year had significantly higher levels of both pro-inflammatory cytokines (IL-2 and IFN-γ) and Th2 cytokines (IL-4 and IL-10) compared with the patients on GFD for more than 1 year (Manavalan et al., 2010). In other studies, serum IL-6 levels have been also found to be significantly increased in patients with ACD compared with controls, and decreased after following GFD for one year (Fornari et al., 1998; Romaldini et al., 2002; as cited in Manavalan et al., 2010). Only serum IL-8 levels remained elevated despite a GFD and remained so even after a year of gluten exclusion (Manavalan et al., 2010). It was in contrast to what has been described in patients with dermatitis herpertiformis, in whom serum IL-8 levels returned to normal levels within 2 years on a GFD (Hall et al., 2007, as cited in Manavalan et al., 2010).

In addition, a statistically significant correlation between levels of TTG IgA titers and serum levels of Th2 cytokines IL-4, IL-10 and inflammatory cytokines such as IL-1α, IL-1β, and IL-8 was observed. Moreover, using linear regression analysis, serum levels of IL-4, IL-6 and IL-8 were found to correlate with the degree of villous atrophy (Manavalan et al., 2010). Higher levels of serum cytokines in patients with severe degrees of villous atrophy suggest a link between local mucosal alterations and systemic immune activation in this disease.

These results suggest that patients with CD have high levels of circulating pro- and anti-inflammatory cytokines, especially during the active phase of the disease, and differ from those of otherwise healthy individuals. Interestingly, most of these cytokines decrease when the patients commence a GFD; however a few cytokines that have been involved in the pathogenesis of tissue damage in CD, such as IFN-γ, persist in the circulation despite GFD. Therefore, the serum cytokine profile does not seem to mirror the cytokine profile of the inflamed small intestinal mucosa of ACD patients. Cytokine elevations have also been reported in other diseases or disorders frequently associated with CD, including autoimmune thyroiditis, diabetes, hepatitis, osteopenia, as well as psychiatric manifestations, especially depression. It is likely that elevated levels of certain serum cytokines might underlie extraintestinal manifestations of CD (Manavalan et al., 2010).

5. Conclusion

In this chapter we have discussed three paradigmatic cases of malnutrition that have a strong immune and inflammatory impact: anorexia nervosa (AN) and bulimia nervosa (BN), obesity, and celiac disease (CD). These patients have dysregulated levels of various inflammation-related molecules, especially during the active phase of the disease, and differ from those of otherwise healthy individuals. It is likely that these alterations might contribute to the onset and maintenance of the systemic inflammation. The failure to control the inflammatory response may be one of the factors underlying forthcoming complications and concomitant development of other diseases or disorders, including autoimmune thyroiditis, diabetes, hepatitis, osteopenia, psychiatric manifestations (especially depression), as well as some types of cancer. Consequently, malnutrition plays a key role in the development of associated systemic inflammation and related pathologies. All these observations collectively underline the complexity of the pathogenic mechanisms of these diseases and suggest that the damage relies on the activation of multiple rather than single cell pathways.

6. References

Allende, L.M.; Corell, A.; Manzanares, J.; Madruga, D.; Marcos, A; Madroño, A.; López-Goyanes, A.; García-Pérez, M.A.; Moreno, J.M.; Rodrigo, M.; Sanz, F. & Arnaiz-Villena, A. (1998). Immunodeficiency associated with anorexia nervosa is secondary and improves after refeeding. *Immunology*, Vol.94, No.4, (August 1998), pp. 543-551, ISSN 0019-2805

Arita, Y.; Kihara, S.; Ouchi, N.; Takahashi, M.; Maeda, K.; Miyagawa, J.; Hotta, K.; Shimomura, I.; Nakamura, T.; Miyaoka, K.; Kuriyama, H.; Nishida, M.; Yamashita, S.; Okubo, K.; Matsubara, K.; Muraguchi, M.; Ohmoto, Y.; Funahashi, T.; Matsuzawa, Y. (1999). Paradoxical decrease of an adipose-specific protein, adiponectin, in obesity. *Biochemical and Biophysical Research Communications*, Vol.257, No.1, (April 1999), pp. 79–83, ISSN 0006-291X

Bessler, H.; Karp, L.; Notti, I.; Apter, A.; Tyano, S.; Djaldetti, M. & Weizman, R. Cytokine production in anorexia nervosa. *Clinical neuropharmacology*, Vol.16, No.3, (June 1993), pp. 237-243, ISSN 0362-5664

Bulló, M.; García-Lorda, P.; Megias, I. & Salas-Salvadó, J. (2003). Systemic inflammation, adipose tissue tumor necrosis factor, and leptin expression. *Obesity Research*, Vol.11, No.4, (April 2003), pp. 525-31, ISSN 1930-7381

Cancello, R.; Tordjman, J.; Poitou, C.; Guilhem, G.; Bouillot, J.L.; Hugol, D.; Coussieu, C.; Basdevant, A.; Bar Hen, A.; Bedossa, P.; Guerre-Millo, M. & Clement, K. (2006). Increased infiltration of macrophages in omental adipose tissue is associated with marked hepatic lesions in morbid human obesity. *Diabetes*, Vol.55, No.6, (June 2006), pp. 1554–1561, ISSN 0012-1797

Caspar-Bauguil, S.; Cousin, B.; Galinier, A.; Segafredo, C.; Nibbelink, M.; André, M.; Casteilla, L. & Pénicaud, L. (2005). Adipose tissues as an ancestral immune organ: Site-specific change in obesity. *FEBS Letters*, Vol.579, No.17, (July 2005), pp. 3487-3492, ISSN 0014-5793

Cleary, B.S.; Gaudiani, J.L. & Mehler, P.S. (2010). Interpreting the complete blood count in anorexia nervosa. *Eating disorders*, Vol.18, No.2, (March 2010), pp. 132-139, ISSN 1064-0266

Coll, T.; Barroso, E.; Alvarez-Guardia, D.; Serrano, L.; Salvadó, L.; Merlos, M.; Palomer, X. & Vázquez-Carrera, M. (2010). The role of peroxisome proliferator-activated receptor beta/delta on the inflammatory basis of metabolic disease. *PPAR Research*, (July 2010), pii: 368467, eISSN 1687-4765

De Nitto, D; Monteleone, I.; Franzè, E.; Pallone, F. & Monteleone, G. (2009). Involvement of interleukin-15 and interleukin-21, two gamma-chain-related cytokines, in celiac disease. *World Journal of Gastroenterology*, Vol.15, No.37, (October 2009), pp. 4609-4614, ISSN 1007-9327

Di Sabatino, A.; Ciccocioppo, R.; Cupelli, F.; Cinque, B.; Millimaggi, D.; Clarkson, M.M.; Paulli, M.; Cifone, M.G. & Corazza, G.R. (2006). Epithelium derived interleukin 15 regulates intraepithelial lymphocyte Th1 cytokine production, cytotoxicity, and survival in coeliac disease. *Gut*, Vol.55, No.4, (August 2005), pp. 469-477, ISSN 0017-5749

Fernández-Real, J.M.; Vendrell, J. & Ricart W. (2005). Circulating adiponectin and plasma fatty acid profile. *Clinical Chemistry*, Vol.51, No.3, (March 2005), pp. 603-609, ISSN 0009-9147

Fessler, M.B.; Rudel, L.L. & Brown J.M. (2009). Toll-like receptor signaling links dietary fatty acids to the metabolic syndrome. *Current Opinion in Lipidology*, Vol.20, No.5, (October 2009), pp. 379-385, ISSN 0957-9672

Gregor, M.F. & Hotamisligil, G.S. (2007). Thematic review series: Adipocyte Biology. Adipocyte stress: the endoplasmic reticulum and metabolic disease. *Journal of Lipid Research*, Vol.48, No.9, (September 2007), pp. 1905-1914, eISSN 1539-7262

Grunfeld, C. & Feingold, K.R. (1991). The metabolic effects of tumor necrosis factor and other cytokines. *Biotherapy*, Vol.3, No.2, (1991), pp. 143-158, ISSN 1573-8280

Halberg, N.; Khan, T.; Trujillo, M.E.; Wemstedt-Asterholm, I.; Attie, A.D.; Sherwani, S.; Wang, Z.V.; Landskroner-Eiger, S.; Dineen, S.; Magalang, U.J.; Brekken, R.A. & Scherer, P.E. (2009). Hypoxia-inducible factor 1α induces fibrosis and insulin resistance in white adipose tissue. *Molecular and Cellular Biology*, Vol.29, No.16, (August 2009), pp. 4467-4483, eISSN 1098-5549

Flierl MA, Gaudiani JL, Sabel AL, Long CS, Stahel PF, Mehler PS. Complement C3 serum levels in anorexia nervosa: a potential biomarker for the severity of disease? *Annals of general psychiatry*, No.10, (May 2011), article 16, ISSN 1744-859X

Forsberg, G.; Hernell, O.; Hammarström, S. & Hammarström, M.L. (2007). Concomitant increase of IL-10 and pro-inflammatory cytokines in intraepithelial lymphocyte subsets in celiac disease. *International Immunology*, Vol.19, No.8, (July 2007), pp. 993-1001, ISSN 0953-8178

Garrote, J.A.; Gómez-González, E.; Bernardo, D.; Arranz, E. & Chirdo, F. (2008). Celiac disease pathogenesis: the proinflammatory cytokine network. *Journal of pediatric gastroenterology and nutrition*, Vol.47, Suppl.1, (August 2008), pp. S27-32, ISSN 0277-2116

Hernández-Morante, J.J.; Milagro, F.; Gabaldon, J.A.; Martínez, J.A.; Zamora, S. & Garaulet, M. (2006). Effect of DHEA-sulfate on adiponectin gene expression in adipose tissue from different fat depots in morbidly obese humans. *European Journal of Endocrinology*, Vol.155, No.4, (October 2006), pp. 593–600, ISSN 0804-4643

Hotamisligil, G. S. (2006). Inflammation and metabolic disorders. *Nature*, Vol.444, No.7121, (December 2006), pp. 860–867, ISSN 0028-0836

Koerner, A.; Kratzsch, J. & Kiess, W. (2005). Adipocytokines: leptin - the classical, resistin - the controversial, adiponectin - the promising, and more to come. *Best Practice & Research Clinical Endocrinology & Metabolism*, Vol.19, No.4, (December 2005), pp. 525-546, ISSN 1521-690X

Lumeng, C.N.; Bodzin, J.L. & Saltiel, A.R. (2007). Obesity induces a phenotypic switch in adipose tissue macrophage polarization. *Journal of Clinical Investigation*, Vol.117, No.1, (January 2007), pp. 175–184, ISSN 0021-9738

León, A.J.; Garrote, J.A.; Blanco-Quirós, A.; Calvo, C.; Fernández-Salazar, L.; Del Villar, A.; Barrera, A. & Arranz, E. (2006). Interleukin 18 maintains a long-standing inflammation in coeliac disease patients. *Clinical and Experimental Immunology*, Vol.146, No.3, (December 2006), pp. 479-85, ISSN 0009-9104

Leoni, M.C.; Pizzo, D. & Marchi, A. (2010). Adipocytokines: potential biomarkers for childhood obesity and anorexia nervosa (Article in Italian). *Minerva pediatrica*, Vol.62, No.2, (April 2010), pp. 171-178, ISSN 0026-4946

Manavalan, J.S.; Hernández, L.; Shah, J.G.; Konikkara, J.; Naiyer, A.J.; Lee, A.R.; Ciaccio, E.; Minaya, M.T.; Green, P.H. & Bhagat, G. (2010). Serum cytokine elevations in celiac disease: association with disease presentation. *Human immunology*, Vol.71, No.1, (January 2010), pp. 50-57, ISSN 0198-8859

Marcos, A. (2000). Eating disorders: a situation of malnutrition with peculiar changes in the immune system. *European journal of clinical nutrition*, Vol.54, Suppl.1, (March 2000), pp. S61-S64, ISSN 0954-3007

Marcos, A.; Nova, E. & Montero, A. (2003). Changes in the immune system are conditioned by nutrition. *European journal of clinical nutrition*, Vol.57, Suppl.1, (September 2003), pp. S66-S69, ISSN 0954-3007

Marcos, A.; Varela, P.; Santacruz, I.; Muñoz-Vélez, A. & Morandé, G. (1993). Nutritional status and immunocompetence in eating disorders. A comparative study. *European journal of clinical nutrition*, Vol.47, No.11, (November 1993), pp. 787-793, ISSN 0954-3007.

Martínez-Gómez, D.; Eisenmann, J.C.; Wärnberg, J.; Gómez-Martinez, S.; Veses, A.; Veiga, O.L. & Marcos, A. (2010). Associations of physical activity, fitness and fatness with low-grade inflammation in adolescents. The AFINOS study. *International journal of obesity (London)*, Vol.34, No.10, (October 2010), pp. 1501-1507, ISSN 0307-0565

Mayer, E.A. (2011). Gut feelings: the emerging biology of gut-brain communication. *Nature reviews - Neuroscience*, Vol.12, No.8, (July 2011), pp. 453-466, ISSN 1471-003X

Mei, M.; Zhao, L.; Li, Q.; Chen, Y.; Huang, A.; Varghese, Z.; Moorhead, J.F.; Zhang, S.; Powis, S.H.; Li, Q. & Ruan, X.Z. (2011). Inflammatory stress exacerbates ectopic lipid deposition in C57BL/6J mice. *Lipids in Health and Disease*, Vol.10, No.1, (June 2011), pp. 110, [Epub ahead of print], ISSN 1476-511X

Mujico, J.R.; Lombardía, M.; Mena, M.C.; Méndez, E. & Albar J.P. (2011). A highly sensitive real-time PCR system for quantification of wheat contamination in gluten-free food for celiac patients. *Food Chemistry*, Vol.10, No.3, (October 2011), pp. 795-801, ISSN 0308-8146

Nogueira, J.P.; Maraninchi, M.; Lorec, A.M.; Corroller, A.B.; Nicolay, A.; Gaudart, J.; Portugal, H.; Barone, R.; Vialettes, B. & Valéro, R. (2010). Specific adipocytokines profiles in patients with hyperactive and/or binge/purge form of anorexia nervosa. *European journal of clinical nutrition*, Vol.64, No.8, (August 2010), pp. 840-844, ISSN 0954-3007

Nova, E.; Gómez-Martínez, S.; Morandé, G. & Marcos, A. (2002). Cytokine production by blood mononuclear cells from in-patients with anorexia nervosa. *The British journal of nutrition*, Vol.88, No.2, (August 2002), pp. 183-138, ISSN 0007-1145

Nova, E. & Marcos, A. (2006). Immunocompetence to assess nutritional status in eating disorders. *Expert review of clinical immunology*, Vol.2, No.3, (May 2006), pp. 433-444, ISSN 1744-666X

Odegaard, J.I.; Ricardo-Gonzalez, R.R.; Goforth, M.H.; Morel, C.R.; Subramanian, V.; Mukundan, L.; Red Eagle, A.; Vats, D.; Brombacher, F.; Ferrante, A.W. & Chawla, A. (2007). Macrophage-specific PPARgamma controls alternative activation and improves insulin resistance. *Nature,* Vol.447, No.7148, (June 2007), pp. 1116–1120, ISSN 0028-0836

Patsouris, D.; Li, P.P.; Thapar, D.; Chapman, J.; Olefsky, J.M. & Neels, J.G. (2008). Ablation of CD11c-positive cells normalizes insulin sensitivity in obese insulin resistant animals. *Cell Metabolism,* Vol.8, No.4, (October 2008), pp. 301–309, ISSN 1550-4131

Pérez de Heredia, F.; Sánchez, J.; Priego, T.; Larqué, E.; Portillo, M.P.; Palou, A.; Zamora, S. & Garaulet, M. (2009). Adiponectin is associated with serum and adipose tissue fatty acid composition in rats. *Journal of Endocrinological Investigation,* Vol.32, No.8, (September 2009), pp. 659-665, ISSN 0391-4097

Pérez de Heredia, F.; Wood, I.S. & Trayhurn, P. (2010). Hypoxia stimulates lactate release and modulates monocarboxylate transporter (MCT1, MCT2, MCT4) expression in human adipocytes. *Pflügers Archive – European Journal of Physiology,* Vol.459, No.3, (February 2010), pp. 509-518, ISSN 0031-6768

Pérez de Heredia, F.; Wood, I.S. & Trayhurn P. (2010). Lactate enhances the inflammatory response in human preadipocytes in vitro. *Obesity Reviews,* Vol.11, Suppl.1, (2010), pp. 122, ISSN 1467-789X [Abstract]

Pietiläinen, K.H.; Róg, T.; Seppänen-Laakso, T.; Virtue, S.; Gopalacharyulu, P.; Tang, J.; Rodriguez-Cuenca, S.; Maciejewski, A.; Naukkarinen, J.; Ruskeepää, A.L.; Niemelä, P.S.; Yetukuri, L.; Tan, C.Y.; Velagapudi, V.; Castillo, S.; Nygren, H.; Hyötyläinen, T.; Rissanen, A.; Kaprio, J.; Yki-Järvinen, H.; Vattulainen, I.; Vidal-Puig, A. & Orešič, M. (2011). Association of lipidome remodeling in the adipocyte membrane with acquired obesity in humans. *Public Library of Science Biology,* Vol.9, No.6, (June 2011), pp-e1000623, eISSN 1545-7885

Poglio, S.; de Toni-Costes, F.; Arnaud, E.; Laharrague, P.; Espinosa, E.; Casteilla, L.; Cousin, B. (2010). Adipose tissue as a dedicated reservoir of functional mast cell progenitors. *Stem Cells,* Vol.28, No.11, (November 2010), pp. 2065-2072, ISSN 1066-5099

Polack, E.; Nahmod, V.E.; Emeric-Sauval, E.; Bello, M.; Costas, M.; Finkielman, S. & Arzt, E. (1993). Low lymphocyte interferon-gamma production and variable proliferative response in anorexia nervosa patients. *Journal of clinical immunology,* Vol.13, No.6, (November 1993), pp. 445-451, ISSN 0271-9142

Romeo, J.; Martinez-Gomez, D.; Diaz, L.E.; Gomez-Martinez, S.; Marti, A.; Martin-Matillas, M.; Puertollano, M.A.; Veiga, O.L.; Martinez, J.A.; Warnberg, J.; Zapatera, B.; Garagorri, J.M.; Morandé, G.; Campoy, C.; Moreno, L.A.; Marcos, A. & EVASYON Study Group. (2011). Changes in cardiometabolic risk factors, appetite-controlling hormones and cytokines after a treatment programme in overweight adolescents: preliminary findings from the EVASYON study. *Pediatric Diabetes,* Vol.12, (June 2011), pp. 372-380, ISSN 1399-543X

Saely, C.H.; Geiger, K. & Drexel, H. (2010). Brown versus white adipose tissue: a mini-review. *Gerontology,* (December 2010), DOI 10.1159/000321319, [Epub ahead of print], ISSN 0304-324X

Samuvel, D.J.; Sundararaj, K.P.; Nareika, A.; Lopes-Virella, M.F. & Huang, Y. (2009). Lactate boosts TLR4 signaling and NF-KB pathway-mediated gene transcription in macrophages via monocarboxylate transporters and MD-2 up-regulation. *The Journal of Immunology,* Vol.182, No.4, (February 2009), pp. 2476-2484, ISSN 0022-1767

Stryjecki, C. & Mutch, D.M. (2011). Fatty acid-gene interactions, adipokines and obesity. *European Journal of Clinical Nutrition*, Vol.65, No.3, (March 2011), pp. 285-297, eISSN 1476-5640

Suganami, T.; Tanimoto-Koyama, K.; Nishida, J.; Itoh, M.; Yuan, X.; Mizuarai, S.; Kotani, H.; Yamaoka, S.; Miyake, K.; Aoe, S.; Kamei, Y. & Ogawa, Y. (2007). Role of the toll-like receptor 4/NF-kappaB pathway in saturated fatty acid-induced inflammatory changes in the interaction between adipocytes and macrophages. *Arteriosclerosis, Thrombosis and Vascular Biology*, Vol.27, No.1, (January 2007), pp. 84–91, ISSN 0276-5047

Terashi, M.; Asakawa, A.; Harada, T.; Ushikai, M.; Coquerel, Q.; Sinno, M.H.; Déchelotte, P.; Inui, A. & Fetissov, S.O. (2011). Ghrelin reactive autoantibodies in restrictive anorexia nervosa. *Nutrition*, Vol.27, No.4, (April 2011), pp. 407-413, ISSN 0899-9007

Tilg, H. & Moschen, A.R. (2006). Adipocytokines: mediators linking adipose tissue, inflammation and immunity. *Nature,* Vol.6, No.10, (October 2006), pp. 772-783, ISSN 0028-0836

Trayhurn, P.; Pérez de Heredia, F.; Wang, B. & Wood, I.S. (2010). Hypoxia - Role in adipocyte function and dysfunction. In: Novel insight into adipose cell functions. Clément et al. (eds); Springer-Verlag Berlin Heidelberg, pp. 45-60, ISBN 9783642135163

Vaisman, N.; Barak, Y.; Hahn, T.; Karov, Y.; Malach, L. & Barak, V. (1996). Defective in vitro granulopoiesis in patients with anorexia nervosa. *Pediatric research,* Vol.40, No.1, (July 1996), pp. 108-111, ISSN 0031-3998

Vaz-Leal, F.J.; Rodríguez-Santos, L.; Melero-Ruiz, M.J.; Ramos-Fuentes, M.I. & García-Herráiz, M.A. (2010). Psychopathology and lymphocyte subsets in patients with bulimia nervosa. *Nutritional neuroscience*, Vol.13, No.3, (Jun 2010), pp. 109-115, ISSN 1028-415X

Villaret, A.; Galitzky, J.; Decaunes, P.; Estève, D.; Marques, M.A.; Sengenès, C.; Chiotasso, P.; Tchkonia, T.; Lafontan, M.; Kirkland, J.L. & Bouloumié, A. (2010). Adipose tissue endothelial cells from obese human subjects: differences among depots in angiogenic, metabolic, and inflammatory gene expression and cellular senescence. *Diabetes*, Vol.59, No.11, (November 2010), pp. 2755-2763, ISSN 0012-1797

Virtue, S. & Vidal-Puig, A. (2010). Adipose tissue expandability, lipotoxicity and the metabolic syndrome—An allostatic perspective. *Biochimica et Biophysica Acta*, Vol.1801, No.3, (March 2010), pp. 338–349, ISSN 0005-2736

Visser, J.; Rozing, J.; Sapone, A.; Lammers, K. & Fasano, A. (2009). Tight junctions, intestinal permeability, and autoimmunity: celiac disease and type 1 diabetes paradigms. *Annals of the New York Academy of Sciences*, No.1165, (May 2009), pp. 195-205, ISSN 0077-8923

Wärnberg, J.; Nova, E.; Moreno, L.A.; Romeo, J.; Mesana, M.I.; Ruiz, J.R.; Ortega, F.B.; Sjöström, M.; Bueno, M.; Marcos, A. & AVENA Study Group. (2006). Inflammatory proteins are related to total and abdominal adiposity in a healthy adolescent population: the AVENA Study. *American Journal of Clinical Nutrition*, Vol.84, No.3, (September 2006), pp. 505-512, ISSN 0002-9165

Weisberg, S.P.; McCann, D.; Desai, M.; Rosenbaum, M.; Leibel, R.L. & Ferrante, A.W., Jr. (2003). Obesity is associated with macrophage accumulation in adipose tissue. *Journal of Clinical Investigation,* Vol.112, No.12, (December 2003), pp. 1796-1808, ISSN 0021-9738

Wellen, K.E. & Hotamisligil, G.S. (2005). Inflammation, stress, and diabetes. *Journal of Clinical Investigation*, Vol.115, No.5, (May 2005), pp. 1111–1119, ISSN0021-9738

16

Inflammation in COPD and New Drug Strategies

Liam Heaney and Izhaq Masih
Queens University, Belfast, Northern Ireland, United Kingdom

1. Introduction

Chronic obstructive pulmonary disease (COPD) is a disease characterized by poorly reversible airflow limitation of the airways that is usually progressive and associated with an abnormal inflammatory response in the lung[1]. The abnormal inflammatory response is usually triggered by smoking[2], or other environmental irritant exposures[3] which interact with genetic factors[4], leading to both airway and systemic inflammation resulting in airway injury and lung damage.

The term COPD is a descriptive term encompassing a heterogeneous subset of clinical syndromes, specifically chronic bronchitis, emphysema and asthma and it is now recognised that there is significant overlap between the previously described clinical syndromes. The term 'overlap syndrome' is often used to describe a patient with fixed airflow obstruction (COPD), but having some asthmatic features[5]. Chronic bronchitis is clinically defined as a cough productive of sputum lasting at least three months for two consecutive years and emphysema is a pathological entity characterised by destruction of the lung parenchyma with resultant enlarged alveolar spaces and loss of alveolar walls[6].

Morbidity and mortality due to COPD are significant and there remains a significant unmet clinical need. Many acute medical admissions to hospital are due to exacerbations of COPD[7] and mortality can be high as many patients with an acute exacerbation of COPD may not fulfil the criteria for admission to intensive care[8] and ward based management including non-invasive ventilation may not be appropriate in all cases due to intolerance or in the terminal stage of the disease[9, 10]. Globally, COPD is on the rise and currently it is ranked as the fifth largest disease to cause death worldwide[11] and estimation by the World Health Organisation is that by 2020, it will be the third largest cause of mortality. Despite this significant level of morbidity, many of the management and prevention targets outlined in the 1998 Global strategy for the diagnosis, management and prevention of Obstructive pulmonary Disease (GOLD) have not been met[12]. A better understanding of the inflammatory pathophysiological mechanisms in COPD is essential to developing novel effective therapies.

2. Pathogenesis

The major risk factors for COPD are tobacco smoking; occupational dust exposure, industrial fumes, and indoor pollution from biomass cooking with inadequate ventilation in poor living conditions and all of these have been directly implicated in the abnormal inflammatory response in the airways[13, 14]. However, not all smokers get COPD, so clearly there are genetic factors which define the 'susceptible smoker'. The best characterised genetic susceptibility factor is homozygous deficiency of α-1 antitrypsin[15] but there are clearly other factors which are poorly understood.

The pathophysiology of COPD involves inflammation of the proximal and peripheral airways and destruction of lung parenchyma with emphysema. The airway damage results in significant physiological derangement with expiratory airflow limitation and abnormal gas exchange[16]. Emphysema contributes to the airflow limitation by reducing the elastic recoil of the lung through parenchymal destruction, as well as by reducing the elastic load applied to the airways inflammation is present in smokers before airflow obstruction is evident with pulmonary function tests[17.]. Persistent and progressive inflammatory changes in the large and smaller airways are the hallmark of the disease process and once established, these changes persist even in ex-smokers[18]. The pathophysiology of COPD involves inflammation of the proximal and peripheral airways and destruction of lung parenchyma with emphysema[19, 20].The airway damage results in significant physiological derangement with expiratory through destruction of alveolar attachments[21]. Inflammation of peripheral airways contributes to the airflow limitation by increasing the thickness of the airway wall which, together with fibrosis and smooth muscle hypertrophy, may cause airway narrowing. The presence of increased quantities of purulent sputum in the airways also contributes to airflow limitation[22]. Functionally, the decrement of FEV1 is due to both the small airways narrowing and mechanical effects of emphysema while the decrease in gas transfer arises from the parenchymal destruction of emphysema. Whilst the inflammatory changes are present in stable COPD, they become more evident in exacerbations of the disease[23] and recurrent exacerbations can accelerate this process with progressive loss of lung function[24]. Recent data has also demonstrated systemic inflammation is also present in COPD, and there is a strong association of increased cardiopulmonary mortality in COPD patients with exaggerated systemic inflammatory markers[25]. COPD is associated with important comorbidities including cardiac failure, metabolic syndrome and the combination of these co-morbidities combined with a systemic inflammatory response has led to the term of 'chronic systemic inflammatory syndrome' [26].

3. Stages of inflammation in COPD

The precise immunological inflammatory mechanisms in COPD have not been totally elucidated but there is mounting evidence to suggest that there is a cascade of evolutionary events involved in the development of disease. Many of the steps in this cascade are similar to those proposed in other chronic inflammatory diseases[27] such as rheumatoid arthritis, atherogenesis, multiple sclerosis, and systemic lupus erythematosus [28].

On the basis of current evidence, it has been suggested that the immunological inflammatory / repair pathway in COPD comprise of three stages[29].

Stage 1: Initial response to the smoke and noxious stimuli

The constant insult due to inhaled irritants to the airways kick starts both innate and adaptive immunological responses. The innate response is a non-selective response while the adaptive response is more selective to specific antigenic stimulation. The innate response results in a non-specific inflammatory response in the airways and lung parenchyma with recruitment and activation of inflammatory cells such as neutrophils and macrophages[30].

Stage 2: T-cell proliferation

There is migration of dendritic cells to regional lymph nodes with resultant significant proliferation of T-lymphocytes during this phase which results in the expression of pro-inflammatory cytokines and interferon-Y positive T-lymphocytes which has a direct link with disease activity[31]. The role of tissue specific chemokines driving an ongoing inflammatory influx becomes more evident by this time[32].

Stage 3: Adaptive immune response

The adaptive response of immunity is the hallmark of this step which leads to the dominance of CD8+ cytotoxic lymphocytes in all parts of the airways and lung parenchyma[33]. The function of these cells involves apoptosis and eventual tissue destruction[34]. However, the CD4 lymphocytes and B lymphocytes are also found abundantly in the airways of patients with COPD[35, 36].

4. Cellular inflammatory response in COPD

The inflammatory process in COPD occurs due to a persistent airways insult (commonly tobacco smoke exposure) and is characterised by abnormal activation of both the innate and adaptive immune responses of the airway tract. The cells which have been most implicated in the pathogenesis of COPD have been the $CD8^+$ T lymphocyte and the macrophage, however, other cells, in both the innate immune system and the adaptive immune response are also likely to have important roles, including neutrophils, airway epithelial cells, endothelial cells, eosinophil and fibroblasts[37].

Cells involved in inflammation in COPD (innate and adaptive immune response)

CD8+ lymphocytes
Macrophages
Neutrophils
CD4+ lymphocytes
Epithelial cells
Endothelial cells
Eosinophil
Fibroblasts

Cytokines and chemokines of inflammation

Interleukin 8(IL-8)
Tumour necrosis factor (TNF-α)
Interleukin 6(IL-6)
Leukotriene-B4 (LTB4)
GRO alpha (GRO- α)
Interleukin 1(IL-1)

Sampling the airway using induced sputum, has demonstrated an airway neutrophilia in patients with COPD, which is also seen in sputum samples of non-obstructed smokers, but to a lesser extent[38]. Bronchial biopsies demonstrate an infiltration of $CD8^+$ T lymphocytes and recent data suggests reduced apoptosis of these $CD8^+$ cells in the airway, which may explain one of the mechanisms of their persistence in the airway[39]. These $CD8^+$ T lymphocytes infiltrate the lung and pulmonary vasculature and it has been hypothesised that this reflects an underlying auto-immune process specifically that lung injury in COPD may occur due to an auto-antigen recognised by the CD8 cytotoxic T cells causing airway damage[40, 41]

In the case of emphysema, alveolar macrophages have been implicated and in bronchoalveolar lavage samples, the numbers of activated macrophages are 5 to 10 fold higher than non-obstructed smokers [42]. These macrophages also produce oxidants and pro-inflammatory cytokines and proteases which collectively potentially drive lung parenchymal destruction[43].

Protease / anti-protease imbalance

As a consequence of activated inflammatory cells in the airway and alveolar compartment, proteases including neutrophil elastase, cathepsins and matrix metalloproteinases (MMP) are released and have been implicated in the patho-physiology of COPD[44]. Bronchoalveolar lavage macrophages from patients with emphysema express more MMP-9 and MMP-1 than cells from control subjects, suggesting that these cells, rather than neutrophils, may be the major cellular source of these proteases[45]. The action of the proteases is inhibited by anti-proteases like, α-1antitrypsin (α-AT), α1- anti-chymotrypsin, secretory leukocyte protease inhibitor (SLPI), and tissue inhibitors of metalloproteinases (TIMPs) [46]. A decrease in anti-protease activity is considered as a potential factor in airway wall and parenchymal destruction causing emphysema[47]. However, given that many smokers with airway inflammation do not develop COPD and those who do develop COPD have varying degrees of emphysematous change, the interaction between protease and anti-protease activity is likely to complex and heterogeneous[48].

Cytokine / chemokine response

As a consequence of the abnormal cellular activation in the airway, pro-inflammatory cytokines including interleukin 8 (IL-8) and tumour necrosis factor (TNF-α) are upregulated[49]. Both IL-8 and TNFα promote neutrophil chemotaxis and activation of adhesion molecules. In parallel, a reduction of the anti-inflammatory cytokine IL-10 promotes a pro-inflammatory environment[50]. Many of the pro-inflammatory abnormalities identified in induced sputum and lung biopsies of COPD patients persist even after smoking cessation[51], suggesting that once the inflammatory process has been activated, and removal of the original inciting insult does not stop a progressive process.

In COPD, the inflammatory process is also augmented by the important chemotactic mediators such as leukotriene-B4 (LTB4) and GRO alpha (GRO-α). Both GRO-α and IL8 recruit neutrophils to the airway and IL8, TNF-α and LBT4 are increased in the sputum of COPD patients[52]. Some patients show evidence of eosinophil recruitment to the airway and increased eosinophil basic proteins (eosinophil cationic proteins and eosinophil peroxidase) have been observed in induced sputum of COPD patients. This may reflect 'overlap' syndrome as described above, and sputum eosinophilia has been shown to predict a better response to steroid treatment in COPD[53].

Oxidative stress

Increased oxidative stress has been suggested to be an important piece in the inflammatory jigsaw of chronic obstructive pulmonary disease[54]. Cigarette smoke causes increased oxidative stress[55]. Smoking produces exogenous stress to the epithelial cells of the airways due to the presence of harmful oxidants in the smoke. Endogenous stress occurs due to the inflammatory process[56] provoked by the increased production of alveolar neutrophils and macrophages and endogenous oxidants like, hydrogen peroxide, ethane, and isoprostane in the exhaled breath condensates from patients with COPD[57].

Oxidative stress may increase mucous secretion, enhance elastase activity and reduce activity of protease inhibitors[58]. Moreover, oxidative stress activates nuclear factor-κB (NF-κB) which increase transcription of important pro-inflammatory genes like, IL-8, Inducible nitric oxide synthase and cyclooxygenase (COX-2) are possible factors[59]. An increase in endothelial dysfunction of peripheral blood vessels together with haemostatic and coagulation markers have also been reported after inhalation of cigarette smoke and particulate matter, again supporting the profound systemic effects of inhaled tobacco smoke[60].

Systemic inflammation in COPD

As well as an inflammatory response in the airways, chronic obstructive pulmonary disease is characterised by systemic inflammation[61]. Evidence exists to support the fact that the systemic inflammation is seen in stable COPD and when there is an exacerbation, systemic inflammatory markers get worse[62, 63].

The precise interaction between systemic inflammation and COPD pathogenesis is unclear. In smokers, increased serum levels of CRP relate to a higher risk of developing COPD[64]. As well as CRP, other serum biomarkers are elevated in COPD including fibrinogen, TNF-α, IL-6 and IL-8. In general, acute phase reactants are strongly induced by IL-6 or TNF-alpha cytokines[65]. Higher concentrations of these markers have been observed in the cases of severe COPD[66]. Plasma CRP and fibrinogen are acute phase proteins which are produced in the liver and are released in the bloodstream and fibrinogen is under the control of IL-6. Raised levels are present in the blood of stable COPD patients but significantly higher levels have been described during exacerbation of COPD which strongly suggest its systemic inflammatory link to airway obstruction[67]. This rise of plasma fibrinogen in patients with COPD can be of further clinical importance since it has been implicated in coronary heart disease[68]. An inverse relationship between systemic inflammatory biomarkers and pulmonary function tests (FEV1) has been described, which may be of a diagnostic value and helpful to determine prognosis[69, 70].

The concept of systemic inflammation in COPD is based upon the theory of 'spill-over'[71]. According to this theory, pulmonary inflammation stimulates the haematopoietic system, releasing increased numbers of leucocytes and platelets into the bloodstream[72, 73]. Lung-derived inflammatory cytokines and other mediators circulate in the bloodstream and then cause a systemic inflammatory effect[74]. However whilst systemic inflammation certainly co-exists with lung inflammation, it has not been proven in studies using the surfactant marker-D (SP-D,) that the inflammatory mediators present in the systemic circulation are actually derived from the lung[75].

Obesity and the metabolic syndrome[76] have been identified as risk factors for COPD, but, their relationship with inflammation and COPD needs further explanation[77]. Hormones including adiponectin and most notably leptin may have a role in mediating systemic inflammation. Leptin has effects on adipose tissue and on the hypothalamus to regulate food intake by satiety but it is also a T-cell modulator and influences inflammation. Leptin levels are influenced by IL-6 and lipopolysaccharide[78]. It is profoundly increased in the sputum of COPD patients and correlates with sputum CRP and TNF-α levels[79]. Conversely, it is well known that cachexia in COPD is a marker of increased mortality and may be due to an increase in lipolysis due to persistent inflammation[80]. Half of COPD patients die with

cardiovascular events in hospital and as the role of systemic inflammation in heart disease is proven, the relationship between COPD and ischaemic heart disease may be important[81]. It has been proposed that systemic inflammation in COPD affects the vascular endothelium causing arterial stiffness and atherosclerosis. The presence of increased CRP and circulating leukocytes in patients with COPD and cardiovascular events supports this theory [82]. Many other inflammatory mediators including tissue factor, FVIIa[83], and nitric oxide have been studied to explore involvement of the coagulation system and oxidative stress in causing systemic inflammation in COPD[84, 85].
Osteoporosis and osteopenia are important disease co-morbidities of COPD[86]. Reduced bone density, resulting in fractures in COPD patients is common and increases as the disease progresses[87]. This is very notable in patients with alpha antitrypsin-1 deficiency. A number of studies have suggested that systemic inflammation is implicated in reduced bone density[88, 89]. Bone remodelling due to increased osteoclastic activity may be related to systemic inflammation, skeletal muscle loss and reduced physical activity, poor nutritional status, hypovitaminosis D, nutritional calcium deficiency and glucocorticoid treatment[90, 91].

Comorbidities in COPD

COPD has significant morbidity and mortality[92]. There are multiple extra-pulmonary manifestations, which are related to the disease and other systemic effects[93], such as weight loss, muscle wasting, osteoporosis, cachexia, atherosclerosis and co-morbid associations such as congestive cardiac failure, depression & chronic fatigue, dementia and cancer. More than 50% of deaths among COPD patients are from the cardiovascular causes[94, 95]. Chronic obstructive pulmonary disease progression not only has important physical effects but also has significant psychological morbidity[66]. Depression is common in COPD and correlates with reduced exercise tolerance, muscle weakness and fatigue[97]. Studies have demonstrated that as COPD gets worse, fatigue and depression leads to a decline in quality of life and ultimately a worse prognosis. TNF-α has also been implicated in the depression seen in COPD patients and an association between systemic markers of inflammation and depression whilst modest, is statistically significant, in comparison to the other co-morbidities[98].

5. COPD and related co-morbidities

Lung:

Pneumonia
Lung cancer
Obstructive sleep apnoea

Heart:

Pulmonary hypertension
Cor-pumonale
Coronary heart disease
Congestive cardiac failure

CNS:

Anxiety
Depression
Stroke

Musculo-skeletal:

Peripheral muscle deconditioning
Peripheral muscle wasting
Steroid myopathy
Osteoporosis and bone fractures

Blood and circulation:

Peripheral vascular disease
Normocytic anaemia

Metabolic and endocrine:

Diabetes
Metabolic syndrome

Degenerative:

Cognitive impairment
Parkinson's disease

Miscellaneous:

Arthritis
Glaucoma
Bowel and prostate cancer

In summary, there is a consensus now that both airway and systemic inflammation play a key role in the pathogenesis of chronic obstructive pulmonary disease[99, 100, 101]. The underlying mechanisms and interactions are likely to be complex and need better description which is an important future research goal[102].

6. Current treatment of COPD

Whilst COPD is a complex disease, current treatments are largely symptomatic and do not significantly alter the natural disease progression[103]. Many countries have formulated their own guidelines and most national and international respiratory societies have taken initiatives to provide training and knowledge to their professionals and act as patient advocates[104].

Conventionally, COPD is treated with both pharmacological and non-pharmacological interventions[105, 106]. Smoking cessation, regular exercise, adequate nutritional support, weight reduction and pulmonary rehabilitation are the important non-pharmacological treatment modalities[107]. Bronchodilators, anti-cholinergic, thioxanthines, steroids and antibiotics for bacterial exacerbation and oxygen therapy are the medical therapeutic options[108]. Smoking cessation and long term home oxygen[109] are the only two treatments which have been demonstrated to improve mortality[110]. The remaining treatments provide symptom control and some improvement in quality of life[111]. Short and long acting beta adrenoceptor agonists have been the gold standard of airways disease in COPD and asthma, and in COPD[112] there has been a move to the earlier introduction of long-acting bronchodilators, and it is probable that multiple combinations of long-acting bronchodilator therapies will become available[113].

Treatment of inflammation in COPD

The concept of targeting inflammation to treat COPD has largely been neglected until relatively recently[114]The mainstay of current anti-inflammatory therapy is steroid therapy, however it is now recognised that these drugs have a minimal effect in established COPD[115]. As stated above, there is a pressing need for a better understanding of the key pathophysiological mechanisms in this disease to allow more targeted therapy.

Steroids

A number of clinical trials in COPD demonstrated that high dose inhaled steroid treatment had no effect in disease progression, measured by progressive loss of FEV1, however there was some improvement in disease specific quality of life[116]. Inhaled steroids reduce exacerbations in COPD and this has been demonstrated in a number of studies examining long-acting β-agonists / inhaled steroid combination therapies[117]. Despite, the predominant neutrophilic and lymphocytic involvement of cells in the pathogenesis of COPD, the presence of some eosinophils[118] in the airways of such patient have provoked a great interest in the non-invasive, easy and reproducible measurement of biomarkers such as the of fractional exhaled nitric oxide (FENO) to identify patients who may respond better to steroid therapy[119, 120]however FeNO is reduced by smoking

Phosphodiesterase 4 (PDE4) inhibitors

There are other therapies which have been investigated to target inflammation in COPD[121]. Roflumilast is the first selective PDE4 inhibitor which has recently been licensed for COPD in Europe and America. It has been advocated in subjects with frequent exacerbations and symptomatic severe COPD patients with productive cough[122]. Roflumilast is an oral preparation which inhibits pulmonary inflammation through the selective inhibition of the iso-enzyme PDE4, which hydrolyses cyclic AMP[123], which is expressed in structural cells of the lung such as, smooth muscle cells, airway epithelium and inflammatory cells such as neutrophils, lymphocytes or macrophages[124]. Despite the concerns regarding dose dependant side effects such as headache, nausea and diarrhoea[125], it may offer some benefit in COPD patients with frequent exacerbations. Recent data have demonstrated that the use of roflumilast decreased the exacerbations and the need for adjuvant steroid therapy. Its use showed improvement in pulmonary function tests and when compared with the placebo, it showed improvement in functional capacity[126, 127]. Further longitudinal studies are warranted to measure the real benefit and effectiveness. However the clinical use of roflumilast has been encouraging so far in reducing exacerbations and improving lung function[128].

Novel treatment strategies for COPD

With better understanding of the pathophysiology of COPD disease process and recognition of inflammation as an important feature, it is anticipated that disease modifying therapy for COPD[129] targeting pulmonary and systemic inflammation, will prove effective. There are a number of specific therapeutic targets against the influx of inflammatory cells into the lung[130]. including inhibitors of p38 mitogen-activated protein kinase (MAPK), nuclear factor-κB (NF-κB), and phosphoinositide-3-kinase (PI3K) [131]. There is also a search for inhibitors of proteinases and matrix metalloproteinases (MMPs) which could prevent lung destruction and emphysema. The immunomodulatory role of macrolides is also one of the potential novel treatments for COPD[132].

Cytokines and chemokines inhibitors

TNF-α TNF-α plays a key role in COPD and acts as a catalyst for chemokine interleukin-8 (IL-8). Infliximab is a monoclonal antibody which neutralizes TNF-α by binding it. Its role has been evaluated in COPD[133] but its use has failed to show any change in sputum neutrophils, FEV1, FEV1/FVC or IL-6[134]. There is also significant toxicity and cost issues and further attempts to use it in COPD have been halted[135].

Antibody against human IL-8

A fully humanised monoclonal IgG_2 antibody directed against human IL-8 (ABX-IL8) blocks binding to IL-8 receptors on neutrophils and neutralizes IL-8–mediated neutrophil activation *in vitro*[136]. It has been shown that pretreatment of sputum supernatant of 20 patients with COPD with an anti–IL-8 antibody led to a concentration-dependent inhibition of neutrophil chemotaxis. Moreover, ABX-IL8 is proposed to block IL-8–induced neutrophil activation and degranulation, preventing release of neutrophil elastase[137].However in a clinical trial, whilst well tolerated and shown to be beneficial in reducing dyspnoea, there was no real added benefits were noted in secondary outcomes (lung function, health status and inflammatory markers) [138].

CXCL1, CXCL8 receptor antagonists

CXCL1 (GRO-α) is produced by structural and inflammatory cells and is chemotactic for neutrophils[139]. Using agents which are CXCL1 and CXCL8 (IL8) receptor antagonists blocks the neutrophilic inflammatory response in the lungs and may help to control COPD[140] and clinical trial data is awaited

CCL2 (MCP-1) and CCR2 antagonists

Bronchoalveolar lavage from patients with COPD contains increased MCP-1 (CCL2) in comparison to healthy non-smokers[141] and it has also been postulated that in COPD, the MCP-1 receptor, CCR2, shows increased expression. These findings relate to disease severity and FEV1. Therefore targeting of CCL2 and its receptor could provide potentially potent and novel anti-inflammatory agents[142]. The study of such products in humans is in the early phase and clinical preparations are probably a long way off currently[143].

5-Leukotriene B_4 / Lipoxygenase inhibitors

Leukotriene B_4 (LTB_4), a pro-inflammatory derivative of arachidonic acid, is both a chemoattractant and activator of neutrophils and may be important in COPD[144]. LTB4 is synthesized by neutrophils and alveolar macrophages, where the conversion of arachidonic acid to the intermediate compound 5-hydroperoxyeicosatetraenoic acid requires both the enzyme 5-lipoxygenase (5-LO) and 5-lipoxygenase activating protein (FLAP). In a preliminary double-blind, randomized, placebo-controlled trial the effects of the FLAP antagonist, BAYx1005, on sputum LTB4 and myeloperoxidase (a marker of sputum neutrophil number and activation) concentrations, and on the chemotactic activity of the secretions in patients with COPD and chronic bronchitis was studied[145]. A modest but significant reduction in sputum LTB4 concentrations in the patients in this trial was observed. However, the reductions in LTB4 concentration were comparable in magnitude to those seen during the resolution of purulent exacerbations of chronic bronchitis. This study have established that a leukotriene synthesis inhibitor may affect neutrophilic bronchial inflammation in patients with stable COPD and chronic bronchitis, and that this class of drug merits further investigation in a larger number of patients. Another Possible way to inhibit leukotriene synthesis pathway is to target is 5-lipoxygenase inhibition[146]. The potential clinical benefits of both of these approaches remain under investigation[147].

Anti-oxidants including N-Acetylcysteine

N-Acetylcysteine is an anti-oxidant which is most commonly used in paracetamol overdose. It targets oxidative stress and causes activation of anti-proteases and reduces expression of IL-8 and TNF-α [148]. Recent data demonstrated an improvement in vital capacity and inspiratory capacity of patients with COPD in an ICU setting[149]. NAC treatment of patients with stable, moderate-to-severe COPD has a beneficial effect on physical performance, probably due to a reduction in air trapping[150] NAC probably exhibits an anti-inflammatory effect by influencing neutrophils and macrophage function[151].

p38 mitogen-activated protein kinase (MAPK) inhibitors

p38 MAPK inhibitors are another novel drug strategy proposed for targeting inflammation in COPD[152]. The p38 MAPK pathway is activated by stress and it regulates a wide variety of inflammatory cytokines including IL-8, TNF-α and MMPs[153]. Corticosteroids partially suppress cytokine production by COPD alveolar macrophages [154, 155] but p38 MAPK activation in alveolar macrophages is corticosteroid insensitive. One study investigated the dose-sparing and efficacy-enhancing effects of combined treatment with a corticosteroid and a p38 MAPK inhibitor, and showed the combination synergistically enhances the anti-inflammatory effects on cytokine production by alveolar macrophages in COPD patients and controls[156]. Another study has demonstrated that SB-681323 is a potent p38 MAPK inhibitor that potentially suppresses inflammation in COPD[157]. But further clinical trials with this class of molecule are starting and are eagerly awaited.

Nuclear factor-κB (NF-κB) inhibitors

Nuclear factor-κB (NF-κB) has been implicated in inflammation in COPD by causing propagation of cytokines and neutrophils[158]. Therefore, this pathway has been targeted to overcome inflammation and airways injury in COPD patients. One approach is to inhibit the IκB kinase (IKK) using glucocorticoids, such as dexamethasone or prednisolone which downregulates the pro-inflammation[159]. Experiments have also been performed using resveratrol, one of the flavonoids naturally occurring in red wine. It inhibits this pathway of inflammation[160] however, there is no evidence of clinical benefit currently.

Phosphoinositide 3-kinases (PI3K) inhibitors

The components of the PI3K pathway play a crucial role in the expression and activation of inflammatory mediators, inflammatory cell recruitment, immune cell function, airway remodelling and corticosteroid insensitivity in COPD and asthma[161].Targeting this pathway has a potential therapeutic role and this may be one of the actions of theophylline[652] The idea for development of PI3K inhibitors would be to ensure greater efficacy in severe steroid-insensitive asthma and COPD where corticosteroids are of limited[163] with a better side effect profile.

7. Anti-proteinases

Neutrophil elastase inhibitors

For nearly two decades, there has been a pursuit to find safe oral inhibitors of neutrophil elastase. Many of the compounds developed have had poor pharmacokinetics and a low therapeutic index. Tripeptidyl trifluoromethyl ketones were the first developed with an improved profile but they have not been fully optimized for oral use yet[164]. Targeting neutrophil elastase may be very useful in COPD since it can cause direct activation of MMPs such as MMP-9, which play a crucial role in airway inflammation[165]. Recent work on the relatively newer compounds like Sivelestat sodium hydrate has not proved to be very encouraging[166].

Matrix metalloproteinases (MMPs) inhibitors

MMPs are a major class of proteolytic enzymes potentially involved in COPD. Bronchoalveolar lavage of patients with emphysema shows high levels of MMP-1 and MMP-9[167]. Drugs such as BMS-561392 and gw3333 which could inhibit the MMPs and TNF-α are in the pre-clinical stage. Their development and potential efficacy in targeting inflammation in COPD has yet to be established[168].

HDAC modifiers

There are 11 classic human HDACs that regulate histone acetylatio[169]. HDAC2 is involved in suppression of NF-κB–mediated inflammatory gene expression by corticosteroids[170] and HDAC2 mRNA and protein expression is significantly reduced in tissue specimens of the peripheral lung and in alveolar macrophages from patients with COPD[171]. This speculated link may have therapeutic implications, because reductions in HDAC activity may be reversible. Theophylline is an activator of HDAC157, and there is evidence to suggest that low concentrations of theophylline completely restore HDAC activity in alveolar macrophages from patients with COPD, with reduced production of inflammatory cytokines and restoration of responsiveness to corticosteroids[172]. It has been reported that theophylline[173] and PI3K inhibitor (LY294002) have a similar effect in lung macrophage cells, increasing HDAC2 expression and re-sensitizing the cells to steroids. Whether this is a mechanism of the therapeutic action of theophylline in COPD is not known.

Macrolides

The hallmark of COPD is the airways inflammation which is primarily neutrophilic in nature and low grade neutrophilic inflammation is often persistent[174]. Treatment with macrolides has been shown to reduce the number of neutrophils and the levels of interleukin-8 (IL-8) protein in bronchoalveolar lavage fluid in COPD[175]. The mechanisms by which macrolides exert a beneficial effect on chronic inflammatory airway disease are thought to be independent of their antibiotic effects but rather due their anti-inflammatory effects[176], through reducing lower airway bacterial colonization may also be beneficial[177] Macrolides in COPD decrease neutrophil counts and inflammatory markers and reduce the number of exacerbations[178]. The role of regular macrolides in COPD[179] needs to be defined more clearly, and there remain concerns about widespread use of these drugs particularly with regard to antibiotic resistance and superadded infections like MRSA and C.difficile[180].

Non-pharmacological treatments - novel strategies

Non-pharmacological treatments will remain important in the future management of COPD and will continue to involve more integrated care[181]. There is compelling evidence of the role of systemic inflammation in decreasing muscle mass, weakness and loss of function in COPD patients[182]and tests to detect early markers of muscle involvement may be clinically beneficial to target patients of greatest risk of losing muscle mass with early rehabilitation interventions[183]. Targeting patients with multiple co-morbidities and provision of early pulmonary rehabilitation and physiotherapy can have a major impact on improving morbidity and decreasing mortality[184]. Identifying which smokers are at risk of development of COPD and which patients will develop more progressive disease may also be important advances in the future[185, 186, 187].

8. Summary

Chronic obstructive pulmonary disease (COPD) is a disease characterized by poorly reversible airflow limitation which is usually progressive and associated with an abnormal inflammatory response in the lung. Cigarette smoking is the major risk factor responsible for the development of COPD, however other environmental exposures, such as combustion of biomass fuels, are major causes in certain countries. A decade since the introduction of the Global strategy for the diagnosis, management and prevention of Obstructive pulmonary Disease (GOLD), the incidence of COPD continues to rise and the World Health Organisation and the World Bank predict that by the 2020, it will be the third leading cause of mortality in the world.

The term chronic obstructive pulmonary disease is a descriptive term encompassing a heterogeneous subset of clinical syndromes, specifically chronic bronchitis, emphysema and asthma and it is now recognised that there is significant overlap between the previously described clinical syndromes. The term 'overlap syndrome' is often used to describe a patient with fixed airflow obstruction (COPD), but having some asthmatic features. Chronic bronchitis is clinically defined as a cough productive of sputum lasting at least three months for two consecutive years and emphysema is a pathological entity characterised by destruction of the lung parenchyma with resultant enlarged alveolar spaces and loss of alveolar walls.

The patho-physiology of COPD involves inflammation of the proximal and peripheral airways and destruction of lung parenchyma with emphysema. The airway damage results in significant physiological derangement with expiratory airflow limitation and abnormal gas exchange. Emphysema contributes to the airflow limitation by reducing the elastic recoil of the lung through parenchymal destruction, as well as by reducing the elastic load applied to the airways through destruction of alveolar attachments. Inflammation of peripheral airways contributes to the airflow limitation by increasing the thickness of the airway wall which, together with fibrosis and smooth muscle hypertrophy, may cause airway narrowing.

The inflammatory process in COPD usually starts with a persistent airways insult (commonly tobacco smoke exposure) which leads to abnormal activation of both the innate and adaptive immune responses of the airway tract. Pathologically, epithelial squamous cell metaplasia, goblet cell hyperplasia, parenchymal destruction (emphysema) and small airway are all consequences of this persistent inflammatory environment. Both, innate and adaptive immune responses are involved in the inflammatory process in COPD. There is evidence that airways inflammation is present in smokers before airflow obstruction is evident with pulmonary function tests. The cells which have been mostly implicated in this inflammatory process $CD8^{+}$ T lymphocytes and macrophages which through the production of LTB4, TNF-α, IL-8, GRO-α recruit neutrophils to the airway, with resultant injury. Increased neutrophils are seen in bronchoalveolar lavage and induced sputum of the patients with COPD compared to smokers without airflow obstruction. Neutrophil myeloperoxidase and human neutrophil lectin are also elevated consistent with neutrophil activation and degranulation. Some patients show evidence of eosinophil recruitment to the airway and increased eosinophil basic proteins (eosinophil cationic proteins and eosinophil peroxidase) have been observed in induced sputum of COPD patients. This may reflect 'overlap' syndrome as described above, and sputum eosinophilia has been shown to predict a better response to steroid treatment in COPD. Exacerbations are significant events in patients with COPD as they cause increased breathlessness and purulent sputum production. In patients with frequent exacerbations, there is accelerated lung function decline, as a consequence of augmented inflammation and injury during exacerbations.

Bronchial biopsies in COPD have shown infiltration of mononuclear cells and $CD8^+$ T lymphocytes. Macrophages are activated by cigarette smoke and other inhaled irritants and may play an important role in driving the inflammatory process in COPD through the release of neutrophil chemotactic factors as well as proteolytic enzymes. More recently, it has been suggested that COPD may represent an 'auto-immune' disease, with failure to regulate the adaptive response to auto-antigens produced as a consequence of tobacco smoke exposure. A subtype of regulatory CD4+ T-cells expressing CD25 (Tregs) are upregulated in COPD, which supports an auto-immune aetiology.

Protease / anti-protease imbalance excessive oxidative stress have also been linked to progressive airway injury in COPD. Neutrophil elastase, cathepsins and matrix metalloproteinases have all been implicated in the patho-physiology of COPD. Bronchoalveolar lavage macrophages from patients with emphysema express more MMP-9 and MMP-1 than cells from control subjects in COPD, suggesting that these cells, rather than neutrophils, may be the major cellular source. There is also evidence for increased oxidative stress in COPD, evidenced by an increase in oxidized or nitrated proteins and peroxidised polyunsaturated fatty acids and their degradation products. Increase in endothelial dysfunction of peripheral blood vessels together with haemostatic and coagulation markers have also been reported after inhalation of cigarette smoke and particulate matter, again supporting the profound systemic effects of inhaled tobacco smoke.

There is growing evidence to suggest that as well as an inflammatory response in the airways, chronic obstructive pulmonary disease is characterised by systemic inflammation. Recent evidence has demonstrated systemic 'spill-over' of this pulmonary inflammation with evidence of elevated systemic inflammatory markers, pro-inflammatory cytokines and lipopolysaccharide binding protein.

Systemic manifestations of COPD may significantly affect patients' quality of life and prognosis of the disease. It has been well recognised that systemic effects may be related to systemic inflammation in COPD. COPD is associated with cachexia, weight loss, osteoporosis, muscle wasting, heart failure, atherosclerosis, dementia, depression, and cancer and these extra- pulmonary manifestations of COPD account for much of the morbidity and mortality in COPD patients. Depression is also a major co-morbidity in COPD and patients with more systemic inflammation as well as more depression or fatigue have been shown to be less physically active and more exercise intolerant. There is evidence to suggest that certain age related conditions like, arthritis, Parkinson's disease and cancer of the prostate and bowel have links with COPD. The risk of developing arthritis, anaemia and glaucoma increases in COPD patients with growing age.

Current anti-inflammatory therapies, particularly steroid therapy, have a minimal effect in established COPD. There is a significant need for a better understanding of the key patho-physiological mechanisms in this disease to allow more targeted therapy. Novel pharmacological strategies are still in the developmental stage. Cytokine and chemokine inhibitors, for example antibodies against human IL-8, CXCL1, CXCL8 antagonists, CCL2, CCR2, lipoxygenase and LB4 inhibitors have shown some promise but there remain issues around safety and efficacy and cost effectiveness. The role of anti-oxidants, MAPK-inhibitors and PI3k inhibitors is still under investigation. The use of macrolides has been the focus of recent attention and recent data has suggested a role in exacerbation prevention.

9. References

[1] Celli BR, MacNee W, ATS/ERS Task Force. Standards for the diagnosis and treatment of patients with COPD: a summary of the ATS/ERS position paper. *Eur Respir J* 2004; 23: 932- 946

[2] Willemse BWM, Postma DS, Timens W, Ten Hacken NHT: The impact of smoking cessation on respiratory symptoms, lung function, airway hyperresponsiveness and inflammation. *Eur Respir J* 2004; 23:464-476

[3] Govender N, U G Lalloo, Naidoo R N. Occupational exposures and chronic obstructive pulmonary disease: a hospital based case-control study. *Thorax* 2011; 66: 597e601

[4] Singh D, Fox S M, Singer R T, Plumb J, Bates S, Broad P, Riley J H,Celli B. Induced sputum genes associated with spirometric and radiological disease severity in COPD ex-smokers. *Thorax* 2011; 66: 489-495

[5] Gibson, PG, Simpson JL. The overlap syndrome of asthma and COPD: what are its features and how important is it? *Thorax* 2009 Aug; 64: 728-35

[6] Puente-Maestu L, Stringer W W. Hyperinflation and its management in COPD. *Int J Chron Obstruct Pulmon Dis* 2006; 1: 38-400

[7] Connolly MJ, Lowe D, Anstey K, et al. Admissions to hospital with exacerbations of chronic obstructive pulmonary disease: effect of age related factors and service organisation. *Thorax* 2006; 61: 843e8

[8] Groarke JD, Gallagher J, Stack J, et al. Use of an admission early warning score to predict patient morbidity and mortality and treatment success. *Emerg Med J* 2008; 25: 803e6

[9] Heitz CR, Gaillard JP, Blumstein H, et al. Performance of the maximum modified early warning score to predict the need for higher care utilization among admitted emergency department patients. *J Hosp Med* 2010; 5: E46e52

[10] Mitchell IA, McKay H, Van Leuvan C, et al. A prospective controlled trial of the effect of a multi-faceted intervention on early recognition and intervention in deteriorating hospital patients. *Resuscitation* 2010; 81: 658e66

[11] Pauwels RA, Rabe KF, Burdon and clinical features of chronic obstructive pulmonary disease (COPD). *Lancet* 2004; 364: 613-620

[12] Rabe K, Hurd S, Anzueto A, et al. Global strategy for the diagnosis, management and prevention of chronic obstructive pulmonary disease. *Am J Respir Crit Care Med.* 2007; 176: 532-55

[13] Peacock J L, Anderson H R, Bremner S A, Marston L, Seemungal T A, Strachan D P, Wedzicha J A. Outdoor air pollution and respiratory health in patients with COPD. *Thorax* 2011; 66: 591e596

[14] Po JY, FitzGerald JM, Carlsten C. Respiratory disease associated with solid biomass fuel exposure in rural women and children: systematic review and meta-analysis. *Thorax* 2011; 66: 232-9

[15] Denden S, Khelil A H, Knani J, Lakhdar R, Perrin P, Lefranc G, Chibani J B. Alpha-1 antitrypsin gene polymorphism in Chronic Obstructive Pulmonary Disease (COPD) *Genet Mol Biol* 2010; 33(1): 23-26

[16] Rodríguez-Roisin R, Drakulovic M, Rodríguez DA, Roca J, Barberà JA, Wagner PD. Ventilation-perfusion imbalance and chronic obstructive pulmonary disease staging severity. *J Appl Physiol* 2009 Jun; 106: 1902-8

[17] Anthonisen NR, Connett JE, Murray RP. Smoking and lung function of Lung Health Study participants after 11 years. *Am J Respir Crit Care Med* 2002 ;16: 675-679

[18] Rutgers SR, Postma DS, ten Hacken NH, et al. ongoing airway inflammation in patients with COPD who do not currently smoke. *Thorax* 2000; 55: 12-18

[19] Hogg JC, Chu F, Utokaparch S, et al. The nature of small-airway obstruction in chronic obstructive pulmonary disease. *N Engl J Med* 2004; 350:2645–2653

[20] Hurst JR, Wilkinson TMA, Perera WR, Donaldson GC, Wedzicha JA. Relationships among bacteria, upper airway, lower airway, and systemic inflammation in COPD. *Chest* 2005; 127: 1219-1226

[21] Lindberg A, Jonsson AC, Ronmark E, Lundgren R, Larsson LG, Lundback B: Prevalence of chronic obstructive pulmonary disease according to BTS, ERS, GOLD and ATS criteria in relation to doctor's diagnosis, symptoms, age, gender, and smoking habits. *Respiration* 2005; 72: 471-9

[22] Vestbo J, Prescott E, Lange P, and the Copenhagen City Heart Study Group. Association of chronic mucus hypersecretion with FEV1 decline and chronic obstructive pulmonary disease morbidity. *Am J Respir Crit Care Med* 1996; 153: 1530-1535

[23] Hurst JR, Perera WR, Wilkinson TM, Donaldson GC, Wedzicha JA. Exacerbation of chronic obstructive pulmonary disease: pan-airway and systemic inflammatory indices. *Proc Am Thorac Soc* 2006 Aug; 3: 481-2

[24] Donaldson GC, Seemungal TAR, Bhowmik A, Wedzicha JA. Relationship between exacerbation frequency and lung function decline in chronic obstructive pulmonary disease. *Thorax* 2002; 57: 847-852

[25] Marquis K, Maltais F, Duguay V et al. "The metabolic syndrome in patients with chronic obstructive pulmonary disease" *Journal of Cardiopulmonary Rehabilitation* 2005; 25: 226- 232

[26] Fabbri L M, K F Rabe. From COPD to chronic systemic inflammatory syndrome? *Lancet* 2007; 370: 797-99

[27] Rose N, Afanasyeva M. Autoimmunity: busting the atherosclerotic plaque. Nat *Med* 2003; 9: 641-2

[28] Steinman L. State of the art: four easy pieces: interconnections between tissue injury, intermediary metabolism, autoimmunity and chronic degeneration. *Proc Am Thorac Soc* 2006; 3: 484-6

[29] Cosio MG, Saetta M, Agusti A. Immunologic aspects of chronic obstructive pulmonary disease. *N Engl J Med* 2009; 360: 2445-54

[30] Barnes PJ, Cosio MG. Cells and mediators of chronic obstructive pulmonary disease. *Eur Respir Monogr* 2006; 38: 130-58

[31] Di Stefano A, Caramori G, Capelli A, et al. STAT4 activation in smokers and patients with chronic obstructive pulmonary disease. *Eur Respir J* 2004; 24: 78-85

[32] Freeman CM, Curtis JL, Chensue SW. CC chemokine receptor 5 and CXC chemokine receptor 6 expression by lung CD8+ cells correlates with chronic obstructive pulmonary disease severity. *AmJ Pathol* 2007; 171: 767-76

[33] Retamales I, Elliott WM, Meshi B, et al. Amplification of inflammation in emphysema and its association with latent adenoviral infection. *Am J Respir Crit Care Med* 2001; 164: 469-73

[34] Calabrese F, Giacometti C, Beghe B, et al. Marked alveolar apoptosis/proliferation imbalance in end-stage emphysema. *Respir Res* 2005; 6: 14

[35] Turato G, Zuin R, Miniati M, et al. Airway inflammation in severe chronic obstructive pulmonary disease: relationship with lung function and radiologic emphysema. *Am J Respir Crit Care Med* 2002; 166: 105-10
[36] van der Strate BW, Postma DS, Brandsma CA, et al. Cigarette smoke-induce emphysema: a role for the B cell? *Am J Respir Crit Care Med* 2006; 173: 751-8
[37] Barnes PJ, Shapiro SD, Pauwels RA: Chronic obstructive pulmonary disease: molecular and cellular mechanisms. *Eur Respir J* 2003; 22:672-688
[38] Cowburn AS, Condliffe AM, Farahi N, Summers C, Chilvers ER. Advances in neutrophil biology: clinical implications. *Chest* 2008; 134: 606-12
[39] Siena L, Gjomarkaj M, Elliot J, Pace E, Bruno A, Baraldo S, Saetta M, Bonsignore MR, James A. Reduced apoptosis of CD8+ T-Lymphocytes in the airways of smokers with mild/moderate COPD. *Respir Med* 2011 May 23: (Epub)
[40] Agustí A, MacNee, W, Donaldson, K, Cosio, M. Hypothesis: Does COPD Have an autoimmune component? *Thorax.* 2003; 58: 832-834
[41] Saetta M, Turato G, Maestrelli P, Mapp CE, and Fabbri LM. Cellular and structural bases of chronic obstructive pulmonary disease. *Am J Respir Crit Care Med.* 2001; 163: 1304-1309
[42] Cowburn AS, Condliffe AM, Farahi N, Summers C, Chilvers ER: Advances In neutrophil biology: clinical implications. *Chest* 2008; 134:606-12
[43] Barnes P J. Mediators of Chronic Obstructive Pulmonary Disease. *Pharmacol Rev* 2004; 56:515-548
[44] Stockley RA. Proteases and antiproteases. *Novartis Found Symp* 2001; 234: 189-199
[45] Belvisi MG, Bottomley KM. The role of matrix metalloproteinases (MMPs) in the pathophysiology of chronic obstructive pulmonary disease (COPD): a therapeutic role for inhibitors of MMPs. *Inflamm Res* 2003; 52: 95-100
[46] Chapman HA Jr. Shi GP. Protease injury in the development of COPD. Thomas A Neill lecture. *Chest* 2000; 117: 2955-95
[47] Turino G M. The origins of a concept: the protease antiprotease imbalance hypothesis. *Chest* 2002; 122: 1058-1060
[48] Betsuyaku T, Takeyabu K, Tanino M, Nishimura M. Role of secretory leukocyte protease inhibitor in the development of subclinical emphysema. *Eur Respir J* 2002; 19: 1051-1057
[49] Hurst J R, Perera W R, Wilkinson T M A, Donaldson G C, Wedzicha J A. Systemic and Upper and Lower Airway Inflammation at Exacerbation of Chronic Obstructive Pulmonary Disease. *Am J Respir Crit Care Med* 2006; 173: 71-78
[50] Barnes PJ. Emerging targets for COPD therapy. *Curr Drug Targets Inflamm Allergy* 2005; 4: 675-83
[51] Saetta M, Turato G, Maestrelli P, Mapp CE, Fabbri LM. Cellular and structural bases of chronic obstructive pulmonary disease. *Am J Respir Crit Care Med.* 2001; 163: 1304-1309
[52] Chung KF. Cytokines as targets in chronic obstructive pulmonary disease. *Curr Drug Targets* 2006; 7: 675-81
[53] Balzano G, Stefanelli F, Iorio C, et al. Eosinophilic inflammation in stable chronic obstructive pulmonary disease. Relationship with neutrophils and airway function. *Am J Respir Crit Care Med* 1999; 160: 1486-1492

[54] Kirkham PA, Caramori G, Casolari P, Papi A, Edwards M, Shamji B, Triantaphyllopoulos K, Hussain F, Pinart M, Khan Y, Heinemann L, Stevens L, Yeadon M, Barnes PJ, Chung KF, Adcock IM. Oxidative Stress-induced Antibodies to Carbonyl-modified Protein Correlate with Severity of COPD. *Am J Respir Crit Care Med* 2011 Jun 16 (Epub ahead of print)
[55] Lin JL, Thomas PS. Current perspectives of oxidative stress and its measurement in chronic obstructive pulmonarydisease. *COPD* 2010; 7: 291-306
[56] Bowler RP, Barnes PJ, Crapo JD. The role of oxidative stress in chronic obstructive pulmonary disease. *COPD* 2004; 1: 255-77
[57] Montuschi P, Collins JV, Ciabattoni G, Lazzeri N, Corradi M, Kharitonov SA, and Barnes PJ. Exhaled 8-isoprostane as an in vivo biomarker of lung oxidative stress in patients with COPD and healthy smokers. *Am J Respir Crit Care Med* 2000; 162: *Care Med* 162: 1175- 1177-Cavalcante AG, de Bruin PF. The role of oxidative stress in COPD: current concepts and perspectives. *J Bras Pneumol* 2009; 35: 1227-37
[58] Rahman I, Adcock M.Oxidative stress and redox regulation of lung inflammation in COPD. *Eur Respir J* 2006; 28: 219–242
[59] Sabit R, Thomas P, Shale D J, Collins P, Linnane S J. The effects of hypoxia on markers of coagulation and systemic inflammation in patients with COPD. *Chest* 2010; 138: 47-5161-Siafakas NM. "In the Beginning" of COPD: is evolution important? *Am J Respir Crit Care Med* 2007; 175: 423-4
[60] Taylor DR. Risk assessment in asthma and COPD: a potential role for biomarkers? *Thorax* 2009; 64: 261-4
[61] Vernooy JH, Kucukaycan M, Jacobs JA, Chavannes NH, Buurman WA, Dentener MA, Wouters EF: Local and systemic inflammation in patients with chronic obstructive pulmonary disease: soluble tumor necrosis factor receptors are increased in sputum. *Am J Respir Crit Care Med* 2002; 166: 1218-1224
[62] Tonstad S, Cowan J L. C-reactive protein as a predictor of disease in smokers: a review. Int J clin pract 2009; 63:1550-3
[63] Polatli M, Cakir A, Cildag O, Bolaman AZ, Yenisey C, Yenicerioglu Y. Microalbuminuria, von Willebrand factor and fibrinogen levels as markers of the severity in COPD exacerbation. *J Thromb Thrombolysis* 2007; 26: 97-102
[64] Higashimoto Y, Iwata T, Okada M, Satoh H, Fukuda K, Tohda Y. Serum biomarkers as predictors of lung function decline in chronic obstructive pulmonary disease. *Respir Med* 2009; 103: 1231-8
[65] Chung KF, Adcock IM Multifaceted mechanisms in COPD: inflammation, immunity, and tissue repair and destruction. *Eur Respir J* 2008; 31: 1334-56
[66] MacCallum PK. Markers of hemostasis and systemic inflammation in heart disease and atherosclerosis in smokers. *Proc Am Thorac Soc* 2005; 2: 34-43
[67] Donaldson G C, Seemungal TAR, Patel IS, Bhowmik A, Wilkinson TMA, Hurst JR, MacCallum PK, Wedzicha JA. Airway and Systemic Inflammation and decline in Lung Function in Patients With COPD. *Chest* 2005; 128: 1995-2004
[68] Gan WQ, Man SF, Senthilselvan A, Sin DD: Association between chronic obstructive pulmonary disease and systemic inflammation: a systematic review and a meta-analysis. *Thorax* 2004, 59:574-80

[69] Wouters EF, Reynaert NL, Dentener MA, Vernooy JH. Systemic and local inflammation in asthma and chronic obstructive pulmonary disease: is there a connection? *Proc Am Thoacic Soc* 2009; 6: 638-47
[70] Wouters EF. Local and systemic inflammation in chronic obstructive pulmonary disease. *Proc Am Thorac Soc* 2005; 2: 26-33
[71] Han MK. Update in chronic obstructive pulmonary disease in 2010. *Am J Respir Crit Care Med* 2011; 183: 1311-5
[72] Barnes PJ. The cytokine network in chronic obstructive pulmonary disease. *Am J Respir Cell Mol Biol* 2009; 41: 631-8
[73] Lomas DA, Silverman EK, Edwards LD, Locantore NW, Miller BE, Horstman DH, Tal-Singer R. Serum surfactant protein D is steroid sensitive and associated with exacerbations of COPD. *Eur Respir J* 2009; 34: 95-102
[74] Hajer GR, van Haeften TW, Visseren FL. Adipose tissue dysfunction in obesity, diabetes, and vascular diseases. *Eur Heart J* 2008; 29: 2959-2971
[75] Sood A. Obesity, adipokines, and lung disease. *J Appl Physiol* 2010; 108: 744-53
[76] Faggioni R, Feingold KR, Grunfeld C. Leptin regulation of the immune response and the immunodeficiency of malnutrition. *FASEB J* 2001; 15: 2565-2571
[77] Broekhuizen R, Vernooy JH, Schols AM, Dentener MA, Wouters EF. Leptin as local inflammatory marker in COPD. *Respir Med* 2005; 99: 70-4
[78] Celli BR, Cote CG, Marin JM, et al. The body-mass index, airflow obstruction, dyspnea, and exercise capacity index in chronic obstructive pulmonary disease. *N Engl J Med* 2004; 350: 1005e12
[79] Ramaraj R. COPD in smokers with atherosclerosis: are we missing the trail? *Am J Respir Crit Care Med* 2009; 179: 35-40
[80] Ross R. Atherosclerosis-an inflammatory disease. *N Engl J Med* 1999; 340: 115-26
[81] Borensztajn KS, von der Thüsen JH, Spek CA. The role of coagulation in chronic inflammatory disorders: a jack of all trades. *Curr Pharm Des* 2011; 17: 9-16
[82] Maestrelli P, Paska A, Saetta M, Turato G, Nowicki Y, Monti S, Formichi B, Miniati M, and Fabbri LM. Decreased haem oxygenase-1 and increased inducible nitric oxide synthase in the lung of severe COPD patients. *Eur Respir J* 2003; 21: 971-976
[83] Agusti AG, Villaverde JM, Togores B, and Bosch M Serial measurements of exhaled nitric oxide during exacerbations of chronic obstructive pulmonary disease. *Eur Respir J* 1999; 14: 523-528
[84] Jorgensen NR, Schwarz P, Holme I, Henriksen BM, Petersen LJ, Backer V. The prevalence of osteoporosis in patients with chronic obstructive pulmonary disease: a cross sectional study. *Respir Med* 2007; 101: 177-185
[85] Vrieze A, de Greef MH, Wijkstra PJ, Wempe JB. Low bone mineral density in COPD patients related to worse lung function, low weight and decreased fat-free mass. *Osteoporos Int* 2007; 18: 1197-1202
[86] Tanaka Y, Nakayamada S, Okada Y. Osteoblasts and osteoclasts in bone remodeling and inflammation. *Curr Drug Targets Inflamm Allergy* 2005; 4: 325-8
[87] Lacativa PG, Farias ML. Osteoporosis and inflammation. *Arq Bras Endocrinol Metabol* 2010; 54: 123-32
[88] Ebeling PR. Clinical practice. Osteoporosis in men. *N Engl J Med* 2008; 358:1474-1482

[89] Lam J, Takeshita S, Barker JE, Kanagawa O, Ross FP, Teitelbaum SL. TNF-α induces osteoclastogenesis by direct stimulation of macrophages exposed to permissive levels of RANK ligand. *J Clin Invest* 2000; 106: 1481-1488

[90] Barnes P J, Celli B R. Systemic manifestations and comorbidities of COPD. *Eur Respir J* 2009; 33: 1165–1185

[91] Spencer S, Calverley PM, Sherwood BP, Jones PW: Health status deterioration in patients with chronic obstructive pulmonary disease. *Am J Respir Crit Care Med* 2001; 163: 122- 128

[92] Feary JR, Rodrigues LC, Smith CJ, Hubbard RB, Gibson JE. Prevalence of Major Comorbidities in Subjects with COPD and Incidence of Myocardial Infarction and Stroke *Thorax* 2010; 65: 956-962

[93] Danesh J, Collins R, Appleby P, Peto R. Association of fibrinogen, C-reactive protein, albumin, or leukocyte count with coronary heart disease: meta analyses of prospective studies. *JAMA* 1998; 279: 1477-1482

[94] Yohannes AM, Baldwin RC, Connolly MJ. Depression and anxiety in elderly patients with chronic obstructive pulmonary disease. *Age Ageing* 2006; 35: 457-459

[95] Hill K, Geist R, Goldstein RS, Lacasse Y. Anxiety and depression in end-stage COPD. *Eur Respir J* 2008; 31: 667-677

[96] Anisman H, Merali Z, Hayley S. Neurotransmitter, peptide and cytokine processes in relation to depressive disorder: comorbidity between depression and neurodegenerative disorders. *Prog Neurobiol* 2008; 85: 1-74

[97] Gan WQ, Man SF, Senthilselvan A, Sin DD. Association between chronic obstructive pulmonary disease and systemic inflammation: a systematic review and a meta-analysis. *Thorax* 2004; 59: 574-580

[98] Barnes PJ. Chronic obstructive pulmonary disease. *N Engl J Med* 2000; 343:269- 280

[99] Spencer S, Calverley PM, Burge PS, Jones PW: Impact of preventing exacerbations on deterioration of health status in COPD. *Eur Respir J* 2004; 23: 698-702

[100] Agusti A: Systemic effects of chronic obstructive pulmonary disease: what we know and what we don't know (but should). *Proc Am Thorac Soc* 2007; 4: 522-525

[101] Alifano M, Cuvelier A, Delage A , Roche N, Lamia B Molano L C , Couderc L-J, Marquette C-H, Devilliere P. Treatment of COPD: from pharmacological to instrumental therapies. *Eur Respir Rev* 2010; 19: 115, 7-23

[102] Tsoumakidou M, Tzanakis N, Voulgaraki O, Mitrouska I, Chrysofakis G, Samiou M, Siafakas NM. Is there any correlation between the ATS, BTS, ERS and GOLD COPD's severity scales and the frequency of hospital admissions? *Respir Med* 2004; 98: 178-83

[103] Sin DD, McAlister FA, Man SF, Anthonisen NR. Contemporary management of chronic obstructive pulmonary disease: scientific review. *JAMA* 2003; 290: 2301-12

[104] Quon BS, Gan WQ, Sin DD. Contemporary management of acute exacerbations of COPD: a systematic review and meta-analysis. *Chest* 2008; 133: 756-766

[105] Rafii R, Albertson TE, Louie S, Chan AL. Update on pharmaceutical and minimally invasive management strategies for chronic obstructive pulmonary disease. *Pulm Med* 2011; 2011: 257496

[106] Wilt TJ, Niewoehner D, MacDonald R, Kane RL. Management of stable chronic obstructive pulmonary disease: a systematic review for a clinical practice guideline. *Ann Int Med* 2007; 147: 639-53

[107] Stoller JK, Panos RJ, Krachman S, Doherty DE, Make B; Long-term Oxygen Treatment Trial Research Group. Oxygen therapy for patients with COPD: current evidence and the long-term oxygen treatment trial. *Chest* 2010; 138: 179-87

[108] Berry CE, Wise RA. Mortality in COPD: causes, risk factors, and prevention. *COPD* 2010; 7: 375-82

[109] Bosse G, Schmidbauer W, Spies CD, Sörensen M, Francis RC, Bubser F, Krebs M, Kerner T. Adherence to Guideline-based Standard Operating Procedures in Pre-hospital Emergency Patients with Chronic Obstructive Pulmonary Disease. *J Int Med Res* 2011; 39: 267-76

[110] Sin DD, Man SF. Corticosteroids and adrenoceptor agonists: the compliments for combination therapy in chronic airways diseases. *Eur J Pharmacol* 2006; 533: 28-35

[111] Schachter EN. New β_2-adrenoceptor agonists for the treatment of chronic obstructive pulmonary disease. *Drugs Today (Barc)* 2010; 46: 911-8

[112] Brusasco V, Crimi E. Airway Inflammation in COPD: Friend or Foe? *Am J Respir Crit Care Med* 2007; 176: 425-429

[113] Brightling CE, McKenna S, Hargadon B, et al. Sputum eosinophilia and the short term response to inhaled mometasone in chronic obstructive pulmonary disease. *Thorax* 2005; 60: 193-198

[114] Brightling CE, Wasrd R, Parker D, Morgan MD, Wardlwa AJ, Pavord AD. Sputum eosinophilia and short-term response to prednisolone in chronic obstructive pulmonary disease: A randomised control trial. *Lancet* 2000; 356:1480-1485

[115] Berry M, Parker D, Monteiro W, Pavord ID, *et al.* Sputum eosinophilia and the short term response to inhaled mometasone in chronic obstructive pulmonary disease. *Thorax* 2005; 60: 193-198

[116] Brightling CE, McKenna S, Hargadon B, Birring S, Green R, Siva R, Berry M, Parker D, Monteiro W, Pavord ID, *et al.* Sputum eosinophilia and the short term response to inhaled mometasone in chronic obstructive pulmonary disease. *Thorax* 2005; 60: 193- 198

[117] Lim KG, Mottram C. The use of fraction of exhaled nitric oxide in pulmonary practice. *Chest* 2008; 133: 1232-42

[118] Barnes PJ, Dweik RA, Gelb AF, Gibson PG, George SC, Grasemann H, Pavord ID, Ratjen F, Silkoff PE, Taylor DR, Zamel N. Exhaled nitric oxide in pulmonary diseases: a comprehensive review. *Chest* 2010; 138: 682-92

[119] Buckley J, Birrell MA, Maher SA et al. EP4 receptor as a new target for bronchodilator therapy. Doi: 10.1136/thx.2010.158568

[120] Rabe KF. Update on roflumilast, a phosphodiesterase 4 inhibitor for the treatment of chronic obstructive pulmonary disease. *Br J Pharmacol* 2011; 163: 53-67

[121] Martorana PA, Beume R, Lucattelli M, Wollin L, Lungarella G. Roflumilast fully prevents emphysema in mice chronically exposed to cigarette smoke. *Am J Respir Crit Care Med* 2005; *172: 848-853*

[122] Grootendorst DC, Gauw SA, Verhoosel RM, et al. Reduction in sputum neutrophil and eosinophil numbers by the PDE4 inhibitor roflumilast in patients with COPD. *Thorax* 2007; 62:1081-1087

[123] Grootendorst DC, Gauw SA, Verhoosel RM, et al. Reduction in sputum neutrophil and eosinophil numbers by the PDE4 inhibitor roflumilast in patients with COPD. *Thorax* 2007; 62: 1081-1087

[124] Vestbo J, Tan L, Atkinson G, Ward J; UK-500,001 Global Study Team. A controlled trial of 6-weeks' treatment with a novel inhaled phosphodiesterase type-4 inhibitor in COPD. *Eur Respir J* 2009; 33:1039-44

[125] Fabbri LM, Calverley PM, Izquierdo-Alonso JL, Bundschuh DS, Brose M, Martinez FJ, Rabe KF. Roflumilast in moderate-to-severe chronic obstructive pulmonary disease treated with long acting bronchodilators: two randomised clinical trials. *Lancet* 2009; 374: 695-703

[126] Bateman ED, Rabe KF, Calverley PM, Goehring UM, Brose M, Bredenbröker D, Fabbri L. Roflumilast with long-acting {beta}2 agonists for COPD: influence of exacerbation history. *Eur Respir J* 2011 Jul 7 [Epub ahead of print]

[127] Donnelly LE, Rogers DF. Novel targets and drugs in inflammatory lung disease. *Curr Opin Pharmacol* 2008; 8: 219-21

[128] Hansel TT, Barnes PJ. New drugs for exacerbations of chronic obstructive pulmonary disease. *Lancet* 2009; 374: 744-55

[129] Barnes PJ. New treatments for chronic obstructive pulmonary disease. *Ann Ist Super Sanita* 2003; 39: 573-82

[130] Rubin BK, Henke MO. Immunomodulatory activity and effectiveness of macrolides in chronic airway disease. *Chest* 2004; 125: 70S-78S

[131] Dentener MA, Creutzberg EC, Pennings HJ, Rijkers GT, Mercken E, Wouters EF. Effect of infliximab on local and systemic inflammation in chronic obstructive pulmonary disease: a pilot study. *Respiration* 2008; 76: 275-82

[134] Van der Vaart H, Koeter GH, Postma DS, et al. First study of infliximab treatment in patients with chronic obstructive pulmonary disease. *Am J Respir Crit Care Med* 2005; 172: 465-469

[135] Rennard SI, Fogarty C, Kelsen S, et al. The safety and efficacy of infliximab in moderate to severe chronic obstructive pulmonary disease. *Am J Respir Crit Care Med* 2007; 175: 926-34

[136] Beeh, KM, Kornmann, O, Buhl, R, et al Neutrophil chemotactic activity of sputum from patients with COPD: role of interleukin 8 and leukotriene B_4. *Chest* 2003; 123: 1240-1247

[137] Nadel, JA Role of neutrophil elastase in hypersecretion during COPD exacerbations, and proposed therapies. *Chest* 2000; 117: 386S-389S

[138] Mahler DA, Huang S, Tabrizi M, Bell GM. Efficacy and safety of a monoclonal antibody recognizing interleukin-8 in COPD: a pilot study. *Chest* 2004; 126: 926-934

[139] Dwyer MP, Yu Y, Chao J, et al. Discovery of 2-Hydroxy-N,N-dimethyl-3- {2- [[(R)-1-(5-methylfuran-2-yl)propyl]amino]-3,4-dioxocyclobut-1 enylamino} benzamide (SCH 527123): A Potent, Orally Bioavailable CXCR2/CXCR1 Receptor Antagonist. *J Med Chem* 2006; 49: 7603-7606

[140] Nicholson GC, Tennant RC, Carpenter DC, et al. A novel flow cytometric assay of human whole blood neutrophil and monocyte CD11b levels: upregulation by chemokines is related to receptor expression, comparison with neutrophil shape change, and effects of a chemokine receptor (CXCR2) antagonist. *Pulm Pharmacol Ther* 2007; 20: 52-59

[141] Capelli A, Di Stefano A, Gnemmi I, et al. Increased MCP-1 and MIP- 1beta in bronchoalveolar lavage fluid of chronic bronchitics. *Eur Respir J* 1999; 14: 160-165

[142] Butora G, Morriello GJ, Kothandaraman S, et al. 4-Amino-2-alkyl-butyramides as small molecule CCR2 antagonists with favorable pharmacokinetic properties. *Bioorg Med Chem Lett* 2006; 16: 4715-4722

[143] Pasternak A, Marino D, Vicario PP, et al. Novel, orally bioavailable gamma-aminoamide CC chemokine receptor 2 (CCR2) antagonists. *J Med Chem* 2006; 49: 4801-4804

[144] Snelgrove RJ. Leukotriene A4 hydrolase: an anti-inflammatory role for a proinflammatory enzyme. *Thorax* 2011; 66: 550-1

[145] Gompertz S, Stockley RA. A randomized, placebo-controlled trial of a leukotriene synthesis inhibitor in patients with COPD. *Chest* 2002; 122: 289-294

[146] Kilfeather S. 5-Lipoxygenase Inhibitors for the Treatment of COPD. *Chest* 2002; 121; 197S-200S

[147] Woodruff PG, Albert RK, Bailey WC, Casaburi R, *et al*. Randomized trial of zileuton for treatment of COPD exacerbations requiring hospitalization. *COPD* 2011; 8:21-9

[148] Stav D, Raz M: Effect of N-acetylcysteine on air trapping in COPD: a randomized placebo-controlled study. *Chest* 2009, 136: 381-386

[149] Bandarupalli U M, Williams G D. Recently published papers: Novel therapies in chronic obstructive pulmonary disease, cardiac chemicals and intensive care outcomes. *Critical Care* 2009; 13: 198

[150] Stav D, Raz M. Effect of N-acetylcysteine on air trapping in COPD: a randomized placebo-controlled study. *Chest* 2009; 136: 381-6

[151] Drost E, Lannan S, Bridgeman MME, *et al*. Lack of effect of *N*-acetylcysteine on the release of oxygen radicals from neutrophils and alveolar macrophages. *Eur Respir J 1991;* 4*:* 723-729

[152] Kumar S, Boehm J, Lee JC. p38 MAP kinases: key signalling molecules as therapeutic targets for inflammatory diseases. Nat Rev Drug Discov 2003; 2:717–726

[153] Renda T, Baraldo S, Pelaia G, et al. Increased activation of p38 MAPK in COPD. *Eur Respir J* 2008; 31: 62-69

[154] Medicherla S, Fitzgerald M, Spicer D, et al. p38a selective MAP kinase inhibitor, SD-282, reduces inflammation in a sub-chronic model of tobacco smoke-induced airway inflammation. *J Pharmacol Exp Ther* 2007; 324: 921-929

[155] Smith SJ, Fenwick PS, Nicholson AG, et al. Inhibitory effect of p38 mitogen- activated protein kinase inhibitors on cytokine release from human macrophages. *Br J Pharmacol* 2006; 149: 393-404

[156] Armstrong J, Harbron C, Lea S, Booth G, Cadden P, Wreggett K, Singh D. Synergistic effects of p38 MAPK inhibition with a corticosteroid in alveolar macrophages from COPD patients. *JPET* 2011

[157] Singh D, Smyth L, Borrill Z, Sweeney L, Tal-Singer R. A Randomized, Placebo-Controlled Study of the Effects of the p38 MAPK Inhibitor SB-681323 on Blood Biomarkers of Inflammation in COPD Patients *J Clin Pharmacol* 2010; 50: 94-100

[158] Baldwin AS Jr. The NF-kappa B and I kappa B proteins: new discoveries and insights. *Annu Rev Immunol* 1996; 14: 649-683

[159] Auphan N, DiDonato JA, Rosette C, et al. Immunosuppression by glucocorticoids: inhibition of NFkappa B activity through induction of kappa B synthesis. *Science* 1995; 270: 286-290

[160] Jazrawi E, Cosio BG, Barnes PJ, et al. Inhibition of IKK2 and JNK differentially regulates GM-CSF and IL-8 release in epithelial cells and alveolar macrophages. *Am J Respir Crit Care Med* 2003; 167: A798
[161] Thomas MJ, Smith A, Head DH, et al. Airway inflammation: chemokine- induced neutrophilia and the class I phosphoinositide 3-kinases. *Eur J Immunol* 2005; 35:1283- 1291
[162] -To Y, Ito K, Kizawa Y, Failla M, Ito M, Kusama T, Elliott W M, Hogg J C, Adcock I M, Barnes P J Targeting Phosphoinositide-3-Kinase-δ with Theophylline Reverses *Am J Respir Crit Care Med* 2010; 182: 897-904
[163] Ito K, Yamamura S, Essilfie-Quaye S, et al. Histone deacetylase 2- mediated deacetylation of the glucocorticoid receptor enables NF-kappaB suppression. *J Exp Med* 2006; 203:7-13
[164] Edwards PD, Andisik DW, Bryant CA, et al. Discovery and biological activity of orally active peptidyl trifluoromethyl ketone inhibitors of human neutrophil elastase. *J Med Chem* 1997; 40: 1876-1885
[165] Ferry G, Lonchampt M, Pennel L, et al. Activation of MMP-9 by neutrophil elastase in an in vivo model of acute lung injury. *FEBS Lett* 1997; 402: 111-115
[166] Iwata K, Doi A, Ohji G, Oka H, Oba Y, Takimoto K, Igarashi W, Gremillion DH, Shimada T. Effect of neutrophil elastase inhibitor (sivelestat sodium) in the treatment of acute lung injury (ALI) and acute respiratory distress syndrome (ARDS): a systematic review and meta-analysis. Intern Med 2010; 49: 2423-32
[167] Belvisi MG, Bottomley KM. The role of matrix metalloproteinases (MMPs) in the pathophysiology of chronic obstructive pulmonary disease (COPD): a therapeutic role for inhibitors of MMPs? *Inflamm Res* 2003; 52: 95-100
[168] Magnussen H, Watz H, Kirsten A, Wang M, Wray H, Samuelsson V, Mo J, Kay R. Safety and tolerability of an oral MMP-9 and -12 inhibitor, AZD1236, in patients with moderate- to-severe COPD: A randomised controlled 6-week trial. *Pulm Pharmacol Ther* 2011 May 23. [Epub ahead of print]
[169] de Ruijter AJ, van Gennip AH, Caron HN, Kemp S, van Kuilenburg AB. Histone deacetylases (HDACs): characterization of the classical HDAC family. Biochem J 2003;370:737-749
[170] Ito K, Barnes PJ, Adcock IM. Glucocorticoid receptor recruitment of histone deacetylase 2 inhibits interleukin-1 beta-induced histone H4 acetylation on lysines 8 and 12. Mol Cell Biol 2000;20:6891-6903
[171] Ito K, Ito M, Elliott W M, Cosio B, Caramori G, Kon O M, Barczyk A Hayashi, S, Adcock I M, Hogg J C, Barnes P J. Decreased Histone Deacetylase Activity in Chronic Obstructive Pulmonary Disease. N Engl J Med 2005; 352: 1967-1976
[172] Rahman I, Marwick J, Kirkham P. Redox modulation of chromatin remodeling: impact on histone acetylation and deacetylation, NF-kappaB and pro-inflammatory gene expression. *Biochem Pharmacol* 2004; 68: 1255-1267
[173] Cosio BG, Tsaprouni L, Ito K, et al. Theophylline restores histone deacetylase activity and steroid responses in COPD macrophages. *J Exp Med* 2004; 200: 689-695
[174] Saraiva-Romanholo BM, Barnabé V, Carvalho AL, Martins MA, Saldiva PH, Nunes Mdo P. Comparison of three methods for differential cell count in induced sputum. *Chest* 2003; 124: 1060-1066

[175] He Z-Y, Ou L-M, Zhang J-Q, Bai J, Liu G-N, *et al*. Effect of 6 months of erythromycin treatment on inflammatory cells in induced sputum and exacerbations in chronic obstructive pulmonary disease. *Respiration* 2010; 80: 445-452

[176] van Eeden SF, Sin DD: Chronic obstructive pulmonary disease: a chronic systemic inflammatory disease. *Respiration* 2008; 75: 224-238

[177] Giamarellos-Bourboulis EJ: Macrolides beyond the conventional antimicrobials: a class of potent immunomodulators. *Int J Antimicrob Agents* 2008; 31: 12-20

[178] Patel IS, Seemungal TA, Wilks M, Lloyd-Owen SJ, Donaldson GC, Wedzicha JA: Relationship between bacterial colonisation and the frequency, character, and severity of COPD exacerbations. *Thorax* 2002; 57: 759-764

[179] Sethi S, Murphy TF: Infection in the pathogenesis and course of chronic obstructive pulmonary disease. *N Engl J Med* 2008; 359: 2355-2365

[180] Kunisaki KN, Niewoehner DE. Antibiotic prophylaxis for chronic obstructive pulmonary disease. Resurrecting an old idea. *Am JRespir Crit Care Med* 2008; 178: 1098-1099

[181] Clini EM, Ambrosino N. Nonpharmacological treatment and relief of symptoms in COPD. *Eur Respir J* 2008; 32: 218-28

[182] Kuzma AM, Meli Y, Meldrum C, Jellen P, Butler-Lebair M, Koczen-Doyle D, Rising P, Stavrolakes K, Brogan F. Multidisciplinary care of the patient with chronic obstructive pulmonary disease. *Proc Am Thorac Soc* 2008 1; 5: 567-71

[183] Soriano J.B, Zieliński J, Price D. Screening for and early detection of obstructive pulmonary disease. *Lancet* 2009; 374: 721-732

[184] Feary JR, Rodrigues LC, Smith CJ, Hubbard RB, Gibson JE. Prevalence of major comorbidities in subjects with COPD and incidence of myocardial infarction and stroke: a comprehensive analysis using data from primary care. *Thorax* 2010; 65: 956-6

[185] Rutgers SR, Postma DS, ten Hacken NH, et al. Ongoing airway inflammation in patients with COPD who do not currently smoke. *Thorax* 2000; 55: 12-18

[186] Verrills NM, Irwin JA, Yan He X, Wood LG, Powell H, Simpson JL, McDonald VM, Sim A, Gibson PG. Identification of novel diagnostic biomarkers for asthma and chronic obstructive pulmonary disease. *Am J Respir Crit Care Med* 2011; 183: 1633-4

[187] Lacoma A, Prat C, Andreo F, Domínguez J. Biomarkers in the management of COPD. *Eur Respir Rev* 2009; 18: 96-104

17

Ocular Involvement in Behçet's Disease

Yonca Aydın Akova and Sirel Gür Güngör
Başkent University Faculty of Medicine
Department of Ophthalmology
Turkey

1. Introduction

Behçet's disease (BD) is a chronic, relapsing inflammatory disorder of unknown etiology and characterized by obstructive vasculitis. It can involve both the arteries and veins of almost any organ and characterized by recurrent oral and genital aphthous ulcers, ocular inflammation, and skin lesions. Behçet's disease frequently involves the joints, the central nervous system, and the gastrointestinal tract as well. Behçet's disease may be the best example of a disorder characterized mainly by its retinal vascular involvement, often with devastating results on the patient's eyesight.

First description of BD has been attributed to Hippocrates in the 5th century BC, in the "Third book of endemic diseases" (Nussenblatt, 2010). In 1937, Hulusi Behçet (1889-1948), a Turkish dermatologist (Behçet, 1937), reported three patients with a triad of symptoms: recurrent intraocular inflammatory episodes with oral and genital ulcerations.

2. Epidemiology

2.1 Geographic and ethnic distribution

Behçet's disease is most common in the countries of the Eastern Mediterranean and in the Eastern rim of Asia, and is very frequently noted between 30^0 and 45^0 north latitude in Asian and European populations, which corresponds to the old Silk Route used by traders from the East to Europe (Ohno, 1986). The exact incidence, prevalence, and family occurrence of the disease are not well known. The highest prevalence being 80-420 cases per 100000 populations in Turkey has been reported (Azizlerli et al., 2003; Yazici, 1994; Yurdakul et al, 1988).

2.2 Sex

Many reports, mainly from Mediterranean basin and the Far East, have shown a preponderance of males to females in BD. Data have shown that men predominate in Japan (2:1), Lebanon (11:1), Greece (7.9:1), Egypt (5:1), Isreal (3:1), Turkey (3:1) and Iran (1.2:1), whereas women predominate in Germany (1:0,9), Brazil (1:0.7), and the United States (1:0.2) (Atmaca, 1989; Chajec & Fainaru, 1975; Hamdi & Abdalla, 1974; Mamo & Baghdassarian, 1964; Ozdal et al., 2002; Shimuzu, 1971).

2.3 Age

Although BD effects primarily young adults more frequently between the second and fourth decade of life and is rarely seen in children, the onset can occur at any age from infants to the elderly (Ghate et al., 1999; Kone-Paut et al., 1998; Önder & Gürer, 2000; Tugal-Tutkun et al., 2004).

2.4 Heredity

Familial occurrence is seen in 8-18 % of Turkish patients with the disease (Onal et al., 2001), 15% of Koreans, 13% of Jews, and 2.6% of Chinese (Fietta, 2005). Additionally, several familial cases (Dundar et al, 1985; Vaiopoulus et al., 1996; Villanueva et al., 1993) and a pair of monozygotic brothers (Hamuryudan et al., 1991) concordant for the disease have been reported, but no consistent inheritance pattern has been confirmed.

3. Clinical features

The diagnosis of BD is based firmly on the presence of a set of clinical findings. The diagnostic criteria were first described in 1969 by Mason & Barnes (Mason & Barnes, 1969). Numerous sets of clinical criteria have been proposed for the diagnosis of BD (O' Duffy, 1974; Zhang, 1980).

The most popular diagnostic system has been suggested by the Behçet's Research Committee of Japan in 1974 (Behçet's Disease Research Committee of Japan, 1974) (Table 1). The committee has revised the diagnostic criteria in 2003 (Kurokawa & Suzuki, 2004). The presence of ocular inflammation is given greater weight in the diagnosis in this system.

Main symptoms: 1-Recurrent aphtous ulcers on oral mucosa; 2-Skin lesions (erythema nodosum, subcutaneous thrombophlebitis, follicular papules, acneiform papules, skin hypersensitivity); 3-Ocular lesions (anterior and/or posterior uveitis); 4-Genital ulcers **Additional symptoms: 1-**Arthritis without deformity or sclerosis; 2-Epididymitis; 3-Gastrointestinal lesion (Ileocecal ulceration); 4-Vascular lesions; 5-Central nervous system lesions *Criteria for diagnosis of disease types:* **Complete type:** Four main symptoms **Incomplete type:** Three of the main symptoms, or two main symptoms and two additional symptoms; typical ocular lesion and another main symptom, or two additional symptoms **BD suspected:** Some main symptoms appear, but the case does not meet the criteria for the incomplete type; typical additional symptom is recurrent or becomes more severe **Special lesions:** Gastrointestinal lesions (abdominal pain and occult blood) Vascular lesions (vasculitis of aorta, artery, large or small veins) Neuronal lesions (headache, paresis, lesions of brain and spinal cord, mental symptoms) *Laboratory data:* 1-Negative or positive pathergy test; 2-Negative or positive prick test for vaccine for streptococci; 3-Inflammatory responses (increase of erythrocyte sedimentation rate, C-reactive protein positive, neutrophilia, increase in complement activity)

Table 1. Revised Diagnostic Criteria proposed by the Behçet's Disease Research Committee of Japan in 2003 (Kurokawa & Suzuki, 2004).

The diagnostic system that has been suggested by the International Study Group by Behçet's Disease (International Study Group for Behçet's Disease, 1990) requires the presence of oral ulceration in all patients plus any 2 of the following findings: genital ulceration, typically defined eye lesions, typically defined skin lesions, or a positive pathery test (Table 2).

Diagnostic criteria of International Study Group for Behçet's disease
RECURRENT ORAL ULCERATION
Minor or major aphthous lesions or herpetiform-like lesions observed by the physician or patient at least three times within a 12-month period.
PRESENCE OF TWO OTHER CRITERIA
Recurrent genital ulceration: Observation by the physician or patient of the aphthous ulceration or scar is required.
Eye lesions: The ocular disease can include anterior and/or posterior uveitis, cells in the vitreous, or the presence of a retinal vasculitis.
Skin lesions: These changes, noted by the physician or patient, include erythema nodosum, pseudofolliculitis, and papulopustular lesions. In addition, lesions would include an acneiform nodule in postadolescent patients not receiving corticosteroid therapy.
Positive pathergy test result: Read by physician at 24-48 hours.

Table 2. Modified from International Study Group for BD. Criteria for diagnosis of BD, Lancet 1990; 335:1078-1080.

3.1 Oral aphthous ulcers

The common clinical finding in Behçet's patients is the presence of recurrent mucocutaneous ulcers. Oral ulcerations are usually the initial symptom, occurring in 98% of the patients (Okada et al., 2004). They are painful, rounded, with surrounding erythema and pseudomembranous covering. The lesions are 3 to 15 mm in diameter and may occur in clusters. The lesions may be located anywhere in the oral cavity: the lips, gums, palate, tongue, uvula, and posterior pharynx. They usually heal in 7-10 days without scarring, but scarring occurs when a particularly large ulcer heal. The lesions may recur every 5 to 10 days, or every month, or even years apart without following any rule. The trauma to the oral mucosa can provoke them to appear strikingly reminiscent of the prick test (Wray et al., 1981) and the lesions can also occur in some individuals after eating certain type of foods.

3.2 Genital ulcers

Genital ulcers occur in 75 to 87% of the BD patients (Smith & Shur, 2005). Genital ulcers can occur on the scrotum or penis in males. In females they can appear on the vulva and vaginal mucosa (Bonfioli & Orefice, 2005). Such ulcers can also be found on the perianal areas. Vulvar lesions frequently occur premenstrually (Nussenblatt, 2010). Genital lesions can be deep or may scar as they heal. Thus an examination of the genital region in a patient with suspected BD can be useful as a sign of old disease may be present. The genital lesions may be more painful in males.

3.3 Skin lesions

Skin lesions occur in 75 to 87% of the patients (Smith & Shur, 2005). Erythema nodosum like painful and recurrent lesions are frequently noted on the anterior surface of the leg but can be also seen on the face, neck, buttocks, and elsewhere. These lesions involute without ulceration and scarring, in several weeks, but they may indeed leave scars.

Acne-like lesions or folliculitis are also common dermatologic lesions. They can appear on the back and face.

Forty present of patients with BD exhibit a cutaneous phenomenon termed pathergy, in which sterile pustules develop at sites of spontaneous or induced trauma (venipuncture, injection of sterile saline). This phenomenon is not pathognomonic of BD, although it is an important criterion that can be used for the diagnosis (International Study Group for Behçet's Disease, 1990). Dermatographia, another dermatologic phenomenon of cutaneous hypersensitivity, can also be found in one third to one half of the patients (Zafirakis & Foster, 2002).

3.4 Ocular involvement (Ocular Behçet's disese)

The frequency of ocular involvement in patients with BD is approximately 70%-90% (Atmaca, 1989; Mochizuki et al., 1996; Verity et al., 1999). The characteristic ocular involvement is a relapsing remitting panuveitis. Table 3 summarizes the ocular findings. The ocular disease manifests approximately in 2-3 years after the initial symptoms noted (Tugal-Tutkun et al., 2004). Morever, eye involvement may be the first presenting manifestation of BD in approximately 10% to 20 % of the patients (Dilsen et al., 1986). The mean age at onset of uveitis is around 30 years. Males are more frequently involved, had an earlier disease onset, and had a more severe disease. Ocular involvement in BD occurs more commonly and severely among Japanese and Turkish patients (Özen, 1999; Tugal-Tutkun et al., 2004; Tursen et al, 2003).

The frequency of bilateral involvement ranges between 78% and 95% in in most of the series (Atmaca, 1989; Barra et al., 1991; Mishima et al., 1979; Tugal-Tutkun et al., 2004). Bilateral but asymmetric ocular inflammation is a characteristic feature (Atmaca, 1989, Bhisitkul & Foster, 1996).

The ocular inflammatory episodes in BD are characteristically associated with a sudden severe onset of visual loss. Severity and number of repeated inflammatory attacks involving the posterior segment determine the extent of permanent structural changes and the resultant rate of irreversible visual loss. Because of that, Behçet panuveitis is a medical emergency, which must be treated immediately. Ocular involvement in patients with BD, especially posterior uveitis presence, is the primary indication of immunosuppressive treatment.

In 1970, Mamo reported that 90% of the untreated patients lost their vision over a mean period of 3.36 years (Mamo 1970). The severity of the visual loss is also correlated with the duration of the disease. Ben Ezra and Cohen (BenEzra & Cohen, 1986) reported that 74% of eyes lost useful visual acuity 6 to 10 years after the onset of uveitis despite intensive follow-up and treatment. In more recent studies, early and aggressive immunosuppressive treatment has been shown to reduce the rate of visual loss (Hamuryudan et al., 1997, Yazici & Ozyazgan, 1999, Kaklamani & Kaklamanis, 2001).

3.4.1 Anterior segment

Iridocyclitis may be isolated finding but is often generally is observed along with posterior- or panuveitis. The recurrent acute iridocyclitis attacks may persist for up to 2 to 3 months. However, the inflammation usually does not resolve completely between attacks. Mild to moderate blurred vision, periorbital pain, photophobia, redness, reactive miosis, and lacrimation occur during acute attacks of anterior uveitis.

Acute ciliary type of conjunctival vasodilatation and injection usually develops over a period of hours or days. In the slit lamp examination, there is an abundant number of floating cells and flare in the anterior chamber which indicates active inflammation. Small keratic precipitates may also be observed, typically in the lower corneal endothelium. The cells in the anterior chamber will move easily and slide over the corneal endothelium if the patient's head is tilted. After the cells have disappeared, persistent flare may ensue in the long standing cases, indicating persistent vascular damage rather than active inflammation that may not merit treatment. In a study from Turkey, which the laser cell flare meter was used and a large number of patients with BD were examined, it was suggested that those eyes with flare measured at ≥6 photons/s had a higher possibility of recurrence (Tugal-Tutkun et al., 2008).

The hypopyon may be a presentation of iridocyclitis which has been described as a characteristic sign. Mamo and Baghdassarian (Mamo & Baghdassarian, 1964) reported that hypopyon has become an uncommon finding, this apparent decline to the advent of steroid management in controlling inflammatory response. It was reported that hypopyon present only in about one-tenth (Tugal-Tutkun et al., 2004) to one-third of BD patients (Ohno et al., 1986; Mishima et al., 1979). However, the development of hypopyon may be provoked by local trauma such as cataract surgery (Kim et al., 2002, Matsuo et al., 2001) or sudden interruption of the treatment in patient with Behçet uveitis. The hypopyon may occur in other types of anterior uveitis but the hypopyon in patients with BD is typical that shifts with gravity as the patient changes his head position. The microhypopyon may not be visible to the naked eye but seen only with the slit lamp or in the angle when gonioscopic examination is performed, called as angle hypopyon.

When the disease is particularly severe and long-standing, cyclitic membranes can form, (Inomata et al., 2003). Peripheral anterior synechia, posterior synechia and iris atrophy may develop during the course of repeated ocular inflammatory attacks. The presence of peripheral anterior synechia or iris bombe from pupillary seclusion may lead to secondary glaucoma. Neovascularization of the iris and secondary glaucoma may occur as a result of posterior segment ischemia and neovascularization. It is also an ominous sign, a prognosticator of poor outcome.

Cellular infiltration also occurs in the anterior vitreous cavity behind the lens. Vitreal cells tend to have more restricted circulation when compared the anterior chamber as a result of viscosity of vitreous gel.

Cataract formation is not unusual, due to either the inflammation or the corticosteroid therapy in these patients. Other less frequent anterior segment findings are episcleritis, scleritis, conjonctivitis, subconjunctival hemorrhage, conjunctival ulcers, filamentary keratitis, and corneal immune ring opacity (Colvard et al., 1977; Dursun et al., 2004; Matsuo et al., 2002; Zamir et al., 2003).

3.4.2 Posterior segment

Posterior segment involvement is a poor prognostic sign of ocular BD and is seen in up to 93% of patients with ocular disease (Atmaca & Batıoglu, 1994). The ocular inflammatory episodes in BD are characteristically assosiciated with a sudden severe onset of visual loss that may gradually improve with remission. Recurrent attacks of posterior segment may lead to severe retinal damage and irreversible visual loss (Atmaca & Batıoglu, 1994).

The most common and universal posterior segment finding are vitritis and retinal perivasculitis involving both the arteries (periarteritis) and veins (periphlebitis). Active periphlebitis is characterized by a fluffy white haziness surrounding the vessel with patchy involvement and irregular outside extensions. Fluorescein angiography has been reported to reveal leakage from retinal vessels even in eyes without clinicallay detectable vasculitis (Atmaca, 1989). Vitritis is characterized by cellular infiltration and its products of the vitreous along with posterior segment involvement. Vitreous haze is usually severe and accompanied by serious posterior segment inflammation. The view of the fundus may be markedly obscured because of the vitreal haze.

Occlusive vasculitic attacks of the retina are the most commonly dreaded complication of posterior segment involvement. Examination of the retina will show areas of hemorrhage and infarction in the retina. If the occlusive vasculitic attack involves the macular region, the visual acuity will reduce.

The retinitis characterized by scattered superficial yellow-white solitary or multifocal infiltrates of the inner retina with indistinct margin, giving the retina a cloudy appearance with obstruction of the retinal vessels. The lesions are usually transient and heal without scarring. Massive deep retinal exudates involve the outer retinal layers and are associated with vascular obliteration. During the resolution of the posterior segment inflammation, that follows severe vitritis and vitreal haze, inflammatuar cells accumulate in the inferior preretinal area, resemble a pearl necklace.

During the active phase, generalized vascular leakage with diffuse retinal or optic disc edema, optic disc hyperemia, venous engorgement, and intraretinal hemorrhages may also be observed.

The most common complication of ocular BD is cystoid macular edema (CME), which observed in approximately in half of the patients with uveitis. It may resolve with appropriate treatment or if untreated progress to persistent chronic macular damage and sequel of CME, with structural changes after recurrences resulting in permanent visual loss. In some cases, it may lead to form a partial or full-thickness macular hole formation (Sheu & Yang, 2004). Macular ischemia due to occlusive vasculitis, scarring, degeneration with pigment epithelial changes, and epiretinal membrane formation may also occur (Yılmaz et al, 2000).

In incomplete treated patients, gliotic inflammatory vessel sheathing, retinal ischemia, retinal atrophy, and retinal tear may occur (Akova et al., 1999). Disc swelling, papillitis, optic atrophy and papilledema due to increased intracranial pressure and dural sinus occlusion are the optic disc findings. In some cases, neovascularization of the iris, retina, or optic disc may develop. Tugal Tutkun et al. reported that intraocular inflammation is more frequent cause of neovascularization of optic disc than retinal vascular occlusion (Tugal-Tutkun et al., 2006). Neovascularization may cause to vitreoretinal hemorrhage and tractional retinal detachment (Elgin et al., 2004; Ghate & Jorizzo, 1999; Lee, 2001; Nussenblatt, 1997).

At the end stage of the ocular disease, the repeated episodes of posterior segment inflammation and complications cause total optic atrophy, vascular attenuation, and sheathing with occluded and sclerozed vessels, diffuse retinal atrophy with variable chorioretinal pigmentation and scarring.

ANTERİOR SEGMENT: 1-Iridocyclitis ± hypopyon; 2-Secondary glaucoma; 3-Secondary cataract
Less frequent findings: 1-Episcleritis; 2-Scleritis; 3-Conjonctivitis; 4-Subconjunctival hemorrhage; 5-Conjunctival ulcers; 6-Filamentary keratitis; 7-Corneal immune ring opacity
POSTERİOR SEGMENT: 1-Vitritis; 2-Retinal perivasculitis; 3-Retinal hemorrhage and infarction due to occlusive vasculitic attacks; 4-Retinitis; 5-Diffuse retinal or optic disc edema; 6-Optic disc hyperemia; 7-Venous engorgement; 8-Cystoid macular edema; 9-Macular ischemia; 10-Macular scarring; 11-Pigment epithelial changes; 12-Epiretinal membrane formation
In incomplete treated patients: 1-Vessel sheathing; 2-Retinal ischemia; 3-Retinal atrophy; 4-Retinal tear; 5-Disc swelling; 6-Papillitis; 7-Optic atrophy; 8-Papilledema; 9-Neovascularization of the iris, retina, or optic disc; 10-Vitreoretinal hemorrhage; 11-Tractional retinal detachment
End stage ocular disease: 1-Optic atrophy; 2-Vascular attenuation and sheathing; 3-Diffuse retinal atrophy

Table 3. The ocular findings.

4. Behçet's disease in children

According to a French nationwide survey in 1993, the estimated prevalence of Behçet's disease in children younger than 15 years of age is one in 600,000 (Kone-Paut et al., 1998). In a more recent study reviewing 761 patients in Turkey, almost 57% of patients with an identifiable diagnosis had BD, with being 10.4% juvenile onset disease (Kazokoglu et al., 2008).

In pediatric uveitis series, the incidence of Behçet's disease has been reported to be 0.5% to 2.2% in countries where the disease is uncommon (Kanski & Shun-Shin, 1984; Pivetti-Pezzi, 1996; Tugal-Tutkun et al., 1996). By comparison, in a study from Turkey, Soylu et al. reported that 11% of children with uveitis had juvenile onset of BD (Soylu et al., 1997).

The study by Tugal -Tutkun from Turkey involving 36 pediatric cases with BD reported that the male patients outnumbered female patients by a ratio of 2.3 to 1. Onset of uveitis was in late childhood. Bilateral panuveitis with retinal vasculitis and retinal infiltrates was the typical presentation. Uveitis was the initial manifestation of the disease in only 8.3% of the patients (Tugal-Tutkun & Urgancıoğlu, 2003).

5. Pathogenesis

The cause of BD is uncommon. It is believed to be due to an autoimmune process triggered by an infectious or environmental agent in a genetically predisposed individual (Pay, 2007; Kulaber, 2007).

5.1 Genetics and human leukocyte antigen (HLA) typing

The sibling ratio has been reported as 11.4-52.5% by Gül et al. Although environmental factors shared by families can influence familiar clustering they cannot account for this risk ratio, which supports a strong genetic background in BD (Gül et al, 2000).

HLA-B51 allele located in the MHC (major histocompatibilty complex) locus, on chromosome 6p has been the most strongly associated risk factor for BD in areas along the Old Silk Route, with a stronger association in Turkish and Japanese patients in comparison to Caucasians (Verity et al, 1999).

On the other hand, HLA-DR1 and HLA-DQw1 have been shown to be significantly decreased in patients with BD. This may indicate that an individual who carries these antigens is resistant to develop the disease. These results suggest that not only disease susceptibility but also resistant genes play an important role in the immunogenetic mechanism of BD (Numaga et al., 1988).

5.2 Environment (Infectious agents, heat shock proteins) and self-antigens

Individuals from endemic areas who have immigrated to areas with low prevalence of the disease have an intermediate risk for developing the disease, which suggest that environment, has some role in development of BD (Sakane et al., 1999, Zouboulis et al., 1997).

Several microorganisms have been implicated in the pathology of BD, especially *herpes simplex virus-1* and *Streptococcus sangius* (Direskeneli, 2001; Lehner, 1997; Verity et al, 1999).

5.3 Immunohistopathology

Immunohistopathologic studies of specimens taken from active inflammatory sites of BD patient support the findings of those found in the peripheral blood and indicate immune-complex mediated disease. Necrotizing, neutrophilic (leukocytoclastic) obliterative perivasculitis (phlebitis) and venous thrombosis with lymphocytic and monocytic cellular infiltration of veins, capillaries and the arteries of all sizes, with and without fibrin deposition in the vessel wall, is the hallmark of BD (George et al., 1997).

6. Diagnosis

There is no pathognomonic or sensitive test and histopathologic finding in BD. Therefore, it is mainly diagnosed on the clinical grounds alone and currently relies on the recognition and grouping together of sufficient clinical features in a patient. The criteria defined either by the International Study Group of Behçet's Disease or the Japanese Research Committee of Behçet's Disease is the most commonly used criteria. Although the clinical diagnosis, some tests may be helpful for evaluation and diagnosis of BD.

6.1 Fundus fluorescein angiography and indocyanine green angiography

Fluorescein angiography and indocyanin green angiography (ICG) can provide diagnostic clues and may be used in the follow-up of cases with Behçet uveitis (Matsuo et al., 1999).Vasculitic ocular changes in BD have been investigated in depth using FA. This technique can reveal dye leakage from retinal arteries, veins, and capillaries and also provides useful information about retinal vasculature. Fluorescein angiography is demonstrative of the retinal vasculitic lesions and reveals perivascular staining of the retina with vascular dye leakage of the dilated retinal capillaries during the acute stage, inflammation, and occlusion of the retinal vessels, even before ophthalmologic signs of detectable retinal perivasculitis clinically appear. The most characteristic fluorescein angiographic signs of Behçet's uveitis are extensive leakage from small and large retinal and optic nerve vessels during early phases and staining in the late phases of the FA.

Eearly and profuse leakage from the optic nerve head during the early phase may be observed and in advanced cases, neovascularization on the optic disc and elsewhere may also be present. In some cases, the neovascularization on the optic disc and elsewhere may be overlooked during the fundus examination and it can be exposed in FA.
Macular alterations including macular ischemia, cystoid macular edema, macular hole and epiretinal membrane can be seen by FA. Cyctoid macular edeme may be distinguished as typical late phase-pooling within the cyctic spaces with a foveal patalloid pattern.
Atmaca reported that FA disclosed vasculitic changes in 6.3% of BD patients who had no abnormal finding on fundus examination (Atmaca, 1989). Fluorescein angiography is very important in the study and longitudinal care of patients with ocular BD.
Fluorescein angiography does not provide adequate information about choroidal circulation. Indocyanine green angiography may be superior to FA by showing hyper- and hypo-fluorescent lesions, choroidal vessel leakage, irregular filling of the choriocapillaris and choriodal filling defects (Gedik et al., 2005). The ICG angiography findings described in the literature include optic disc hyperfluorescence, segmental staining of the retinal and choroidal vessels, choroidal fuzziness and hyperfluorescence, delayed perfusion of choriocapillaries, hypofluorescent plaques, and hyperfluorescent spots (Bozzoni-Pantaleoni et al., 2001; Klaeger et al., 2000).

6.2 Ocular tests

Optical coherence tomography may be useful in detecting and monitoring the foveal thickness anatomically in BD patients with CME. The laser cell flare meter may be used in Behçet uveitis since eyes with flare measurements is related with a higher possibility of recurrence (Tugal-Tutkun et al., 2008).

6.3 Serologic studies

The erythrocyte sedimentation rate, C-reactive protein, and other acute-phase reactants, such as properdin factor b and α1-acid glycoprotein, may be shown elevated during the acute phase of BD (Özoran et al., 1996). An elevation in the level of β2-microglobulin (Aygündüz et al., 2002) and myeloperoxidase (Accardo-Palumbo et al., 2000), generated by activated neutrophils, have been reported. Serum levels of several cytokines, including TNF-α, IFN-γ, IL-1β, IL-6, IL-8 may be also elevated.

7. Treatment

The primary goals of management are symptom control, early suppression of inflammation and prevention of end-organ damage. Even though therapy of acute disease is essential, to prevent or at least to decrease the number of repetitive ocular and systemic inflammatory episodes is important. Drugs are frequently used in combination in order to maximize the efficacy while minimizing side effects. The choice of medication is based on the severity of the disease. In general, treatment should be more aggressive whenever the following are present: complete BD, involvement of CNS, vascular involvement, retinal and bilateral involvement, male sex, and a geographic origin as the Mediterranean basin or Far East (Mishima et al., 1979).
In general, the duration of treatment should be at least 6 months followed by a close monitoring of possible relapse afterwards; tough treatment courses may need to span a

number of years. Many treatment modalities have been tried in ocular BD with varying claims of success. For the time being, the most commonly used agents are corticosteroids, cytotoxic drugs, colchicine, Cyc-A and tacrolimus (FK-506). Table 4 summarizes the treatment modalities.

7.1 Corticosteroids

Systemic or topical corticosteroids have a beneficial effect on the acute ocular inflammation of BD but their long term use is limited as a result of significant side effects, which requires the simultaneous use of other is drugs.

The application principal of corticosteroids, by whatever route, should initially be given at a large dose, and then tapered as quickly as possible over several weeks once the inflammation comes under control. Because of the inflammation may recur in reduction period, the corticosteroid treatment may be continued in a small dose for a long period.

7.1.1 Topical corticosteroids for ocular disease

Similar to other types of uveitis, in Behçet uveitis, strong steroids (prednisolone 1%, dexamethasone 0.1%, betamethasone) should be preferred to weaker ones. Since the solutions penetrates the cornea better than the suspensions or ointment, during the day the solutions should be preferred. The ointments may be used at bedtime.

Topical short-acting mydriatic and cycloplegic agents (e.g., tropicamide 1%, or cyclopentolate 1%) along with sympathomimetics such as phenylephrine 2.5-10% should simultaneously added to local corticosteroids to prevent photophobia and pain by relieving the spasm of the ciliary muscle and pupillary sphincter, thus promoting patient comfort. Additionally, these agents also prevent the development of new posterior synechia formation in cases with iridocyclitis.

7.1.2 Periocular corticosteroid injections

In severe anterior uveitis and hypopyon unresponsive to frequent topical ophthalmic drops, periocular route (subconjunctival, anterior parabulbar sub-Tenon capsule, or trans-septal orbital floor injections) can also be effective. Water soluble preparations (methylprednisolone sodium succinate), which diffuse from the depot more rapidly, are short-acting, even when steroids with a prolonged biological $t^{1/2}$ (dexamethasone sodium phosphate are used.

Acute attacks of vitritis, intermediate uveitis, CME, and mild posterior uveitis, especially if unilateral, can be treated with posterior parabulbar sun-Tenon capsule corticosteroid injections (under topical anesthesia) with or without systemic administration. Depot agents should be preferred such as triamcinolone acetonide or methylprednisolone acetate to achieve long-lasting effect.

7.1.3 Intravitreal corticosteroid injection

The intravitreal triamcinolone acetonide injection may be used as an adjunctive therapy for the treatment of panuveitis attacks and CME in patients with BD who are unresponsive or intolerant to systemic medications.

Sustained release intravitreal implants, including the fluocinolone acetonide implant and dexamethasone drug delivery system, offer an alternative therapy for chronic, recalcitrant posterior uveitis and CME. Studies in CME developed in retinal vein occlusion show promising results that this treatment options may be effective in uveitis associated CME (Coscas et al., 2011; Haller JA et al., 2010).

7.1.4 Systemic corticosteroids for ocular Behçet's disease

Acute and severe disease exacerbations of anterior uveitis, posterior, or panuveitis should be treated with higher dosages of systemic corticosteroid to offer a rapid response. Oral prednisolone 1-2 mg/kg/day given in a single morning dose after meals or intravenous pulse methylprednisolone 1 g/day for 3 consecutive days is preferred in concurrence with calcineurin inhibitors or other immunosuppressive drugs as steroid-sparing agents (Kaklamani & Kaklamanis, 2001, Toker et al., 2002). After remission of the disease has been obtained, it is gradually tapered to the maintenance dosage of 5-10 mg daily. Although oral corticosteroid monotherapy has palliative effect on ocular attacks, long-term treatment should be avoided since especially in patients with posterior segment involvement, it does not improve the visual prognosis and does not prevent the recurrent attacks of inflammation (Tugal-Tutkun et al, 2004).

7.2 Antimetabolites

7.2.1 Azathioprine

In a large randomized, placebo-controlled trial, azathioprine 2.5 mg/kg/day in a dosage reduced the incidence, frequency, and severity of eye disease (Yazıcı et al., 1990). Early treatment with azathioprine is effective in controlling the attacks of posterior ocular inflammation and vasculitis, preventing recurrences, and improving the long-term visual prognosis of the disease (Greenwood et al., 1998; Nussenblatt, 1997).

7.2.2 Mycophenolate mofetil

Initial evidence for mycophenolate mofetil's efficacy has been reported in animal models of ocular inflammation (Chanaud et al, 1995; Dick et al, 1998). Previous literature on mycophenolate mofetil in patients with ocular inflammation, including patients with BD, consists of prospective pilot studies in refractory uveitis (Kilmartin et al., 1998; Larkin G & Lightman 1999; Zierhut et al., 2001) and retrospective case series (Baltatzis et al., 2003; Choudhary et al., 2006; Doycheva et al., 2007; Greiner et al., 2002; Lau et al., 2003; Siepmann et al., 2006; Thorne et al., 2005). This relatively large series makes a significant contribution to the literature on mycophenolate mofetil therapy for uveitis and confirms that mycophenolate mofetil is both effective and well tolerated. Additionally, it was reported that mycophenolate mofetil is an effective agent also in the treatment for uveitis in children, with marked steroid-sparing potential and an acceptable side effect profile (Doycheva et al. 2007).

There is not a prospective study on mycophenolate mofetil in patients with Behçet uveitis. Since mycophenolate mofetil is effective in the other type of uveitis, it may be suggested that this agent is cures Behçet uveitis.

7.3 Calcineurin inhibitors

7.3.1 Cyclosporine-A

Cyclosporin-A (5 mg/kg/day in 2 divided doses) is effective in the treatment in most of BD features, especially in posterior segment disease. Cyclosporine-A, when used in combination with corticosteroids, has a corticosteroid-sparing effect, permitting the use of lower dosages

of corticosteroids. In ocular disease, it has been shown to decrease the frequency and severity of acute uveitis most rapidly (Binder et al, 1987; Kaklamani & Kaklamanis, 2001) and combined therapy with azathioprine is more effective than monotherapy with a better outcome in ocular disease (Sakane & Takeno, 2000; Yazici, 2002; Yazici & Özyazgan, 1999). If combined therapy is applied, lesser dosage of both agents is possible.
Cyclosporine-A is a cytostatic agent, and therefore the inflammation may recur when the therapy is tapered or on withdrawn (rebound phenomenon). Because of that, patients generally need to continuous treatment for several years.

7.3.2 Tacrolimus

Tacrolimus (FK-506) has also been used to treat refractory posterior uveitis in BD with limited experience (PO 0.05-0.20 mg/kg/day b.i.d) (Kilmartin et al, 1998). In comparison with CycA, tacrolimus has different side effect profiles, which may be an important issue in the choice of this therapy (Tanabe, 2003). Tacrolimus is less frequently associated hyperlipidemia, hirsutizm, gingival hypertrophy, but it may induce diabetes mellitus (Marshall, 2004).

7.4 Alkylating agents

7.4.1 Chlorambucil

Chlorambucil was the first immunosuppressive drug to be used in patients with ocular BD (Zafirakis & Foster, 2002). The use of this agent is not preferred in Behçet uveitis since its side effects and slow acting characteristic. Tabbara (Tabbara, 1983) reported long term results with chlorambucil that were disappointing, with 755 of eyes in patients treated with chlorambucil as monotherapy having visual acuity of 20/200 or less. These results could be explained by the fact that chlorambucil, a slow acing agent, suppresses the immune system slowly, which would be a disadvantage, as rapid immunosuppression is usually desirable for BD patients.

7.4.2 Cyclophosphamide

Cyclophosphamide is even more toxic than chlorambucil and it should be reserved for very refractory sight-threatening ocular BD patients. Cyclophosphamide has been utilized widely in Japan with favorable results in controlling uveitis, preventing ocular attacks, and maintain good visual acuity for long periods in BD patients (Hijikata & Masuda, 1978). It has been shown that cyclophosphamide is superior to steroids in suppressing ocular inflammation in BD patients in the acute phase (Gills & Buckley, 1970; Oniki et al., 1976). Foster et al (Foster et al., 1991) have shown that both cyclophosphamide and chlorambucil were superior to Cyc-A in the management of the posterior segment manifestations of BD. In contrary, Ozyazgan et al reported (Ozyazgan et al., 1992) that intravenous cyclophosphamide was less effective than oral CycA, especially during the first 6 months of the treatment.

7.5 Current concepts

7.5.1 Interferon-α

Clinical trials on IFN-α have shown encouraging results in the treatment of severe refractory uveitis in BD combined with corticosteroid and immunosuppressive therapy. Initial treatment modalities and doses are ranging from three to nine million IU daily versus

thrice-a-week regimen, as well as duration of IFN-α2a administration and corticosteroid therapy tapering; vary widely, among reported studies.
Kötter et al demonstrated in their open-label prospective study that recombinant human IFN-α2a at a daily dosage of 6 million IU for at least 14 days is effective in ocular BD (Kötter et al., 2003), leading to significant improvement of visual acuity with complete remission of ocular retinal vasculitis in the majority of the patients. Sight-threatening ocular disease has responded to IFN-α2a in 92% of the cases.
Tugal-Tutkun et al. reported that IFN-α2a was effective for the treatment of Behçet's patients with NVD, who were treated with intensive anti-inflammatory drugs, conventional immunosuppressive treatment and retinal laser photocoagulation without success (Tugal - Tutkun et al., 2006).
Recently a retrospective report of IFN-α2a use in 7 children with corticosteroid dependent Behçet uveitis with clinical improvement was published, allowing corticosteroid dose reduction in 5 patients (Guillaume-Czitrom et al., 2007).

7.5.2 Anti-TNF-α biological agents

TNF-α is a fundamental cytokine in the establishment and maintenance of the inflammatory response. At present, there are 3 TNF-α inhibitors available: infliximab, are recombinant chimeric monoclonal antibody; adalimumab, a humanized monoclonal antibody; and the fusion protein human p75 TNF-α receptor IgG1 etanercept (Ehrlich, 1997).

7.5.2.1 Infliximab

Infliximab is a human-murine chimeric anti TNF IgG1 monoclonal antibody. It binds to human TNF-α and neutralized its activity (Saravanan & Hamilton, 2002).
In an open label trial by Tugal-Tutkun et al., they investigated the efficacy of infliximab in 13 BD patients with uveitis resistant the combination therapy of azathioprine, Cyc-A, and corticosteroids. Following 4 infusions of infliximab (5mg/kg) administrated at weeks 0, 2, 4, and 14, combined with azathioprine and corticosteroids, 4 patients remained attacks-free for 22 weeks. The mean number of uveitis attacks and daily corticosteroid doses were significantly lower during the infusion period than the previous-treatment period (Tugal-Tutkun et al, 2005).
In a recent study (Tabbara et al., 2008) the outcome of retinal vasculitis in BD treated with conventional immunosuppressive therapy (prednisone, azathioprine, cyclosporine, or methotrexate) was compared to ones treated with infliximab. The authors reported that infliximab (5mg/kg per infusion) induced a mean remission period of 17 months in BD compared to a mean remission period of 5 months in patients treated with conventional immunosuppressive agents. These results suggest that TNF-α blocking agent should be considered for the prevention of vision-threatening retinal vasculitis caused by BD. In this study 60% of the patients developed optic atrophy in the conventional therapy group compared to 30% in the infliximab group. Prevention of the optic nerve vasculitis by infliximab may be desirable in order to prevent optic atrophy.
Retinal vasculitis in BD requires multiple infliximab infusion. Relapses have been reported to occur with complete cessation of infliximab infusion (Tognon et al., 2007; Toubi et al., 2005). The clinical results obtained from these studies suggest that infiliximab is effective in suppressing the inflammatory episodes of retinal vasculitis and preserves visual function in BD patients. The exact dosage and frequency of infliximab therapy remain undetermined.

Treatment	**Effects**		**Side effects**	**Indications**
Corticosteroids	Inhibition of cyclo-oxygenase and lipo-oxygenase pathways. By inhibition of phospholipase A2, corticosteroids reduce arachidonic acid formation, and inhibit prostaglandins, leukotriens, and thromboxane.	Decreases lymphocyte migration and chemotaxis, circulating monocytes, macrophage activity, the levels of complement and interleukins. Broad and non-selective suppression of the immune system	Hypertension, hyperglycemia, weight gain, fluid retention, electrolyte disturbance, peptic ulcers, Cushing syndrome, osteoporosis, mental status changes and growth retardation in the pediatric group. Local side effects; secondary cataract and intraocular pressure elevation.	Acute ocular and systemic inflammation
Antimetabolites				
Azathioprine	Converted to – mercaptopurine which is converted to 6-thioguanine nucleotides and inhibits purine ring synthesis and, consequently, DNA and RNA synthesis	Inhibits the proliferation of T and B lymphocytes	Gastrointestinal intolerance, bone marrow suppression, infection, and azoospermia	Posterior ocular inflammation, arthritis, oral and genital ulceration
Methotrexate	Foliate analog and interferes with its action		Hepatotoxicity, renal toxicity, gastrointestinal toxicity and bone morrow depression	Neuro-BD, severe mucocutaneous involvement, and anterior uveitis
Mycophenolate mofetil	Converted to mycophenolic acid, which prevents replication of T and B lymphocytes by selectively inhibiting inosine-5-monophosphate	Does not inhibit the early production of IL-2 or the production cytokines of T-helper-cell clones belonging to the Th0 and Th2 subsets. Because mycophenolate mofetil works at a later stage in the T-		Posterior ocular inflammation

Treatment	Effects		Side effects	Indications
	dehydrogenase and consequently de novo purine synthesis, and also immune trafficking through the inhibition of vascular endothelial adhesion molecule expression	cell cycle, it acts synergistically with other immunosuppressive agents		
Calcineurin inhibitors				
Cyclosporine-A	Interfere with the activation and recruitment of T lymphocytes	Selectively suppresses CD4+ T lymphocytes	Neurotoxicity, hepatotoxicity, nephrotoxicity, hypertension, hirsutism, paraesthesia, gastrointestinal manifestations, hyperlipidemia, and gingival hyperplasia	Posterior ocular inflammation and most of the BD features
Tacrolimus	Interfere with the activation and recruitment of T lymphocytes	Selectively suppresses CD4+ T lymphocytes	Diabetes mellitus	Posterior ocular inflammation
Alkylating agents				
Chlorambucil	Interferes with DNA replication by cross-link, and causes decreased B and T cell functions	Slow acing agent	Bone marrow suppression	Neuro-BD
Cyclophosphamide	Similar with chlorambucil	Fast acting agent	Pulmonary fibrosis, renal toxicity, and hemorrhagic cystitis	Refractory sight-threatening ocular BD patients
Colchicine	Inhibits neutrophil migration by interfering with microtubule formation		Gastrointestinal intolerance, alopecia and bone marrow suppression	Mucocutaneous and articular involvement

Treatment	Effects		Side effects	Indications
Dapsone	Modifying neutrophil chemotaxis with antioxidant properties			Oragenital ulcers and cutaneous manifestations
Thalidomide	Diminishes TNF production and activity and decreases neutrophil migration		Teratogenicity, peripheral neuropathy, sedation, dizziness, headache, nausea, and weight gain	Oragenital ulcers, skin lesions, neurological and gastrointestinal involvement
Interferon-α	Reduces the number of circulating γδ-T cells, to increase HLA1 expression on peripheral monocytes in BD patients and to inhibits T cell adhesion to endothelial cells		Flu-like illness, leukopenia, thrombocytopenia, agranulocytopenia, bone marrow fibrosis, alopecia, pruritus, and depression	Refractory posterior uveitis
Anti-TNF-α biological agents				
Infliximab	Binds to human TNF-α and neutralized its activity		Infections, reactivation of tuberculosis, anaphylaxis, demyelination, lymphoma, and a development of auto-antibodies against double-stranded deoxyribonucleic acid	All manifestations of both systemic and ocular BD
Etanercept	Binds to human TNF-α and neutralized its activity			Mucocutaneous manifestations
Adalimumab	Binds to human TNF-α and neutralized its activity			Refractory sight-threatening ocular BD patients

Table 4. The treatment modalities.

7.5.2.2 Etanercept

Etanercept is a dimeric fusion protein of the p75 kD TNF-α receptor and Fc portion of human IgG1 (Maini & Taylor, 2000). It is produces by recombinant DNA technology, has a good tolerability, and is administered by subcutaneous injection (Thomas-Golbanov & Sridharan, 2001). A recent experimental study from Turkey has demonstrated that etanercept has a definite effect on the treatment of endotoxin-induced uveitis in rats (Avunduk et al., 2004). Clinically, beneficial effects have been observed with etanercept in maintaining visual acuity in BD patients with refractory uveitis, although the effect was not sustained in the post-treatment follow-up (Melikoglu et al., 2002).

7.5.2.3 Adalimumab

This agent has maintained disease remission in 3 patients with uveitis with no recurrences and stable visual acuity during the follow-up after whom being switched from infliximab to adalimumab (Mushtaq et al., 2007). Van Laar Jam et al reported that 6 patients with refractory disease (2 of them uveitis) were treated with adalimumab (with or without other therapies) and showed clinical improvement (Van Laar et al., 2007). A recent study involving 11 patients reported that adalimumab has been shown to improve visual acuity and also to have a corticosteroid and immunosuppressive sparing effect. It can induce and maintain sustained remission of the disease (Bawazeer et al., 2010).

7.6 Management of ocular complications

Cataract formation is especially common, both because of the recurrent inflammation and as a consequence of the steroid treatment. Cataract surgery should be delayed until uveitis has been quiescent for at least 3 months. Perioperative anti-inflammatory therapy, including topical, periocular, intracamaral, intravitreal, or even systemic corticosteroid, should be aggressively employed with intensive pre-, intra and post-surgery. Immunosuppressive drugs should be continued during the pre- and postoperative period. During the surgery minimum trauma should be given to the eye and minimal corneal incision should be performed. Complete removal of cortical material is important and a posterior chamber intraocular lens should be placed into the capsular bag. Intense fibrinoid reaction may still develop postoperatively. Nd:YAG laser capsulotomy may be needed in many cases for secondary posterior capsule opacifications which are frequently seen in the eyes with uveitis. With appropriate preoperative and postoperative suppression of inflammation, phacoemulsification and intraocular lens implantation are safe procedures leading to visual improvement in patients with BD without preexisting fundus lesions (Berker et al., 2004; Ciftci & Ozdemir, 1996; Gungor et al., 2008).

Secondary and neovascular glaucoma may be responsible for vision loss in BD patients. Initial therapy with topical and systemic antiglaucoma medications may not suffice. Secondary glaucomas in BD with or without pupillary block and angle-closure glaucoma, if present, may be treated with Nd:YAG-laser iridotomy or surgical peripheral iridectomy, diode-laser cyclodestruction, trabeculectomy with antimetabolites or aqueous drainage implants, as indicated (Elgin et al., 2004; Yalvaç et al., 2004). Cyclocryotherapy may be indicated for neovascular glaucoma and enucleation for cosmetic reasons or painful eyes.

Pars plana vitrectomy may be indicated in case of epiretinal membrane, macular hole, or vitreous hemorrhage along with retinal photocoagulation in cases of retinal tears. Retinal

detachment is therefore common in the later stages of the disease. Phthisis bulbi with or without iris neovascularization usually follows retinal detachment.
Development of retinal and optic disc neovascularization is a major complication of the repeated attacks on the retinal vasculature. This neovascularization is attributed to the BD vasculopathy leading to retinal hypoxia. Meticulous evaluation of retina is very important for the early diagnosis of neovascularization. Control of the inflammation is important; additionally laser photocoagulation of the ischemic area is helpful. Intravitreal anti- vascular endothelial growth factor agent might be applied.

8. Prognosis

BD has a variable course characterized by relapses and remissions. Prognosis depends on the clinical involvement. Loss of visual acuity and neurological disease are major causes of morbidity and mortality.
Prognosis of BD improved in the last decade due to the use of modern therapy modalities, including IFN-α and anti TNF-α blockers, and a more aggressive treatment strategy. Despite modern treatment, the disease still carries a poor visual prognosis with one-quarter of the patients blind (Kump et al., 2008; Yoshida et al., 2004).
Sakomato et al (Sakamoto et al., 1995) did try to determine prognostic factors for visual outcome. They concluded that skin lesions, arthritis and posterior uveitis attacks were linked to loss of vision, whereas female sex, disease free interval, and anterior attacks were related to retention of vision. Demiroğlu et al (Demiroglu et al., 1997) reported that age of 30 years or less, male sex, vascular thrombosis, and CNS involvement were risk factors for ocular disease.
Recently, Kaçmaz et al. conducted a study to estimate the risk of structural ocular complications and loss of visual acuity in cases with BD. They reported that loss of visual acuity and ocular complications might occur in patients with ocular inflammation associated with BD, even with aggressive therapy. Ongoing inflammation during follow-up, presence or occurrence of posterior synechia, hypotony, and elevated IOP were associated with an increased risk of loss of visual acuity (Kaçmaz et al., 2008).

9. Conclusions

Behçet's disease is a multi-system inflammatory disease, characterized by relapsing inflammation. Although intraocular inflammation may involve anterior or posterior segment, the hallmark of BD is the presence of panuveitis and vasculitis, and the sequela of the posterior segment inflammation appears to be sight-threatening. Corticosteroids are used to control acute inflammation, but have little effect in controlling recurrences. Conventional immunosuppression agents (most frequently azathioprine and Cyc-A) are the most frequently used agents in preventing recurrences in BD. However conventional immunosuppressive agents may take several weeks to show significant clinical effect and induce remission. In cases resistant to these agents, IFN-α2a and anti-TNF agents (esp. infliximab) give promising results in the treatment of Behçet uveitis. However, controlled randomized studies are necessary to determine the optimum doses and duration of therapy and specify the role of these immunomodulatary agents in the therapeutic regimen. In addition to this, new treatment agents are still needed.

10. References

Accardo-Palumbo A, Triolo G, Carbone MC, Ferrante A, Ciccia F, Giardina E & Triolo G. (2000). Polymorphonuclear leukocyte myeloperoxidase levels in patients with Behçet's disease. Clin Exp Rheumatol. Vol.18, No.4, pp.495-498.

Akova YA, Yilmaz G & Aydin P. (1999). Retinal tears associated with panuveitis andBehçet's disease. Ophthalmic Surg Lasers. Vol. 30, No.9, pp.62-65.

Arayssi T, Hamra R, Homeidan F, Uthman I, Awwad ST, Mroue K, Mansour W & Bashshur ZF. (2005) The efficacy of a single dose of infliximab in the treatment of Behçet's disease uveitis. Clin Exp Rheumatol. Vol.23, No.3, pp.427.

Atmaca LS. (1989). Fundus changes associated with Behçet's disease. Graefes Arch Clin Exp Ophthalmol. Vol.227, No.4, pp.340-344.

Atmaca LS. (1990). Experience with photocoagulation in Behçet's disease. Ophthalmic Surg. Vol.21, No.8, pp.571-576.

Atmaca LS & Batioğlu F. (1994). The efficacy of cyclosporin-a in the treatment of Behçet's disease. Ophthalmic Surg. Vol.25, No.5, pp.321-327.

Avunduk MC, Avunduk AM, Oztekin E, Baltaci AK, Ozyazgan Y & Mogolkoc R. (2004). Etanercept treatment in the endotoxin-induced uveitis of rats. Exp Eye Res. Vol.79, No.3, pp.357-365.

Aygündüz M, Bavbek N, Oztürk M, Kaftan O, Koşar A & Kirazli S. Serum beta 2-microglobulin reflects disease activity in Behçet's disease. Rheumatol Int. Vol.22, No.1, pp.5-8.

Azizlerli G, Köse AA, Sarica R, Gül A, Tutkun IT, Kulaç M, Tunç R, Urgancioğlu M & Dişçi R. (2003). Prevalence of Behçet's disease in Istanbul, Turkey. Int J Dermatol. Vol.42, No.10, pp.803-806.

Baltatzis S, Tufail F, Yu EN, Vredeveld CM & Foster CS. (2003). Mycophenolate mofetil as an immunomodulatory agent in the treatment of chronic ocular inflammatory disorders. Ophthalmology. Vol.110, No.5, pp.1061-1065.

Barra C, Belfort Júnior R, Abreu MT, Kim MK, Martins MC & Petrilli AM. (1991). Behçet's disease in Brazil--a review of 49 cases with emphasis on ophthalmic manifestations. Jpn J Ophthalmol. Vol.35, No.3, pp.339-346.

Bawazeer A, Raffa LH & Nizamuddin SH. (2010). Clinical experience with adalimumab in the treatment of ocular Behçetdisease. Ocul Immunol Inflamm. Vol.18, No.3,pp.:226-332.

Behçet H. (1937). Uber rezidivierende aphthose, durch ein virus verursachte Geshwure am Mund, am Auge, und an den Genitalien. Derm Wochenschr. Vol.36, pp.1152-1157.

BenEzra D & Cohen E. (1986). Treatment and visual prognosis in Behçet's disease. Br J Ophthalmol. Vol.70, No.8, pp.589-592.

Behçet's Disease Research Committee of Japan. (1974) . Behçet's disease: Guide to diagnosis of Behçet's disease. Jpn J ophthalmol. Vol.18 , pp.291-294.

Bhisitkul RB & Foster CS. (1996). Diagnosis and ophthalmological features of Behçet's disease. Int Ophthalmol Clin.Vol.;36, No.1, pp.127-134.

Binder AI, Graham EM, Sanders MD, Dinning W, James DG & Denman AM. (1987). Cyclosporin A in the treatment of severe Behçet's uveitis. Br J Rheumatol. Vol.26, No.4, pp.285-291.

Bonfioli AA & Orefice F. (2005). Behçet's disease. Semin Ophthalmol. Vol. 20, No.3, pp.199-206.

Bozzoni-Pantaleoni F, Gharbiya M, Pirraglia MP, Accorinti M & Pivetti-Pezzi P. (2001). Indocyanine green angiographic findings in Behçet's disease. Retina. Vol.21, No.3, pp.230-236.

Buckley CE 3rd & Gills JP Jr. (1970). Oral cyclophosphamide in the treatment of uveitis. Trans Am Acad Ophthalmol Otolaryngol. Vol.74, No.3, pp.505-508.

Chajek T & Fainaru M. (1975). Behçet's disease. Report of 41 cases and a review of the literature. Medicine (Baltimore). Vol.54, No.3, pp.179-196.

Chavis PS, Antonios SR & Tabbara KF. (1992). Cyclosporine effects on optic nerve and retinal vasculitis in Behçet's disease.Doc Ophthalmol. Vol.80, No.2, pp.133-142.

Choudhary A, Harding SP, Bucknall RC & Pearce IA. (2006). Mycophenolate mofetil as an immunosuppressive agent in refractory inflammatory eye disease. J Ocul Pharmacol Ther. Vol.22, No.3, pp.168-175.

Colvard DM, Robertson DM & O'Duffy JD. (1977). The ocular manifestations of Behçet's disease. Arch Ophthalmol. Vol.,95, No.10, pp.1813-11817.

Demiroğlu H, Barişta I & Dündar S. (1997). Risk factor assessment and prognosis of eye involvementn Behcet's disease in Turkey. Ophthalmology. Vol.104, No.4. pp.701-705.

Doycheva D, Deuter C, Stuebiger N, Biester S & Zierhut M. (2007). Mycophenolate mofetil in the treatment of uveitis in children. Br J Ophthalmol. Vol.91, No.2,pp.180-184.

Dursun D, Akova Y, Yücel E. (2004). Myositis and scleritis associated with Behcet's disease: an atypical presentation. Ocul Immunol Inflamm. 2004 Vol.12, No.4, pp.329-332.

Dündar SV, Gençalp U & Simşek H. (1985). Familial cases of Behcet's disease. Br J Dermatol. Vol.113, No.3, pp.319-321.

Elgin U, Berker N & Batman A. (2004). Incidence of secondary glaucoma in behcet disease. J Glaucoma. Vol.13, No.6, pp.441-444.

Erdoğru T, Koçak T, Serdaroğlu P, Kadioğlu A & Tellaloğlu S. (1999). Evaluation and therapeutic approaches of voiding and erectile dysfunction in neurological Behçet's syndrome. J Urol. Vol.162, No.1, pp:147-153.

Erkan F & Cavdar T. (1992). Pulmonary vasculitis in Behçet's disease. Am Rev Respir Dis. Vol.146, No.1, pp.232-239.

Evereklioglu C. (2004) Managing the symptoms of Behçet's disease. Expert Opin Pharmacother. Vol.5, No.2, pp.317-328.

Evereklioglu C. (2005).Current concepts in the etiology and treatment of Behçet's disease. Surv Ophthalmol. Vol.50, No.4, p.297-350.

Fietta P. (2005). Behçet's disease: familial clustering and immunogenetics. Clin Exp Rheumatol. Vol.23, pp.96-105.

Gedik S, Akova Y, Yilmaz G& Bozbeyoğlu S. (2005). Indocyanine green and fundus fluorescein angiographic findings in patients with active ocular Behcet's disease. OculImmunol Inflamm. Vol.13, No.1, pp.51-58.

Greenwood AJ, Stanford MR & Graham EM.(1998) The role of azathioprine in the management of retinal vasculitis. Eye. Vol.12, No.5, pp.783-788.

Guillaume-Czitrom S, Berger C, Pajot C, Bodaghi B, Wechsler B & Kone-Paut I. (2007). Efficacy and safety of interferon-alpha in the treatment of corticodependent uveitis of paediatric Behcet's disease. Rheumatology (Oxford). Vol.46, No.10, pp.1570-1573.

Gül A, Inanç M, Ocal L, Aral O & Koniçe M. (2000). Familial aggregation of Behçet's disease in Turkey. Ann Rheum Dis. Vol.59, No.8, pp.622-625.

Güngör SG, Akova YA. (2008). Clinical results of intraoperative triamsinolone acetonide injection during phacoemulsification in patients with uveitis. ASCRS ASOA 2008 Symposium& Congress, Chicago, USA, April 2008.

Hamdi M & Abdalla MI. (1974). Ocular manifestations of Behcet's disease. Bull Ophthalmol Soc Egypt.Vol. 67, pp.73-83.

Hamuryudan V, Yurdakul S, Ozbakir F, Yazici H & Hekim H. (1991). Monozygotic twins concordant for Behçet's syndrome. Arthritis Rheum. Vol.34, No.8, pp.1071-1072.

Hamuryudan V, Yurdakul S, Moral F, Numan F, Tüzün H, Tüzüner N, Mat C, Tüzün Y, Ozyazgan Y & Yazïci H. (1994). Pulmonary arterial aneurysms in Behçet's syndrome: a report of 24 cases. Br J Rheumatol. Vol.33, No.1, pp.48-51.

Hamuryudan V, Ozyazgan Y, Hizli N, Mat C, Yurdakul S, Tüzün Y, Senocak M & Yazici H. (1997). Azathioprine in Behcet's syndrome: effects on long-term prognosis. Arthritis Rheum. Vol.40, No.4, pp.769-774.

Inomata H, Yoshikawa H&Rao NA. (2003). Phacoanaphylaxis in Behçet'sdisease: a clinicopathologic and immunohistochemical study. Ophthalmology.Vol. 110, No. 10, pp. 1942-1945.

International Study Group for Behçet's Disease. (1990). Criteria for diagnosis of Behçet's disease. Lancet. Vol. 335, pp.1078-1080.

Kaklamani VG & Kaklamanis PG. (2001). Treatment of Behçet's disease--an update. Semin Arthritis Rheum. Vol.30, No.5, pp.299-312.

Kanski JJ & Shun-Shin GA. (1984). Systemic uveitis syndromes in childhood: an analysis of 340 cases. Ophthalmology. Vol.91, No.10, pp.:1247-1252.

Kazokoglu H, Onal S, Tugal-Tutkun I, Mirza E, Akova Y, Ozyazgan Y, Soylu M, Batioglu F & Apaydin C. (2008). Demographic and clinical features of uveitis in tertiary centers in Turkey. Ophthalmic Epidemiol. Vol. 15, No. 5, pp. 285-293.

Kesen MR, Goldstein DA & Tessler HH. (2008).Uveitis associated with pediatric Behçet's disease in the american midwest. Am J Ophthalmol. Vol.146, No.6, pp.819-827.

Kilmartin DJ, Forrester JV & Dick AD. (1998). Rescue therapy with mycophenolate mofetil in refractory uveitis. Lancet. Vol.4, No.352, pp.35-36.

Kilmartin DJ, Forrester JV & Dick AD. (1998). Tacrolimus (FK506) in failed cyclosporin A therapy in endogenous posterior uveitis. Ocul Immunol Inflamm. Vol.6, No.2, pp.101-109.

Klaeger A, Tran VT, Hiroz CA, Morisod L & Herbort CP. (2000). Indocyanine green angiography in Behçet's uveitis. Retina. Vol.20, No.3, pp.309-314.

Koné-Paut I, Yurdakul S, Bahabri SA, Shafae N, Ozen S, Ozdogan H & Bernard JL. (1998). Clinical features of Behçet's disease in children: an international collaborative study of 86 cases. J Pediatr. Vol.132, No.4, pp.721-725.

Kötter I, Dürk H, Eckstein A, Zierhut M, Fierlbeck G & Saal JG. (1996). Erosive arthritis and posterior uveitis in Behçet's disease: treatment with interferon alpha and interferon gamma. Clin Exp Rheumatol. Vol.14, No.3, pp.313-315.

Kulaber A, Tugal-Tutkun I, Yentür SP, Akman-Demir G, Kaneko F, Gül A & Saruhan-Direskeneli G. (2007). Pro-inflammatory cellular immune response in Behçet's disease. Rheumatol Int. Vol.27, No.12, pp.1113-1118.

Kump LI, Moeller KL, Reed GF, Kurup SK, Nussenblatt RB & Levy-Clarke GA. (2008). Behçet's disease: comparing 3 decades of treatment response at the National Eye Institute. Can J Ophthalmol. Vol.43, No.4, pp.468-472.

Kural-Seyahi E, Fresko I, Seyahi N, Ozyazgan Y, Mat C, Hamuryudan V, Yurdakul S & Yazici H. (2003). The long-term mortality and morbidity of Behçet syndrome: a 2-decade outcome survey of 387 patients followed at a dedicated center. Medicine (Baltimore). Vol.82, No.1, pp.60-76.

Kurokawa MS & Suzuki N. (2004). Behçet's Disease. Clin Exp Med. Vol.3, pp.10-20.

Larkin G & Lightman S. (1999). Mycophenolate mofetil. A useful immunosuppressive in inflammatory eye disease. Ophthalmology. Vol.106, No.2, pp.370-374.

Lee LA. (2001). Behçet's disease. Semin Cutan Med Surg. Vol.20, No., pp.153-157.

Lehner T, Batchelor JR, Challacombe SJ, Kennedy L. (1979). An immunogenetic basis for the tissue involvement in Behçet's syndrome. Immunology. Vol.37, No.4, pp.895-900.

Maini RN & Taylor PC. (2000). Anti-cytokine therapy for rheumatoid arthritis. Annu Rev Med. Vol.51, pp.207-229.

Mamo JG & Baghdassarian A. (1964). Behcet's disease; a report of 28 cases. Arch Ophthalmol. Vol.71, pp.4-14.

Mason RM, Barnes CG. (1969). Behçet's syndrome with arthritis. Ann Rheum Dis. Vol.28, No.2, pp.,95-103.

Marshall SE.(2004). Behçet's disease. Best Pract Res Clin Rheumatol. Vol.18, No.3, pp.291-311.

Masuda K, Nakajima A, Urayama A, Nakae K, Kogure M & Inaba G. (1989). Double-masked trial of cyclosporin versus colchicine and long-term open study of cyclosporin in Behçet's disease. Lancet Vol.20, No.1, pp.1093-1096.

Matsuo T, Sato Y, Shiraga F, Shiragami C & Tsuchida Y. (1999). Choroidal abnormalities in Behçet's disease observed by simultaneous indocyanine green and fluorescein angiography with scanning laser ophthalmoscopy. Ophthalmology. Vol.106, No.2, pp.295-300.

Matsuo T, Itami M, Nakagawa H & Nagayama M.(2002). The incidence and pathology of conjunctival ulceration in Behçet's syndrome. Br J Ophthalmol. Vol.86, No.2, pp.140-143.

Melikoglu M, Özyazgan, Y & Fresko I. (2002). The response of treatment resistant uveitis in Behçet's syndrome (BS) to a TNF-α blocker, etanercept: an open study. Arthritis Rheum. Vol.46, pp.181.

Mendes D, Correia M, Barbedo M, Vaio T, Mota M, Gonçalves O &Valente J. (2009). Behçet's disease--a contemporary review. J Autoimmun, Vol. 32, No. 3-4, (January 2009), pp. 178-188.

Mishima S, Masuda K & Izawa Y. (1979). Behçet's disease in Japan: Ophthalmologic aspects. Trans Am Ophthalmol Soc. Vol. 76, pp. 225-279.

Mizushima Y. (1991). Behçet's disease. Curr Opin Rheumatol. Vol.3, No.1, pp.32-35.

Mochizuki M, Akduman L, Nussenblatt RB. (1996). Behçet's disease. In: Pepose J.S., Holland G.N., Wilhelmus K.R. (Eds.), Ocular infection and immunity. Mosby, St. Louis, pp.663-675.

Mushtaq B, Saeed T, Situnayake RD & Murray PI. (2007). Adalimumab for sight-threatening uveitis in Behçet's disease. Eye (Lond). Vol.21, No.6, pp.824-825.

Müftüoğlu AU, Yazici H, Yurdakul S, Tüzün Y, Pazarli H, Güngen G & Deniz S. (1986). Behçet's disease. Relation of serum C-reactive protein and erythrocyte sedimentation rates to disease activity. Int J Dermatol. Vol.25, No.4, pp.:235-239.

Numaga J, Matsuki K, Mochizuki M, Minami M & Juji T. (1988). An HLA-D region restriction fragment associated with refractory Behçet's disease. Am J Ophthalmol. Vol.15, No.10, pp.528-533.

Nussenblatt RB. (2010). Behçet's Disease, In: Uveitis Fundamentals and Clinical Practice, R.B. Nussenblatt & S.M. Whitcup, (Ed.), 332-354, Mosby ,ISBN 978-1-4377-0677-3, St.Louis.

O'Duffy. (1984). Suggested criteria for diagnosis of Behçet's disease. J Rheumatol. Vol. 1, pp.18.

O'Duffy JD, Robertson DM & Goldstein NP. (1984). Chlorambucil in the treatment of uveitis and meningoencephalitis of Behçet's disease. Am J Med. Vol.76, N.1, pp.75-84.

Ohno S. (1986). Behçet's Disease in the world. In: Recent Advances in Behçet's Disease, Lehnet T, Barnes C.G. (Eds), Royal Society of Medicine Service, London.

Ohno S, Nakamura S, Hori S, Shimakawa M, Kawashima H, Mochizuki M, Sugita S, Ueno S, Yoshizaki K & Inaba G. (2004). Efficacy, safety, and pharmacokinetics of multiple administration of infliximab in Behçet's disease with refractory uveoretinitis. J Rheumatol. Vol.31, No.7, pp.1362-1368.

Okada AA, Rao NA, Usui M. (2004). Behçet's disease. In: Yanoff M, Duker JS (Eds), Ophthalmology, 2nd ed, Mosby, London.

Onal S, Tugal-Tutkun I, Urgancioglu M & Gul A. (2001). Clinical course of ocular Behçet's disease in siblings. Ocul Immunol Inflamm. Vol.9, No.2, pp.111-124.

Onder M & Gürer MA. (1999). Behçet's disease: an enigmatic vasculitis. Clin Dermatol. Vol.17, No.5, pp.571-576.

Ozdal PC, Ortaç S, Taşkintuna I & Firat E. (2002). Posterior segment involvement in ocular Behçet's disease. Eur J Ophthalmol. Vol.12, No.5, pp.424-431.

Ozoran K, Düzgün N, Tutkak H, Gürler A & Tokgöz G. (1996). Fibronectin and circulating immune complexes in Behet's disease. Rheumatol Int. Vol.15, No.6, pp.221-224.

Ozyazgan Y, Yurdakul S, Yazici H, Tüzün B, Işçimen A, Tüzün Y, Aktunç T, Pazarli H, Hamuryudan V & Müftüoğlu A. (1992). Low dose cyclosporin A versus pulsed cyclophosphamide in Behçet's syndrome: a single masked trial. Br J Ophthalmol.Vol. 76, No.4, pp.241-243.

Ozen S. (1999). Vasculopathy, Behçet's syndrome, and familial Mediterranean fever. Curr Opin Rheumatol. Vol.11, No.5, pp.393-398.

Pay S, Simşek I, Erdem H & Dinç A. (2007). Immunopathogenesis of Behçet's disease with special emphasize on the possible role of antigen presenting cells. Rheumatol Int. Vol.27, No.5, pp417-424.

Pivetti-Pezzi P. (1996). Uveitis in children. Eur J Ophthalmol. Vol.6, No.3, pp.293-298.

Ramsay A & Lightman S. (2001). Hypopyon uveitis. Surv Ophthalmol. Vol. 46, No: 1, pp. 1-18.

Sakamoto M, Akazawa K, Nishioka Y, Sanui H, Inomata H & Nose Y. (1995). Prognostic factors of vision in patients with Behçet's disease. Ophthalmology. Vol.102, No.2, pp.317-321.

Sakane T, Takeno M, Suzuki N & Inaba G. (1999). Behçet's disease. N Engl J Med. Vol.21, No.341, pp.1284-1291.

Sakane T & Takeno M. (2000). Current therapy in Behcet's disease. Skin Therapy Lett. Vol.5, No.6, pp.3-5.

Saravanan V & Hamilton J. (2002). Advances in the treatment of rheumatoid arthritis: old versus new therapies. Expert Opin Pharmacother. Vol.3, No.7, pp.845-856.

Sarica R, Azizlerli G, Köse A, Dişçi R, Ovül C &Kural Z. (1996).Juvenile Behçet's disease among 1784 Turkish Behçet's patients. Int J Dermatol. Vol.35, No.2, pp.109-111.

Sfikakis PP. (2002). Behçet's disease: a new target for anti-tumour necrosis factor treatment. Ann Rheum Dis. Vol.61, pp.51-53.

Shek LP & Lim DL. (2002). Thalidomide in Behçet's disease. Biomed Pharmacother. Vol.56, No.1, pp.31-35.Sheu SJ & Yang CA. (2004). Macular hole in Behcet's disease. Kaohsiung J Med Sci. Vol.20, No.11, pp.558-562.

Shimizu T. (1971). Behcet's syndrome. Naika. Vol.27, No.3pp.520-521.

Siepmann K, Huber M, Stübiger N, Deuter C & Zierhut M. (2006). Mycophenolate mofetil is a highly effective and safe immunosuppressive agent for the treatment of uveitis : a retrospective analysis of 106 patients. Graefes Arch Clin Exp Ophthalmol. Vol.244, No.7, pp.788-794.

Smith EL & Schur PH. (2005). Clinical manifestations and diagnosis of Behçet's disease. www.uptodateonline.com. UpToDate ®

Tabbara KF. (1983). Chlorambucil in Behçet's disease. A reappraisal. Ophthalmology. Vol.90, No.8, pp.906-908.

Tabbara KF & Al-Hemidan AI. (2008). Infliximab effects compared to conventional therapy in the management of retinal vasculitis in Behçet's disease. Am J Ophthalmol. Vol.146, No.6, pp.845-850.

Tekeli O &Ozdemir O. (2004). Heidelberg retina tomograph in ocular Behçet'sdisease.Eye. Vol.18, No.2, pp.143-146.

Thomas-Golbanov C & Sridharan S. (2001). Novel therapies in vasculitis. Expert Opin Investig Drugs. Vol.10, No.7, pp.1279-1289.

Thorne JE, Jabs DA, Qazi FA, Nguyen QD, Kempen JH & Dunn JP. (2005). Mycophenolate mofetil therapy for inflammatory eye disease. Ophthalmology. Vol.112, No.8, pp.1472-1477.

Tognon S, Graziani G & Marcolongo R. (2007). Anti-TNF-alpha therapy in seven patients with Behcet's uveitis: advantages and controversial aspects. Ann N Y Acad Sci. Vol.1110, pp.474-484.

Toubi E, Kessel A, Mahmudov Z, Hallas K, Rozenbaum M & Rosner I. (2005). Increased spontaneous apoptosis of CD4+CD25+ T cells in patients with active rheumatoid arthritis is reduced by infliximab. Ann N Y Acad Sci. Vol.1051, pp.506-514.

Tugal-Tutkun I, Havrlikova K, Power WJ & Foster CS. (1996). Changing patterns in uveitis of childhood. Ophthalmology. Vol.10, No.3, pp.375-383.

Tugal-Tutkun I & Urgancioglu M. (2003). Childhood-onset uveitis in Behçet's disease:a descriptive study of 36 cases. Am J Ophthalmol. Vol.136, No.6, pp.1114-1119.

Tugal-Tutkun I, Onal S, Altan-Yaycioglu R, Huseyin Altunbas H & Urgancioglu M. (2004). Uveitis in Behçet's disease: an analysis of 880 patients. Am J Ophthalmol.Vol. 138, No. 3, (March 2004), pp. 373-380.

Tugal-Tutkun I, Mudun A, Urgancioglu M, Kamali S, Kasapoglu E, Inanc M & Gül A. (2005). Efficacy of infliximab in the treatment of uveitis that is resistant to treatment with the combination of azathioprine, cyclosporine, and corticosteroids in Behçet's disease: an open-label trial. Arthritis Rheum. Vol.52, No.8, pp.2478-2484.

Tugal-Tutkun I, Onal S, Altan-Yaycioglu R, Kir N & Urgancioglu M. (2006). Neovascularization of the optic disc in Behçet's disease. Jpn J Ophthalmol. Vol.50, No.3, pp.256-265.

Tugal-Tutkun I, Cingü K, Kir N, Yeniad B, Urgancioglu M & Gül A. (2008). Use of laser flare-cell photometry to quantify intraocular inflammation in patients with Behçet uveitis. Graefes Arch Clin Exp Ophthalmol. Vol. 246, No.8, pp.1169-1177.

Tursen U, Gurler A & Boyvat A. Evaluation of clinical findings according to sex in 2313 Turkish patients with Behçet's disease. Int J Dermatol. Vol.,42, No.5, pp.346-351.

Vaiopoulos G, Sfikakis PP, Hatzinikolaou P, Stamatelos G & Kaklamanis P. (1996). Adamantiadis-Behçet's disease in sisters. Clin Rheumatol. Vol.15, No.4, pp.382-384.

van Laar JA, Missotten T, van Daele PL, Jamnitski A, Baarsma GS & van Hagen PM. (2006). Adalimumab: a new modality for Behçet's disease? Ann Rheum Dis. Vol.66, No.4, pp.565-566.

Verity DH, Marr JE, Ohno S, Wallace GR, Stanford MR. (1999). Behçet's disease, the Silk Road and HLA-B51: historical and geographical perspectives. Tissue Antigens. Vol.4, No.3, pp.213-220.

Wray D, Graykowski EA & Notkins AL. (1981). Role of mucosal injury in initiating recurrent aphthous stomatitis. Br Med J (Clin Res Ed). Vol.12, No.283, pp.1569-1570.

Yalvac IS, Sungur G, Turhan E, Eksioglu U & Duman S. (2004). Trabeculectomy with mitomycin-C in uveitic glaucoma associated with Behçet's disease. J Glaucoma. Vol.13, No.6, pp.450-453.

Yazici H, Pazarli H, Barnes CG, Tüzün Y, Ozyazgan Y, Silman A, Serdaroğlu S, Oğuz V, Yurdakul S & Lovatt GE. (1990). A controlled trial of azathioprine in Behçet's syndrome. N Engl J Med. Vol.1, No.322, pp.281-285.

Yazici H. (1994). Behçet's syndrome. In: Klippel J.H., Dieppe P.A. (Eds.), Rheumotology, 6.20.1.-6.20.6, Mosby, London.

Yazici H & Ozyazgan Y. (1999). Medical management of Behçet's syndrome. Dev Ophthalmol. Vol.31, pp.118-131.

Yilmaz G, Akova Y & Aydin P. (2000). Macular ischaemia in Behçet's disease. Eye. Vol.14, No. 5, pp.717-720.

Yoshida A, Kawashima H, Motoyama Y, Shibui H, Kaburaki T, Shimizu K, Ando K, Hijikata K, Izawa Y, Hayashi K, Numaga J, Fujino Y, Masuda K & Araie M. (2004). Comparison of patients with Behçet's disease in the 1980s and 1990s. Ophthalmology. Vol.111, No.4, pp.810-815.

Yurdakul S, Günaydin I, Tüzün Y, Tankurt N, Pazarli H, Ozyazgan Y & Yazici H. (1988). The prevalence of Behçet's syndrome in a rural area in northern Turkey. J Rheumatol. Vol.15, No.5,pp.820-822.

Yurdakul S, Hamuryudan V &Yazici H. (2004). Behçet syndrome. Curr Opin Rheumatol. Vol.16, No.1, pp.38-42.

Zafirakis P & Foster C.S. (2002). Adamantiades-Behçet's disease, In: Diagnosis and Tretment of Uveitis, C.S. Foster& A.T. Vitale, (Ed.), 632-653, W.B. Saunders, ISBN 0-7216-6338-9, Philadelphia, Pennsylvania.

Zhang XQ. (1980). Criteria for Behçet's disease. Chin J Intern Med. Vol.19, pp.1-20.

Zierhut M, Stübiger N, Aboalchamat W, Landenberger H, Bialasiewicz AA & Engelmann K. (2001). Immunosuppressive therapy with mycophenolate mofetil (CellCept) in treatment of uveitis. Ophthalmologe. Vol.98, No. 7, pp.647-651.Zouboulis CC, Kötter I, Djawari D, Kirch W, Kohl PK, Ochsendorf FR, Keitel W, Stadler R, Wollina U, Proksch E, Söhnchen R, Weber H, Gollnick HP, Hölzle E, Fritz K, Licht T & Orfanos CE. (1997). Epidemiological features of Adamantiades-Behçet's disease in Germany and in Europe. Yonsei Med J. Vol.38, No.6, pp.411-422.

18

Anti-CXCL13 and Anti-TNFα Monoclonal Antibodies Combinatorial Treatment Inhibits Autoimmune Disease in a Murine Model of Systemic Lupus Erythematosus

Debra B. Gardner, Patricia Rafferty, Peter Bugelski and Bailin Liang
Centocor Research and Development
USA

1. Introduction

Systemic lupus erythematosus (SLE) is an autoimmune disorder characterized by the involvement of multiple organ systems with alternating clinical exacerbations and remissions. Circulating immune complexes and autoantibodies can cause tissue damage and organ dysfunction with manifestations involving the skin, serosal surfaces, central nervous system, and kidneys (Rahman & Isenberg, 2008).

B cells are believed to play an important role in SLE. B cells can function as APCs, produce cytokines and chemokines contributing to lymphoid regulation, and can respond to stimuli in the microenvironment at local tissues (Ramanujam & Davidson, 2008). Pathogenic autoantibodies produced by autoreactive B cells are believed to play an important role in the pathogenesis of SLE.

CXCL13 has been shown to be a key mediator of organization of lymphoid tissues. CXCL13 is a B cell chemoattractant that is expressed by peritoneal macrophages and follicular dendritic cells in secondary lymphoid organs, such as the follicles of Peyer's patches, the spleen and lymph nodes. Through interaction with CXCR5, a G-protein coupled receptor, CXCL13 attracts B lymphocytes and promotes migration of small numbers of T helper follicular cells and macrophages (Gunn et al., 1998). CXCL13 is critical for B cell homing and follicle formation in lymph node and spleen, and it is required for the development of lymph nodes and Peyer's patches (Ansel et al., 2000). CXCL13 protein level is elevated in ectopic B cell follicles formed in the inflamed tissues of multiple chronic diseases, and plays an important role in maintaining inflammation by actively recruiting B cells (Carlsen et al., 2004; Magliozzi et al., 2004; Salolonsson et al., 2002; Shi et al., 2001;). CXCL13 has been shown to have increased expression in the thymus and kidney of aged NZB/W F1 mice, and may play a role in breaking immune tolerance in the thymus of autoimmune prone mice (Ishikawa et al., 2001). Treatment with anti-CXCL13 has shown efficacy in animal models of RA and EAE (Bagaeva et al. 2006; Zheng et al., 2005). Because of its function and presence in various pathological conditions, CXCL13 and CXCL13 dependent pathways are thought to be instrumental in the pathogenesis of a variety of diseases where B cells may play a significant role, including RA, OA, UC, and SLE, and could be potential targets for autoimmune therapy (Table 1).

Human Disease	Potential role of B cell	Reference
Systemic Lupus Erythematosus	Antibody production, T cell activation, Antigen presentation, cytokine production, lymphoid neogenesis	Lipsky, 2001
Rheumatoid arthritis	Cytokine production, lymphoid neogenesis, T cell activation	Panayi, 2005
Sjogren's Syndrome	Antibody production, lymphoid neogenesis	Liang, 2007
Autoimmune thyroiditis	Antibody production, lymphoid neogenesis	Yu, 2008
Multiple Sclerosis	Lymphoid neogenesis, T cell activation	Hirotani, 2010
Myasthenia Gravis	Lymphoid neogenesis, antibody production	Meraouna, 2006

Table 1. Role of B cells in human autoimmune diseases.

NZB/W F1 mice develop an autoantibody response against DNA and chromatin antigens, a polyclonal hypergammaglobulinemia and ultimately, severe immune complex mediated glomerulonephritis (Aringer & Smolen, 2008). These mice have been widely used as a model to study lupus nephritis. TNFα is a pleiotropic cytokine produced by many cell types that plays a key role in the pathogenesis of multiple autoimmune disorders, as well as a controversial role in SLE (Aringer & Smolen, 2008; Kollias, 1999).
Although individual therapies with anti-TNFα or anti-CXCL13 mAb for additional inflammatory diseases have been explored with limited success, there has not been any attempt to combine the two mabs for the treatment of any disease (Bagaeva et al., 2006; Dick et al., 1996; Ruddle et al., 1990; Zheng et al., 2005). This study was designed to investigate the effect of anti-CXCL13 and anti-TNFα mAbs treatment on disease development in NZB/W F1 mice.

2. Materials and methods

2.1 Antibodies and reagents

RPMI media, heat-inactivated fetal bovine serum, gentamycin and L-glutamine were purchased from Invitrogen (Carlsbad, CA). Neutralizing rat anti-CXCL13 mAb (MAB4701) was purchased from R&D Systems (Minneapolis, MN) with an endotoxin level of 1.2 EU/mg. Anti-TNFα was made at Centocor, and had an endotoxin level of 0.262 EU/mg.

2.2 Animals and experimental protocol

NZB/W F_1 mice aged 10-12 weeks were obtained from Jackson Laboratories (Bar Harbor, ME). On day 0, the study animals were randomly assigned to control or treatment groups (n = 15/group). An intraperitoneal injection of saline, anti-mCXCL13 mAb (0.5 mg/mouse, 2 times a week, weeks 16-34), anti-TNFα mAb (0.5 mg/mouse, 2 times a week, weeks 16-18, then 0.25 mg/mouse, 2 times a week, weeks 19-34) or a combination of anti-CXCL13 plus anti-TNFα mabs were administered weekly from 16 to 34 weeks of age. Animal were monitored weekly. Urine was collected via free catch (once every 3 weeks starting from 12 weeks of age) and stored at -80°. Blood was collected every three weeks starting from 16 weeks of age, and serum was stored at -80°. At the final harvest, spleen, lymph nodes, and kidneys were harvested into appropriate storage buffers before further analysis by in vitro functional assays. This study protocol was reviewed and approved by Centocor's Institutional Animal Care and use Committee.

2.3 Flow cytometry analysis of B cell activation status

Mice were killed at 34 weeks of age and their spleens were removed. A portion of the spleen was placed in cold RPMI-1640 medium supplemented with 10% fetal bovine serum, 10 mg/ml gentamycin, 2 mM L-glutamine, 0.1 mM 2-mercaptoethanol. Red blood cells were lysed in red blood cell lysing buffer (Biowhittaker) on ice for 5 minutes. Splenocytes were stained with optimal concentrations of fluorochrome conjugated mAbs (5 x 10^5 cells in 200 µl of phosphate buffered saline, 1% bovine serum albumin, 0.1% sodium azide) in U-shaped microtiter plates at 4° C for 30 min, and fixed with 1% paraformaldehyde. Samples were analyzed on a FACSCalibur Instrument (Becton Dickinson, Mountain View, CA). Anti-murine CD23 PE (clone B3B4) and anti-murine CD24 FITC (clone M1/69) were purchased from BD Biosciences (Chicago, IL) and used for analysis of B cell activation.

2.4 Autoantibody analysis

Anti-dsDNA autoantibodies were determined by ELISA. Double stranded-DNA coated plates were purchased from DiaSorin (Stillwater, MN). 1:100 diluted serum samples were incubated at room temperature for 2 hours on the plates. Alkaline phosphatase conjugated anti-murine IgG (Southern Biotechnology Associates, Birmingham, AL) was added to the plate for 1 hour followed by incubation with p-nitrophenylphosphate substrate (Sigma, St. Louis, MO) for 30 minutes and the plates were read at OD405 nm. OD values from separate assays were normalized to a single MRL lpr/lpr MRL/MpJ-Fas^{lpr}/J positive control serum.

2.5 Proliferation assays

B cell proliferation was assessed using 1 x 10^6 splenocytes stimulated with 2 µg/ml each of anti IgM F(ab') (Pierce Biotechnology) and 5 µg/ml anti-CD40 (BD Pharmingen, Sacramento CA) for 72 hours. Proliferation was assessed using BrDU (Roche Applied Science, Indianapolis, IN) and counting luminescence singles on a TopCount (PerkinElmer, Shelton, CT).

2.6 Urine total protein/creatinine analysis

Urine samples were collected from mice via free catch and frozen at -80° C for subsequent analysis of urine total protein/creatinine ratio determined by Ace Analyzer (Alpha Wasserman, West Caldwell, NJ). Urine total protein was measured in undiluted urine and creatinine was measured using urine diluted 1:10 in deionized distilled H_2O.

2.7 Histologic analysis of kidney pathology

Kidneys were harvested and immediately immersed in 0.7% periodate lysine paraformaldehyde (PLP) buffer, composed of 0.1 M phosphate buffer, 0.7% paraformaldehyde, 75 mM L-lysine and 10 mM $NaIO_4$. The kidneys were processed for microscopic examination and embedded in paraffin by routine methods after overnight fixation in PLP buffer. The 5 µm thick sections were stained with haematoxylin & eosin (H&E) for general morphology. Samples were examined and scored for disease severity in a blinded fashion. Pathology was assessed using the World Health Organization (WHO) classifications (Weening et al., 2004).

2.8 Immunohistochemical staining

Spleens were harvested, cut in half along its vertical axis, and one half was suspended in OCT and frozen in 2-methyl-butane cooled with dry ice. Spleen sections were prepared, fixed in acetone and incubated in PBS (no azide), then in 0.3% H_2O_2 to quench endogenous peroxidase activity. The sections were blocked using PBS/5% normal goat serum/0.1% Tween 20 and stained with biotinylated peanut agglutinin (Vector Labs) and B220 FITC (BD Biosciences). Streptavidin-Horseradish peroxidase (HRP, Southen Biotchnologies) and anti-FITC-alkaline phosphatase (AP, Southern Biotechnologies) were used as secondary antibodies. HRP and AP were developed using 3-amino-9-ethyl-carbazole and Fast-Blue BB base (Sigma Chemical Co., St. Louis, MO) respectively. Samples were examined in a blinded fashion.

2.9 Chemotaxis of purified B cells

B cells were purified by negative selection using the B cell isolation kit from Miltenyi Biotec (Auburn CA). B cell purity was determined by staining for CD19-positive cells and was >95%. Purified murine B cells (4 x 10^7 cells in 10 ml RPMI/10% FBS) were loaded with calcein dye (1 mg/ml in dry DMSO, Molecular Probes, Invitrogen) for one hour at 37° C. Cells were centrifuged at 1200 rpm for 7 min, then resuspended in PBS/2%FBS to a final concentration of 1 x 10^6 cells/ml. CXCL13 (R&D Systems, Minneapolis, MN) was diluted in PBS/2%FBS to a final concentration of 750 ng/ml and aliquoted to a 5 µm Neuroprobe (Neuroprobe, Gaithersburg, MD) 96 well chemotaxis apparatus, and 50 µl of cells were loaded onto the filter. The chemotaxis plate was incubated for one hour at 37° C, then washed and centrifuged briefly to bring the cells to the bottom of the well. Fluorescence at the bottom of the well was read on the Tecan (Tecan, Mannedorf, Switzerland).

2.10 Statistical analysis

Cell surface marker expression, anti-dsDNA levels, B cell proliferation and chemotaxis were expressed as mean ± SE and statistical significance was determined by two tailed analysis of variance by standard t test. For statistical analysis on kidney pathologies, the incidence of severe disease was compared across groups by Fisher Exact test with a Bonferroni adjustment of the nominal type I error to determine the variance among the treatment groups. Rank order histological data was analyzed by ANOVA with Dunn's correction for multiple comparisons. p values < 0.05 were accepted as significant.

3. Results

3.1 Anti-CXCL13/Anti-TNFα treatment increased follicular B cell and reduced transitional B cells in spleen

We first examined the phenotype of B cells harvested from the treated mice. Spontaneous autoreactive B cell development occurs in NZB/W F1 mice with decreasing follicular B cells and increasing transitional B cells over time. At 34 weeks, follicular B cells in mice treated with anti-CXCL13/anti-TNFα mAbs were significantly increased as compared to that in mice treated with saline, (Fig. 1), while transitional B cells were significantly decreased (Fig. 2) by treatment with anti-CXCL13/anti-TNFα mAbs. These observations suggested that anti-CXCL13/anti-TNFα mAbs treatment helps to maintain a relatively normal B cell repertoire in NZB/W F1 mice, potentially interfering with the spontaneous autoreactive B cell development.

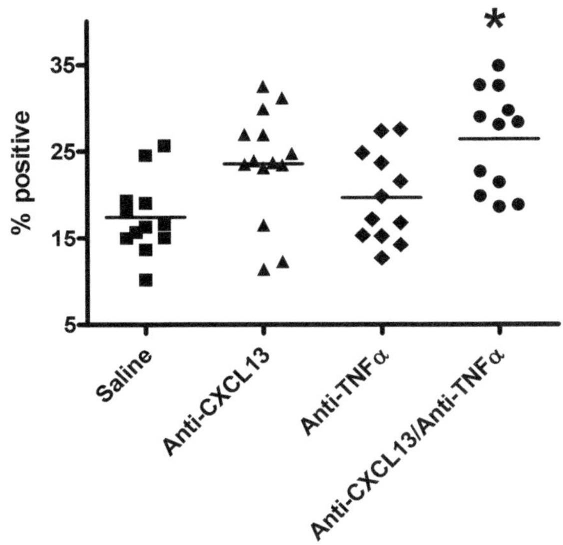

Fig. 1. Anti-CXCL13/anti-TNFα mAbs treatment increased the number of follicular B cells. Total splenocytes were gated on CD19+ B cells and were analyzed with anti-CD23 and anti-CD24 antibodies by flow cytometry to determine the population of CD23+CD24- follicular B cells at 34 weeks of age.. * indicates $p<0.05$ vs saline treated control.

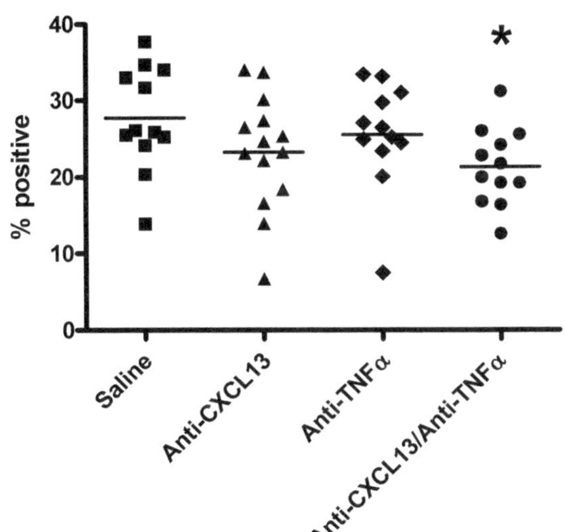

Fig. 2. Anti-CXCL13/anti-TNFα mAbs treatment decreased the number of transitional B cells. Total splenocytes were gated on CD19+ B cells and were analyzed with anti-CD23 and anti-CD24 antibodies by flow cytometry to determine the population of CD23-CD24+ transitional B cells (b) at 34 weeks of age. * indicates $p<0.05$ vs saline treated control.

3.2 Anti-CXCL13/Anti-TNFα mAb treatment inhibited anti-dsDNA autoantibody production in the serum

Since the presence of autoantibodies against dsDNA is a marker of SLE, the effect of anti-CXCL13/anti-TNFα mAbs treatment on anti-dsDNA autoantibody production was examined in the serum samples (Fig. 3). Serum anti-dsDNA autoantibody levels increased over the course of the study, and anti-TNFα or anti-CXCL13 mAb treatment alone did not significantly affect the overall anti-dsDNA production as compared to the control treatment with saline. However, anti-dsDNA production in the animals receiving the combination of anti-CXCL13/anti-TNFα mAbs was significantly decreased as compared to the anti-TNFα treatment group (Fig. 3).

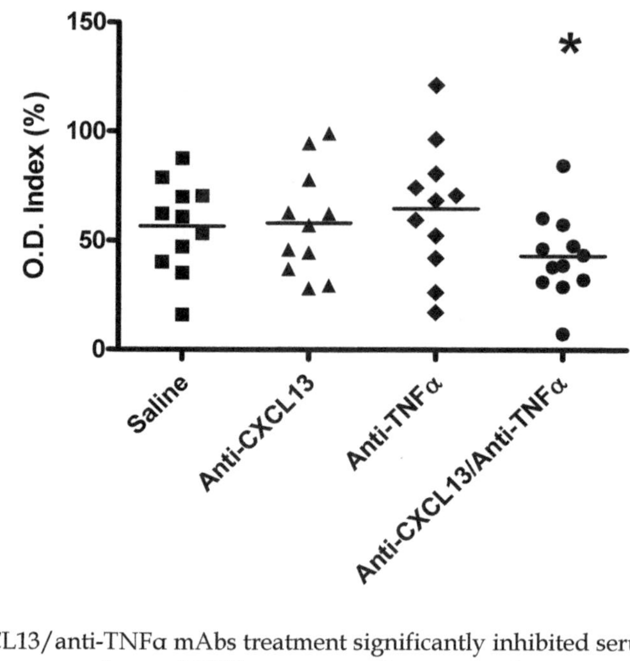

Fig. 3. Anti-CXCL13/anti-TNFα mAbs treatment significantly inhibited serum anti-dsDNA autoantibody as compared to anti-TNFα treatment. Serum samples were analyzed for anti-dsDNA autoantibody levels by ELISA at 34 weeks of age. O.D. index values represent individual data point normalized throughout the studies to a single positive control serum with anti dsDNA. * indicates $p < 0.05$ vs. anti-TNFα mAb treated group.

3.3 Anti-CXCL13/Anti-TNFα mAb treatment decreased B cell proliferation

To further investigate whether anti-CXCL13/anti-TNFα mAbs treatment affects the functions of B cells, antibody induced in vitro proliferation was performed to determine B-cell responses using splenocytes isolated from various treatment groups. Ex vivo B-cell proliferation stimulated with anti-CD40/anti-IgM mAbs was significantly depressed by in vivo anti-CXCL13/anti-TNFα mAbs treatment as compared to the saline and single anti-TNFα or anti-CXCL13 antibody treatments when mice were 34 weeks old (Fig. 4). These data demonstrated that B cells from animals treated with anti-CXCL13/anti-TNFα mAbs were more resistant to ex vivo stimulation and activation.

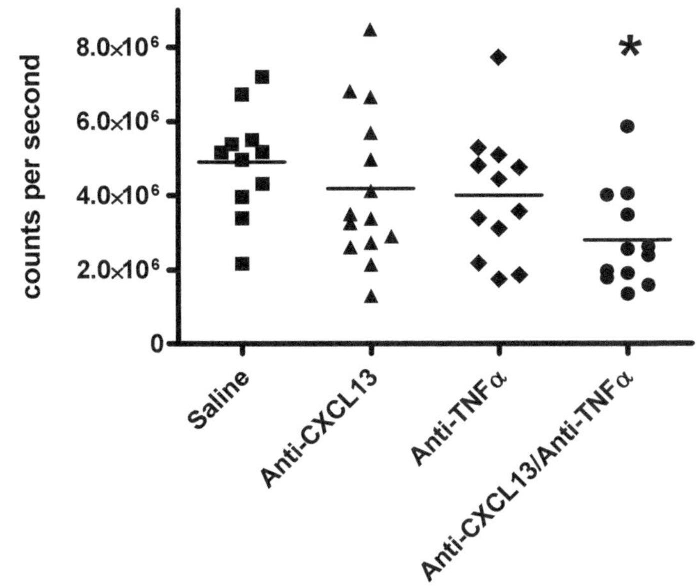

Fig. 4. B cell proliferation is decreased in NZB/W mice treated with anti-CXCL13/anti-TNFα mAbs. Cell Proliferation ELISA using BrDU was performed to determine B cell proliferation and results are expressed as counts per second. * indicates $p<0.05$ vs saline control treated groups.

3.4 Anti-CXCL13/Anti-TNFα mAb treatment suppressed kidney pathology

Glomerulonephritis is another feature of SLE. To determine the effects of anti-CXCL13/anti-TNFα mAbs treatment on kidney function and pathology, we examined urine total protein/creatinine ratios and renal histopathology. Treatment with anti-CXCL13/anti-TNFα mAbs significantly decreased urine total protein/creatinine ratios compared to the anti-TNFα, anti-CXCL13, or saline treatment groups (Fig.5).

At 34 weeks of age, periarterial lymphocytic infiltration at the hilus and along the major branches of the renal artery was observed in the PBS control group. There was also evidence of glomerular disease characterized by an increase in mesangial cellularity, collapse of capillary lumina, thickened basement membranes and the presence of amorphous hyaline deposits. These histological changes were associated with an increase in urinary total protein/creatinine ratio (Fig. 5).

Anti-TNFα or anti-CXCL13 mAb treatment alone did not significantly affect the glomerular disease development at week 34 as compared to the control treatment with saline. The beneficial effect of anti-CXCL13/anti-TNFα mAbs treatment on decreasing renal disease severity was reflected by the rank score of disease severity across the groups for glomerular disease (Fig. 6).

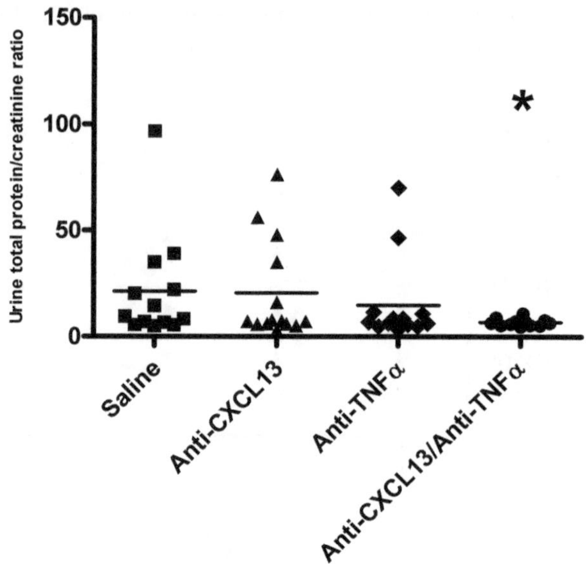

Fig. 5. Anti-CXCL13/anti-TNFα mAbs treatment significantly inhibited urine total protein/creatinine ratios. Urine total protein/creatinine ratios were determined at 34 weeks. * indicates $p<0.05$ vs. saline control treated group.

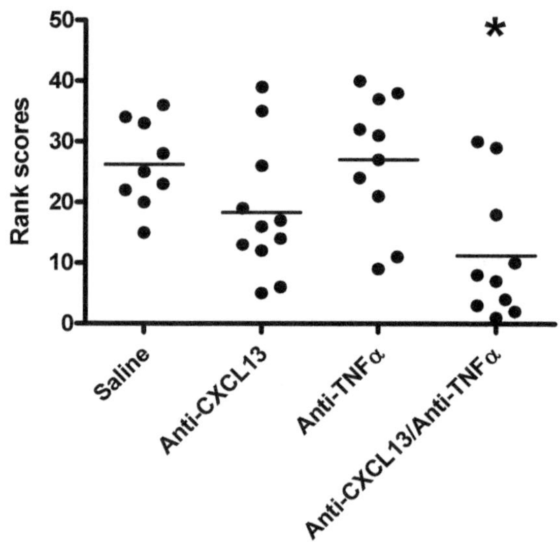

Fig. 6. Anti-CXCL13/anti-TNFα mAbs treatment reduced kidney disease in NZB/W F1 mice. Samples were examined and scored for disease severity in a blinded fashion. Pathology was assessed using the WHO Classifications. * indicates $p<0.05$ vs. saline control treated group.

3.5 Anti-CXCL13/Anti-TNFα mAb treatment decreased germinal center formation

In the splenic germinal center, B cell activation is triggered by ligation with sufficient antigen that has been captured by follicular dendritic cells in a complement and antibody-dependent process. B cell activation leads to migration of B cells towards the T cell zone. B cells then receive help from primed T-helper cells also expressing CXCR5 to form follicles and propagate GCs (Fazilleau et al., 2009). In the GCs, immunoglobulin class switching and somatic hypermutation as well as subsequent selection of centrocytes expressing BCR of increased affinity and specificity for the antigen result in the generation of affinity matured, long-lived plasma cells and memory cells.

To investigate the mechanism by which anti-CXCL13/anti-TNFα mAbs treatment has suppressed autoimmune responses in murine SLE, we examined the spleens for germinal center formation. Immunohistochemical staining for germinal center formation reveals that NZB/W mice treated with anti-CXCL13/anti-TNFα mAbs have decreased germinal center formation (Fig. 7). The reduction of the germinal center formation most likely resulted in a decrease of B cell stimulation and activation which subsequently led to suppressed anti-dsDNA autoAb production and glomerular disease development in mice treated with the anti-CXCL13/anti-TNFα mAbs. Mice treated with either mAb alone had germinal center formation similar to that of the saline treated mice in both number and size.

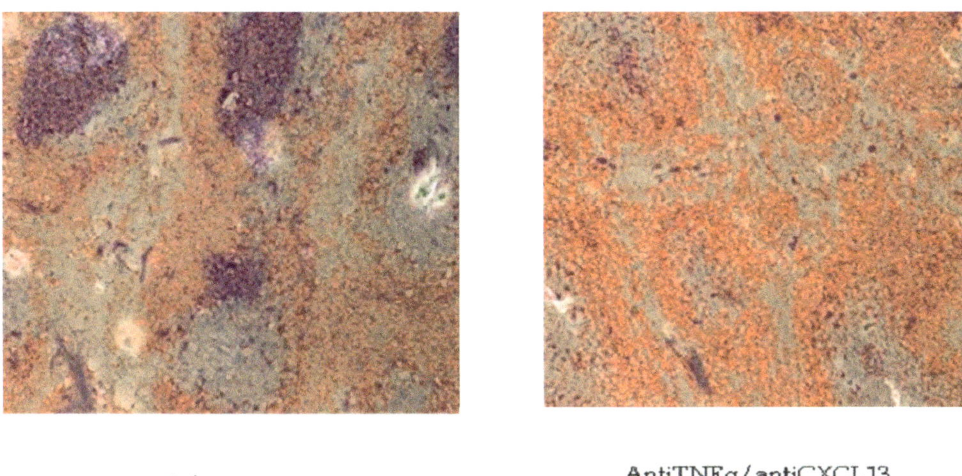

Fig. 7. Anti-CXCL13/anti-TNFα mAbs treatment decreased germinal center formation in NZB/W mouse spleen. (a) Saline or (b) Anti-CXCL13/anti-TNFα mAb treated spleen sections were stained with peanut agglutinin (blue) and anti-B220 (red) to identify germinal center and B cell zones. (Original magnification 20X).

3.6 Anti-CXCL13/Anti-TNFα treatment increased chemotactic activity of naive B cells

By treating NZB/W F1 mice with anti-CXCL13/anti-TNFα mAbs, we were able to inhibit autoimmune disease progression in NZB/W F1 mice. CXCL13 has been shown to be a very specific mature B cell chemoattractant. Expression of CXCR5 in mature naïve B cells is high, but after activation and differentiation, B cells lose CXCR5 expression (Hargreaves et al.,

2001). Thus naïve mature B cells would be more responsive to chemotatic migration induced by CXCL13. We investigated the effect of antibody treatment on B cell chemotaxis in our study. After treatment with anti-TNFα alone or the combination treatment of anti-CXCL13/anti-TNFα mAbs, the B cells purified from splenocytes were significantly more responsive to in vitro chemotactic stimulation induced by CXCL13 as compared to the B cells from animals treated with saline, or anti-CXCL13 mAb alone (Fig. 8).

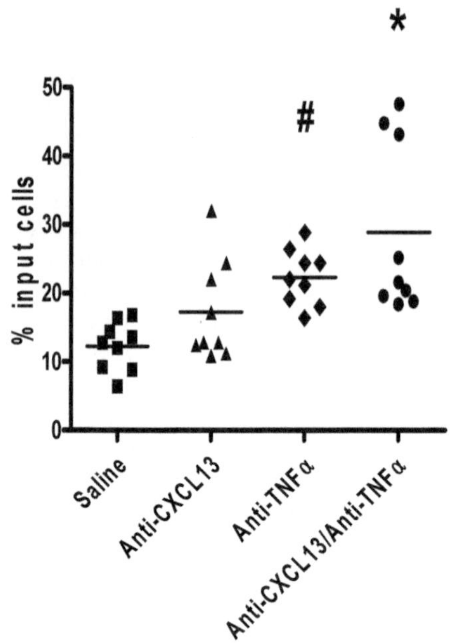

Fig. 8. Anti-CXCL13/anti-TNFα or anti-TNFα mAbs treatment significantly increased chemotaxis of B cells. B cells purified by negative selection over an AutoMacs column were loaded onto a 5 μM 96 well chemotaxis apparatus and exposed to 750 ng/ml CXCL13 for one hour. The cells in the bottom well were counted and expressed as a fraction of the cells loaded onto the apparatus. * and # indicates $p<0.05$ vs saline treated control.

A logical explanation for this observation is that in the saline or anti-CXCL13 mAb treated mice, there are an increased number of activated and differentiated B cells and decreased number of naïve B cells. Activated or differentiated B cells express fewer CXCR5 receptors and thus responded poorly in the chemotaxis assay. In contrast, there are more naïve B cells, which have normal expression of CXCR5 receptors, in the anti-TNFα and anti-CXCL13/anti-TNFα mAbs treated mice. This result is highly consistent with the B cell phenotype described earlier.

4. Discussion and conclusion

Systemic lupus erythematosus (SLE) is a complex autoimmune disease characterized by hyperactivity of autoreactive T and B cell responses against a variety of organs and can have widely varying degrees of severity(Ardoin & Pisetsky, 2008). Traditional therapies include steroids, mycophenolate, azathioprine, cyclophosphamide and hydroxychloroquine, which utilize various mechanisms of action resulting in global immune suppression and significant side effects (Wallace & Hahn, 2007).

There is a pressing need in the lupus field to find efficacious drugs with more specific immunosuppression. It has been shown by many investigators that various chemokines and cytokines play a role in the progression and pathogenesis of this complex disease (Dorner et al., 2009). It is generally accepted that treatments that would inhibit specific immune cell functions that are responsible for development of SLE may be beneficial for patients. The current study was designed to investigate the effect and mechanism of simultaneous application of two antibodies specific for B cells and inflammation in the inhibition of disease development in a murine model of lupus.

This study shows novel findings that can have applications for potential treatment of autoimmune disease. TNFα is increased in the blood and inflamed kidneys of SLE patients and correlates with disease activity (Ernandez & Mayadas, 2009; Studnicka-Bencke et al., 1996). TNF expression was also shown to be increased in aged NZB/W mice (Shiffer et al., 2008; Studnicka-Bencke et al., 1996). However, other literature addressing the role of TNFα in SLE suggests that it has a complex function. Administration of TNFα reduces incidence of SLE in young NZB/W F1 mice (Jacob et al., 1991). In NZB/W F1 mice, TNFα deficiency accelerates autoimmune disease and the mice develop severe lupus-like disease including autoantibodies to dsDNA and immune complex glomerulonephritis (Aringer & Smolen, 2008). TNFα seems to check autoimmunity in some paradigms, and foster inflammation in others, suggesting that other factors not yet identified may contribute to the role played by TNFα in SLE. This actually in part accounts for why we did not observe significant inhibition of autoimmune responses by anti-TNFα treatment alone in the current study.

Anti-dsDNA autoantibody levels in the serum were sometimes associated with disease activity and immune complex formation as well as glomerulonephritis in patients and mice. In our study, treatment with anti-CXCL13/anti-TNFα mAbs resulted in decreased anti-dsDNA autoantibody levels in the serum of NZB/W F1 mice, as compared with that of the TNFα alone treated mice (Fig 3). This result showed that blocking TNFα alone is not enough to suppress the autoimmune responses in this model as it did in other models. The likely reason could be the heavy involvement of B cells in such responses. The combination therapy with blockade of both TNFα and CXCL13 is superior to just the TNFα blockade alone due probably to the simultaneous suppression of both autoreactive B cells and TNFα.

CXCL13 participates in the follicular compartmentalization of B cells in GC and the induction of lymphotoxin ($LT\alpha_1\beta_2$) expression on B cells (Ansel et al., 2000). GCs support the differentiation of memory B cells and long-lived antibody secreting plasma cells. CXCL13 plays an important role in attracting naïve B cells to form germinal centers and can initiate lymphoid neogenesis when expressed aberrantly in mice (Cyster, 1999; Melchers et al., 1999; Takemura et al., 2001). Ectopic CXCL13 was expressed in aged NZB/w mice developing lupus nephritis (Ito et al., 2004). CXCL13 was enhanced in the thymus and kidney of aged NZB/w F1 mice (Ishikawa et al., 2001). There was a decreased number of CXCL13 producing peritoneal macrophages in aged NZB/w mice and the ectopic high expression of CXCL13 results in abnormal B1 cell trafficking during the development of murine lupus (Ito et al., 2004). As expected, treatment of NZB/w mice with a combination of anti-CXCL13 and anti-TNFα mAbs resulted in decreased germinal center formation in spleen sections in our study (Fig. 7). Combined treatment with anti-CXCL13/anti-TNFα mAbs significantly inhibited ex vivo IgM/CD40 stimulated B cells proliferation (Fig. 4), increased the frequency of follicular B cells (Fig. 1), and decreased the frequency of transitional B cells in the spleen (Fig. 2), when the total spleen cell number was not changed (data not shown) in our study. These novel results demonstrate that the combination therapy significantly dampens the autoimmune response in this model by maintaining a relatively normal lymphoid structure as well as B cell repertoire and lowering the activation status of the B cells, resulting in a higher threshold for hypereactivity.

Glomerulonephritis is a consequence of immune complex deposition and subsequent inflammatory cell infiltration and is a pathological hallmark feature of murine SLE. TNFα is highly expressed in glomeruli in all forms of lupus nephritis and the degree of TNFα expression correlates with renal inflammatory activity (Aringer & Smolen, 2003; Herrerra-Esparza et al., 1998). Administration of anti-CXCL13/anti-TNFα mAbs in our study significantly decreased the disease severity of glomerulonephritis in NZB/w F1 mice (Fig. 5 & 6), as reflected in decreased protein/creatinine ratios and kidney disease scores. In addition to the impact on B cells, neutralization of TNFα and CXCL13 could also result in decreased DC recruitment in the circulation and decreased DC differentiation and maturation into CXCL13 producing DC which has been suggested to play a pivotal role in the development of SLE (Ishikawa, 2002). In addition, treatment of NZB/W F1 mice with anti-TNFα or a combination of anti-CXCL13/anti-TNFα mAbs in our study resulted in a significant increase of mature B cell chemotactic response mediated by CXCL13. In the saline treated group, there were a large number of activated and differentiated B cells in the spleen, which do not express CXCR5 and therefore cannot respond to CXCL13 mediated chemotaxis. Treatment with anti-TNFα or anti-CXCL13 mAb alone did not result in significant inhibition of autoimmune responses and kidney nephritis in this particular murine lupus model. Treatment with anti-CXCL13 only affects naive mature B cell migration to the germinal center. The activated and memory B cells that contribute significantly to the autoimmune responses and disease development in this animal model were not significantly impacted by the anti-CXCL13 mAb, which limited subsequent efficacy. Furthermore, TNFα can interact and signal through two different receptors: TNFR1 and TNFR2, which can also bind LTα. LTα links with two LTβ molecules to form a heterotrimer that signals through LTβR (Browning et al., 1997). Both of these receptor pathways have been shown to activate expression of many genes, including CXCL13 (Ngo et al., 1999). Treatment with anti-TNFα mAb alone may only block the biologic activity of TNFα in symptoms driven by chronic inflammation, but not necessarily the autoimmune responses mediated by autoreactive B cells and LTβR with LTα. LTα would still be able to signal through TNFR or LTβR and contribute to increased CXCL13 expression and enhanced chemotaxis which may account for normal GC formation in the spleen of the TNFα mAb alone treated mice in our study. Simultaneously blocking both TNFα and CXCL13 allowed interruption of complementary inflammatory pathways, suppressed CXCL13 production and FDC maturation that contributes to the ultimate autoimmune disease development in this murine lupus model.

Further characterization of the effect of neutralization of CXCL13 and TNFα in this disease model might be achieved by use of an anti-CXCL13 antibody with increased potency, to ensure complete neutralization of CXCL13. Also neutralization of LT to evaluate the complete shutdown of the TNFα signaling pathway on the development of disease would be useful to characterize its contribution to disease development. An investigation of the effect of the combination of anti-CXCL13 and anti-TNFα in a therapeutic format could determine pathways essential in established disease. Additional studies to further characterize the mechanism of action of anti-CXCL13/anti-TNFα combinatorial treatment could include the contribution of cells from the innate immune system. Specifically, findings have been linked to mast cell stabilization including normalization of the B cell antibody profile for the promotion of innate as well as adaptive immunity during developmental phases of inflammation-induced immune dysfunction (Khatami, 2008, 2011)

In conclusion, this study demonstrated that combined administration of anti-TNFα and anti-CXCL13 mAbs significantly inhibited autoimmune responses and autoimmune disease progression in the NZB/W F1 murine model of systemic lupus erythematosus. This combined therapy could provide added benefit for advanced lupus patients that have advanced autoimmune disease.

5. Acknowledgements

We are very grateful to Dr. Meera Ramanujam for her scientific discussions and helpful comments.

6. References

Ansel, K.M., Ngo, V.N., Hyman, P.L., Luther, S.A., Forster, R., Sedgwick, J.D., Browning, J.L., Lipp, M., & Cyster, J.G. (2000). A chemokine-driven positive feedback loop organizes lymphoid follicles. *Nature* ,Vol.406, No. No.6793, (July 2000), pp. 309-314, ISSN 0028-0836

Ardoin, S.P., & Pisetsky, D.S. (2008). Developments in the scientific understanding on lupus. *Arthritis Research and Therapy,*Vol.10, No.5, (October 2008), pp.218-225, ISSN 1478-6354

Aringer, M., & Smolen, J.S. (2003). SLE-Complex cytokine effects in a complex autoimmune disease: tumor necrosis factor in systemic lupus erythematosus. *Arthritis Research and Therapy,* Vol.5, No.4, (May 2003), pp.172-177, ISSN 1478-6354

Aringer, M., & Smolen, J.S. (2008). Efficacy and safety of TNF-blocker therapy in systemic lupus erythematosus. *Expert Opinion on Drug Safety,* Vol.7, No.4, (July 2008), pp.411-419, ISSN 1474-0338

Bagaeva, L.V., Rao, P., Powers, J.M., & Segal, B. (2006). CXC chemokine ligand 13 plays a role in experimental autoimmune encephalomyelitis. *Journal of Immunology,* Vol.176, No.12, (June 2006), pp.7676-7685, ISSN 0022-1767

Browning, J.L., Sizing, I.D., Lawton, P., Bourdon, P., Rennert, P., Majeau, g., Ambrose, C., Hession, C., Miatkowski, K., Griffiths, D., Ngam-ek, A., Meier, W., Benjamin, C., & Hochman, P. (1997). Characterization of Lymphotoxin-αβ complexes on the surface of murine lymphocytes. *Journal of Immunology,* Vol.159, No.7, (October 1997), pp.3288-3298, ISSN 0022-1767

Carlsen, H., Baekkevoid, E., Morton, H.C., Haraldsen, G., & Brandtzaeg, P. (2004). Monocyte-like and mature macrophages produce CXCL13 (B cell-attracting chemokine-1) in inflammatory lesions with lymphoid neogenesis. *Blood,* Vol.104, No.10, (November 2004), pp. 3021-3027, ISSN 0006-4971

Cyster, J.G. (1999). Chemokines and cell migration in secondary lymphoid organs. *Science,* Vol.286, No.5447, (December 1999), pp.2098-2102, ISSN 0036-8075

Dick, A.D., McMenamin, P.G., Korner, H., Scallon, B.J., Ghrayeb, .J, Forrester, J.V., & Sedgwick JD. (1996). Inhibition of tumor necrosis factor activity minimizes target organ damage in experimental autoimmune uveoretinitis despite quantitatively normal activated T cell traffic to the retina. *European Journal of Immunology,* Vol.26, No.5, (May 1996), pp.1018-1025, ISSN 0014-2980

Dorner, T., Jacobi, A.M., & Lipsky, P.E. (2009). B cells in autoimmunity. *Arthritis Research and Therapy,* Vol. 11, No. 5, (October 2009), pp.247-257, ISSN 0004-3591

Ernandez, T., & Mayadas, T.N. (2009). Immunoregulatory role of TNFα in inflammatory kidney diseases. *Kidney International,* Vol.76, No.3, (August 2009), pp.262-276, ISSN 0085-2538

Fazilleau, N., Mark, L., McHeyzer-Williams, L.J., & McHeyzer-Williams, M.G. (2009). Follicular helper T cells: lineage and location. *Immunity* Vol.30, No.3, pp.324-335, (March 2009), ISSN 1074-7613

Gunn, M.D., Ngo, V.N., Ansel, M., Ekland, E.H., Cyster, J.G., & Williams, L.T. (1998). A B-cell-homing chemokine made in lymphoid follicles activated Burkitt's lymphoma receptor-1. *Nature,* Vol. 391,No.6669, (February 1998), pp.799-803, ISSN 0028-0836

Hargreaves, D.C., Hyman, P.L., Lu, T., Ngo, V., Bidgol, A., Suzuki, G., Zou, Y., Littman, D., & Cyster, J. (2001). A coordinated change in chemokine responsiveness guides plasma cell movements. *Journal of Experimental Medicine,*Vol.194, No.1, (July 2001), pp.45-56, ISSN 0022-1007

Herrera-Esparza, R., Barbosa-Cisneros, O., Villalobos-Hurtado, R., & Avalos-Diaz, E. (1998). Renal expression of IL-6 and TNFα genes in lupus nephritis. *Lupus,* Vol.7, No.3, (March 1998), pp.154-158, ISSN 0961-2033

Hirotani, M., Niino, M., Sasaki, H. (2010). The role of B cells in Multiple Sclerosis: Implications for B-cell-Targeted Therapy. *Current Medicinal Chemistry,* Vol. 17, No. 28, (September 2010), pp.3215-3222, ISSN 0929-8673

Ishikawa, S., Sato, T., Abe, M., Nagai, S., Onai, N., Yoneyama, H., Zhang, Y., Suzuki, T., Hashimoto, S., Shirai, T., Lipp, M., & Matsushima, K. (2001). Aberrant High Expression of B Lymphocyte Chemokine (BLC/CXCL13) by CD11b+CD11c+ Dendritic cells in murine lupus and preferential chemotaxis of B1 cells toward BLC. *Journal of Experimental Medicine,* Vol.193, No.12, (June 2001), pp.1393-1402, ISSN 0022-1007

Ishikawa, S., Nagai, S., Sato, T., Akadegawa, K., Yoneyama, H., Zhang, Y., Onai, N., & Matsushima, K. (2002). Increased circulating CD11b+CD11c+ dendritic cells (DC) in aged BWF1 mice which can be matured by TNFα into BLC/CXCL13-producing DC. *European Journal of Immunology,* Vol.32, No.7, (July 2002), pp.1881-1887, ISSN 0014-2980

Ito, T., Ishikawa, S., Sato, T., Akadegawa, K., Yurino, H., Kitabatake, M., Hontsu, S., Ezaki, T., Kimura, H., & Matsushima, K. (2004). Defective B1 cell homing to the peritoneal cavity and preferential recruitment of B1 cells in the target organs in a murine model for systemic lupus erythematosus. *Journal of Immunology,* Vol.172, No.6, (March 2004), pp.3628-3634, ISSN 0022-1767

Jacob, C.O., Hwang, F., Lewis, G.D., & Stall, A.M. (1991). Tumour necrosis factor alpha in murine systemic lupus erythematosus disease models: Implications for genetic predisposition and immune regulation. *Cytokine,* Vol.3, No.6, (November 1991), pp.551-561, ISSN 1043-4666

Khatami, M. (2008). 'Yin and Yang' in inflammation: duality in innate immune cells function and tumorigenesis. *Expert Opinion on Biological Therapy,* Vol.8, No.10, (October 2008), pp.1461-1472, ISSN 1471-2598

Khatami, M. (2011). Unresolved inflammation: 'immune tsunami' or erosion of integrity in immune-privileged and immune-responsive tissues and acute and chronic inflammatory diseases or cancer, In: *Expert Opinion on Biological Therapy,* June 2011, Available from: http://informahealthcare.com/toc/ebt/0/0

Kollias, G., Douni, E., Kassiotis, G., & Kontoyiannis, D. (1999). The function of tumor necrosis factor and receptors in models on multi-organ inflammation, rheumatoid arthritis, multiple sclerosis and inflammatory bowel disease. *Annals of the Rheumatic Diseases,*Vol.58, No.Suppl I, (November 1999), pp.I32-I39, ISSN 0003-4967

Liang, B., Eaton-Bassiri, A., Bugelski, P. (2007). B cells and beyond, therapeutic opportunities targeting inflammation. *Innflammation and Allergy-Drug Targets,* Vol.6, No.3, (September 2007), pp.142-149, ISSN 1871-5281

Lipsky, P. (2001). Systemic lupus erythematosus: an autoimmune disease of B cell hyperactivity. *Nature Immunology,* Vol.2, No.9, (September 2001), pp.764-766, ISSN 1529-2908

Magliozzi, R., Columba-Cabezas, S., Serafini, B., & Aloisi, F. (2004). Intracerebral expression of CXCL13 and BAFF is accompanied by formation of lymphoid follicle-like structures in the meninges of mice with relapsing experimental autoimmune encephalomyelitis. *Journal of Neuroimmunology,*Vol.148, No.1, pp.11-23, ISSN 0165-5728

Melchers, F., Rolink, A.G., & Schaniel, C. (1999). The role of chemokines in regulating cell migration during humoral immune responses. *Cell,* Vol.99, No.4, (November 1999), pp.351-354, ISSN 0092-8674

Meraouna, A., Cizeron-Clairac, G., Le Panse, R., Bismuth, J., Truffault, F., Tallaksen, C., Berrih-Aknin, S. (2006). The chemokine CXCL13 is a key molecule in autoimmune myasthenia gravis. *Blood,* Vol. 108, No.2, (July 2006), pp.432-440, ISSN 0006-4971

Ngo, V.N., Korner, H., Gunn, M.D., Schmidt, K., Riminton, D., Cooper, M., Browning, J., Sedgwick, J., & Cyster, J.G. (1999). Lymphotoxin alpha/beta and tumor necrosis factor are required for stromal cell expression of homing chemokines in B and T cell areas of the spleen. *Journal of Experimental Medicine,* Vol.189, No.2, (January 1999), pp.403-412, ISSN 0022-1007

Panayi, G. (2005). B cells: a fundamental role in the pathogenesis of rheumatoid arthritis? *Rheumatology,* Vol.44, Suppl.2, (May 2005), pp. 113-ii7, ISSN 0315-162X

Rahman, A., & Isenberg, D. (2008). Systemic Lupus Erythematosus. *New England Journal of Medicine,* Vol.358, No.9, (February 2008), pp.929-939, ISSN 0028-4793

Ramanujam, M., & Davidson, A. (2008)., Targeting of the immune system in systemic lupus erythematosus. *Expert Reviews in Molecular Medicine,* Vol.10, No.2, (January 2008), pp.1-27,ISSN 1226-3613

Ruddle, N.H., Bergman, C.M., McGrath, K.M., Lingenheld, E.G., Grunnet, M.L., Padula, S.J.,& Clark, R.B. (1990). An antibody to lymphotoxin and tumor necrosis factor prevents transfer of experimental allergic encephalomyelitis. *Journal of Experimental Medicine,*Vol.172, No.4, (October 1990), pp.1193-1200, ISSN 0022-1007

Salomonsson, S., Larsson, P., Tengner, P., Mellquist, E., Hjelmstrom, P., & Wahren-Herlenius, M. (2002). Expression of the B cell-attracting chemokine CXCL13 in the target organ and autoantibody production in ectopic lymphoid tissue in the chronic inflammatory disease Sjogren's syndrome. *Scandanavian Journal of Immunology,* Vol.55, No.4, (April 2002), pp.336-342, ISSN 0300-9475

Schiffer, L., Bethunaickan, R., Ramanujam, M., Huang, W., Schiffer, M., Tao, H., Madaio, M., Bottinger, E., & Davidson, A. (2008). Activated renal macrophages are markers of disease onset and disease remission in lupus nephritis. *Journal of Immunology,* Vol.180, No.3, (February 2008), pp.1938-1947, ISSN 0022-1767

Shi, K., Hayashida, K., Kaneko, M., Hashimoto, J., Tomita, T., Lipsky, P.E., Yoshikawa, H., & Ochi, T. (2001). Lymphoid Chemokine B cell-attracting chemokine-1 (CXCL13) is expressed in germinal center of ectopic lymphoid follicles within the synovium of chronic arthritis patients. *Journal of Immunology* Vol.166, No. 1, (January 2001), pp.650-655, ISSN 0022-1767

Studnicka-Benke, A., Steiner, G., Petera, P., & Smolen, J.S. (1996). Tumor necrosis factor alpha and its soluble receptors parallel clinical disease and autoimmune activity in systemic lupus erythematosus. *British Journal of Rheumatology,*Vol.35, No.11, (November 1996), pp.1067-1074, ISSN 0263-7103

Takemura, S., Braun, A., Crowson C., Kurtin P., Cofield, R., O'Fallon, W., Goronzy, J., & Weyand, C. (2001). Lymphoid neogenesis in Rheumatoid Synovitis. (2001). *Journal of Immunology,*Vol.167, No.2, (July 2001), pp.1072-1080, ISSN 0022-1767

Wallace, D.J., & Hahn B. (2007). *DuBois Lupus Erythematosus, 7th edn.* Lippincott Williams & Wilkins, ISBN 978-0-7817-9394-0, Philadelphia,PA

Weening, J.J., D'Agati, V.D., Schwartz, Seshan, S., Alpers, C., Appel, G., Balow, J., Bruijn, J., Cook, T., Farrario, F., Fogo, A., Ginzler, E., Hebert, L., Hill, G., Hill, P., Jennette, J., Kong, N., Lesavre, P., Lockshin, M., Looi, L., Makino, H., Moura, L., & Nagata, M. (2004). The classification of glomerulonephritis in systemic lupus erythematosus revisited. *Kidney International,* Vol.65, No.2, (February 2004), pp.521-530, ISSN 0085-2538

Yu, S., Dunn, R., Kehry, M., Braley-Mullen, H. (2008). B cell depletion inhibits spontaneous autoimmune thyroiditis in NOD.H-2h4 mice. *Journal of Immunology,* Vol.180, No.11, (June 2008), pp.7706-7713, ISSN0022-1767

Zheng, B., Ozen, Z., Zhang, X., De Silva, S., Marinova, E., Guo, L., Wansley, D., Huston, D., West, M., & Han, S. (2005). CXCL13 neutralization reduces the severity of collagen-induced arthritis. *Arthritis and Rheumatism,* Vol.52, No.2, (February 2005), pp.620-626, ISSN 0004-3591

19

Biologic Agents for Inflammatory Bowel Disease (The Current, the Future and the Controversy)

Iyad A. Issa
Lebanese American University
Lebanon

1. Introduction

Inflammatory bowel conditions (IBD) are chronic relapsing diseases. Crohn's disease (CD) is characterised by transmural inflammation due to an imbalance between pro- and anti-inflammatory molecules. Ulcerative colitis (UC) is only a mucosal disease, however one quarter of patients develop fulminating disease and 20% require surgery. Treatment objectives usually include steroid-free remission, decrease in hospitalization and surgery and sustained clinical remission and mucosal healing as well as reduction in the risk of dysplasia and cancer.

The description of the cell signalling cascade over the past 20 years has led to a surge in potential treatments for IBD. It was initially thought that since CD is mediated through the T helper 1 cascade, using specific molecules to block it would be a reasonable approach to potential cure. A multitude of medications and trials later proved this theory to be true. In addition, UC which was thought to be mediated through a different inflammatory cascade (T helper 2) was soon discovered to respond to these newer molecules. In fact several trials showed T helper 1 cells to be prevalent in the serum, stool and mucosa of patients with active UC. The better knowledge of the inflammatory pathways in IBD lead to the development of new targeted therapies with a multitude of actions including inhibition of leukocytes trafficking, inhibition of T cell activation or polarization and inhibition of pro-inflammatory cytokines. Additionally a new technique called humanization was developed through advances in protein engineering and lead to the production of partially humanized and finally fully humanized antibodies.

2. Anti-TNFs

Development of Tumour Necrosis Factor (TNF) agents dramatically changed the course of IBD. They block both soluble and membrane TNF but also fix complement.

2.1 Infliximab

Infliximab is a partially human chimeric molecule introduced in the market before 2000. It was shown to be adequately effective in inducing and maintaining remission in patients with moderate to severe disease (ACCENT 1 & 2). It is a chimeric monoclonal anti-TNF IgG1 antibody and able to block both soluble and membrane TNF and also fix complement. It is also capable of inducing apoptosis of T-cells and monocytes in a caspase dependant manner [Ten Hove et al. 2002]. It has a proven efficacy in induction and maintenance of remission in patients with refractory luminal and fistulising CD [Hanauer et al. 2002; Present et al. 1999; Targan et al. 1997]. It has also been shown to induce rapid and profound mucosal healing. In the ACCENT 1 trial [Hanauer et al. 2002], IFX induced a clinical response at 5 mg/Kg administered at weeks 0, 2 and 6. It was given every 8 weeks afterwards and assessed at week 54 where a remission rate of 29% was demonstrated compared to the 5% induced in the placebo group. Moreover, mucosal healing was obtained in 44% of patients compared to 18% in the placebo group. The ACCENT 2 study showed that IFX (similar loading and maintenance regimen) improved fistulising disease in 55% and 38% of patients treated respectively with 10 and 5 mg/Kg compared to the placebo group (13%) [Sands et al. 2004]. At week 54, a sustained response was observed in 69% and 46% of patients of the 2 groups compared to placebo (23%).

There is some controversy as to wether the addition of immune-modulators alters the response to IFX. The original ACCENT 1 and 2 trials did not establish the benefit of concomitant therapy. Similarly, the COMMIT study evaluating the addition of methotrexate to IFX regimens for CD failed to demonstrate any benefit [Feagan B et al. 2008]. Others did observe that the addition of immune-modulators prior to IFX does help to maintain duration of response, especially if started more than 3 months before [Rudolph et al. 2008].

The efficacy of IFX in inducing and maintaining remission in 110 children with a diagnosis of CD has been shown in the REACH trial [Hyams et al. 2007] with 88% response and 59% remission rate at week 10 and 64% and 56% at 1 year.

Subsequent to the marketing of IFX for CD in the United States in 1998 there were several reports of "open label" use of IFX for refractory, moderate to severe UC in out-patients settings [Gornet et al. 2003; Su et al. 2002; Chey et al. 2001]. There were no standardized administration schedules and most patients received a single infusion. The first randomized placebo controlled trial was reported in 2003; it enrolled patients with corticosteroid refractory disease to receive IFX at 5 mg/Kg at weeks 0 and 2. Results showed no statistical difference with placebo regarding clinical or endoscopic remission [Probert et al. 2003]. However, two large multi-center, placebo-controlled randomized trials were performed to clarify the role of IFX in refractory UC. The ACT 1 and 2 were designed to evaluate both induction and maintenance effect. They studied the efficacy of IFX at a dose of 5 mg or 10 mg/Kg administered at week 0, 2 and 6 in moderate to severe UC compared to placebo during 54 weeks (ACT 1) or 30 weeks (ACT 2) [Rutgeert et al. 2005]. Week 8 clinical response was 61 and 69% in patients treated with 5 mg and 10 mg/Kg respectively versus 29 and 37% in the placebo group. At the conclusion of 54 weeks in ACT 1 and 30 weeks in ACT 2, clinical remissions were observed in 35% in the IFX group compared to 15% in the placebo group. Furthermore, additional pre-defined end-points including "mucosal healing" and "steroid free remissions" were reported with significant benefit. Follow up of these cohorts also reported a drop in the rate of colectomy (67%) versus placebo (27%) [Janerot et al. 2005].

Clinical series in pediatric patients with moderate to severe refractory UC have described very similar results to series enrolling adult patients with approximately 50% of patients avoiding colectomy within 5 years of initiating IFX [Hyams et al. 2010; Russo et al. 2009; Wilhelm et al. 2008; Jakobovits et al. 2007].

In the settings of severe-fulminant UC, cyclosporine has been (although controversial) described as salvage therapy for patients who have failed a course of intravenous steroids

[McDonald et al. 2005; Hanauer et al. 2005]. A placebo controlled trial comparing IFX to placebo in hospitalized patients with severe UC not responding to conventional therapy was conducted [Janerot et al. 2005]. Patients admitted, who didn't respond to IV steroids within 4 or 7 days (depending on their initial status) received a single infusion of IFX, 4-5 mg / Kg or placebo with the primary endpoint of colectomy 3 months after randomization. 7 out of 14 patients in the IFX group versus 14 out of 21 in the placebo group underwent colectomy. The debate between uses of cyclosporine or IFX for patients with fulminant UC has been complicated by the complexity of monitoring cyclosporine IV compared to the ease of giving IFX [Janerot et al. 2006].

Additional questions remain regarding the need for long term dosing after anti-TNF induction therapy as ACT studies did not evaluate the long term responses and one may speculate that doses may need adjustment on the long term [Danese et al. 2008; Kohn et al. 2007].

Some patients were noted to develop anti-drug antibodies and this increased the risk of potential hypersentivity reactions (acute and delayed) as well as secondary loss of response [Hanauer et al. 2004; Baert et al. 2003]. Episodic treatment was coupled with a higher rate of anti-drug antibodies (30 - 60%) compared to patients receiving a scheduled protocol (7 - 10%) [Hanauer et al. 2004]. This risk seems to be lower if patients are treated with concomitant immune-suppressive agents. ACCENT 1 and 2 showed and acceptable tolerability profile with a low rate of serious side effects. Development of active tuberculosis in patients with latent tuberculosis was observed [Keane et al. 2001]. Therefore the presence of latent tuberculosis has to be evaluated before treatment [Rutgeerts et al. 2004]. The TREAT trial showed similar mortality rates in IFX and placebo group [Lichtenstein et al. 2006].

This drug received FDA approval in 1998 for use in patients with moderate to severe CD and in those with fistulising disease. Currently we have a decade of experience with it and a massive number of patients and trials detailing its efficacy, long term benefits and adverse effects. The use in UC was advocated later, it received FDA approval for use in moderate to severe disease patients in 2006.

2.2 Adalimumab

Adalimumab (ADA) is a fully humanized monoclonal anti-TNF and therefore immunogenicity is very low. The CLASSIC 1 trial was the first multi-center randomized double blind controlled trial studying the response to ADA in 299 moderate-severe CD patients naïve to anti-TNF therapy [Hanauer et al. 2006). They received induction therapy with ADA 40 mg/20 mg, 80 mg/40 mg, 160 mg/80 mg or placebo, at weeks 0 and 2. The primary endpoint was remission at week 4. Rates seen in the 160 mg/80 mg group was 36% versus 12% for the placebo group. Clinical response was significantly higher in both groups of ADA with higher dosing regimen. 55 patients from the CLASSIC 1 trial were enrolled in the CLASSIC 2 study [Sandborn et al. 2007]. This study showed remission maintained at week 54 in 74%, 83% and 44% of the patients treated respectively with ADA 40 mg every 2 weeks, every week and placebo. Data from the CHARM trial [Colombel et al. 2007], conducted in CD patients with the same clinical characteristics, randomized to receive ADA 40 mg QOW, 40 mg weekly or placebo after an open label induction regimen of ADA 80 mg/40 mg, support in a large cohort (854 patient) the fact that this drug is more effective than placebo for maintaining clinical remission at week 26 (40%, 47% versus 17% in placebo). No significant difference was found between the dosage of 40 mg QOW and 40 mg QW. Interestingly, the response rate was higher in patients who had never received other anti-TNFs before. There is no randomized controlled trial studying ADA in fistulizing CD, but the presence of a fistula was not an exclusion criteria in the CHARM trial and post hoc data have been published. Complete fistula closure was seen in 36% of patients treated with ADA every other week, 46% in those treated weekly and 14% in the placebo group [Colombel et al. 2009]. In an open label single arm trial , the CHOICE, 673 CD patients who were IFX primary non-responders (17%) or initial responders (83%), were enrolled and treated with ADA (induction dose 160/80 mg and maintenance dose 40 mg QOW). At baseline 88 patients (13%) had at least one draining cutaneous fistula. Complete fistula healing was achieved by 34 patients (39%) at the last visit (dates from week 4 to week 36) [Lichtiger et al. 2010]. Improvements in quality of life and work productivity were sustained all throughout, as well as the group of non-responders. The GAIN study reported the first data on ADA use in IFX intolerant or secondary non-responder patients [Sandborn et al. 2007]. 301 patients enrolled showed remission in 21% at week 4 (standard induction and maintenance doses) compared to only 7% in the placebo group. The safety of ADA was comparable to that of IFX. Remission rate was 39% at 6 months and 29% at one year. Data on the efficacy of ADA on primary non-responders to IFX are limited. In the large cohort of the open label CARE study, about one quarter of patients were primary non-responders to IFX [Lofberg et al. 2011]. The percentage of patients in remission was 43% at week 4 and increased to 52% at week 20. Remission was significantly different between IFX-naïve compared to IFX-exposed patients (62% vs 42%). A systematic review including all open-label cohorts that evaluated the efficacy of ADA in IFX primary and secondary non-responders was published. Among the 15 studies included, 1810 CD patients with previous IFX exposure were identified. Short term clinical response (week 4) ranged from 41% to 83%. Long term clinical remission (12 months) ranged from 19% to 68%. The authors concluded that the variability was because of differences in the study design and baseline characteristics of the patients included in the studies [Ma et al. 2009].

Regarding "mucosal healing", the EXTEND study included 135 patients with moderate-severe ileo-colonic CD and baseline mucosal ulceration [Colombel et al. 2010]. After induction 129 patients enrolled were randomized to maintenance. The primary endpoint was deep remission and mucosal healing as evidenced by the absence of mucosal ulceration at week 12 and 52. A highly statistical difference was noted at 52 weeks between the 2 groups (19% vs 0%).

The RESEAT trial is the largest multi-center experience using ADA for pediatric CD [Rosh et al. 2009]. 115 children included were shown to have clinical response rates at 3, 6 and 12 months of 65%, 71% and 70%. Similarly, clinical remission was 32%, 43% and 49%.

Preliminary data from open-label trials showed efficacy of ADA in mild-moderate UC with loss of response or poor tolerability to IFX [Trinder and Lawrance 2009]. Until now, the only randomized placebo-controlled double blind trial was an 8 week multi-center study, conducted in North America and Europe, it included patients with moderately to severely active UC [Reinisch et al. 2011]. All patients were naïve to IFX and failed or didn't tolerate conventional treatment. Standard ADA dosing was used and the primary endpoint was clinical remission at week 8. No significant difference was found in clinical remission, response and mucosal healing in the three arms. However, a difference was noted regarding rectal bleeding score and physician global assessment. Recently a small randomized trial assessed the long term efficacy of ADA in patients with UC. Clinical response and remission were assessed at weeks 4 and 12. The proportion of patients who continued on ADA and those who remained colectomy free were noted over the long term. Clinical response was achieved in 53% and 60% at week 4 and 12 respectively and remission in 10% and 27%. After a 48 week follow up, 50% of patients were still on ADA and only 20% underwent

colectomy. All patients who achieved clinical response at week 12 were colectomy free at 1 year [Taxonera et al. 2011]. Data on efficacy should be confirmed by large prospective trials.
The safety profile of ADA in global clinical trials in CD patients was comparable to that of IFX. Analysing the largest trial of ADA in CD, the types and frequency of adverse events and serious adverse events were similar to placebo in both induction and maintenance phases [Colombel et al. 2009]. In the all exposed patients from the main trials, 56 patients (1.8%) had opportunistic infections. The most frequently reported serious adverse event was serious infection (5.8%). Low incidences of malignancies were reported in the CD trials. Four deaths were recorded, in particular only one of these was related to ADA therapy [Colombel et al. 2009].
This medication was rewarded FDA approval for use in patients with CD in 2007. Although data from the open label trials showed it is also efficacious in UC but large prospective trials results are still pending and so is the FDA approval.

2.3 Certolizumab Pegol

Certoluzimab Pegol is the third medication in this family and involves the addition of two polyethylene glycols to the antibody fragment rendering its plasma half-life longer. The preliminary placebo-controlled phase II trial studied certolizumab at different doses (100, 200 and 400 mg) at weeks 1, 4 and 8 in patients with moderate - severe CD [Schreiber et al. 2005]. All doses produced benefit at week 2 but at week 10 the optimal dose was discovered to be 400 mg. The PRECISE 1 and 2 trials used an induction dose of 400 mg at week 0, 2 and 4 and then every 4 weeks. The trial showed response by two thirds of patients at week 6 in comparison to placebo but no significant improvement in remission at weeks 6 and 26 [Sandborn et al. 2007; Schreiber et al. 2007].

3. Adhesion molecules

In CD there is continuous release of pro-inflammatory cytokines and persistent recruitment of leukocytes into the gastrointestinal tissue. Interference with the mechanism of regulation of this trafficking would reasonably be an attractive therapeutic strategy. Much of this leukocyte trafficking is mediated through a large family of transmembrane proteins including integrins, selectins, chemokines and their associated ligands [Springer et al. 1994]. This on-going and persistent recruitment of leukocytes into gut tissue is of paramount importance in maintaining and perpetuating the inflammation associated with IBD. Adhesion molecules are located at the surface of endothelial cells and play a crucial role in the migration of leukocytes from blood vessels to intestinal tissues.

3.1 Natalizumab

Natalizumab is a humanized monoclonal antibody inhibiting the migration and adhesion of leukocytes into inflamed tissues. This humanization resulted in an antibody that is 95% human, with a potential for lower immunogenicity, increased half-life, and the ability for repeated administration while maintaining potency [Kent et al. 1995; Leger et al. 1997].
In CD, the initial pilot study was a small, randomized, placebo-controlled trial conducted in 30 patients with mild to moderate active disease, randomized to receive either Natalizumab 3 mg/Kg as a single intravenous infusion, or placebo [Gordon et al. 2001]. At week 2 the mean drop in CDAI (Crohn's disease activity index) was significantly higher in the treatment group compared to placebo. The phase III study program consisted of evaluating

Natalizumab as induction therapy for CD [Sandborn et al. 2005]. The ENACT 1 trial randomized patients to receive either Natalizumab 300 mg of placebo at weeks 0, 4 and 8. Both response and remission were not statistically significant between the 2 groups, which was disappointing. However, subgroup analysis showed a significant difference in patients with baseline elevated CRP and those on concomitant immune-modulators. Similarly there was also a significant difference in both endpoints in patients previously treated with anti-TNFs. The mixed results of the ENACT 1 trial lead to the design of a second induction trial, ENCORE [Targan et al. 2007]. It involved only patients with elevated CRP and moderate - severe CD. The primary endpoint was response through week 12. Both rates of response and remission were significantly higher in the Natalizumab group (48% and 26%) compared to the placebo group (32% and 16%). These rates were substantially higher starting week 4, thus demonstrating the efficacy of Natalizumab for induction of remission in selected CD patients. The ENACT 2 involved 339 patients who had a response in ENACT 1, they were randomized to receive 300 mg of natalizumab or placebo every 4 weeks for 12 months [Sandborn et al. 2005]. 61% of patients treated with Natalizumab had a sustained response through week 36 compared to 28% in the placebo group. The remission rate was 44% versus 26%. Serious adverse events were similar in both groups.

A pilot study of Natalizumab in UC showed no major adverse events [Gordon et al. 2002].

In phase I and II trials, the occurrence of adverse events ranged from 9% - 12%, with the most frequent being headache and abdominal pain [Gordon et al. 2001; Ghosh et al. 2003]. Similarly in the ENACT 1 and 2 trials adverse events were reported in comparable frequency between both groups. Influenza like symptoms were reported more frequently in patients receiving Natalizumab. Acute infusion reactions were reported in 11% and 7% in both trials and antibody detected were less than 10%. Although deemed safe Natalizumab was associated with progressive multifocal leukoencephalopathy (PML), a fatal opportunistic infectious brain disorder induced by the JC virus [Van Assche et al. 2005]. This complication has also been described in six patients treated for multiple sclerosis. A follow up of more than 3000 patients who received Natalizumab in different clinical trials showed no additional cases. As of June 2007, more than 10,000 patients had received the drug for multiple sclerosis with no new reports of PML.

In January 2008, the FDA approved the use of Natalizumab in the treatment of patients with moderate - severe CDwho have failed or cannot tolerate available therapies including anti-TNFs.

3.2 Vedolizumab

Due to the major adverse events associated with Natalizumab, newer selective adhesion molecules inhibitors are in development. Vedolizumab (MLN-02) is one of those new agents; it is a humanized antibody directed against integrin $\alpha 4\beta 7$. It has been studied in 181 patients with active ulcerative colitis [Feagan et al. 2005]. The difference in clinical response at week 6 was significantly different between groups: 33% (0.5 mg/Kg), 32% (2 mg/Kg), and 14% (placebo). The phase II, double blind, placebo-controlled, dose finding trial has been reported [Feagan et al. 2003]. 185 patients were randomized to receive either one of 2 doses (0.5 mg/Kg or 2 mg/Kg) Vedolizumab or placebo at day 1 and 29. The study failed to show a difference in response between the groups, however remission rate on day 57 in the 2 mg/Kg group (37%) was statistically superior than both groups. But since dynamic data showed that the receptors were not completely saturated, it is possible that the appropriate dose was not studied yet.

4. New molecules

Interleukin 12 is one of those many cytokines that drive the inflammatory response. It is found in high amounts and concentrations in the bowel walls of patients with CD [Gately et al. 1998]. Administration of recombinant anti-IL 12 has been shown to inhibit colitis in mice [Davidson et al. 1998]. Currently two fully humanized IgG1 monoclonal antibodies have been developed: ABT-874 and CNTO 1275 (Ustekinumab). A randomized controlled study of 79 moderate - severe CD patients treated with ABT-874 (1 or 3 mg/Kg) was done. Response was 75% in the group with the higher dose compared to 25% in the placebo group [Mannon et al. 2004]. A high proportion of patient included developed injection-site reactions, but only 3 out of 79 patients developed anti-drug antibodies. Recently a double blind trial studied the efficacy of ustekinumab [Sandborn et al. 2008]. Response rates versus placebo were 53% and 30% respectively at weeks 4 and 49% and 40% respectively at week 8. In the subgroup of patients exposed previously to IFX, clinical response to ustekinumab was again significantly higher than placebo.

Visiluzimab is a humanized anti-CD3 monoclonal antibody. An open label phase I trial included 32 severe steroid-refractory UC patients. They received Visiluzimab at 10 or 15 µg/Kg, intravenously on 2 consecutive days. The remission rate (66%) and response rate (87%) were both acceptable as well as the adverse events. However, development of this compound has been halted due to transient elevation of blood EBV-DNA noted in some patients [Plevy et al. 2007].

IL-6 is a molecule that promotes inflammation by playing a key role in the apoptosis resistance of T cells in CD, it acts in synergy with IL-12 [Yen et al. 2006]. Preliminary studies for blocking IL6 showed potential in decreasing colitis in mice. Tocilizumab a recombinant anti-IL 6 showed efficacy at week 12 both in induction of response and remission in 36 patients with moderate-severe CD. Intravenous doses of 8 mg/Kg every 2 weeks and every 4 weeks were given. The response was higher in the group treated every 2 weeks, no major adverse events were noted [Ito et al. 2004].

Il-10 is an anti-inflammatory cytokine whose production is reduced in patients with CD. IL-10 deficient mice develop transmural inflammation of the gut. This can be prevented by administering recombinant IL-10 [Kuhn et al. 1993]. However, when tested clinically no efficacy was observed and multiple side effects occurred [Fedorak et al. 2000].

Problems caused by epithelial permeability have been implicated in the pathophysiology of CD. This is usually threatened during inflammation because of severe damage to the bowel wall. Epidermal growth factor (EGF) has been suggested to be involved in preserving mucosal integrity and the regeneration of cells [Beck and Podolsky 1999]. Initially a recombinant EGF was formulated and tested in 24 patients with moderate - severe UC. This randomized placebo-controlled trial showed remission in 83% of patients versus 8% in the placebo group [Sinha et al. 2003].

Granulocyte-macrophage colony stimulating factor (GM-CSF) can be used for the treatment of disorders due to neutrophil dysfunction. A phase II trial included 124 CD patients and showed Sargramostin (GM-CSF) to be effective in inducing remission, the actual mechanism is still unknown [Korzenik et al. 2005]

5. The controversy

In general biologic agents have succeeded where conventional therapy has failed; they have changed the natural history of inflammatory bowel disease. Several prospective trials have already shown a decrease in hospitalization and surgery in these patients over time. A new marker of response has been gaining more momentum and significance: mucosal healing was discovered to be of prime importance in the prognosis of IBD patients. For instance in UC the presence of mucosal healing 1 year after diagnosis was associated with a significant decrease in the rate of colectomies up to 5 years later. In CD patients it was associated with a substantial drop in the need for corticosteroids. In IBD, mucosal healing data are available for steroids, azathioprine, methotrexate, infliximab, certoluzimab pegol and adalimumab. Evidence points clearly to the superiority of biologic agents in that respect.

With this new era of treatment options dawning, the clinicians are faced with the dilemma of rightfully placing these new medications in the conventional protocol of standards of care. When should we start these drugs? Which patients should be selected to receive them? How can we stratify patients to receive them? All of these questions are covered by evidence, however the answers so far are not very clear. The therapeutic approach to patients with CD depends on the clinical presentation and the potential for complications. Several tools are available, mainly through retrospective studies that may aid in predicting a more aggressive course of disease. These parameters include a younger age at diagnosis, active smoking, extensive small bowel disease, deep colonic ulcers, perianal disease and the initial need for corticosteroids. Many clinicians still apply a stepwise approach in managing CD starting from mesalamine, antimicrobials or budesonide moving to more toxic medications like corticosteroids and immuno-suppressants (azathioprine, 6MP, tacrolimus and methotrexate). Biologic agents have generally been used only after intolerance to or failure of this therapy. This escalating approach is called the "step up approach". However, there is increasing evidence that a strategy of earlier use of potent immuno-suppressants and namely biologic agents maybe the optimal approach in selected patients. The key to understanding this theory lies in the natural history of CD. Patients usually evolve in a steady progressive fashion from easily treatable inflammatory lesions towards irreversible fibrotic disease such as strictures and fistulae. A large load of evidence is currently present to support what is now called the "top down therapy" ranging from randomized trials (SONIC, CHARM) to sub-analysis (REACH, ACCENT, PRECISE). Unlike CD where longer duration usually means problems for patients, the same cannot be said for UC. One important long term issue here is dysplasia prevention. Theoretically the premise still holds, however although evidence does support the use of amino-salicylates in this regard, it is still lacking for biologics and therefore at present there is little rationale for a top down approach in managing UC.

A third factor playing a major role in the confusion for the use of biologics is their side effects. A multitude of cohorts have shown their potential for serious adverse events ranging from severe infections to life threatening allergic reactions and anaphylaxis. Although they fare well in comparison to conventional immuno-suppressants and corticosteroids, mounting evidence has shown that combination therapy may carry a dramatic toll on the patients. In a CD registry in the US (TREAT); that involved more than 6000 patients it was found that steroid treatment was associated with increased risk of serious infection and mortality, OR of 2.5 and 1.9 respectively. This was statistically significant when compared to both IFX and immune-suppressants [Lichtenstein, 2006]. Another study examined wether treatment of CD or UC patients with immune-suppressant medications was associated with an increased risk of death in the era prior to anti-TNF treatment. It showed that patient with IBD, particularly those with CD, have an increased mortality risk that may be even higher among those receiving steroids [Lewis, 2008]. One of their most controversial effects is their theoretical potential for increasing the risk for cancer.

We already know that IBD per say increases the chance of developing colon cancer; for instance based on stratified pooled data the risk of developing colon cancer in UC patients increases steadily with the length of disease. It is 2% by 10 years, 8% by 20 and an exponential 18% by 30 years of disease [Eaden, 2001]. Another prospective, observational, non-randomized, parallel-group, post-marketing safety surveillance registry (ENCORE) was launched in 8 European countries to collect long-term (5-year) safety data in patients with CD treated with infliximab (IFX) or non-biologic therapies. Additionally, data on efficacy and health economics were also obtained. As of May 2007, 842 patients received non-biologic therapy, and 1166 received IFX with a median follow-up of 12.7 and 13.2 months, respectively. A total of 122 subjects switched from non-biologic therapy to IFX therapy. Follow-up patient years were 1016 for patients on non-biologic therapy and 1506 for patients on IFX therapy. Mean disease time since first diagnosis was 8 years for patients in the non-biologic therapy group and 9.1 years in the IFX group. The number of hospitalizations, need for narcotic analgesics, and treatment with methotrexate and azathioprine were greater at baseline for patients in the IFX group. More corticosteroids, sulfasalazine/5-ASA, and other Crohn's disease medications were used in the non-biologic therapy group at baseline. Patients placed in the IFX group initially had a higher mean Harvey-Bradshaw severity score (8.4 compared to 6.3 in the non-biologic therapy group), more infections requiring antibiotics, and/or (draining) fistulae. This indicates that patients in the IFX group had more active and severe disease at baseline compared to those on non-biologic treatment. The incidence of overall adverse events was 53.7% in the IFX group compared to 41.2% in the non-biologic therapy group and the occurrence of Crohn's disease related AEs was higher in the IFX group than in non-biologic group (12.9% *vs* 8.05%). As previously shown, the incidence of serious infections was slightly higher in the IFX group than in the non-biologic therapy group (2.8% *vs* 1.7 %). Events like congestive heart failure, malignancies, and death were observed at an event rate of less than 1 percent, and treatment with IFX was not a predictor of risk for these events. No new safety signals in those treated with IFX were presented in this interim data analysis of the 5 year ENCORE registry, long-term follow-up on approximately 2000 Crohn's Disease patients [Colombel 2008]. A 4-fold increased risk in lymphoproliferative disorders (LPD) was reported in a recent meta-analysis of IBD patients receiving thiopurines that pooled data mainly originating from tertiary centers. The main objective of the cross-sectional, nationwide French CESAME cohort was to determine prospectively the risk of LPD associated with the use of immunosuppressive therapy (IT) in IBD, at a population level. Between May 2004 and May 2005, 821 French gastroenterologists (322 and 497 in hospital and private practice, respectively) included 20,802 IBD patients (60% with CD and 40% with UC or indeterminate colitis (IC)) into the cohort. At inclusion, 35.3% of the patients were receiving an IT (thiopurines (AZA, 29.8%), and/or methotrexate (3.5%), and/or an anti-TNF agent (4.8%)), 10.0% had previously been treated with IT, and 54.7% were naïve to any IT. Investigators had to report up to December 2007 the incident cases of cancers. Only LPD with a minimal 3-month interval between the inclusion and the time of histologic diagnosis were taken into account. Clinical and histologic characteristics of LPD were reviewed for validation. LPD were considered as EBV-associated in the case of high systemic EBV viral load (by PCR) and/or presence of viral RNA or proteins in neoplastic tissues. One case of Hodgkin's disease and 16 cases of non-Hodgkin's LPD (NH-LPD) were reported. Compared with the general population, the standardized incidence ratio (SIR) of LPD was 1.86 (95% CI 1.08–2.97; p=0.03). For Hodgkin's disease and NH-LPD, respectively, SIR were 0.7 (95% CI 0.01–3.92; p=0.82) and 2.07 (1.2–3.3; p=0.01). Among the

16 cases of NH-LPD, 3 occurred in patients naïve to IT. One fatal case occurred in a patient who previously received AZA. The 12 remaining cases (5 deaths) occurred in patients receiving AZA at the time of diagnosis of NH-LPD. Among these, 11 could be tested for EBV; 7 were EBV-associated, including 1 fatal case of brain LPD, 1 fatal case of intestinal large ß-cell lymphoma, and 2 fatal cases of early post-mononucleosis LPD. These interim results of the CESAME cohort suggest an overall increased risk of LPD in IBD. The excess risk appears to be related to immunosuppressive therapy since 13 of the incident cases of LPD occurred in patients receiving AZA, with a fatal issue in almost half of the cases, and a frequent association with EBV infection [Kandiel, 2005 & Beaugerie 2008]. There is concern that anti-TNF agents may be associated with an increased risk of lymphoma: This study aimed to determine the rate of non-Hodgkin's lymphoma (NHL) in adult CD patients who have received anti-TNF therapy, and to compare this to the expected rate in the Surveillance Epidemiology & End Results (SEER) registry and to estimates from a meta-analysis of patients with IBD treated with immunomodulators. This meta-analysis included randomized controlled trials, cohort studies, or case series of consecutive adult CD patients, with a minimum median follow-up time of 48 weeks, reporting adverse effects of treatment with infliximab, adalimumab, or certolizumab pegol. Twenty-six studies involving 8843 patients were included. Ten cases of NHL were reported for a rate of 5.5 per 10,000 patient-years for anti-TNF-treated patients. Compared to the expected rate of NHL in the SEER database, the incidence rate ratio (IRR) was 2.88 (95% CI 1.19–6.50). Compared to the rate of NHL in CD patients treated with immunomodulators alone, the IRR was 1.50 (95% CI 0.43–6.57). Excluding studies with a high drop-out rate yielded a rate of lymphoma of 9.4 per 10,000 patient-years. When compared to the general population or to CD patients treated with immunomodulators alone, patients treated with anti-TNF agents were found to have an increased risk of NHL. This increased risk could be a result of the anti-TNF treatment, the severity of the underlying disease, or other factors. While the absolute event rate is low, understanding this increased risk will assist providers and patients in making decisions about anti-TNF treatment for CD [Siegel 2008]. Cohorts from European and American polls are still on-going to report incidences of adverse events but so far physicians are still moderately cautious with their use.

6. Conclusion

In general the last 10 years have seen a significant surge in new medications and options for treatment. This coincided with a parallel change in protocols and patient approach. The future management to IBD will be based on accurate risk assessment and secondary phenotypic predictions based on clinical, serologic and genetic profiling. In defining the potential therapeutic benefit of each new biologic agent, it will be important to further delineate risk profiles so that the benefits can be fairly weighed against the potential unwanted effects. Undoubtedly, the number of new strategies will continue to expand, the years ahead will be exciting for investigators and enormously promising for patients.

7. References

Baert, F., M. Noman, et al. (2003). "Influence of immunogenicity on the long-term efficacy of infliximab in Crohn's disease." *N Engl J Med* 348(7): 601-608.

Beaugerie L, Carrat F, Bouvier A-M, et al, for the CEAME Study Group. Excess risk of lymphoproliferative disorders in inflammatory bowel diseases: Interim results of the CESAME cohort. Presented at DDW 2008, May 17–28, 2008; San Diego, CA; Abstract 818.

Chey, W. Y. (2001). "Infliximab for patients with refractory ulcerative colitis." *Inflamm Bowel Dis* 7 Suppl 1: S30-33.

Chey, W. Y., A. Hussain, et al. (2001). "Infliximab for refractory ulcerative colitis." *Am J Gastroenterol* 96(8): 2373-2381.

Colombel, J. F., W. J. Sandborn, et al. (2007). "Adalimumab for maintenance of clinical response and remission in patients with Crohn's disease: the CHARM trial." *Gastroenterology* 132(1): 52-65.

Colombel, J. F., W. J. Sandborn, et al. (2009). "Adalimumab safety in global clinical trials of patients with Crohn's disease." *Inflamm Bowel Dis* 15(9): 1308-1319.

Danese, S. (2008). "Mechanisms of action of infliximab in inflammatory bowel disease: an anti-inflammatory multitasker." *Dig Liver Dis* 40 Suppl 2: S225-228.

D'Haens, G., F. Baert, et al. (2008). "Early combined immunosuppression or conventional management in patients with newly diagnosed Crohn's disease: an open randomised trial." *Lancet* 371(9613): 660-667.

Eaden JA, et al. (2001) “Cumulative risk of colorectal cancer in UC patients” *Gut* 48: 526-533

Feagan, B. G., G. R. Greenberg, et al. (2008). "Treatment of active Crohn's disease with MLN0002, a humanized antibody to the alpha4beta7 integrin." *Clin Gastroenterol Hepatol* 6(12): 1370-1377.

Feagan, B. G., G. R. Greenberg, et al. (2005). "Treatment of ulcerative colitis with a humanized antibody to the alpha4beta7 integrin." *N Engl J Med* 352(24): 2499-2507.

Feagan, B. G., R. Panaccione, et al. (2008). "Effects of adalimumab therapy on incidence of hospitalization and surgery in Crohn's disease: results from the CHARM study." *Gastroenterology* 135(5): 1493-1499.

Feagan, B. G. and A. Parikh (2010). "Response to Baumgart review." *Inflamm Bowel Dis* 16(9): 1449.

Fedorak, R. N., A. Gangl, et al. (2000). "Recombinant human interleukin 10 in the treatment of patients with mild to moderately active Crohn's disease. The Interleukin 10 Inflammatory Bowel Disease Cooperative Study Group." *Gastroenterology* 119(6): 1473-1482.

Gately, M. K., L. M. Renzetti, et al. (1998). "The interleukin-12/interleukin-12-receptor system: role in normal and pathologic immune responses." *Annu Rev Immunol* 16: 495-521.

Ghosh, S. (2003). "Therapeutic value of alpha-4 integrin blockade in inflammatory bowel disease:the role of natalizumab." *Expert Opin Biol Ther* 3(6): 995-1000.

Ghosh, S., E. Goldin, et al. (2003). "Natalizumab for active Crohn's disease." *N Engl J Med* 348(1): 24-32.

Gordon, F. H., M. I. Hamilton, et al. (2002). "A pilot study of treatment of active ulcerative colitis with natalizumab, a humanized monoclonal antibody to alpha-4 integrin." *Aliment Pharmacol Ther* 16(4): 699-705.

Gordon, F. H., C. W. Lai, et al. (2001). "A randomized placebo-controlled trial of a humanized monoclonal antibody to alpha4 integrin in active Crohn's disease." *Gastroenterology* 121(2): 268-274.

Gornet, J. M., S. Couve, et al. (2003). "Infliximab for refractory ulcerative colitis or indeterminate colitis: an open-label multicentre study." *Aliment Pharmacol Ther* 18(2): 175-181.

Hanauer, S. B., B. G. Feagan, et al. (2002). "Maintenance infliximab for Crohn's disease: the ACCENT I randomised trial." *Lancet* 359(9317): 1541-1549.

Hanauer, S. B. (2004). "Efficacy and safety of tumor necrosis factor antagonists in Crohn's disease: overview of randomized clinical studies." *Rev Gastroenterol Disord* 4 Suppl 3: S18-24.

Hanauer, S. B. (2005). "Infliximab or cyclosporine for severe ulcerative colitis." *Gastroenterology* 129(4): 1358-1359; author reply 1359.

Hanauer, S. B., W. J. Sandborn, et al. (2006). "Human anti-tumor necrosis factor monoclonal antibody (adalimumab) in Crohn's disease: the CLASSIC-I trial." *Gastroenterology* 130(2): 323-333; quiz 591.

Hanauer, S. B., C. L. Wagner, et al. (2004). "Incidence and importance of antibody responses to infliximab after maintenance or episodic treatment in Crohn's disease." *Clin Gastroenterol Hepatol* 2(7): 542-553.

Hyams, J., W. Crandall, et al. (2007). "Induction and maintenance infliximab therapy for the treatment of moderate-to-severe Crohn's disease in children." *Gastroenterology* 132(3): 863-873; quiz 1165-1166.

Hyams, J. S., T. Lerer, et al. (2010). "Outcome following infliximab therapy in children with ulcerative colitis." *Am J Gastroenterol* 105(6): 1430-1436.

Ito, H., M. Takazoe, et al. (2004). "A pilot randomized trial of a human anti-interleukin-6 receptor monoclonal antibody in active Crohn's disease." *Gastroenterology* 126(4): 989-996; discussion 947.

Jakobovits, S. L., D. P. Jewell, et al. (2007). "Infliximab for the treatment of ulcerative colitis: outcomes in Oxford from 2000 to 2006." *Aliment Pharmacol Ther* 25(9): 1055-1060.

Jarnerot, G. (2006). "Infliximab or cyclosporine for severe ulcerative colitis." *Gastroenterology* 130(1): 286; author reply 287.

Jarnerot, G., E. Hertervig, et al. (2005). "Infliximab as rescue therapy in severe to moderately severe ulcerative colitis: a randomized, placebo-controlled study." *Gastroenterology* 128(7): 1805-1811.

Kandiel A, Fraser AG, Korelitz BI, et al. Increased risk of lymphoma among inflammatory bowel disease patients treated with azathioprine and 6-mercaptopurine. Gut 2005; 54(8): 1121–5

Keane, J., S. Gershon, et al. (2001). "Tuberculosis associated with infliximab, a tumor necrosis factor alpha-neutralizing agent." *N Engl J Med* 345(15): 1098-1104.

Kent, S. J., S. J. Karlik, et al. (1995). "A monoclonal antibody to alpha 4-integrin reverses the MR-detectable signs of experimental allergic encephalomyelitis in the guinea pig." *J Magn Reson Imaging* 5(5): 535-540.

Kohn, A., M. Daperno, et al. (2007). "Infliximab in severe ulcerative colitis: short-term results of different infusion regimens and long-term follow-up." *Aliment Pharmacol Ther* 26(5): 747-756.

Kuhn, R., J. Lohler, et al. (1993). "Interleukin-10-deficient mice develop chronic enterocolitis." *Cell* 75(2): 263-274.

Leger, O. J., T. A. Yednock, et al. (1997). "Humanization of a mouse antibody against human alpha-4 integrin: a potential therapeutic for the treatment of multiple sclerosis." *Hum Antibodies* 8(1): 3-16.

Lewis, J. D. (2008). "Will 2008 mark the start of a new clinical trial era in gastroenterology?" *Gastroenterology* 134(5): 1289.

Lichtenstein, G. R., B. G. Feagan, et al. (2006). "Serious infections and mortality in association with therapies for Crohn's disease: TREAT registry." *Clin Gastroenterol Hepatol* 4(5): 621-630.

Lichtiger, S., D. G. Binion, et al. (2010). "The CHOICE trial: adalimumab demonstrates safety, fistula healing, improved quality of life and increased work productivity in patients with Crohn's disease who failed prior infliximab therapy." *Aliment Pharmacol Ther* 32(10): 1228-1239.

Lofberg, R., E. V. Louis, et al. (2011). "Adalimumab produces clinical remission and reduces extraintestinal manifestations in Crohn's disease: Results from CARE." *Inflamm Bowel Dis.*

Ma, C., R. Panaccione, et al. (2009). "Systematic review: the short-term and long-term efficacy of adalimumab following discontinuation of infliximab." *Aliment Pharmacol Ther* 30(10): 977-986.

Mannon, P. J., I. J. Fuss, et al. (2004). "Anti-interleukin-12 antibody for active Crohn's disease." *N Engl J Med* 351(20): 2069-2079.

McDonald, J. W., B. G. Feagan, et al. (2005). "Cyclosporine for induction of remission in Crohn's disease." *Cochrane Database Syst Rev*(2): CD000297.

Panaccione, R., J. F. Colombel, et al. (2010). "Adalimumab sustains clinical remission and overall clinical benefit after 2 years of therapy for Crohn's disease." *Aliment Pharmacol Ther* 31(12): 1296-1309.

Plevy, S., B. Salzberg, et al. (2007). "A phase I study of visilizumab, a humanized anti-CD3 monoclonal antibody, in severe steroid-refractory ulcerative colitis." *Gastroenterology* 133(5): 1414-1422.

Podolsky, D. K. (2009). "Beyond tumor necrosis factor: next-generation biologic therapy for inflammatory bowel disease." *Dig Dis* 27(3): 366-369.

Present, D. H. (1999). "Review article: the efficacy of infliximab in Crohn's disease--healing of fistulae." *Aliment Pharmacol Ther* 13 Suppl 4: 23-28; discussion 38.

Present, D. H., P. Rutgeerts, et al. (1999). "Infliximab for the treatment of fistulas in patients with Crohn's disease." *N Engl J Med* 340(18): 1398-1405.

Probert, C. S., S. D. Hearing, et al. (2003). "Infliximab in moderately severe glucocorticoid resistant ulcerative colitis: a randomised controlled trial." *Gut* 52(7): 998-1002.

Reinisch, W., W. J. Sandborn, et al. (2011). "Adalimumab for induction of clinical remission in moderately to severely active ulcerative colitis: results of a randomised controlled trial." *Gut* 60(6): 780-787.

Rosh, J. R., T. Lerer, et al. (2009). "Retrospective Evaluation of the Safety and Effect of Adalimumab Therapy (RESEAT) in pediatric Crohn's disease." *Am J Gastroenterol* 104(12): 3042-3049.

Rudolph, S. J., D. I. Weinberg, et al. (2008). "Long-term durability of Crohn's disease treatment with infliximab." *Dig Dis Sci* 53(4): 1033-1041.

Russo, E. A., A. W. Harris, et al. (2009). "Experience of maintenance infliximab therapy for refractory ulcerative colitis from six centres in England." *Aliment Pharmacol Ther* 29(3): 308-314.

Rutgeerts, P., G. Van Assche, et al. (2004). "Optimizing anti-TNF treatment in inflammatory bowel disease." *Gastroenterology* 126(6): 1593-1610.

Rutgeerts, P., W. J. Sandborn, et al. (2005). "Infliximab for induction and maintenance therapy for ulcerative colitis." *N Engl J Med* 353(23): 2462-2476.

Sandborn, W. J., J. F. Colombel, et al. (2005). "Natalizumab induction and maintenance therapy for Crohn's disease." *N Engl J Med* 353(18): 1912-1925.

Sandborn, W. J., J. F. Colombel, et al. (2005). "Natalizumab induction and maintenance therapy for Crohn's disease." *N Engl J Med* 353(18): 1912-1925.

Sandborn, W. J., B. G. Feagan, et al. (2008). "A randomized trial of Ustekinumab, a human interleukin-12/23 monoclonal antibody, in patients with moderate-to-severe Crohn's disease." *Gastroenterology* 135(4): 1130-1141.

Sandborn, W. J., B. G. Feagan, et al. (2007). "Certolizumab pegol for the treatment of Crohn's disease." *N Engl J Med* 357(3): 228-238.

Sandborn, W. J., S. B. Hanauer, et al. (2007). "Adalimumab for maintenance treatment of Crohn's disease: results of the CLASSIC II trial." *Gut* 56(9): 1232-1239.

Sandborn, W. J., P. Rutgeerts, et al. (2007). "Adalimumab induction therapy for Crohn disease previously treated with infliximab: a randomized trial." *Ann Intern Med* 146(12): 829-838.

Sands, B. E., M. A. Blank, et al. (2004). "Long-term treatment of rectovaginal fistulas in Crohn's disease: response to infliximab in the ACCENT II Study." *Clin Gastroenterol Hepatol* 2(10): 912-920.

Schreiber, S., M. Khaliq-Kareemi, et al. (2007). "Maintenance therapy with certolizumab pegol for Crohn's disease." *N Engl J Med* 357(3): 239-250.

Schreiber, S., P. Rutgeerts, et al. (2005). "A randomized, placebo-controlled trial of certolizumab pegol (CDP870) for treatment of Crohn's disease." *Gastroenterology* 129(3): 807-818.

Siegel C, Marden SM, Persing SM, et al. Risk of lymphoma associated with anti-TNF agents for the treatment of Crohn's disease. *Gastroenterology* 2008; 134: A-144 (Abstract 970).

Springer, T. A. (1994). "Traffic signals for lymphocyte recirculation and leukocyte emigration: the multistep paradigm." *Cell* 76(2): 301-314.

Su, C., B. A. Salzberg, et al. (2002). "Efficacy of anti-tumor necrosis factor therapy in patients with ulcerative colitis." *Am J Gastroenterol* 97(10): 2577-2584.

Targan, S. R., B. G. Feagan, et al. (2007). "Natalizumab for the treatment of active Crohn's disease: results of the ENCORE Trial." *Gastroenterology* 132(5): 1672-1683.

Targan, S. R., S. B. Hanauer, et al. (1997). "A short-term study of chimeric monoclonal antibody cA2 to tumor necrosis factor alpha for Crohn's disease. Crohn's Disease cA2 Study Group." *N Engl J Med* 337(15): 1029-1035.

Taxonera, C., J. Estelles, et al. (2011). "Adalimumab induction and maintenance therapy for patients with ulcerative colitis previously treated with infliximab." *Aliment Pharmacol Ther* 33(3): 340-348.

Ten Hove, T., C. van Montfrans, et al. (2002). "Infliximab treatment induces apoptosis of lamina propria T lymphocytes in Crohn's disease." *Gut* 50(2): 206-211.

Trinder, M. W. and I. C. Lawrance (2009). "Efficacy of adalimumab for the management of inflammatory bowel disease in the clinical setting." *J Gastroenterol Hepatol* 24(7): 1252-1257.

Van Assche, G., S. Vermeire, et al. (2005). "Medical treatment of inflammatory bowel diseases." *Curr Opin Gastroenterol* 21(4): 443-447.

Wilhelm, S. M., K. A. McKenney, et al. (2008). "A review of infliximab use in ulcerative colitis." *Clin Ther* 30(2): 223-230.

Yen, D., J. Cheung, et al. (2006). "IL-23 is essential for T cell-mediated colitis and promotes inflammation via IL-17 and IL-6." *J Clin Invest* 116(5): 1310-1316.

Permissions

The contributors of this book come from diverse backgrounds, making this book a truly international effort. This book will bring forth new frontiers with its revolutionizing research information and detailed analysis of the nascent developments around the world.

We would like to thank Mahin Khatami, Ph.D, for lending her expertise to make the book truly unique. She has played a crucial role in the development of this book. Without her invaluable contribution this book wouldn't have been possible. She has made vital efforts to compile up to date information on the varied aspects of this subject to make this book a valuable addition to the collection of many professionals and students.

This book was conceptualized with the vision of imparting up-to-date information and advanced data in this field. To ensure the same, a matchless editorial board was set up. Every individual on the board went through rigorous rounds of assessment to prove their worth. After which they invested a large part of their time researching and compiling the most relevant data for our readers. Conferences and sessions were held from time to time between the editorial board and the contributing authors to present the data in the most comprehensible form. The editorial team has worked tirelessly to provide valuable and valid information to help people across the globe.

Every chapter published in this book has been scrutinized by our experts. Their significance has been extensively debated. The topics covered herein carry significant findings which will fuel the growth of the discipline. They may even be implemented as practical applications or may be referred to as a beginning point for another development.

The editorial board has been involved in producing this book since its inception. They have spent rigorous hours researching and exploring the diverse topics which have resulted in the successful publishing of this book. They have passed on their knowledge of decades through this book. To expedite this challenging task, the publisher supported the team at every step. A small team of assistant editors was also appointed to further simplify the editing procedure and attain best results for the readers.

Our editorial team has been hand-picked from every corner of the world. Their multi-ethnicity adds dynamic inputs to the discussions which result in innovative outcomes. These outcomes are then further discussed with the researchers and contributors who give their valuable feedback and opinion regarding the same. The feedback is then collaborated with the researches and they are edited in a comprehensive manner to aid the understanding of the subject.

Apart from the editorial board, the designing team has also invested a significant amount of their time in understanding the subject and creating the most relevant covers. They scrutinized every image to scout for the most suitable representation of the subject and create an appropriate cover for the book.

The publishing team has been involved in this book since its early stages. They were actively engaged in every process, be it collecting the data, connecting with the contributors or procuring relevant information. The team has been an ardent support to the editorial, designing and production team. Their endless efforts to recruit the best for this project, has resulted in the accomplishment of this book. They are a veteran in the field of academics and their pool of knowledge is as vast as their experience in printing. Their expertise and guidance has proved useful at every step. Their uncompromising quality standards have made this book an exceptional effort. Their encouragement from time to time has been an inspiration for everyone.

The publisher and the editorial board hope that this book will prove to be a valuable piece of knowledge for researchers, students, practitioners and scholars across the globe.

List of Contributors

Mahin Khatami
National Cancer Institute (NCI), The National Institutes of Health (NIH), Bethesda, Maryland, USA

Luis Chávez-Sánchez, Karina Chávez-Rueda, María Victoria Legorreta-Haquet, Eduardo Montoya-Díaz and Francisco Blanco-Favela
Unidad de Investigación Médica en Inmunología de la UMAE, Hospital de Pediatría, Centro Médico Nacional SXXI, Instituto Mexicano de Seguro Social, México

Julia Schumann
Institute of Physiological Chemistry, Faculty of Veterinary Medicine, University of Leipzig, Germany

Tamar Aprahamian
Boston University School of Medicine, USA

Omar L. Esponda
Internal Medicine Department, University Hospital Dr. Ramón Ruiz Arnaú, Bayamón, Puerto Rico, USA

Yaliz Loperena, Gladiany Ramos and A. Valance Washington
Laboratory of Anatomy and Cell Biology, Universidad Central del Caribe, Bayamón, Puerto Rico, USA

Joshua Jabaut and Karina Ckless
State University of New York at Plattsburgh (SUNY Plattsburgh), Chemistry Department, USA

Tanya LeRoith and S. Ansar Ahmed
Virginia Tech, USA

Gustavo P. Garlet
Department of Biological Sciences, School of Dentistry of Bauru, Universidade de São Paulo, Brazil

Andreza M.F. Aranha, Elcia M. Silveira and Andreia Espindola Vieira
Department of Biological Sciences, School of Dentistry of Bauru, Universidade de São Paulo, Brazil

Celso M. Queiroz-Junior, Mila F.M. Madeira and Tarcilia A. Silva
Department of Oral Pathology and Surgery, Faculty of Dentistry, Universidade Federal de Minas Gerais, Brazil

Sandra Y. Fukada
Department of Physics and Chemistry, School of Pharmaceutical Sciences of Ribeirão Preto, Universidade de São Paulo, Brazil

Priyanka Pundir
Institute for Nutrisciences and Health, National Research Council, Charlottetown, PE, Canada
Department of Biomedical Sciences, Atlantic Veterinary College, University of Prince Edward Island, Charlottetown, PE, Canada

Marianna Kulka
Institute for Nutrisciences and Health, National Research Council, Charlottetown, PE, Canada
Allergy-Immunology Division, Northwestern University, Feinberg School of Medicine, Chicago, IL, USA

Joziana M.P. Barçante, Ana Paula Peconick and Luciano J. Pereira
Departamento de Medicina Veterinária, Universidade Federal de Lavras, Brazil

Thales A. Barçante
ICBS, Pontifícia Universidade Católica de Minas Gerais, Brazil

Walter S. Lima
Departamento de Parasitologia, Universidade Federal de Minas Gerais, Brazil

Hiroshi Nakanishi
Department of Aging Science and Pharmacology, Faculty of Dental Science, Kyushu University, Fukuoka, Japan
Japan Science and Technology Agency, CREST, 5, Sanbancho, Chiyoda-ku, Tokyo, Japan

Berit Carow and Martin E. Rottenberg
Dept. of Microbiology, Tumor and Cell Biology, Karolinska Institutet, Stockholm, Sweden

C. E. Pang
Singapore National Eye Centre, Singapore

Sabrina Bréchard, Véronique Schenten and Eric J. Tschirhart
University of Luxembourg, Luxembourg

Jorge R. Mujico, Fátima Pérez-de-Heredia, Sonia Gómez-Martínez and Ascensión Marcos
Institute of Food Science, Technology and Nutrition (ICTAN-CSIC), Spain

Liam Heaney and Izhaq Masih
Queens University, Belfast, Northern Ireland, United Kingdom

Yonca Aydın Akova and Sirel Gür Güngör
Başkent University Faculty of Medicine, Department of Ophthalmology, Turkey

Debra B. Gardner, Patricia Rafferty, Peter Bugelski and Bailin Liang
Centocor Research and Development, USA

Iyad A. Issa
Lebanese American University, Lebanon